Optimal Design for Nonlinear Response Models

Chapman & Hall/CRC Biostatistics Series

Chapman & Hall/CRC Biostatistics Series

Adaptive Design Methods in Clinical Trials, Second Edition
Shein-Chung Chow and Mark Chang

Adaptive Design Theory and Implementation Using SAS and R
Mark Chang

Advanced Bayesian Methods for Medical Test Accuracy
Lyle D. Broemeling

Advances in Clinical Trial Biostatistics
Nancy L. Geller

Applied Meta-Analysis with R
Ding-Geng (Din) Chen and Karl E. Peace

Basic Statistics and Pharmaceutical Statistical Applications, Second Edition
James E. De Muth

Bayesian Adaptive Methods for Clinical Trials
Scott M. Berry, Bradley P. Carlin,
J. Jack Lee, and Peter Muller

Bayesian Analysis Made Simple: An Excel GUI for WinBUGS
Phil Woodward

Bayesian Methods for Measures of Agreement
Lyle D. Broemeling

Bayesian Methods in Health Economics
Gianluca Baio

Bayesian Missing Data Problems: EM, Data Augmentation and Noniterative Computation
Ming T. Tan, Guo-Liang Tian,
and Kai Wang Ng

Bayesian Modeling in Bioinformatics
Dipak K. Dey, Samiran Ghosh,
and Bani K. Mallick

Biostatistics: A Computing Approach
Stewart J. Anderson

Causal Analysis in Biomedicine and Epidemiology: Based on Minimal Sufficient Causation
Mikel Aickin

Clinical Trial Data Analysis using R
Ding-Geng (Din) Chen and Karl E. Peace

Clinical Trial Methodology
Karl E. Peace and Ding-Geng (Din) Chen

Computational Methods in Biomedical Research
Ravindra Khattree and Dayanand N. Naik

Computational Pharmacokinetics
Anders Källén

Confidence Intervals for Proportions and Related Measures of Effect Size
Robert G. Newcombe

Controversial Statistical Issues in Clinical Trials
Shein-Chung Chow

Data and Safety Monitoring Committees in Clinical Trials
Jay Herson

Design and Analysis of Animal Studies in Pharmaceutical Development
Shein-Chung Chow and Jen-pei Liu

Design and Analysis of Bioavailability and Bioequivalence Studies, Third Edition
Shein-Chung Chow and Jen-pei Liu

Design and Analysis of Bridging Studies
Jen-pei Liu, Shein-Chung Chow,
and Chin-Fu Hsiao

Design and Analysis of Clinical Trials with Time-to-Event Endpoints
Karl E. Peace

Design and Analysis of Non-Inferiority Trials
Mark D. Rothmann, Brian L. Wiens,
and Ivan S. F. Chan

Difference Equations with Public Health Applications
Lemuel A. Moyé and Asha Seth Kapadia

DNA Methylation Microarrays: Experimental Design and Statistical Analysis
Sun-Chong Wang and Arturas Petronis

DNA Microarrays and Related Genomics Techniques: Design, Analysis, and Interpretation of Experiments
David B. Allison, Grier P. Page, T. Mark Beasley, and Jode W. Edwards

Dose Finding by the Continual Reassessment Method
Ying Kuen Cheung

Elementary Bayesian Biostatistics
Lemuel A. Moyé

Frailty Models in Survival Analysis
Andreas Wienke

Generalized Linear Models: A Bayesian Perspective
Dipak K. Dey, Sujit K. Ghosh, and Bani K. Mallick

Handbook of Regression and Modeling: Applications for the Clinical and Pharmaceutical Industries
Daryl S. Paulson

Interval-Censored Time-to-Event Data: Methods and Applications
Ding-Geng (Din) Chen, Jianguo Sun, and Karl E. Peace

Joint Models for Longitudinal and Time-to-Event Data: With Applications in R
Dimitris Rizopoulos

Measures of Interobserver Agreement and Reliability, Second Edition
Mohamed M. Shoukri

Medical Biostatistics, Third Edition
A. Indrayan

Meta-Analysis in Medicine and Health Policy
Dalene Stangl and Donald A. Berry

Monte Carlo Simulation for the Pharmaceutical Industry: Concepts, Algorithms, and Case Studies
Mark Chang

Multiple Testing Problems in Pharmaceutical Statistics
Alex Dmitrienko, Ajit C. Tamhane, and Frank Bretz

Optimal Design for Nonlinear Response Models
Valerii V. Fedorov and Sergei L. Leonov

Randomized Clinical Trials of Nonpharmacological Treatments
Isabelle Boutron, Philippe Ravaud, and David Moher

Randomized Phase II Cancer Clinical Trials
Sin-Ho Jung

Sample Size Calculations in Clinical Research, Second Edition
Shein-Chung Chow, Jun Shao and Hansheng Wang

Statistical Design and Analysis of Stability Studies
Shein-Chung Chow

Statistical Evaluation of Diagnostic Performance: Topics in ROC Analysis
Kelly H. Zou, Aiyi Liu, Andriy Bandos, Lucila Ohno-Machado, and Howard Rockette

Statistical Methods for Clinical Trials
Mark X. Norleans

Statistics in Drug Research: Methodologies and Recent Developments
Shein-Chung Chow and Jun Shao

Statistics in the Pharmaceutical Industry, Third Edition
Ralph Buncher and Jia-Yeong Tsay

Translational Medicine: Strategies and Statistical Methods
Dennis Cosmatos and Shein-Chung Chow

Chapman & Hall/CRC Biostatistics Series

Optimal Design for Nonlinear Response Models

Valerii V. Fedorov
Sergei L. Leonov

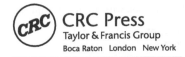

CRC Press
Taylor & Francis Group
Boca Raton London New York

CRC Press is an imprint of the
Taylor & Francis Group, an **informa** business

A CHAPMAN & HALL BOOK

CRC Press
Taylor & Francis Group
6000 Broken Sound Parkway NW, Suite 300
Boca Raton, FL 33487-2742

First issued in paperback 2019

© 2014 by Taylor & Francis Group, LLC
CRC Press is an imprint of Taylor & Francis Group, an Informa business

No claim to original U.S. Government works

ISBN-13: 978-1-4398-2151-0 (hbk)
ISBN-13: 978-0-367-37980-3 (pbk)

Visit the Taylor & Francis Web site at
http://www.taylorandfrancis.com

and the CRC Press Web site at
http://www.crcpress.com

Contents

List of Figures   xiii

List of Tables   xix

Preface   xxi

Introduction   xxiii

1 **Regression Models and Their Analysis**   1
  1.1 Linear Model, Single Response   2
      1.1.1 Least squares estimator   4
      1.1.2 Information matrix   6
  1.2 More about Information Matrix   10
  1.3 Generalized Versions of Linear Regression Model   12
      1.3.1 Heterogeneous but known variance   12
      1.3.2 Unknown parameters in variance   13
      1.3.3 Multivariate response   15
  1.4 Nonlinear Models   17
      1.4.1 Least squares estimator   17
      1.4.2 Variance-covariance matrix   18
      1.4.3 Iterative estimation   19
  1.5 Maximum Likelihood and Fisher Information Matrix   20
      1.5.1 Examples of Fisher information matrix   21
  1.6 Generalized Regression and Elemental Fisher Information Matrices   23
      1.6.1 Univariate distributions   24
      1.6.2 Two multivariate distributions   25
  1.7 Nonlinear Regression with Normally Distributed Observations   30
      1.7.1 Iterated estimators and combined least squares   32
      1.7.2 Examples of iterated estimators   36
          1.7.2.1 Multiresponse linear model with constant covariance matrix   36
          1.7.2.2 Multiresponse linear model with random coefficients   37
          1.7.2.3 Separation of response and variance parameters   39

1.7.3   Simulations 41

2 Convex Design Theory   **49**
2.1 From Optimal Estimators to Optimal Designs 49
2.2 Optimality Criteria 52
    2.2.1 Optimality criteria related to parameter space 52
    2.2.2 Criteria related to variance of predicted response . . . 57
    2.2.3 Criteria that include unknown parameters 59
    2.2.4 Compound criteria 60
2.3 Properties of Optimality Criteria 61
2.4 Continuous Optimal Designs 62
    2.4.1 Information matrix and optimal designs 64
    2.4.2 Necessary and sufficient conditions for optimality . . . 65
2.5 Sensitivity Function and Equivalence Theorems 67
2.6 Equivalence Theorem: Examples 71
2.7 Optimal Designs with Prior Information 77
2.8 Regularization 79
2.9 Optimality Criterion Depends on Estimated Parameters or Unknown Constants 80
2.10 Response Function Contains Uncontrolled and Unknown Independent Variables 84
2.11 Response Models with Random Parameters 85
    2.11.1 Known population mean and variance parameters . . 86
    2.11.2 Known variance parameters 89
    2.11.3 Estimation of population mean parameters 91

3 Algorithms and Numerical Techniques   **93**
3.1 First-Order Algorithm: D-Criterion 93
    3.1.1 Forward iterative procedure 94
    3.1.2 Some useful recursive formulae 95
    3.1.3 Convergence of algorithms 96
    3.1.4 Practical numerical procedures 100
3.2 First-Order Algorithm: General Case 101
3.3 Finite Sample Size 105
3.4 Other Algorithms 108

4 Optimal Design under Constraints   **111**
4.1 Single Constraint 111
    4.1.1 One-stage designs 111
    4.1.2 Two-stage designs 116
4.2 Multiple Constraints 117
4.3 Constraints for Auxiliary Criteria 120
4.4 Directly Constrained Design Measures 122

5 Nonlinear Response Models   **127**
  5.1 Bridging Linear and Nonlinear Cases 128
  5.2 Mitigating Dependence on Unknown Parameters 129
  5.3 Box and Hunter Adaptive Design 131
  5.4 Generalized Nonlinear Regression: Use of Elemental Informa-
       tion Matrices 136
  5.5 Model Discrimination 141

6 Locally Optimal Designs in Dose Finding   **151**
  6.1 Comments on Numerical Procedures 151
  6.2 Binary Models 154
  6.3 Normal Regression Models 156
      6.3.1 Unknown parameters in variance 157
      6.3.2 Optimal designs as a benchmark 160
  6.4 Dose Finding for Efficacy-Toxicity Response 161
      6.4.1 Models 163
      6.4.2 Locally optimal designs 165
  6.5 Bivariate Probit Model for Correlated Binary Responses . . 170
      6.5.1 Single drug 172
      6.5.2 Drug combination 180

7 Locally Optimal Designs in PK/PD Studies   **187**
  7.1 Introduction 188
  7.2 PK Models with Serial Sampling: Estimation of Model Param-
       eters 191
      7.2.1 Study background 191
      7.2.2 Two-compartment population model 192
      7.2.3 Single dose 195
      7.2.4 Repeated dose administration 197
  7.3 Estimation of PK Parameters 199
      7.3.1 Problem setting and model-based designs 200
      7.3.2 PK metrics and their estimation 203
          7.3.2.1 Model-based (parametric) approach 204
          7.3.2.2 Empirical (nonparametric) approach 206
          7.3.2.3 Average PK metrics for one-compartment
                model 210
      7.3.3 Sampling grid 211
      7.3.4 Splitting sampling grid 215
      7.3.5 MSE of AUC estimator, single and split grids 218
  7.4 Pharmacokinetic Models Described by Stochastic Differential
       Equations 221
      7.4.1 Stochastic one-compartment model I 222
      7.4.2 Stochastic one-compartment model II: systems with
          positive trajectories 224
      7.4.3 Proof of Lemma 7.1 228

7.5   Software for Constructing Optimal Population PK/PD Designs 230

    7.5.1   Regression models 231

    7.5.2   Supported PK/PD models 232

    7.5.3   Software inputs 232

    7.5.4   Software outputs 234

    7.5.5   Optimal designs as a reference point 236

    7.5.6   Software comparison 241

    7.5.7   User-defined option 245

8 Adaptive Model-Based Designs   **251**

8.1   Adaptive Design for E_{max} Model 253

    8.1.1   Study background 254

    8.1.2   Model 254

    8.1.3   Adaptive dose selection with constraints 256

    8.1.4   Simulation studies 257

    8.1.5   Generalized E_{max} model 266

    8.1.6   Extensions 268

    8.1.7   Technical details 272

8.2   Adaptive Designs for Bivariate Cox Model 275

    8.2.1   Progress of the trial: single simulation 277

    8.2.2   Multiple simulations 278

8.3   Adaptive Designs for Bivariate Probit Model 282

    8.3.1   Single drug 282

    8.3.2   Combination of two drugs 287

9 Other Applications of Optimal Designs   **293**

9.1   Methods of Selecting Informative Variables 293

    9.1.1   Motivating example 295

    9.1.2   Principal component analysis 297

    9.1.3   Direct selection of variables 298

    9.1.4   Model with measurement errors 301

    9.1.5   Clinical data analysis 304

9.2   Best Intention Designs in Dose-Finding Studies 312

    9.2.1   Utility and penalty functions 313

    9.2.2   Best intention and adaptive D-optimal designs 315

    9.2.3   Discrete design region $\mathfrak{X}$ 328

10 Useful Matrix Formulae   **331**

10.1 Matrix Derivatives 332

10.2 Partitioned Matrices 333

10.3 Equalities 333

10.4 Inequalities 334

Bibliography   **337**

Index   **369**

Symbol Description

$y, \boldsymbol{y}$	response or independent or observed variable	r_i, n_i	number of observations at $\mathbf{x}_i$
$\eta, \boldsymbol{\eta}$	response function	p_i, w_i	weight of observations at $\mathbf{x}_i$
$x, \mathbf{x}$	independent or control or design or regressor variables, predictors	n	number of support points
		N	total number of observations
		$\mathbf{M}, \mathbf{M}(\xi)$	normalized information matrix
$z, \mathbf{z}$	uncontrolled regressor variables, covariates	$\underline{\mathbf{M}}$	nonnormalized information matrix
$\theta, \boldsymbol{\theta}$	parameters	$\boldsymbol{\mu}(\mathbf{x}, \boldsymbol{\theta})$	Fisher information matrix
m	number of parameters	$\mathbf{D}, \underline{\mathbf{D}}$	dispersion matrix of estimators $\hat{\boldsymbol{\theta}}$
$\boldsymbol{\Theta}$	parameter space		
$\mathbf{f}(\mathbf{x})$	vector of basis functions	$d(\mathbf{x}, \xi)$	normalized variance of predicted response $\eta(\mathbf{x}, \hat{\boldsymbol{\theta}})$
$\eta(\mathbf{x}, \boldsymbol{\theta})$	response function		
$\varepsilon, \boldsymbol{\varepsilon}$	(response) error	$\Psi, \Psi(\mathbf{M})$	optimality criterion
σ^2	variance of the error	$\boldsymbol{\Omega}$	variance-covariance matrix of random parameters
ξ_n	discrete design		
$\xi, \xi(d\mathbf{x})$	continuous design	$\varphi(\mathbf{x}, \xi)$	sensitivity function for design ξ at $\mathbf{x}$
ξ^*	optimal design		
Ξ	set of designs	$\phi(\mathbf{x})$	penalty/cost function at $\mathbf{x}$
$x_i, \mathbf{x}_i$	design support points	$\Phi(\xi)$	total penalty/cost for design ξ
$\mathfrak{X}$	support (design) region		

List of Figures

1.1 Ellipsoids of concentration, $m = 2$; here $\mathbf{A} \leq \mathbf{B}$, and $\mathcal{E}_{\mathbf{A}} \supseteq \mathcal{E}_{\mathbf{B}}$. Dashed and dotted lines correspond to principal axes of ellipsoids $\mathcal{E}_{\mathbf{A}}$ and $\mathcal{E}_{\mathbf{B}}$, respectively. 7

1.2 Example 1.1: $\eta(x,\theta) = S(x,\theta) = e^{\theta x}$, 20 points per set. Top – CIRLS, middle – MIRLS, bottom – IRLS. 42

1.3 Example 1.1: Isolines of functions $V(\theta,\theta')$ (CIRLS, top) and $\bar{V}(\theta,\theta')$ (MIRLS, bottom), CIRLS-divergent set. 44

1.4 Example 1.1: Isolines of functions $V(\theta,\theta')$ (top, CIRLS) and $\bar{V}(\theta,\theta')$ (bottom, MIRLS), CIRLS-convergent set. 45

1.5 Example 1.2: $\eta(x,\theta) = S(x,\theta) = e^{\theta x}$, 80 points per set. 47

1.6 Example 1.3: $\eta(x,\theta) = \theta x$, $S(x,\theta) = e^{\theta x}$, 20 points per set. . 48

2.1 Ellipsoid of concentration (2.10) with $R = 1$; nondiagonal matrix. Dash-dotted and dashed lines correspond to the largest and the smallest principal axes, respectively. 55

2.2 Individual and global (shrinkage) estimators. Top panel: observed random effects $\mathbf{y}_i$. Bottom panel: true random effects $\boldsymbol{\gamma}_i$. 87

6.1 D-optimal designs for logistic and probit models, $x = (z - \theta_0)/\theta_1$.   Upper panel: logistic model, $z = -3 + 1.81x$. Lower panel: probit model, $z = -1.66 + x$. 155

6.2 Plots for Example 6.1. Upper left panel: response function $\eta(x,\boldsymbol{\theta})$. Lower left panel: sensitivity function $d(x,\xi_2,\boldsymbol{\theta})$ for twofold serial dilution design; circles denote serial dilution ξ_2. Lower right: sensitivity function $d(x,\xi^*,\boldsymbol{\theta})$ for optimal design; triangles denote optimal design ξ^*. 159

6.3 Cox model with parameter $\boldsymbol{\theta} = (3,3,4,2,0,1)$. Top left: response probabilities. Top right: penalty function (6.26) with $C_E = C_T = 1$. Bottom: penalty function with $C_E = 1$, $C_T = 0$ (left) and $C_E = 0$, $C_T = 1$ (right). 167

6.4 Locally optimal designs for Cox model with $\boldsymbol{\theta} = (3,3,4,2,0,1)$. Top left: traditional. Top right: penalized with penalty function (6.26) with $C_E = 1, C_T = 1$. Bottom left: restricted. Bottom right: up-and-down design. 168

6.5 Response probabilities and locally D-optimal designs for the bivariate probit model with $\boldsymbol{\theta} = (-0.9, 10, -1.2, 1.6)$; traditional locally optimal (left) and restricted locally optimal (right). . . . 173

6.6 Response probabilities for the bivariate probit model with $\boldsymbol{\theta} = (-0.9, 10, -1.2, 1.6)$ and penalized locally D-optimal designs; penalty function (6.26) with $C_E = 0, C_T = 1$ (top), $C_E = 1, C_T = 0$ (bottom left), and $C_E = 1, C_T = 1$ (bottom right). 175

6.7 Probabilities, penalty functions and corresponding penalized locally optimal designs for $\boldsymbol{\theta}_3$ (left) and $\boldsymbol{\theta}_8$ (right). 178

6.8 Traditional locally D-optimal design (left) and penalized locally D-optimal design (right); ρ is an unknown parameter. Top panel: $\rho = -0.8$; middle panel: $\rho = 0$; bottom panel: $\rho = 0.8$. . 179

6.9 Response probability surfaces for the drug combination bivariate probit model. 181

6.10 Contour plot for p_{10} in the restricted region. 182

6.11 Locally optimal design and restricted region. 183

6.12 Penalty functions and penalized locally optimal designs for drug combinations. Top panel: $C_E = 0, C_T = 1$; middle panel: $C_E = 1, C_T = 0$; bottom panel: $C_E = 1, C_T = 1$. 184

7.1 Diagram of two-compartment model. 191

7.2 Sensitivity function for cost-based design. 198

7.3 Schematic presentation of type II AUC estimators; see (7.33). See (7.32) for method M2 (parametric) and (7.38) for method E2 (nonparametric). 207

7.4 Uniform grid with respect to values of response (left) and AUC (right). Inverted triangles: odd samples on the mean response curve; circles: odd samples on the scaled AUC curve. Triangles: even samples on the mean response curve; diamonds: even samples on the scaled AUC curve. 210

7.5 Type III population curve $\eta(x, \boldsymbol{\gamma}^0)$, solid line. Type II population curves $\bar{\eta}(x) = E_{\gamma}[\eta(x, \boldsymbol{\gamma})]$ for different values of coefficient of variation CV: 15% (dashed), 30% (dash-dotted), and 50% (dotted). 212

7.6 Example of cubic spline overfitting. 213

7.7 Estimation of Type II AUC metric: 10,000 runs, 16 sampling times, $N=20$, $AUC_2=1.836$ (marked by vertical line). Left panel – single grid, right panel – split grid. Upper plots – model-based, middle plots – empirical (hybrid), lower plots – spline. 215

7.8 Estimation of Type II T_{max} metric, same setting as in Figure 7.7, $T_2 = 0.0521$. 216

7.9 Method 2: estimation of Type II C_{max} metric, same setting as in Figure 7.7, $C_2 = 7.210$. 217

7.10 MSE as a function of N and k, $u = 2.4$, $\sigma = 9$, $25 \leq N \leq 40$. 220

7.11 Three sources of variability in SDE models. 224

7.12 Sampling times and examples of optimal designs for stochastic PK model. 226

7.13 Typical input screen: one-compartment model with first-order absorption and linear elimination. 235

7.14 Input screen for one-compartment PK model and E_{max} PD model. 238

7.15 Sensitivity function for optimal two-sequence design. 241

7.16 Mean response curves: first-order approximation (solid line), computed at mean values of log-normal distribution (dashed), and Monte Carlo average (dotted). Locations of circles and diamonds correspond to sampling times from the sequence $\mathbf{x}$ in (7.84). 246

7.17 User-defined option, input screens: parameters and dosing regimen. 247

7.18 User-defined option, input screens: specifying differential equations and measured compartments. 248

8.1 Screenshot, E_{max} model. 258

8.2 Sensitivity function, D-optimal design. 259

8.3 Simulations, single run: selected doses. Log-dose is shown on the y-axis as a multiple of $x_{MIN} = 0.001$. Dashed horizontal lines correspond to optimal doses, with dash-dotted lines showing true values of ED_{10} and ED_{90}. Short dotted lines give estimated ED_{10} and ED_{90} for each cohort. 260

8.4 Simulations, single run: estimated dose-response curves, after four (top) and eight (bottom) cohorts. Vertical dashed lines correspond to the optimal doses. The true dose-response curve is shown with a heavy gray dashed line. 261

8.5 Selected doses after 1000 simulations, cohort 7 (top) and cohort 8 (bottom). Vertical dashed lines correspond to the optimal doses. 262

8.6 Histogram of estimates of ED_{90}. Top left – fixed design, top right – adaptive, bottom left – composite, bottom right – D-optimal. The dashed vertical line represents the true value of ED_{90}. 264

8.7 Screenshot of the tool to compare models (8.4) and (8.12). . 267

8.8 Screenshot, multiparameter binary logistic model. 269

8.9 Histograms of estimates of ED_{80}, 1000 simulations, model (8.15). Vertical dashed line represents the true value; dotted line – median; solid line – boundaries of empirical 90% confidence interval; dash-dotted lines – boundaries of empirical 80% confidence interval. 270

8.10 Screenshot, four-parameter E_{max} model. 271

8.11 Histograms of selected doses, model (8.17). Vertical dashed lines correspond to optimal doses: $d_2 = 0.5$, $d_4 = 2$, $d_5 = 5$. 272

8.12 Convergence of the three performance measures for the three designs: PAD (left column), modified PAD (middle column), and PLD (right column). Cox model with parameter $\theta = (3, 3, 4, 2, 0, 1)$. Penalty function (6.26) with parameters $C_E = C_T = 1$. Top row – criterion (6.33); middle row – (6.32); bottom row – criterion (6.34). 276

8.13 Graphical summary of the progress of the trial. 277

8.14 Four scenarios for multiple simulations. 278

8.15 Scenario 1: Cox model with parameters $\theta = (3, 3, 4, 2, 0, 1)$. Dose allocation (top) and selection of the optimal safe dose (bottom) for the PAD and up-and-down design. 280

8.16 Scenario 2: Cox model, parameters $\theta = (0, 2, 0.5, 1, -0.5, 1)$. . 281

8.17 Scenario 3: Cox model, parameters $\theta = (1, 4, 1, 2, -1, 2)$. . . . 281

8.18 Scenario 4: Cox model, parameters $\theta = (4, 4, 0, 0.5, -2, 0.5)$. . 282

8.19 Progress of adaptive designs under bivariate probit model. . . 283

8.20 Dose allocation distribution for adaptive designs; 1000 runs. Top panel – after 30 patients; middle panel – after 70 patients; bottom panel – after 100 patients. 284

8.21 Histograms of parameter estimates, fully adaptive designs. . . 286

8.22 Histograms of parameter estimates, composite designs. 288

8.23 Adaptive design, restricted design region. 289

8.24 Composite design for drug combination study; initial design utilizes single drugs only. 290

8.25 Composite design for drug combination study; initial design includes drug combinations. 291

9.1 Logs of eigenvalues versus logs of sorted diagonal elements. . 305

9.2 Variance of prediction based on principal components (diamonds) and principal variables (stars), first 15 sorted variables. 307

9.3 Sorted variables, homogeneous error variance, $\sigma_0^2/N = 1$. Optimal continuous design (top); variance of prediction for continuous design (middle); variance of prediction for discrete design (bottom), optimal variables marked by asterisks. 308

9.4 Top: error variance (9.20), $\gamma = 1$, $\sigma_0^2/N = 0.1$; variance of prediction for discrete design, optimal variables marked by asterisks. Middle and bottom: error variance (9.21), $\beta = 2$, $\sigma_0^2/N = 0.1$. Optimal continuous design (middle), variance of prediction (bottom); original ordering of variables. 310

9.5 Illustration of various response probabilities: efficacy without toxicity (solid line), efficacy (dashed), and toxicity (dash-dotted). 314

9.6 Illustration of Robbins-Monro procedure (9.29). 317

9.7 Sample trajectories of naive ARM, type I dose-finding, linear model (left) and quadratic model (right). 318

9.8   Histograms of predicted best doses for the linear model (9.27): ARM (left panel) and PAD (right panel); initial cohort sizes of 2 (top rows) and 8 (bottom rows). Left columns: after 100 observations; right columns: after 400 observations. 320

9.9   Scatterplots of estimates $\hat{\theta}_1$ vs $\hat{\theta}_2$ for the linear model (9.27), same setting as in Figure 9.8. 323

9.10 Histograms of predicted best doses for the quadratic model (9.36): BI (left panel) and PAD (right panel); initial cohort sizes of 3 (top rows) and 12 (bottom rows). Left columns: after 100 observations; right columns: after 400 observations. . . . 326

9.11 Scatterplots of estimates $\hat{\theta}_1$ vs $\hat{\theta}_2$ for the quadratic model (9.36), same setting as in Figure 9.10. 327

List of Tables

1.1 Elemental information for single-parameter distributions . . .   25

1.2 Transformed elemental information for single-parameter distributions   26

1.3 Elemental information matrices for two-parameter distributions   27

1.4 Transformed elemental information matrices for two-parameter distributions   28

2.1 Sensitivity function $\varphi(\mathbf{x}, \xi)$ for various criteria Ψ; $\mathbf{D} = \mathbf{M}^{-1}$.   69

5.1 Sensitivity function for transformations; $\mathbf{D} = \mathbf{M}^{-1}$; λ_i are eigenvalues of the matrix $\mathbf{M}$ 137

6.1 Performance measures for locally optimal designs   170

6.2 Locally D-optimal designs for the bivariate probit model with $\theta = (-0.9, 10, -1.2, 1.6)$.   173

6.3 Parameter values used in sensitivity study.   176

6.4 Relative deficiency of penalized locally D-optimal designs ξ_{pi} with the penalty function (6.26), $C_E = 1$ and $C_T = 1$; deficiency defined in (6.48).   177

6.5 Locally optimal designs for two-drug combination.   185

6.6 Parameter values used in the sensitivity analysis   186

7.1 Single dose, D-efficiency of k-point designs.   196

7.2 Bias, standard deviation and square root of MSE for Type II estimators for model (7.24) – (7.26).   218

8.1 Sample statistics of 1000 simulation runs.   263

8.2 Empirical vs. analytical variance from 1000 simulations. . . .   265

8.3 Performance measures for penalized adaptive D-optimal and up-and-down designs: simulation results for Cox model under Scenarios 1 – 4   280

8.4 Composite traditional and penalized designs with the penalty function (6.26).   287

9.1 Ranking of 35 laboratory tests using mean/variance structure.   296

9.2 Percent of predicted best dose sequences stuck to the boundaries   319

9.3 Risks for different customers 321

9.4 Total penalty $\sum_{i=1}^{n}(x_i - x^*)^2 + nc$ for $c = 0.1$ and $n = 400$. 322

Preface

Our main intent is to introduce the reader to the statistical area that in rather loose terms can be called "model-based optimal design of experiments." The word "design" implies that there exist some variables, the values of which can be chosen in the planning stage. We focus our exposition on cases when a researcher can describe the relation between these variables and responses (response variables) by means of a mathematical model that describes the observed system. Often the system description is based on the deterministic model while the observational component is modeled via stochastic mechanisms. However, it is not always the case: biological systems or clinical trials are good examples of when stochastic models can be used for system description as well. See, for instance, examples in Section 7.4 where stochastic differential equations are used to model intrinsic patient variability in pharmacokinetic studies. Regression models with random parameters provide another example of such a setting.

Both authors spent more than a decade in the pharmaceutical industry developing the optimal design machinery for earlier phases of clinical studies. This explains why the majority of examples are related to biopharmaceutical applications; see earlier survey papers by Fedorov and Leonov (2005) [144], Fedorov et al. (2007) [133]. Nevertheless, we would like to emphasize that the potential applications are much wider. The main distinction of this monograph from many others published recently is the strong emphasis on nonlinear with respect to unknown parameters models. Still, the exposition of key ideas of optimal experimental design is much simpler and more transparent for linear models. That is why the reader will find rather extensive introductory material that is devoted to the linear case.

The book is intended for graduate students and researchers who are interested in the theory and applications of model-based experimental design. The main body of the book requires a modest formal background in calculus, matrix algebra and statistics. Thus the book is accessible not only to statisticians, but also to a relatively broad readership, in particular those with backgrounds in natural sciences and engineering.

We would like to express our gratitude to the many colleagues with whom we have collaborated on various optimal design problems over recent years, in particular Alexander Aliev, Vladimir Anisimov, Anthony Atkinson, Brian McHugh, Vladimir Dragalin, Nancy Flournoy, Bob Gagnon, David Gruben, Agnes Herzberg, Byron Jones, Mindy Magee, Sam Miller, Viacheslav Vasiliev,

Yuehui Wu, Rongmei Zhang, and Anatoly Zhigljavsky. The second author would like to thank members of the PODE (Population Optimum Design of Experiments) community for many fruitful discussions of population optimal design methods and software, in particular Barbara Bogacka, Caroline Bazzoli, Steve Duffull, Andy Hooker, France Mentré, Joakim Nyberg, and Kay Ogungbenro.

We would like to acknowledge two anonymous reviewers for their helpful comments on the draft version of the manuscript.

We are extremely grateful to members of the CRC Press Team for their continuous help during our work on this book, in particular, to David Grubbs for his ultimate patience and support while working with us, to Mimi Williams for her excellent proofreading, and to Marcus Fontaine for his efficient help with our last minute LATEX questions.

Valerii V. Fedorov
Sergei L. Leonov

Introduction

Over the next few pages we provide a rather sketchy and likely subjective overview of the evolution of optimal experimental design. With advances of the Internet, more facts can be found online. As far as authors' preferences are concerned, the first author would "Google" the Web, while the second author would be "Yahooing."

Stigler (1974) [368] provides exciting reading on the early "formalized" attempts of optimal design of experiments. The first well-documented contribution to optimal design theory was made by Kirstine Smith (1918) [364]. She explored the regression problem for univariate polynomials of order up to six, with the control variable varying between −1 and 1. The observational errors were independent, identically distributed and additive. Smith found designs that minimize the maximum variance of prediction over the design region (later called G-optimal). Other designs were considered, for example uniform designs, and the effect of nonconstant variance was investigated. Smith's paper thus had all the components needed to specify an optimal design: a response model, a design region, a design criterion, specification of observational errors and a comparison of optimal designs with designs that are popular among practitioners. Smith's paper was all but forgotten for nearly 40 years.

Wald (1943) [391] started the comparison of designs using values of noncentrality parameters for tests of hypotheses about parameters defining a response model. This problem led him to the necessity of comparing the determinants of the information matrix, i.e., to D-optimality. The close relation of the D-criterion with Shannon's information was explored by Lindley (1956) [258] in the Bayesian setting. Very soon this criterion became one of the most used (and sometimes abused) criteria in design theory. Guest (1958) [184] showed that support points of the G-optimal design for the polynomial of order m coincide with roots of the derivatives of the $(m - 1)$-th Legendre polynomial together with the end points. Hoel (1958) [201] constructed D-optimal designs and commented that his designs were the same as those of Guest. Two years later Kiefer and Wolfowitz (1960) [232] proved the equivalence of G- and D-optimality and started to treat experimental design as a particular area of convex optimization theory. The latter direction was explored by Karlin and Studden (1966) [225] and by Fedorov (1969, 1972) [125], [127].

Jack Kiefer undoubtedly was the main contributor to the development of the core of optimal design theory in the 1950s and 1960s. For a survey and collection of his papers on optimal design, see Wynn (1984) [418] and Brown et al. (1985) [57].

Elfving (1952) [114] gave a geometrical interpretation of optimal designs and introduced a criterion that became known as A-optimality (average variance of regression parameter estimators). He found that the points of the optimum design lie on the smallest ellipsoid that contains the design region, an insight further developed by Silvey and Titterington (1973) [361]. Elfving's results were almost immediately extended to D-optimality by Chernoff (1953) [70] who also introduced the concept of locally optimal design for nonlinear regression models; see Chernoff (1972) [71]. This concept will be used rather extensively in our book.

Box and Lucas (1959) [54] used the results of Chernoff, Elfving, and Wald to find locally D-optimal designs for nonlinear models arising in chemical kinetics. Box and Hunter (1965) [53] developed an adaptive strategy for updating the design one trial at a time as observations become available. They extended Lindley's result [258] for the Bayesian justification of D-optimality and provided a derivation of the best conditions for the next trial. The approach based on the use of the Shannon information measure was further developed by Klepikov and Sokolov (1961) [234] and elaborated by Fedorov and Pazman (1968) [150], Caselton and Zidek (1984) [63], Caselton et al. (1992) [62], and revisited by Sebastiani and Wynn (2000) [354].

Box and Hunter (1965) [53] proved that to maximize the decrement of the determinant of the variance-covariance matrix of estimated parameters, observation(s) should be done at the point where the variance of prediction of the linearized model attains its maximum. It is a short step to consider the same "adaptive" procedure for linear models and to observe that optimal designs are independent of parameter values, and so to obtain the algorithm for the iterative construction of optimal designs. This idea was earlier introduced by Klepikov and Sokolov (1961, 1963) [234], [365], [366] who used the term "continuous" design, which in the modern setting corresponds to the first-order algorithm with constant (but very small) step length. The further development of iterative construction of optimal designs was accomplished by Fedorov (1971, 1972) [126], [127], Wynn (1970, 1972) [416], [417], Fedorov and Malyutov (1972) [148], Atwood (1973) [25], Tsay (1976) [385], Wu and Wynn (1978) [409], Wu (1978) [408]. These results triggered a series of publications on numerical methods of optimal design construction; cf. Mitchell (1974) [286], Fedorov and Uspensky (1975) [151], Titterington (1976) [375], Silvey et al. (1978) [362], Torsney (1983) [380], Nachtsheim (1987) [293], Atkinson and Donev (1992) [19], Gaffke and Mathar (1992) [166], Atkinson et al. (2007) [24].

If several models are of interest, the standard criteria can be extended to compound criteria that are weighted linear combinations of standard criteria and to which the standard convex design theory applies; see Atkinson and Cox (1974) [18], Läuter (1974) [249]. If interest lies solely in choosing one model out of two or more competing models, the T-optimum designs of Atkinson and

Fedorov (1975a,b) [21], [20] address the discrimination problem in the "frequentist" setting. Equivalence between model discrimination problems and parameter estimation problems was initially discussed in Wald (1943) [391]; Fedorov and Khabarov (1986) [140] proved the equivalence of these problems for a range of different criteria. Box and Hill (1967) [51] described a Bayesian procedure for discriminating between models that leads to the sequential updating of the prior probabilities of the models. Fedorov and Pázman (1968) [150] developed an adaptive Bayesian procedure for simultaneous model discrimination and parameter estimation.

Special types of optimal design problems arise in environmental studies, with spatial- and longitudinal-type experiments. In both cases the assumption of independence does not hold, and one has to take into account the dependence between observations introducing various models for covariance functions. Problems of optimal allocations or optimal sampling in the case of correlated observations happened to be mathematically rather difficult. First attempts at constructing optimal sampling schemes in the optimal design setting were done by Sacks and Ylvisacker (1966, 1968a,b) [347], [348], [349] in a series of publications where they proposed asymptotically optimal allocations. Cambanis (1985) [59], Matérn (1986) [270], Megreditchan (1979) [274], Micchelli and Wahba (1981) [282] developed various aspects of optimal spatial allocations. Summaries of results in that area can be found in Fedorov (1996) [131], Guttorp et al. (1993) [185], Martin (1996) [268], Fedorov and Hackl (1997) [135], Müller (2007) [291].

The first comprehensive volume on the theory of optimal experimental design was written by Fedorov (1969, 1972) [125], [127]. Silvey (1980) [360] gave a very compact description of the theory of optimal design for estimation in linear models. Other systematic monographs were published by Bandemer et al. (1977) [30], Ermakov (1983) [115], Pázman (1986) [306], Ermakov and Zhigljavsky (1987) [116], Pilz (1991) [309], Atkinson and Donev (1992) [19], Pukelsheim (1993) [328], Schwabe (1996) [353], Fedorov and Hackl (1997) [135], Wu and Hamada (2002) [414], Melas (2006) [275], Atkinson et al. (2007) [24], Berger and Wong (2009) [44], Morris (2010) [289], Goos and Jones (2011) [180], Rasch et al. (2011) [335], Pronzato and Pázman (2013) [322].

We do not discuss factorial experiments in this book. While there are a lot of intersections between "model-based design of experiments" and "design of factorial experiments," the differences are mainly in models and methods of optimal design construction. In the latter case, these are primarily combinatorial and algebraic methods; see Fisher (1971) [157], Wu and Hamada (2002) [414], Bailey (2008) [29].

While the focus of our monograph is on nonlinear models, we always start the exposition of key ideas for linear with respect to unknown parameters models. Then we move toward linearization of models, locally optimal estimators and designs, and after that proceed to multi-stage and adaptive designs. In discussing adaptive procedures, we use those that are stopped when the sample size (number of observations) reaches the predetermined value. Often this stopping rule is called "noninformative stopping" compared to "informative stopping" when the rule depends on the observed responses and/or current values of estimators.

Models and optimization problems. In the description of experiments we distinguish between *dependent*, or *response* variables that are altered by the change in the experimental conditions, and *independent*, or *predictor* variables that describe the conditions under which the response is obtained. The former variables are usually denoted by y. For the latter we distinguish between variables x that are controlled by the experimenter, and variables z, often called *covariates* that are not, such as weather conditions in meteorology or some of a patient's physical and physiological characteristics in clinical studies. Dependent and independent variables are often vectors that we highlight by using a boldface font, as in $\mathbf{y}$, $\mathbf{x}$ and $\mathbf{z}$.

The set of values of control variables at which the response variable may be observed is called a design region $\mathfrak{X}$. Usually, $\mathfrak{X}$ is a finite set with a dimension corresponding to the number of design variables. More generally, $\mathfrak{X}$ can be a set in the functional space. The structure of $\mathfrak{X}$ is often not essential for major theoretical results in optimal design theory, while the computational aspects can be quite challenging.

Various design constraints are often encountered in practice. In a time-series context, it is typically not possible to have multiple observations at the same time point. Similar restrictions may be imposed due to geographical conditions, mixing constraints, etc. Among the most common causes for constraints are cost limitations and ethical concerns. For instance, the number of patients enrolled in a clinical study of a new drug depends on the study budget. In pharmacokinetic studies the number of drawn blood samples is often limited, in particular when drugs are investigated in special populations (e.g., in pediatric studies). Ethical, cost or any other constraints are quantified by the introduction of respective penalty functions together with inequalities that define their admissible values.

Once the response, control variables, and a model that links them are selected, a researcher should quantify the study objectives and constraints. Typically, objectives are described by a utility function and a particular criterion of optimality. In dose-finding studies, probability of efficacy without toxicity provides an example of the utility function, while the variance of the estimator of a dose that maximizes this probability may be selected as an optimality criterion. In classical design theory, a standard objective is the estimation of unknown parameters that define the response model; optimality criteria are scalar functions of the variance-covariance matrix of parameter estimates. Cost is proportional to the number of observations and has an upper bound.

Through decades of evolution optimal design theory extended in many directions adding more complex models and new types of problems to the traditional regression models and parameter estimation problem. We start the exposition with standard regression models and then proceed with various extensions, which include, among others, multiresponse regression, regression models with random coefficients, and models described by stochastic differential equations. The latter two types of models add an intrinsic component of variability to the observational errors. Selection of the most informative variables discussed in Chapter 9 provides an example where traditional methods of optimal experimental design are applied to problems arising in observational studies.

Illustrating Examples

As noted earlier, the main ideas of optimal experimental design may be applied to a large number of problems in which both response and control variables have rather complicated structures. Here we outline a few examples; for details, see Chapters 6 – 9.

Dose-response studies. Dose-response models arise in clinical trials, either with a categorical outcome (e.g., success – failure as a response to the new experimental treatment, or disease progress on an ordinal scale) or continuous response (e.g., studies of pain medications when patients mark their pain level on a visual analog scale). In these examples, x represents the dose of a drug administered to the patient. The design problem may be formulated as finding those doses, within the admissible range, that provide the most accurate estimation of model parameters or utility functions given the sample size; see Chapters 6 and 8. In a more complex setting, the design variable x represents a dosing regimen (e.g., drug amount and frequency of drug administration).

Bioassay studies. Multiparameter logistic models with continuous response, sometimes referred to as the $E_{\max}$ or Hill models, are widely used in bioassay studies. Examples include models that relate the concentration of an experimental drug to the percentage/number of surviving cells in cell-based assays or models that quantify the concentration of antigens/antibodies in enzyme-linked immunosorbent assays (ELISA). In this context, the design variable x represents the drug concentration level; see Sections 6.3, 6.3.1, 8.1 for details.

Clinical PK studies. Multiple blood samples are taken in virtually all clinical studies, and the collected data are analyzed by means of various PK compartmental models. This leads to quite sophisticated nonlinear mixed effects models, which are discussed in Chapter 7. In these models $\mathbf{x}$ and $\mathbf{y}$ are k-dimensional vectors that represent sequences of k sampling times and respective observations for a particular patient.

Penalized or cost-based designs. In the previous example (PK studies) it is quite obvious that each extra sample provides additional information.

On the other hand, the number of samples that may be drawn from each patient is restricted because of blood volume limitations and other logistic and ethical reasons. Moreover, the analysis of each sample is associated with monetary cost. Thus, it makes sense to incorporate costs and other constraints in the design; see Chapter 4. In dose-finding studies exposure to high doses of an experimental drug may increase chances of toxicity, while exposure to low doses may deprive the patient of a potential cure. Both outcomes are associated with medical ethics. The objective of optimal design is to provide a quantified compromise between the ethics and the informativeness of the study. Examples of cost-based and constrained designs are provided in Sections 6.4, 6.5, 7.2, 7.3, 8.2, 8.3, and 9.2.

The structure of the book is as follows. In Chapter 1 we start with linear regression and least squares estimation and introduce relevant objects and problems of optimal design. At the end of Chapter 1 we focus on the maximum likelihood estimator and discuss estimation methods for nonlinear regression models. Convex design theory is the subject of Chapter 2. Numerical methods of the construction of optimal designs are dealt with in Chapter 3, and constrained/cost-based designs are considered in Chapter 4. In Chapter 5 we bridge earlier results to the case of nonlinear regression models where optimal designs depend on values of unknown parameters. In Chapters 6 – 9 we discuss the application of optimal design theory in biopharmaceutical problems. Chapter 6 is devoted to dose-response models while Chapter 7 addresses the application of optimal design in pharmacokinetic (PK) and pharmacodynamic (PD) studies and includes a description of the MATLAB®-based library for the construction of optimal sampling schemes for PK/PD models. Adaptive model-based designs are discussed in Chapter 8. Chapter 9 presents several examples of nontraditional applications of optimal experimental design. A list of potentially useful formulae from matrix algebra and matrix differential calculus is given in Chapter 10.

Computations for all examples were performed using various software platforms: MATLAB, SAS®, and R. For further details, see Chapters 6 – 9.

Chapter 1

Regression Models and Their Analysis

1.1 Linear Model, Single Response 2
    1.1.1 Least squares estimator 4
    1.1.2 Information matrix 6
1.2 More about Information Matrix 10
1.3 Generalized Versions of Linear Regression Model 12
    1.3.1 Heterogeneous but known variance 12
    1.3.2 Unknown parameters in variance 13
    1.3.3 Multivariate response 15
1.4 Nonlinear Models 17
    1.4.1 Least squares estimator 17
    1.4.2 Variance-covariance matrix 18
    1.4.3 Iterative estimation 19
1.5 Maximum Likelihood and Fisher Information Matrix 20
    1.5.1 Examples of Fisher information matrix 21
1.6 Generalized Regression and Elemental Fisher Information Matrices 23
    1.6.1 Univariate distributions 24
    1.6.2 Two multivariate distributions 25
1.7 Nonlinear Regression with Normally Distributed Observations 30
    1.7.1 Iterated estimators and combined least squares 32
    1.7.2 Examples of iterated estimators 36
        1.7.2.1 Multiresponse linear model with constant covariance matrix 36
        1.7.2.2 Multiresponse linear model with random coefficients ... 37
        1.7.2.3 Separation of response and variance parameters 39
    1.7.3 Simulations 41

In Sections 1.1 and 1.2 we consider a linear regression model with homogeneous errors and introduce the least squares estimator and the information, or "moment" matrix. In Section 1.3 the linear regression model with nonhomogeneous errors is discussed. A distinction is made between the case where the error variance is known and, therefore, a simple transformation reduces this case to the one discussed in Sections 1.1 and 1.2, and the case where unknown parameters enter the variance function. In the latter case iterative procedures are needed to estimate model parameters, so we outline the heuristics behind such procedures. Nonlinear regression models are introduced in Section 1.4, and a rather simple parallel is drawn between linear regression models and the first-order approximation of nonlinear models in the vicinity of true parameter values. It is worth noting that in Sections 1.1 to 1.4 we do not impose any distributional assumptions on measurement errors beyond the existence of the first two moments. Then in Section 1.5 the maximum likelihood estimator (MLE) and the Fisher information matrix are introduced when observations have probability density function; we formulate, again in a rather heuristic fashion, results about the link between the Fisher information matrix and the variance-covariance matrix of the MLE. Section 1.6 presents examples of generalized regression models and elemental information matrices.

Section 1.7 deals with parameter estimation in a nonlinear model with normally distributed observations. In Section 1.7.1 we formally describe several iterated estimators, including iteratively reweighted least squares (IRLS) and combined iteratively reweighted least squares (CIRLS), and then formulate Theorem 1.1 about the equivalence of the CIRLS and the MLE. Section 1.7.2 presents several examples where the general formulae of Section 1.7.1 can be simplified. In Section 1.7.3 we discuss results of simulation studies that illustrate the differences between various iterative procedures.

Compared to Sections 1.1 – 1.5, Section 1.7 has a weaker link to optimal design problems and, therefore, may be skipped during the first reading. Nevertheless, we feel that the reader may benefit from going through the description of various iterative procedures in Section 1.7.1 and a simple example of separation of response and variance parameters in Section 1.7.2.3. Note also that an example of a multiresponse linear model with random coefficients in Section 1.7.2.2 has close ties with population pharmacokinetic/pharmacodynamic models, which are discussed later in the book in Chapter 7.

1.1   Linear Model, Single Response

We start with the linear regression model, which makes the exposition relatively simple, but still allows us to introduce all relevant objects and notations that are used throughout the book. We assume that observations $\{y_{ij}\}$ satisfy

$$y_{ij} = \boldsymbol{\theta}_t^T \mathbf{f}(\mathbf{x}_i) + \varepsilon_{ij}, \ i = 1, 2, \ldots, n; \ \ j = 1, \ldots, r_i, \ \sum_{i=1}^{n} r_i = N, \qquad (1.1)$$

where $\boldsymbol{\theta}_t = (\theta_1, \theta_2, \ldots, \theta_m)^T$ is a vector of unknown parameters; $\mathbf{f}(\mathbf{x}) = [f_1(\mathbf{x}), f_2(\mathbf{x}), \ldots, f_m(\mathbf{x})]^T$ is a vector of known "basis" functions; ε_{ij} are uncorrelated random variables with zero mean and constant variance σ^2,

$$\mathrm{E}\varepsilon_{ij} = 0, \ \ \mathrm{E}\varepsilon_{ij}^2 \equiv \sigma^2, \ \ \mathrm{E}[\varepsilon_{ij}\varepsilon_{i'j'}] = 0 \ \ \text{if } i \neq i' \text{ or } j \neq j'. \qquad (1.2)$$

The subscript "t" in $\boldsymbol{\theta}_t$ indicates the true values of the unknown parameters and will be omitted when this does not lead to ambiguity. Such practice will be extended to other subscripts and superscripts whenever the interpretation remains clear. At this point no assumptions are made about the distribution of random variables $\{\varepsilon_{ij}\}$ except the existence of the first two moments.

The variable y is called the response (dependent, or observed) variable. In this text the lowercase y is used for both the random variable (response) or its realization (observed response) without any additional comments if the meaning is clear from the context. The variable $\mathbf{x}$ is called a predictor (independent, control, or design) variable or covariate. Points $\mathbf{x}_i$ are called design or support points, and r_i stands for the number of observations taken at $\mathbf{x}_i$, $i = 1, \ldots, n$. By an "experiment" we mean the collection of N observations, i.e., design points $\mathbf{x}_i$, number of their replications r_i, and responses y_{ij}. The collection

$$\xi_N = \left\{ \begin{array}{c} \mathbf{x}_1, \ldots, \mathbf{x}_n \\ p_1, \ldots, p_n \end{array} \right\} = \{\mathbf{x}_i, \ p_i\}_1^n, \quad \text{where} \quad p_i = r_i/N, \tag{1.3}$$

is called the design of the experiment, or sometimes exact design, as opposed to continuous designs, which are discussed in detail in Chapter 2. Predictors $\mathbf{x}_i$ can be vectors, matrices, or even elements of a functional space; see examples in Section 1.7.2 and Chapter 6.

In (1.1) the response function $\eta(\mathbf{x}, \boldsymbol{\theta}) = \boldsymbol{\theta}^T \mathbf{f}(\mathbf{x})$ is linear with respect to (unknown) parameters $\boldsymbol{\theta}$. Popular examples of basis functions include

- Polynomial regression: $\mathbf{f}(x) = \left(1, x, \ldots, x^{m-1}\right)^T$, i.e., $f_i(x) = x^{i-1}, i = 1, \ldots, m$.

- Trigonometric regression: $\mathbf{f}(x) = \left(1, \sin x, \ \cos x, \ldots, \sin kx, \cos kx\right)^T$, where $m = 2k + 1$.

- Multivariate linear regression when a scalar predictor x is replaced by the vector $\mathbf{x} = (1, x_1, \ldots, x_{m-1})^T$ and $f_i(\mathbf{x}) = 1$, $f_i(\mathbf{x}) = x_{i-1}$ for $i = 2, \ldots, m$.

Alternative presentation of model (1.1). The model (1.1) may be written in the matrix form that is used in many texts on linear regression; e.g., see Rao (1973) [334], Chapter 4, or Draper and Smith (1998) [106], Chapter 5:

$$\mathbf{Y} = \mathcal{F}^T \boldsymbol{\theta} + \boldsymbol{\varepsilon}, \tag{1.4}$$

where $\mathcal{F}$ is an $m \times N$ matrix, and $\mathbf{Y}$ and $\boldsymbol{\varepsilon}$ are $N \times 1$ column vectors,

$$
\mathcal{F}^T = \begin{bmatrix} f_1(\mathbf{x}_1) & f_2(\mathbf{x}_1) & \cdots & f_m(\mathbf{x}_1) \\ \cdots & \cdots & \cdots & \cdots \\ f_1(\mathbf{x}_1) & f_2(\mathbf{x}_1) & \cdots & f_m(\mathbf{x}_1) \\ \\ f_1(\mathbf{x}_2) & f_2(\mathbf{x}_2) & \cdots & f_m(\mathbf{x}_2) \\ \cdots & \cdots & \cdots & \cdots \\ f_1(\mathbf{x}_2) & f_2(\mathbf{x}_2) & \cdots & f_m(\mathbf{x}_2) \\ \\ \cdots & \cdots & \cdots & \cdots \\ \\ f_1(\mathbf{x}_n) & f_2(\mathbf{x}_n) & \cdots & f_m(\mathbf{x}_n) \\ \cdots & \cdots & \cdots & \cdots \\ f_1(\mathbf{x}_n) & f_2(\mathbf{x}_n) & \cdots & f_m(\mathbf{x}_n) \end{bmatrix}, \quad \mathbf{Y} = \begin{bmatrix} y_{11} \\ \cdots \\ y_{1r_1} \\ \\ y_{21} \\ \cdots \\ y_{2r_2} \\ \\ \cdots \\ \\ y_{n1} \\ \cdots \\ y_{nr_n} \end{bmatrix}, \quad \boldsymbol{\varepsilon} = \begin{bmatrix} \varepsilon_{11} \\ \cdots \\ \varepsilon_{1r_1} \\ \\ \varepsilon_{21} \\ \cdots \\ \varepsilon_{2r_2} \\ \\ \cdots \\ \\ \varepsilon_{n1} \\ \cdots \\ \varepsilon_{nr_n} \end{bmatrix}.
$$

$$(1.5)$$

We prefer the presentation (1.1) because it naturally allows us to introduce "good" statistical estimators of unknown parameters $\boldsymbol{\theta}$ via the key object of model-based optimal design, namely the information matrix; see Sections 1.5 and 1.7.

1.1.1 Least squares estimator

Based on the observations $\{y_{ij}\}$ at support points $\{\mathbf{x}_i\}$, the least squares estimator (LSE) $\hat{\boldsymbol{\theta}}_N$ of $\boldsymbol{\theta}$ is defined as

$$
\hat{\boldsymbol{\theta}}_N = \arg \min_{\boldsymbol{\theta} \in \mathbf{R}^m} \tilde{v}_N(\boldsymbol{\theta}), \tag{1.6}
$$

where

$$
\tilde{v}_N(\boldsymbol{\theta}) = \sum_{i=1}^{n} \sum_{j=1}^{r_i} \left[y_{ij} - \boldsymbol{\theta}^T \mathbf{f}(\mathbf{x}_i) \right]^2. \tag{1.7}
$$

Let

$$
\overline{y}_i = r_i^{-1} \sum_{j=1}^{r_i} y_{ij}. \tag{1.8}
$$

Then the inner sum on the right-hand side of (1.7) may be rewritten as

$$
\sum_{j=1}^{r_i} \left[(y_{ij} - \overline{y}_i) + \left(\overline{y}_i - \boldsymbol{\theta}^T \mathbf{f}(\mathbf{x}_i) \right) \right]^2 = \sum_{j=1}^{r_i} (y_{ij} - \overline{y}_i)^2 + r_i \left[\overline{y}_i - \boldsymbol{\theta}^T \mathbf{f}(\mathbf{x}_i) \right]^2,
$$

where the first term on the right-hand side does not depend on $\boldsymbol{\theta}$. Therefore, the optimization problem (1.6), (1.7) is equivalent to the following optimization problem:

$$
\hat{\boldsymbol{\theta}}_N = \arg \min_{\boldsymbol{\theta}} v_N(\boldsymbol{\theta}), \quad \text{where } v_N(\boldsymbol{\theta}) = \sum_{i=1}^{n} r_i \left[\overline{y}_i - \boldsymbol{\theta}^T \mathbf{f}(\mathbf{x}_i) \right]^2. \tag{1.9}
$$

Using formula (10.6) and setting the first derivative of the function $v_N(\boldsymbol{\theta})$ in (1.9) to zero gives the "normal equations"

$$\underline{\mathbf{M}}(\xi_N)\,\boldsymbol{\theta} \;=\; \mathcal{Y}, \tag{1.10}$$

where

$$\underline{\mathbf{M}}(\xi_N) \;=\; \sigma^{-2} \sum_{i=1}^{n} r_i \mathbf{f}(\mathbf{x}_i) \mathbf{f}^T(\mathbf{x}_i) \tag{1.11}$$

and

$$\mathcal{Y} = \sigma^{-2} \sum_{i=1}^{n} r_i\, \overline{y}_i \mathbf{f}(\mathbf{x}_i). \tag{1.12}$$

It is obvious that $\hat{\boldsymbol{\theta}}_N$ may be uniquely determined if the matrix $\underline{\mathbf{M}}(\xi_N)$ is regular, i.e., if $\mathrm{rank}[\underline{\mathbf{M}}(\xi_N)] = m$ and the inverse matrix $\underline{\mathbf{M}}^{-1}(\xi_N)$ exists. In this case

$$\hat{\boldsymbol{\theta}}_N = \underline{\mathbf{M}}^{-1}(\xi_N)\,\mathcal{Y}. \tag{1.13}$$

It is worthwhile noting that the estimator $\hat{\boldsymbol{\theta}}_N$ in (1.13) will not change if the multiplier σ^{-2} is dropped in the definition of $\underline{\mathbf{M}}(\xi_N)$ and $\mathcal{Y}$ on the right-hand side of (1.11) and (1.12), respectively. The main reason for the introduction of this multiplier is that for normally distributed observations the Fisher information matrix is proportional to σ^{-2}; see (1.21), (1.90).

Since $\overline{y}_i$'s are uncorrelated for different i, the equality $\mathrm{Var}[r_i\overline{y}_i\mathbf{f}(x_i)] = r_i\mathbf{f}(\mathbf{x}_i)\mathbf{f}^T(\mathbf{x}_i)\sigma^2$ implies that

$$\mathrm{Var}[\hat{\boldsymbol{\theta}}_N] = \underline{\mathbf{M}}^{-1}(\xi_N) = \underline{\mathbf{D}}(\xi_N). \tag{1.14}$$

Alternative presentation of the LSE. The optimization problem (1.6), (1.7) can be written as

$$\hat{\boldsymbol{\theta}}_N = \arg\min_{\boldsymbol{\theta}} ||\mathbf{Y} - \mathcal{F}^T\boldsymbol{\theta})||^2, \tag{1.15}$$

where $\mathbf{Y}$ and $\mathcal{F}$ are defined in (1.5), and $||\mathbf{z}|| = \left(\sum_{i=1}^{m} z_i^2\right)^{1/2}$ is the Euclidean norm; see Rao (1973) [334], Chapter 4a, or Draper and Smith (1998) [106]. The normal equations take the form

$$\mathcal{F}\,\mathcal{F}^T\,\boldsymbol{\theta} = \mathcal{F}\mathbf{Y}, \tag{1.16}$$

and the solution of (1.15) is given by

$$\hat{\boldsymbol{\theta}}_a = (\mathcal{F}\mathcal{F}^T)^{-1}\mathcal{F}\mathbf{Y}, \quad \text{with} \quad \mathrm{Var}[\hat{\boldsymbol{\theta}}_a] = \sigma^2(\mathcal{F}\mathcal{F}^T)^{-1}, \tag{1.17}$$

which obviously coincides with $\hat{\boldsymbol{\theta}}_N$ and $\mathrm{Var}[\hat{\boldsymbol{\theta}}_N]$ from (1.13) and (1.14), respectively. As noted earlier, we prefer the presentation (1.11) because it illuminates the additivity of information from independent observations.

The LSE is the best linear unbiased estimator (BLUE), i.e.,

$$E[\hat{\boldsymbol{\theta}}_N] = \boldsymbol{\theta}_t \text{ and } \text{Var}[\hat{\boldsymbol{\theta}}_N] \leq \text{Var}[\tilde{\boldsymbol{\theta}}], \tag{1.18}$$

for an arbitrary linear unbiased estimator $\tilde{\boldsymbol{\theta}}$; cf. the Gauss-Markov Theorem; see Rao (1973) [334], Chapter 4a. The ordering of nonnegative definite matrices, or Loewner ordering, is understood as

$$\mathbf{A} \leq \mathbf{B}, \text{ if } \mathbf{A} = \mathbf{B} + \mathbf{C}, \ \mathbf{C} \geq 0,$$

where the latter inequality means that the square $m \times m$ matrix $\mathbf{C}$ is nonnegative definite, i.e., $\mathbf{z}^T \mathbf{C} \mathbf{z} \geq 0$ for any vector $\mathbf{z}$; see Harville (1997) [195], Chapter 14.2. Note that the set

$$\mathcal{E}_{\mathbf{A}} = \mathcal{E}_{\mathbf{A}}(R) = \{\mathbf{z} \in \mathbf{R}^m : \mathbf{z}^T \mathbf{A} \mathbf{z} \leq R^2\} \tag{1.19}$$

defines an ellipsoid of concentration in $\mathbf{R}^m$; see Cramèr (1946) [83], Chapter 21.10; Klepikov and Sokolov (1961) [234], Appendix 1. The ellipsoid of concentration generates confidence regions for normal linear models; e.g., see Pukelsheim (1993) [328], Chapter 3. Geometrically, the inequality $\mathbf{A} \leq \mathbf{B}$ means that $\mathcal{E}_{\mathbf{A}} \supseteq \mathcal{E}_{\mathbf{B}}$; see Figure 1.1 for an illustration in two-dimensional space, $m = 2$. For more details on ellipsoids of concentration, see Section 2.2.

The existence of the variance-covariance (dispersion) matrix $\underline{\mathbf{D}}(\xi_N)$ implies that the design ξ_N is "good enough" for the unique estimation of all components of the vector $\boldsymbol{\theta}$. Optimal design theory addresses the selection of the design ξ_N in such a way that the variance-covariance matrix $\underline{\mathbf{D}}(\xi_N)$ is the "smallest," in some sense. Indeed, the quality of estimators, or their precision, is traditionally measured by the variance-covariance matrix, and practitioners may want to select a design that is "better" than others in terms of $\text{Var}[\hat{\boldsymbol{\theta}}_N]$. The criteria that evaluate the quality of designs and algorithms for selecting "good" designs are among the main topics of this book.

1.1.2 Information matrix

The matrix $\underline{\mathbf{M}}(\xi_N)$ defined in (1.11) is usually called the "information matrix" of the design ξ_N. It is also often labeled a "moment," or "precision" matrix; e.g., see Pukelsheim (1993) [328], Chapter 3.10. The information matrix $\underline{\mathbf{M}}(\xi_N)$ is determined by the design ξ_N and does not depend upon the observations $\{y_{ij}\}$. An important property of linear models is that the information matrix does not depend on parameter values either.

Two important properties of the information matrix are worth mentioning from the start:

1. The information matrix is a symmetric nonnegative definite matrix. Indeed, it follows from (1.11) that

$$\mathbf{z}^T \underline{\mathbf{M}}(\xi_N) \mathbf{z} = \sigma^{-2} \sum_i r_i [\mathbf{z}^T \mathbf{f}(\mathbf{x}_i)]^2 \geq 0 \tag{1.20}$$

for any vector $\mathbf{z} \in \mathbf{R}^m$.

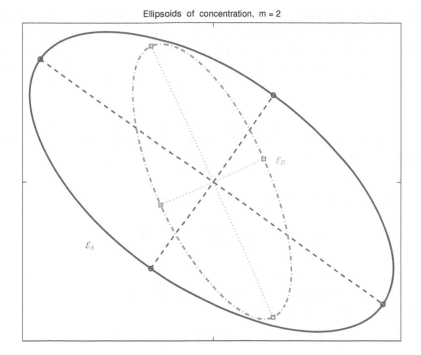

FIGURE 1.1: Ellipsoids of concentration, $m = 2$; here $\mathbf{A} \leq \mathbf{B}$, and $\mathcal{E}_{\mathbf{A}} \supseteq \mathcal{E}_{\mathbf{B}}$. Dashed and dotted lines correspond to principal axes of ellipsoids $\mathcal{E}_{\mathbf{A}}$ and $\mathcal{E}_{\mathbf{B}}$, respectively.

2. The information matrix is additive, i.e., it is the sum of information matrices that corresponds to the individual observations:

$$\underline{\mathbf{M}}(\xi_N) = \sum_{i=1}^{n} r_i \boldsymbol{\mu}(\mathbf{x}_i), \text{ where } \boldsymbol{\mu}(\mathbf{x}) = \sigma^{-2}\mathbf{f}(\mathbf{x})\mathbf{f}^T(\mathbf{x}). \qquad (1.21)$$

Therefore, adding an extra independent observation leads to the increase of the information matrix. The additivity of the information matrix is crucial for optimal design theory. In the case of normally distributed observations, $\boldsymbol{\mu}(\mathbf{x})$ coincides with the Fisher information matrix as described in Section 1.5; see (1.90). Note also that the matrix $\boldsymbol{\mu}(\mathbf{x})$ introduced in (1.21) has rank one.

Remark 1.1 Since the number of observations N for a particular experiment is fixed and $p_i = r_i/N$, one can use p_i instead of r_i in the definition of $v_N(\boldsymbol{\theta})$ in (1.9), i.e., define

$$v_N(\boldsymbol{\theta}) = \sum_{i=1}^{n} p_i \left[\overline{y}_i - \boldsymbol{\theta}^T \mathbf{f}(\mathbf{x}_i) \right]^2 ,$$

without affecting the solution of the optimization problem (1.9). We keep r_i's in the definition of the majority of objects in Chapter 1, to underline the additivity of the information from the individual observations. However, once the concept of "continuous" designs is introduced in Section 2.4, we will use weights p_i instead of r_i and allow p_i to vary continuously in [0,1].

Singular cases. If the information matrix is singular, i.e., $\text{rank}[\mathbf{M}(\xi_N)] = m' < m$, then unique LSEs do not exist for all components of $\boldsymbol{\theta}$. However, a number of linear functions

$$\boldsymbol{\gamma} = \mathbf{L}^T \boldsymbol{\theta} \tag{1.22}$$

may still be uniquely estimated if the solution

$$\hat{\boldsymbol{\gamma}}_N = \arg \min_{\boldsymbol{\gamma} = \mathbf{L}^T \boldsymbol{\theta}} \sum_{i=1}^{n} r_i \left[\overline{y}_i - \boldsymbol{\theta}^T \mathbf{f}(\mathbf{x}_i) \right]^2 \tag{1.23}$$

is unique; see Rao (1973) [334], Chapter 4a. The maximum number of components in $\boldsymbol{\gamma}$ is m'. For these functions, which are called "estimable under ξ_N," the estimator and its variance are

$$\hat{\boldsymbol{\gamma}}_N = \mathbf{L}^T \underline{\mathbf{M}}^-(\xi_N) \mathcal{Y} \quad \text{and} \quad \text{Var}[\hat{\boldsymbol{\gamma}}_N] = \mathbf{L}^T \underline{\mathbf{M}}^-(\xi_N) \mathbf{L}, \tag{1.24}$$

where $\underline{\mathbf{M}}^-$ stands for any g-inverse of $\underline{\mathbf{M}}$; see Harville (1997) [195], Chapter 14.4. Another way to determine $\hat{\boldsymbol{\gamma}}_N$ and its variance is to use the regularized version of (1.13) and (1.14):

$$\hat{\boldsymbol{\gamma}}_N = \lim_{\alpha \to 0} \left[\mathbf{L}^T \underline{\mathbf{M}}(\xi_N) + \alpha \mathbf{P} \right]^{-1} \mathcal{Y} \tag{1.25}$$

and

$$\text{Var}[\hat{\boldsymbol{\gamma}}_N] = \lim_{\alpha \to 0} \mathbf{L}^T \left[\mathbf{M}(\xi_N) + \alpha \mathbf{P} \right]^{-1} \mathbf{L}, \tag{1.26}$$

where $\mathbf{P}$ is any positive definite matrix; see Albert (1972) [5]. Similar to $\hat{\boldsymbol{\theta}}_N$, the estimator $\hat{\boldsymbol{\gamma}}_N$ is the BLUE .

Whenever possible, we avoid cases with singular $\underline{\mathbf{M}}(\xi_N)$. When singularity is essential for a specific problem, regularization similar to (1.25) and (1.26) may be used to overcome difficulties related to the pseudo-inverse.

Combined estimators. Let us assume that q experiments have been performed, such that

$$y_{ij,l} = \boldsymbol{\theta}^T \mathbf{f}_l(\mathbf{x}_{i,l}) + \varepsilon_{ij,l}, \ i = 1, 2, \ldots, n_l; \ j = 1, \ldots, r_{i,l}; \ l = 1, \ldots, q, \tag{1.27}$$

and $\sum_{i=1}^{n_l} r_i = N_l$, $\sum_{l=1}^{q} N_l = N$. The basis functions in different experiments may be, in general, different, which we address by adding the subscript "l" in $\mathbf{f}_l$. Thus, the model structure may be different for the individual experiments but still all of them contain the same parameters. For instance, in some experiments only the first few components of $\boldsymbol{\theta}$ can be estimated, while the rest of the components may be estimated in complementary experiments. Of course, if a particular model does not contain a specific parameter, then the information matrix for that experiment must be extended by corresponding rows and columns of zeros, and generalized inverse is needed to obtain individual LSEs $\hat{\boldsymbol{\theta}}_{N_l}$. We assume that the observations in different experiments are uncorrelated. What is the best way to combine the information of all experiments into a single estimator?

A straightforward extension of (1.9) is

$$\hat{\boldsymbol{\theta}}_{tot} = \arg\min_{\boldsymbol{\theta}} \sum_{l=1}^{q} v_{N_l}(\boldsymbol{\theta}), \text{ where } v_{N_l}(\boldsymbol{\theta}) = \sum_{i=1}^{n} r_{i,l} \left[\overline{y}_{i,l} - \boldsymbol{\theta}^T \mathbf{f}_l(\mathbf{x}_{i,l}) \right]^2. \tag{1.28}$$

The combined estimator $\hat{\boldsymbol{\theta}}_{tot}$ is the BLUE due to the Gauss-Markov theorem. The normal equations become

$$\sum_{l=1}^{q} \left[\sum_{i=1}^{n_l} r_{i,l}\, \overline{y}_{i,l}\, \mathbf{f}_l(\mathbf{x}_{i,l}) - \sum_{i=1}^{n_l} r_{i,l}\, \mathbf{f}_l(\mathbf{x}_{i,l})\, \mathbf{f}_l^T(\mathbf{x}_{i,l})\, \boldsymbol{\theta} \right] = 0, \tag{1.29}$$

cf. (1.10), and the routine algebra leads to the combined estimator

$$\hat{\boldsymbol{\theta}}_{tot} = \underline{\mathbf{M}}^{-1}(\xi_{tot}) \sum_{l=1}^{q} \mathcal{Y}_l, \text{ or} \tag{1.30}$$

$$\hat{\boldsymbol{\theta}}_{tot} = \underline{\mathbf{M}}^{-1}(\xi_{tot}) \sum_{l=1}^{q} \mathbf{M}(\xi_{N_l}) \hat{\boldsymbol{\theta}}_{N_l}, \tag{1.31}$$

where

$$\underline{\mathbf{M}}(\xi_{tot}) = \sum_{l=1}^{q} \mathbf{M}(\xi_{N_l}), \quad \mathbf{M}(\xi_{N_l}) = \sigma^{-2} \sum_{i=1}^{n_l} r_{i,l}\, \mathbf{f}_l(\mathbf{x}_{i,l})\, \mathbf{f}_l^T(\mathbf{x}_{i,l}),$$

and

$$\mathcal{Y}_l = \sigma^{-2} \sum_{i=1}^{n_l} r_{i,l}\, \overline{y}_{i,l}\, \mathbf{f}_l(\mathbf{x}_{i,l}).$$

By ξ_{tot} we denote the design that comprises the support points and the corresponding weights of all individual designs: $\xi_{tot} = \bigcup_{l=1}^{q} \xi_{N_l}$. The variance-covariance matrix of $\hat{\boldsymbol{\theta}}_{tot}$ is

$$\text{Var}[\hat{\boldsymbol{\theta}}_{tot}] = \underline{\mathbf{M}}^{-1}(\xi_{tot}). \tag{1.32}$$

The additivity of the information matrix for combined experiments is analogous to the additivity of individual observations that are combined within a single experiment.

Obviously, the matrix $\underline{\mathbf{M}}(\xi_{tot})$ must be nonsingular for (1.30) – (1.32) to be used. In this case, the expression on the right-hand side of (1.31) is well defined even if some individual information matrices $\underline{\mathbf{M}}(\xi_{N_l})$ are singular. Indeed, even in the case of non-unique LSE $\hat{\boldsymbol{\theta}}_{N_l}$, the product $\underline{\mathbf{M}}(\xi_{N_l})\hat{\boldsymbol{\theta}}_{N_l}$ is invariant because of the normal equations (1.10).

Use of prior information. Let us assume that in the model (1.1) or, equivalently, (1.4), the value of σ^2 is known. Suppose that the prior information about the parameter $\boldsymbol{\theta}$ is available and that $\boldsymbol{\theta}$ has mean $\hat{\boldsymbol{\theta}}_0$ and variance-covariance matrix $\mathbf{D}_0$, where the $m \times m$ matrix $\mathbf{D}_0$ is known and non-singular. Then the posterior distribution of $\boldsymbol{\theta}$ has mean

$$\boldsymbol{\theta}^* = \left(\mathbf{D}_0^{-1} + \sigma^{-2}\mathcal{F}\mathcal{F}^T\right)^{-1} \left(\mathbf{D}_0^{-1}\hat{\boldsymbol{\theta}}_0 + \sigma^{-2}\mathcal{F}\mathbf{Y}\right)$$

$$= \left[\mathbf{D}_0^{-1} + \underline{\mathbf{M}}(\xi_N)\right]^{-1} \left[\mathbf{D}_0^{-1}\hat{\boldsymbol{\theta}}_0 + \underline{\mathbf{M}}(\xi_N)\,\hat{\boldsymbol{\theta}}_N\right], \qquad (1.33)$$

cf. (1.30), and the covariance matrix $\mathbf{D}_B$, where

$$\mathbf{D}_B = \left(\mathbf{D}_0^{-1} + \sigma^{-2}\mathcal{F}\mathcal{F}^T\right)^{-1} = \left(\mathbf{D}_0^{-1} + \underline{\mathbf{M}}(\xi_N)\right)^{-1}, \qquad (1.34)$$

see Tanner (1996) [371], Chapter 2.1. It is worthwhile noting that if a preliminary independent experiment is performed, with the matrix $\mathbf{D}_0^{-1}$ as its information matrix, and a new experiment is performed according to model (1.1), then the information matrix of the combined two-stage experiment is exactly $\mathbf{D}_B^{-1}$, where $\mathbf{D}_B$ is defined in (1.34); see Fedorov (1972), Gladitz and Pilz (1982) [177], Chaloner (1984) [64], Section 1, Pilz (1991) [309], Chaloner and Verdinelli (1995) [65], Section 2.1. For a discussion of Bayesian optimal designs, see Section 2.7. See also Draper and Hunter (1967) [105].

1.2   More about Information Matrix

The variance-covariance matrix $\underline{\mathbf{D}}(\xi_N)$, as defined in (1.14), is traditionally considered a measure of the uncertainty of the estimator $\hat{\boldsymbol{\theta}}_N$, or a measure of the uncertainty of our "knowledge" of $\boldsymbol{\theta}$. The word "certainty" must be substituted for "uncertainty" in the last sentence when we discuss the matrix $\underline{\mathbf{M}}(\xi_N)$ in (1.14). This is one of the reasons why $\underline{\mathbf{M}}(\xi_N)$ is called the information matrix.

Local behavior of sum of squares. Let us rewrite the expression for $v_N(\boldsymbol{\theta})$ in (1.9) by adding and subtracting $\hat{\boldsymbol{\theta}}_N^T \mathbf{f}(x_i)$ inside the square brackets:

$$v_N(\boldsymbol{\theta}) = \sum_i r_i \left[\bar{y}_i - \hat{\boldsymbol{\theta}}_N^T\mathbf{f}(\mathbf{x}_i)\right]^2 + \sum_i r_i \left[(\hat{\boldsymbol{\theta}}_N - \boldsymbol{\theta})^T\mathbf{f}(\mathbf{x}_i)\right]^2$$

$$+ 2 \sum_i r_i \left[\overline{y}_i - \hat{\boldsymbol{\theta}}_N^T \mathbf{f}(\mathbf{x}_i) \right] (\hat{\boldsymbol{\theta}}_N - \boldsymbol{\theta})^T \mathbf{f}(\mathbf{x}_i),$$

It follows from (1.11) that the second term on the right-hand side of the last equality is equal to

$$(\hat{\boldsymbol{\theta}}_N - \boldsymbol{\theta})^T \sum_i r_i \mathbf{f}(\mathbf{x}_i) \mathbf{f}^T(\mathbf{x}_i) \, (\hat{\boldsymbol{\theta}}_N - \boldsymbol{\theta}) = \sigma^2 (\hat{\boldsymbol{\theta}}_N - \boldsymbol{\theta})^T \underline{\mathbf{M}}(\xi_N)(\hat{\boldsymbol{\theta}}_N - \boldsymbol{\theta}),$$

and the third term vanishes because of the normal equations (1.10). Therefore

$$v_N(\boldsymbol{\theta}) = \sum_i r_i \left[\overline{y}_i - \hat{\boldsymbol{\theta}}_N^T \mathbf{f}(\mathbf{x}_i) \right]^2 + \sigma^2 (\hat{\boldsymbol{\theta}}_N - \boldsymbol{\theta})^T \underline{\mathbf{M}}(\xi_N)(\hat{\boldsymbol{\theta}}_N - \boldsymbol{\theta}), \quad (1.35)$$

which reveals the relation between the information matrix and $v_N(\boldsymbol{\theta})$. While the estimator $\hat{\boldsymbol{\theta}}_N$ minimizes the function $v_N(\boldsymbol{\theta})$, the information matrix $\underline{\mathbf{M}}(\xi_N)$ determines its shape that does not depend on observations $\{y_{ij}\}$.

Let $\mathbf{U}$ be a unit-length vector in $\mathbf{R}^m$, i.e., $\mathbf{U}^T \mathbf{U} = 1$. If in the parameter space one moves the distance d from $\hat{\boldsymbol{\theta}}_N$ in the direction of the vector $\mathbf{U}$, then $v_N(\boldsymbol{\theta})$ increases by $\sigma^2 d^2 \mathbf{U}^T \underline{\mathbf{M}}(\xi_N)\mathbf{U}$. The increase is the largest along the principal axis of the ellipsoid $\mathbf{U}^T \underline{\mathbf{M}}(\xi_N)\mathbf{U} \leq 1$, which corresponds to the maximal eigenvalue of the matrix $\underline{\mathbf{M}}(\xi_N)$:

$$\lambda_{\max} = \max_{\mathbf{U}} \mathbf{U}^T \underline{\mathbf{M}}(\xi_N)\mathbf{U}; \qquad (1.36)$$

therefore, the vector $\mathbf{U}_{max}$ defined as

$$\mathbf{U}_{\max} = \arg \max_{\mathbf{U}} \mathbf{U}^T \underline{\mathbf{M}}(\xi_N)\mathbf{U} \qquad (1.37)$$

is the corresponding eigenvector. The smallest increase will be observed along the direction

$$\mathbf{U}_{\min} = \arg \min_{\mathbf{U}} \mathbf{U}^T \underline{\mathbf{M}}(\xi_N)\mathbf{U}, \qquad (1.38)$$

and, correspondingly,

$$\lambda_{\min} = \min_{\mathbf{U}} \mathbf{U}^T \underline{\mathbf{M}}(\xi_N)\mathbf{U} \qquad (1.39)$$

is the minimal eigenvalue of $\underline{\mathbf{M}}(\xi_N)$. Of course, if $\lambda_{\min} = 0$, we have infinitely many solutions for (1.6) or (1.9).

Another useful presentation of the information matrix can be derived by differentiating the sum of squares $v_N(\boldsymbol{\theta})$ in (1.35):

$$\underline{\mathbf{M}}(\xi_N) = \frac{1}{2} \frac{\partial^2 v_N(\boldsymbol{\theta})}{\partial \boldsymbol{\theta} \, \partial \boldsymbol{\theta}^T}, \quad \text{where} \quad \left(\frac{\partial v}{\partial \boldsymbol{\theta}} \right)^T = \frac{\partial v}{\partial \boldsymbol{\theta}^T} = \left(\frac{\partial v}{\partial \theta_1}, \dots, \frac{\partial v}{\partial \theta_m} \right). \quad (1.40)$$

Sensitivity of the LSE with respect to observational errors. Let us formally take the derivative of the LSE $\hat{\boldsymbol{\theta}}_N$ in (1.13) with respect to $\varepsilon_{ij} = y_{ij} - \boldsymbol{\theta}^T f(\mathbf{x}_i)$. This derivative,

$$\frac{\partial \hat{\boldsymbol{\theta}}_N}{\partial \varepsilon_{ij}} = \sigma^{-2} \underline{\mathbf{M}}^{-1}(\xi_N) \mathbf{f}(\mathbf{x}_i), \tag{1.41}$$

defines the relation between the LSE $\hat{\boldsymbol{\theta}}_N$ and ε_{ij}; cf. Cook's distance, which measures the effect of deleting a given observation; see Cook (1979) [78]. An aggregate sensitivity measure is

$$\sigma^2 \sum_{i=1}^{n} \sum_{j=1}^{r_i} \frac{\partial \hat{\boldsymbol{\theta}}_N}{\partial \varepsilon_{ij}} \left(\frac{\partial \hat{\boldsymbol{\theta}}_N}{\partial \varepsilon_{ij}} \right)^T = \underline{\mathbf{M}}^{-1}(\xi_N). \tag{1.42}$$

Alternative decomposition of the sum of squares. If one uses the alternative notation for the linear model as in (1.4), (1.5) and (1.15) – (1.17), then the sum of squares in (1.35) may be presented as

$$||\mathbf{Y} - \mathcal{F}^T \boldsymbol{\theta}||^2 = ||\mathbf{Y} - \mathcal{F}^T \hat{\boldsymbol{\theta}}_N||^2 + (\hat{\boldsymbol{\theta}}_N - \boldsymbol{\theta})^T \mathcal{F} \mathcal{F}^T (\hat{\boldsymbol{\theta}}_N - \boldsymbol{\theta}). \tag{1.43}$$

Throughout the entire book the information matrix is the main object of our discussion. Formulae (1.35), (1.40), and (1.42) give, in some sense, a deterministic motivation for the use of the information matrix. The reader may interpret the results on the basis of this deterministic view. However, we will formulate all subsequent results in the "statistical language," i.e., assuming that the observational errors are random.

1.3   Generalized Versions of Linear Regression Model

1.3.1   Heterogeneous but known variance

In practice, the variance of the observational error may change for different levels of the predictor, i.e.,

$$E[\varepsilon^2 | \mathbf{x}] = \lambda^{-1}(\mathbf{x}) \sigma^2. \tag{1.44}$$

If the weight function $\lambda(\mathbf{x})$ is known, the corresponding regression model may be reduced to the standard case by transformations

$$y_{new} = \sqrt{\lambda(\mathbf{x})}\, y, \quad \mathbf{g}(x) = \sqrt{\lambda(\mathbf{x})}\, \mathbf{f}(x). \tag{1.45}$$

The LSE that results from (1.9) for the transformed data is

$$\hat{\boldsymbol{\theta}}_N = \arg \min_{\boldsymbol{\theta}} \sum_{i=1}^{n} \lambda(\mathbf{x}_i)\, r_i \left[\overline{y}_i - \boldsymbol{\theta}^T \mathbf{f}(\mathbf{x}_i) \right]^2. \tag{1.46}$$

As pointed out by Davidian and Giltinan (1995) [90], Chapter 2.3.2, in the sum of squared deviations, "each deviation is weighted in inverse proportion to the magnitude of uncertainty in the associated response." The solution of (1.46) is given by the formula (1.13), where

$$\underline{\mathbf{M}}(\xi_N) = \sigma^{-2} \sum_{i=1}^{n} \lambda(\mathbf{x}_i) \ r_i \mathbf{f}(\mathbf{x}_i) \mathbf{f}^T(\mathbf{x}_i) \tag{1.47}$$

and

$$\mathcal{Y} = \sigma^{-2} \sum_{i=1}^{n} \lambda(\mathbf{x}_i) \ r_i \mathbf{f}(\mathbf{x}_i) \overline{y}_i; \tag{1.48}$$

see also Beal and Sheiner (1988) [39], Section 2.2; Carroll and Ruppert (1988) [61], Chapter 2.1. The simplicity of transformations that are needed to handle such a general case allows us to assume everywhere, with some occasional exceptions, that $\lambda(\mathbf{x}) \equiv 1$ and to work with the shorter and simpler formulae.

In the case of univariate response the value of variance σ^2 is often unknown; its unbiased estimate is

$$\hat{\sigma}^2 = (N - m)^{-1} v_N(\hat{\boldsymbol{\theta}}_N). \tag{1.49}$$

Note that σ^2 enters both $\underline{\mathbf{M}}^{-1}(\xi_N)$ and $\mathbf{y}$ in (1.13) as a multiplicative constant; see (1.11) and (1.12), or (1.47) and (1.48). Therefore, because of (1.35) the sum of squares $v_N(\hat{\boldsymbol{\theta}}_N)$ does not depend on the actual value of σ^2.

1.3.2 Unknown parameters in variance

Often the weight function has a known functional form, but, unlike the situation discussed in the previous section, it depends on unknown parameters, i.e., $\lambda(\mathbf{x}) = \lambda(\mathbf{x}, \boldsymbol{\beta})$, where a vector of parameters $\boldsymbol{\beta}$ may include some (or all) of parameters in the vector $\boldsymbol{\theta}$ and also may include additional "variance" parameters. A Poisson regression model provides an example where the vector $\boldsymbol{\beta}$ coincides with $\boldsymbol{\theta}$:

$$\mathrm{E}[y|\mathbf{x}] = \boldsymbol{\theta}^T \mathbf{f}(\mathbf{x}) = \mathrm{Var}[y|\mathbf{x}] = \lambda^{-1}(\mathbf{x}, \boldsymbol{\theta}). \tag{1.50}$$

Note that $\lambda(\mathbf{x}, \boldsymbol{\theta})$ must be positive for all $\boldsymbol{\theta}$. Otherwise, one needs to impose constraints on the estimator of $\boldsymbol{\theta}$.

We address the general situation in Sections 1.5 and 1.7 where the maximum likelihood (ML) and iteratively reweighted least squares (IRLS) methods are formally introduced, while in this section we outline the approach in a rather heuristic fashion. Note that models with unknown parameters in the variance function have received considerable attention in the literature; see, for example, Davidian and Carroll (1987) [89], Sections 3.1.1, 3.1.2; Carroll and Ruppert (1988) [61], Chapter 2; Beal and Sheiner (1988) [39], Section 2.5;

Davidian and Giltinan (1995) [90], Chapter 2.3; Vonesh and Chinchilli (1997) [388], Chapter 9.2.

If guesses λ_{0i} for $\lambda(\mathbf{x}_i, \boldsymbol{\theta})$ are available, say $\lambda_{0i} = (\overline{y}_i)^{-1}$ for the Poisson regression (1.50), then a "reasonable" estimate of $\boldsymbol{\theta}$ may be calculated as

$$\boldsymbol{\theta}_{0,N} = \arg\min_{\boldsymbol{\theta}} \sum_{i=1}^{n} \lambda_{0i} \, r_i \left[\overline{y}_i - \boldsymbol{\theta}^T \mathbf{f}(\mathbf{x}_i) \right]^2. \tag{1.51}$$

An obvious extension of (1.51) is the iterative estimation procedure based on

$$\boldsymbol{\theta}_{s,N} = \arg\min_{\boldsymbol{\theta}} \sum_{i=1}^{n} \lambda(\mathbf{x}_i, \boldsymbol{\theta}_{s-1,N}) \, r_i \left[\overline{y}_i - \boldsymbol{\theta}^T \mathbf{f}(\mathbf{x}_i) \right]^2, \tag{1.52}$$

for $s \geq 1$. Two questions arise immediately: (1) Does the iterative procedure (1.52) converge, i.e., does the limit

$$\hat{\boldsymbol{\theta}}_N = \lim_{s \to \infty} \boldsymbol{\theta}_{s,N} \tag{1.53}$$

exist in some sense? and (2) What are the statistical properties of $\hat{\boldsymbol{\theta}}_N$ in (1.53) if the limit exists? The answer to both questions has the "asymptotic flavor," unlike the simpler model with the constant variance as in (1.2). Under certain regularity conditions, the probability P_N that the limit (1.53) exists becomes close to 1 for large N. Moreover, the limiting value of $\hat{\boldsymbol{\theta}}_N$ coincides with the true value $\boldsymbol{\theta}_t$; one of the sufficient conditions of almost sure (a.s.) convergence is the existence of the regular matrix $\mathbf{M}$ such that

$$\lim_{N \to \infty} N^{-1} \underline{\mathbf{M}}(\xi_N) = \mathbf{M}. \tag{1.54}$$

Asymptotically, as $N \to \infty$, the iterated estimator has the same variance-covariance matrix as the LSE (1.46) with the known weight function $\lambda(\mathbf{x})$, i.e.,

$$N^{-1}\mathrm{Var}[\hat{\boldsymbol{\theta}}_N] \simeq N^{-1} \sum_{i=1}^{n} \lambda(\mathbf{x}_i, \boldsymbol{\theta}_t) \, r_i \mathbf{f}(\mathbf{x}_i)\mathbf{f}^T(\mathbf{x}_i). \tag{1.55}$$

It should be emphasized that if one attempts the direct optimization, without the intermediate step of "freezing" the estimate of $\boldsymbol{\theta}$ in the weight function as in (1.52), and considers instead the following problem,

$$\tilde{\boldsymbol{\theta}}_N = \arg\min_{\boldsymbol{\theta}} \sum_{i=1}^{n} \lambda(\mathbf{x}_i, \boldsymbol{\theta}) \, r_i \left[y_i - \boldsymbol{\theta}^T \mathbf{f}(\mathbf{x}_i) \right]^2, \tag{1.56}$$

then the minimization in (1.56) leads, in general, to an inconsistent estimate of $\boldsymbol{\theta}$. Note that the estimation procedure (1.51), (1.52) does not utilize any information that can be extracted from the observed variability of responses at different $\mathbf{x}$'s. In general, this may lead to a considerable loss of precision in $\hat{\boldsymbol{\theta}}$; see Sections 1.7.1, 1.7.3 for further discussion.

1.3.3 Multivariate response

Let us assume that the experimenter observes several, say $k > 1$ response variables. Then the model (1.1) must be extended to

$$\mathbf{y}_{ij} = \mathbf{F}^T(\mathbf{x}_i)\boldsymbol{\theta} + \boldsymbol{\varepsilon}_{ij}, \tag{1.57}$$

where $\mathbf{y}_{ij}$ and $\boldsymbol{\varepsilon}_{ij}$ are $k \times 1$ vectors, and $m \times 1$ vectors $\mathbf{f}_l(\mathbf{x})$ form the columns of the $m \times k$ matrix $\mathbf{F}(\mathbf{x})$:

$$\mathbf{F}(\mathbf{x}) = [\mathbf{f}_1(\mathbf{x}), \dots, \mathbf{f}_k(\mathbf{x})].$$

Similar to the single-response case, we assume that random vectors $\boldsymbol{\varepsilon}_{ij}$ have zero mean, constant variance-covariance matrix and are uncorrelated:

$$\mathrm{E}[\boldsymbol{\varepsilon}_{ij}] = \mathbf{0}, \ \mathrm{E}[\boldsymbol{\varepsilon}_{ij} \, \boldsymbol{\varepsilon}_{ij}^T] = \mathbf{S} > \mathbf{0}, \ \mathrm{E}[\boldsymbol{\varepsilon}_{ij} \, \boldsymbol{\varepsilon}_{i'j'}^T] = \mathbf{0} \ \text{ if } i \neq i' \text{ or } j \neq j'. \tag{1.58}$$

The LSE of $\boldsymbol{\theta}$ is now defined via

$$\hat{\boldsymbol{\theta}}_N = \arg\min_{\boldsymbol{\theta}} \ v_N(\boldsymbol{\theta}, \mathbf{S}), \tag{1.59}$$

where

$$v_N(\boldsymbol{\theta}, \mathbf{S}) = \sum_{i=1}^{n} \sum_{j=1}^{r_i} \left[\mathbf{y}_{ij} - \mathbf{F}^T(\mathbf{x}_i)\boldsymbol{\theta}\right]^T \mathbf{S}^{-1} \left[\mathbf{y}_{ij} - \mathbf{F}^T(\mathbf{x}_i)\boldsymbol{\theta}\right]; \tag{1.60}$$

cf. (1.7). The minimization results in the direct analog of (1.13),

$$\hat{\boldsymbol{\theta}}_N = \underline{\mathbf{M}}^{-1}(\xi_N)\mathcal{Y}, \tag{1.61}$$

where

$$\underline{\mathbf{M}}(\xi_N) = \sum_{i=1}^{n} r_i \mathbf{F}(\mathbf{x}_i)\mathbf{S}^{-1}\mathbf{F}^T(\mathbf{x}_i), \tag{1.62}$$

$$\mathcal{Y} = \sum_{i=1}^{n} r_i \ \mathbf{F}(\mathbf{x}_i)\mathbf{S}^{-1}\bar{\mathbf{y}}_i^T, \ \text{ and } \ \bar{\mathbf{y}}_i = \frac{1}{r_i} \sum_{j=1}^{r_i} \mathbf{y}_{ij}. \tag{1.63}$$

Similar to the univariate response case, the information matrix $\underline{\mathbf{M}}(\xi_N)$ may be written as a weighted sum of information matrices of the individual observations:

$$\underline{\mathbf{M}}(\xi_N) = \sum_{i=1}^{n} r_i \ \boldsymbol{\mu}(\mathbf{x}_i), \ \text{ where } \ \boldsymbol{\mu}(\mathbf{x}) = \mathbf{F}(\mathbf{x})\mathbf{S}^{-1}\mathbf{F}^T(\mathbf{x}). \tag{1.64}$$

However, now $1 \leq \mathrm{rank}[\boldsymbol{\mu}(\mathbf{x}_i)] \leq k$, unlike the case of the single-response model (1.1), (1.2); see comments after (1.21).

Unknown variance-covariance matrix S. In contrast to the single response model (1.1), (1.2), in the multiresponse case, knowledge of the variance-covariance matrix $\mathbf{S}$, up to a multiplicative constant, is essential for the construction of the LSE; cf. (1.61) – (1.63). Similar to Section 1.3.2, here we provide a heuristic outline of an iterative estimator that asymptotically coincides with the BLUE with known $\mathbf{S}$; cf. (1.51), (1.52). For a detailed discussion of this and more general cases, see Section 1.7.

(i) Start with some initial matrix $\mathbf{S}_{0,N}$ of rank k. The matrix

$$\mathbf{S}_{0,N} = \frac{1}{n} \sum_{i=1}^{n} \frac{1}{r_i} \sum_{j=1}^{r_i} (\mathbf{y}_{ij} - \bar{\mathbf{y}}_i)(\mathbf{y}_{ij} - \bar{\mathbf{y}}_i)^T$$

seems to be a natural choice.

(ii) For $s \geq 1$: given $\mathbf{S}_{s-1,N}$, find

$$\boldsymbol{\theta}_{s,N} = \underline{\mathbf{M}}_s^{-1}(\xi_N)\mathcal{Y}_s,$$

where $\underline{\mathbf{M}}_s(\xi_N)$ and $\mathcal{Y}_s$ are defined as in (1.61), with $\mathbf{S}_{s-1,N}$ replacing the matrix $\mathbf{S}$ in (1.62) and (1.63).

(iii) Calculate

$$\mathbf{S}_{s,N} = \frac{1}{n} \sum_{i=1}^{n} \frac{1}{r_i} \sum_{j=1}^{r_i} \left[\mathbf{y}_{ij} - \mathbf{F}^T(\mathbf{x}_i)\boldsymbol{\theta}_{s,N} \right] \left[\mathbf{y}_{ij} - \mathbf{F}^T(\mathbf{x}_i)\boldsymbol{\theta}_{s,N} \right]^T. \quad (1.65)$$

(iv) Repeat steps (ii) – (iii) until a suitable stopping rule is satisfied.

If the limit matrix

$$\mathbf{M} = \lim_{N \to \infty} \frac{1}{N} \underline{\mathbf{M}}(\xi_N)$$

exists and is regular, then it may be established, under rather mild assumptions about moments of random errors $\{\varepsilon_{ij}\}$, that estimators $\hat{\boldsymbol{\theta}}_N$ and $\hat{\mathbf{S}}_N$,

$$\hat{\boldsymbol{\theta}}_N = \lim_{s \to \infty} \boldsymbol{\theta}_{s,N}, \ \hat{\mathbf{S}}_N = \lim_{s \to \infty} \mathbf{S}_{s,N}, \quad (1.66)$$

are strongly consistent estimators of $\boldsymbol{\theta}$ and $\mathbf{S}$, respectively. It may be of interest that the iterative procedure (i) – (iv) minimizes the determinant $|\mathbf{S}(\boldsymbol{\theta})|$ in (1.65). For more details on the estimation procedures, including those for models where the variance parameters $\boldsymbol{\beta}$ differ from the vector $\boldsymbol{\theta}$, cf. Section 1.3.2, see Jobson and Fuller (1980) [215]; Davidian and Carroll (1987) [89], Section 3.1.1 on pseudolikelihood methods; Carroll and Ruppert (1988) [61], Chapter 3; Davidian and Giltinan (1995) [90], Chapter 2.3.3 on pseudolikelihood and restricted maximum likelihood estimation; Vonesh and Chinchilli (1997) [388], Chapter 6.2.1.

1.4 Nonlinear Models

In this section we generalize the linear model (1.1), (1.2) by replacing the linear response $\boldsymbol{\theta}^T \mathbf{f}(\mathbf{x})$ in (1.1) with a nonlinear response function $\eta(\mathbf{x}, \boldsymbol{\theta})$. For more details on nonlinear models, see Section 1.7.

1.4.1 Least squares estimator

Similar to (1.9), the LSE may be defined as

$$\hat{\boldsymbol{\theta}}_N = \arg \min_{\boldsymbol{\theta} \in \boldsymbol{\Theta}} \sum_{i=1}^{n} r_i \left[\bar{y}_i - \eta(\mathbf{x}_i, \boldsymbol{\theta}) \right]^2, \tag{1.67}$$

where $\boldsymbol{\Theta}$ is a compact set in $\mathbf{R}^m$. In general, it is not possible to find a closed form expression for $\hat{\boldsymbol{\theta}}_N$ like (1.13) in the linear case, and one has to resort to various optimization algorithms.

To assess the quality of the estimator $\hat{\boldsymbol{\theta}}_N$, one needs to characterize the "closeness" of the estimator to the true value $\boldsymbol{\theta}_t$. Unlike the estimator (1.13), $\hat{\boldsymbol{\theta}}_N$ from (1.67) is generally biased, i.e., $\mathrm{E}[\hat{\boldsymbol{\theta}}_N] \neq \boldsymbol{\theta}_t$. Except for rare special cases, it is impossible to find an analytical expression for the variance-covariance matrix $\mathrm{Var}[\hat{\boldsymbol{\theta}}_N]$. Most of the results about $\hat{\boldsymbol{\theta}}_N$ have asymptotic character.

Consistency of $\hat{\boldsymbol{\theta}}_N$. Under rather mild assumptions the estimator $\hat{\boldsymbol{\theta}}_N$ is strongly consistent; cf. Seber and Wild (1989) [357], Chapter 12:

$$\lim_{N \to \infty} \hat{\boldsymbol{\theta}}_N = \boldsymbol{\theta}_t \quad a.s. \tag{1.68}$$

The proof of consistency is based mainly on three assumptions:

(A) The response function $\eta(\mathbf{x}, \boldsymbol{\theta})$ is continuous with respect to $\boldsymbol{\theta} \in \boldsymbol{\Theta}$ for all $\mathbf{x}$.

(B) Introduce

$$v_N(\boldsymbol{\theta}, \boldsymbol{\theta}_t, \xi_N) = \sum_{i=1}^{n} p_{iN} [\eta(\mathbf{x}_i, \boldsymbol{\theta}) - \eta(\mathbf{x}_i, \boldsymbol{\theta}_t)]^2, \quad p_{iN} = r_i/N.$$

The limit
$$v(\boldsymbol{\theta}, \boldsymbol{\theta}_t) = \lim_{N \to \infty} v_N(\boldsymbol{\theta}, \boldsymbol{\theta}_t, \xi_N) \tag{1.69}$$

exists uniformly in $\boldsymbol{\Theta}$.

(C) The function $v(\boldsymbol{\theta}, \boldsymbol{\theta}_t)$ has a unique minimum at $\boldsymbol{\theta} = \boldsymbol{\theta}_t$, where $\boldsymbol{\theta}_t$ is the internal point in $\boldsymbol{\Theta}$.

Let us comment on the above assumptions. When $\eta(\mathbf{x}, \boldsymbol{\theta})$ is given explicitly, verification of assumption (A) is straightforward. Verification of assumption (B) is simple if, for example, all observations are allocated at a finite number n of points $x_1, \ldots, x_n$, i.e., $\lim_{N\to\infty} p_{i_N} = p_i$ for $i = 1, \ldots, n$; of course, n must be greater than the number of parameters to be estimated. Note that in the linear case

$$v_N(\boldsymbol{\theta}, \boldsymbol{\theta}_t, \xi_N) = \sigma^2 N^{-1}(\boldsymbol{\theta} - \boldsymbol{\theta}_t)^T \underline{\mathbf{M}}(\xi_N)(\boldsymbol{\theta} - \boldsymbol{\theta}_t); \tag{1.70}$$

cf. (1.35). Thus to satisfy assumption (B), it is sufficient that the limit matrix

$$\lim_{N\to\infty} \sigma^2 N^{-1} \underline{\mathbf{M}}(\xi_N) = \mathbf{M} \tag{1.71}$$

exists and is regular. The consistency of $\hat{\boldsymbol{\theta}}_N$ in the linear case is determined entirely by the behavior of ξ_N; the value of $\boldsymbol{\theta}_t$ is not involved in the analysis.

1.4.2 Variance-covariance matrix

To provide a heuristic hint on the derivation of the variance-covariance matrix $\text{Var}[\hat{\boldsymbol{\theta}}_N]$, we use the Taylor expansion to approximate $\eta(\mathbf{x}, \boldsymbol{\theta})$ in the vicinity of $\boldsymbol{\theta}_t$:

$$\eta(\mathbf{x}, \boldsymbol{\theta}) \cong \eta(\mathbf{x}, \boldsymbol{\theta}_t) + (\boldsymbol{\theta} - \boldsymbol{\theta}_t)^T \mathbf{f}(\mathbf{x}, \boldsymbol{\theta}_t), \quad \text{where} \quad \mathbf{f}(\mathbf{x}, \boldsymbol{\theta}) = \frac{\partial \eta(\mathbf{x}, \boldsymbol{\theta})}{\partial \boldsymbol{\theta}}. \tag{1.72}$$

If $\boldsymbol{\theta}$ is "close enough" to $\boldsymbol{\theta}_t$, then the sum on the right-hand side of (1.67) may be approximated as

$$\sum_{i=1}^{n} r_i \left[\bar{y}_i - \eta(\mathbf{x}_i, \boldsymbol{\theta}_t) - (\boldsymbol{\theta} - \boldsymbol{\theta}_t)^T \mathbf{f}(\mathbf{x}_i, \boldsymbol{\theta}_t) \right]^2, \tag{1.73}$$

which mimics $v_N(\boldsymbol{\theta})$ in (1.9), with two minor differences: now $\bar{y}_i - \eta(\mathbf{x}_i, \boldsymbol{\theta}_t)$ replaces $\bar{y}_i$, and $\boldsymbol{\theta} - \boldsymbol{\theta}_t$ replaces $\boldsymbol{\theta}$. Thus, the direct comparison of (1.73) with (1.9) and (1.13) results in

$$\hat{\boldsymbol{\theta}}_N - \boldsymbol{\theta}_t \simeq \underline{\mathbf{M}}^{-1}(\xi_N, \boldsymbol{\theta}_t)\mathcal{Y}(\xi_N, \boldsymbol{\theta}_t), \tag{1.74}$$

where

$$\underline{\mathbf{M}}(\xi_N, \boldsymbol{\theta}_t) = \sigma^{-2} \sum_{i=1}^{n} r_i \mathbf{f}(\mathbf{x}_i, \boldsymbol{\theta}_t) \mathbf{f}^T(\mathbf{x}_i, \boldsymbol{\theta}_t) \tag{1.75}$$

and

$$\mathcal{Y}(\xi_N, \boldsymbol{\theta}_t) = \sigma^{-2} \sum_{i=1}^{n} r_i \left[\bar{y}_i - \eta(\mathbf{x}_i, \boldsymbol{\theta}_t) \right]. \tag{1.76}$$

Therefore, similar to (1.14),

$$\text{Var}[\hat{\boldsymbol{\theta}}_N] \cong \underline{\mathbf{M}}^{-1}(\xi_N, \boldsymbol{\theta}_t). \tag{1.77}$$

Of course, (1.77) is valid only to the extent by which the first-order approximation (1.72) is justified. Note that the matrix $\underline{\mathbf{M}}(\xi_N, \boldsymbol{\theta}_t)$ depends on the unknown parameters $\boldsymbol{\theta}_t$. At best, $\boldsymbol{\theta}_t$ can be replaced by $\hat{\boldsymbol{\theta}}_N$, so that

$$\text{Var}[\hat{\boldsymbol{\theta}}_N] \cong \underline{\mathbf{M}}^{-1}(\xi_N, \hat{\boldsymbol{\theta}}_N). \tag{1.78}$$

1.4.3 Iterative estimation

The formula (1.74) suggests the following recursion:

$$\boldsymbol{\theta}_{s+1,N} = \boldsymbol{\theta}_{s,N} + \underline{\mathbf{M}}^{-1}(\xi_N, \boldsymbol{\theta}_{s,N})\, \mathcal{Y}(\xi_N, \boldsymbol{\theta}_{s,N}). \tag{1.79}$$

A modified recursion that mitigates extreme oscillations is

$$\boldsymbol{\theta}_{s+1,N} = \boldsymbol{\theta}_{s,N} + \alpha_s\, \underline{\mathbf{M}}^{-1}(\xi_N, \boldsymbol{\theta}_s)\, \mathcal{Y}(\xi_N, \boldsymbol{\theta}_{s,N}), \tag{1.80}$$

where α_s is chosen in such a way that the existence of the limit

$$\hat{\boldsymbol{\theta}}_N = \lim_{s \to \infty} \boldsymbol{\theta}_{s,N} \tag{1.81}$$

is guaranteed. For example, α_s can be found as the solution of a one-dimensional optimization problem

$$\alpha_s = \arg\min_\alpha \sum_{i=1}^n p_i \left[\bar{y} - \eta(\mathbf{x}_i, \boldsymbol{\theta}_s(\alpha))\right]^2, \tag{1.82}$$

where $\boldsymbol{\theta}_s(\alpha) = \boldsymbol{\theta}_{s,N} + \alpha\, \underline{\mathbf{M}}^{-1}(\xi_N, \boldsymbol{\theta}_s)\, \mathcal{Y}(\xi_N, \boldsymbol{\theta}_{s,N})$; cf. (1.80).

If, in addition to assumptions (A) – (C), the existence of the derivatives $\{\partial^2 \eta(\mathbf{x}, \boldsymbol{\theta})/\partial\theta_\alpha \partial\theta_\beta, \, \alpha, \beta = 1, \ldots, m\}$ is assumed, then one can prove that

$$\lim_{N \to \infty} \sigma^{-2} N \text{Var}[\hat{\boldsymbol{\theta}}_N] = \mathbf{M}^{-1}(\boldsymbol{\theta}_t), \tag{1.83}$$

where

$$\mathbf{M}(\boldsymbol{\theta}_t) = \lim_{N \to \infty} \sigma^2 N^{-1} \underline{\mathbf{M}}(\xi_N, \boldsymbol{\theta}_t).$$

It is worthwhile to emphasize once again that in the nonlinear case the information matrix $\underline{\mathbf{M}}(\xi_N, \boldsymbol{\theta}_t)$ and, as a consequence, $\text{Var}[\hat{\boldsymbol{\theta}}_N]$ depend on the unknown $\boldsymbol{\theta}_t$.

The iterative procedures (1.79) and (1.80) are two instances of numerous numerical procedures for computing the LSE; cf. Seber and Wild (1989) [357]. We prefer these two procedures because they explicitly bridge the linear and nonlinear cases.

1.5 Maximum Likelihood and Fisher Information Matrix

In the earlier sections of this chapter we discussed relatively simple linear models like (1.1), (1.2) or its nonlinear version in Section 1.4. To derive least squares estimators (LSEs), no assumptions were imposed on the probability distribution of observations beyond the existence of first and second moments. This fact allows for addressing a variety of problems when a practitioner does not have exact knowledge of the distribution of observed responses. However, in general, the LSEs are less efficient, in terms of their variance-covariance matrices, than estimators that use distributional assumptions. One of the most popular types of such estimators is the maximum likelihood estimator (MLE). The MLE for the regression models described in this chapter does not yield closed-form solutions, except in the simplest of cases. It is necessary, therefore, to resort to iterative procedures and to rely on the convergence and asymptotic properties of these procedures for estimation and inference.

As in Section 1.1, suppose that r_i independent observations are taken at design points $\mathbf{x}_i$, and $\sum_{i=1}^{n} r_i = N$. Let the probability density function of observations $\mathbf{y}_{ij}$ be $p(\mathbf{y}_{ij}|\mathbf{x}_i, \boldsymbol{\theta})$. The log-likelihood function $\mathcal{L}_N(\boldsymbol{\theta})$ for N independent observations $\{\mathbf{y}_{ij}, \ i = 1, \ldots, n; \ j = 1, \ldots, r_i\}$ is

$$\mathcal{L}_N(\boldsymbol{\theta}) = \frac{1}{N} \sum_{i=1}^{n} \sum_{j=1}^{r_i} \ln p(\mathbf{y}_{ij}|\mathbf{x}_i, \boldsymbol{\theta}). \tag{1.84}$$

The score function is defined as a vector of derivatives of log-density $\ln p(\mathbf{y}|\mathbf{x}, \boldsymbol{\theta})$,

$$\mathbf{R}(\mathbf{y}|\mathbf{x}, \boldsymbol{\theta}) = \frac{\partial \ln p(\mathbf{y}|\mathbf{x}, \boldsymbol{\theta})}{\partial \boldsymbol{\theta}}, \tag{1.85}$$

and the Fisher information matrix of a single observation at a "point" $\mathbf{x}$ may be introduced as the variance of the score function:

$$\boldsymbol{\mu}(\mathbf{x}, \boldsymbol{\theta}) = \mathrm{Var}[\mathbf{R}(\mathbf{y}|\mathbf{x}, \boldsymbol{\theta})] = \mathrm{E}\left[\frac{\partial \ln p}{\partial \boldsymbol{\theta}} \frac{\partial \ln p}{\partial \boldsymbol{\theta}^T}\right] = -\mathrm{E}\left[\frac{\partial^2 \ln p}{\partial \boldsymbol{\theta} \, \partial \boldsymbol{\theta}^T}\right]. \tag{1.86}$$

The Fisher information matrix $\boldsymbol{\mu}(\mathbf{x}, \boldsymbol{\theta})$ of a single "observational unit" is the key object for the construction of optimal designs. The Fisher information matrix $\underline{\mathbf{M}}(\xi_N, \boldsymbol{\theta})$ of the design ξ_N is additive, i.e.,

$$\underline{\mathbf{M}}(\xi_N, \boldsymbol{\theta}) = \sum_i r_i \, \boldsymbol{\mu}(\mathbf{x}_i, \boldsymbol{\theta}). \tag{1.87}$$

Any vector $\boldsymbol{\theta}_N$ that maximizes the log-likelihood function $\mathcal{L}_N(\boldsymbol{\theta})$ in (1.84) is called a maximum likelihood estimator (MLE),

$$\boldsymbol{\theta}_N = \arg \max_{\boldsymbol{\theta} \in \Theta} \mathcal{L}_N(\boldsymbol{\theta}). \tag{1.88}$$

Note that for the MLE we use the term "Fisher information matrix" (FIM) while the term "information matrix" is reserved for the LSE. In general, these two matrices are different, with some rare exceptions; see an example in Section 1.5.1 of linear regression models with normally distributed responses with known variances.

Under rather mild regularity assumptions on density p and design ξ_N it can be proved that for large samples the variance-covariance matrix of the MLE $\boldsymbol{\theta}_N$ is approximated by the inverse of the Fisher information matrix,

$$\text{Var}[\boldsymbol{\theta}_N] = \mathbf{D}(\xi_N, \boldsymbol{\theta}) \approx \underline{\mathbf{M}}^{-1}(\xi_N, \boldsymbol{\theta}), \tag{1.89}$$

and that the variance of the MLE attains the lower bound in Cramèr-Rao inequality; e.g., see Jennrich (1969) [212]; Rao (1973) [334], Chapter 5; Seber and Wild (1989) [357].

Similar to least squares estimation, we keep the "underline" notations for the information matrix $\underline{\mathbf{M}}(\xi_N, \boldsymbol{\theta})$ and variance-covariance matrix $\underline{\mathbf{D}}(\xi_N, \boldsymbol{\theta})$ of exact designs ξ_N. When we move to normalized designs ξ, we drop the "underline" and use $\mathbf{M}(\xi, \boldsymbol{\theta})$ and $\mathbf{D}(\xi, \boldsymbol{\theta})$ instead; see Section 2.4.

Once the estimator is specified, one can consider the optimal design problem, i.e., such selection of predictors that leads to the minimization, in some sense, of the variance-covariance matrix $\underline{\mathbf{D}}(\xi_N, \boldsymbol{\theta})$. Since for nonlinear models the information matrix $\boldsymbol{\mu}(\mathbf{x}, \boldsymbol{\theta})$ and, consequently, the variance-covariance matrix $\underline{\mathbf{D}}(\xi_N, \boldsymbol{\theta})$ depend on values of parameters $\boldsymbol{\theta}$, this dependence creates a formidable problem. Several approaches to tackle this problem are addressed in Chapter 5.

In Section 1.7 we focus on estimation procedures for rather general nonlinear normal models, and then in Chapter 2 we formulate and address various optimization problems related to minimization of $\underline{\mathbf{D}}(\xi_N, \boldsymbol{\theta})$. Meanwhile in this section we provide examples of the Fisher information matrix $\boldsymbol{\mu}(\mathbf{x}, \boldsymbol{\theta})$ for several popular probabilistic models.

1.5.1 Examples of Fisher information matrix

Single-response normal linear model. Let y be normally distributed with the mean $\boldsymbol{\theta}^T \mathbf{f}(\mathbf{x})$ and variance σ^2, where $\boldsymbol{\theta} \in \mathbf{R}^m$ and σ^2 is a known constant (not a parameter). Since

$$\ln p(y|\mathbf{x}, \boldsymbol{\theta}) = -\frac{1}{2} \ln(2\pi\sigma^2) - \frac{1}{2\sigma^2} [y - \boldsymbol{\theta}^T \mathbf{f}(\mathbf{x})]^2,$$

then using formula (10.6), one gets

$$\mathbf{R}(y|\mathbf{x}, \boldsymbol{\theta}) = -\frac{[y - \boldsymbol{\theta}^T \mathbf{f}(\mathbf{x})]\mathbf{f}(\mathbf{x})}{\sigma^2}$$

and

$$\boldsymbol{\mu}(\mathbf{x}, \boldsymbol{\theta}) = \sigma^{-4} \, \mathrm{E}[y - \boldsymbol{\theta}^T \mathbf{f}(\mathbf{x})]^2 \mathbf{f}(\mathbf{x})\mathbf{f}^T(\mathbf{x}) = \sigma^{-2} \, \mathbf{f}(\mathbf{x})\mathbf{f}^T(\mathbf{x}). \tag{1.90}$$

Recall that in (1.21) we presented the information matrix of the LSE of the linear model (1.1), (1.2) as the sum of individual information matrices $\boldsymbol{\mu}(x_i)$. Comparison of (1.21) and (1.90) reveals that for normal observations with known constant variance the LSE and MLE coincide. Of course, this is also obvious from the formal definition of the MLE since for the normal errors

$$\mathcal{L}_N(\boldsymbol{\theta}) = -\frac{1}{2}\ln(2\pi\sigma^2) - \frac{1}{2N\sigma^2}\sum_{i=1}^{n}\sum_{j=1}^{r_i}[y_{ij} - \boldsymbol{\theta}^T\mathbf{f}(\mathbf{x}_i)]^2 \qquad (1.91)$$

and, therefore, the maximization of $\mathcal{L}_N(\boldsymbol{\theta})$ in (1.91) is equivalent to the minimization of the sum of squares in (1.7).

Binary response model. In a binary model, a response variable y is defined as

$$y = y(\mathbf{x}) = \left\{ \begin{array}{ll} 1, & \text{a response is present at level } \mathbf{x}, \\ 0, & \text{no response}, \end{array} \right.$$

and the probability of observing a response is modeled as

$$\Pr\{y = 1|\mathbf{x}\} = \eta(\mathbf{x}, \boldsymbol{\theta}),$$

where $0 \leq \eta(\mathbf{x}, \boldsymbol{\theta}) \leq 1$ is a given function and $\boldsymbol{\theta}$ is a vector of m unknown parameters. It is often assumed that

$$\eta(\mathbf{x}, \boldsymbol{\theta}) = \pi(z), \quad \text{with} \quad z = \boldsymbol{\theta}^T\mathbf{f}(\mathbf{x}), \qquad (1.92)$$

and $\pi(z)$ is selected as a nondecreasing function, e.g., a probability distribution function. The probability distribution of y at a point $\mathbf{x}$ and the score function can be written as

$$p(y|\mathbf{x}, \boldsymbol{\theta}) = \pi(z)^y[1 - \pi(z)]^{1-y}$$

and

$$\mathbf{R}(y|\mathbf{x}, \boldsymbol{\theta}) = \mathbf{f}(\mathbf{x})\left\{ \begin{array}{ll} \dot{\pi}/\pi, & y = 1 \\ -\dot{\pi}/(1 - \pi), & y = 0 \end{array} \right.,$$

respectively. It follows from (1.85) and (1.86) that

$$\begin{aligned} \boldsymbol{\mu}(\mathbf{x}, \boldsymbol{\theta}) &= \mathbf{f}(\mathbf{x})\mathbf{f}^T(\mathbf{x})\,\dot{\pi}^2\left[\frac{1}{\pi^2}\pi + \frac{1}{(1-\pi)^2}(1-\pi)\right] \\ &= \frac{\dot{\pi}^2}{\pi[1-\pi]}\,\mathbf{f}(\mathbf{x})\mathbf{f}^T(\mathbf{x}). \end{aligned} \qquad (1.93)$$

For more details on binary models, see Wetherill (1963) [396], Wu (1988) [413], Torsney and Musrati (1993) [384], Cramer (2003) [84].

1.6 Generalized Regression and Elemental Fisher Information Matrices

The reader may have noticed that the derivation of Fisher information matrices for both examples of Section 1.5.1 follows a similar path. In this section we emphasize such similarity and provide the collection of results that allow us to treat the wide class of regression models in a rather routine manner. More detailed exposition can be found in Atkinson et al. (2012) [23].

The results rely on the following simple fact from calculus about transformations of parameters. Let $\boldsymbol{\zeta}$ and $\boldsymbol{\theta}$ be $m' \times 1$ and $m \times 1$ vectors, respectively, and let a transformation

$$\boldsymbol{\zeta} = \boldsymbol{\zeta}(\boldsymbol{\theta}) : \ \mathbf{R}^m \to \mathbf{R}^{m'}$$

be differentiable with the Jacobian matrix $\mathbf{F}$ of order $m \times m'$:

$$\mathbf{F} = \frac{\partial \boldsymbol{\zeta}^T}{\partial \boldsymbol{\theta}} = \begin{pmatrix} \frac{\partial \zeta_1}{\partial \theta_1} & \cdots & \frac{\partial \zeta_{m'}}{\partial \theta_1} \\ \cdots & \cdots & \cdots \\ \frac{\partial \zeta_1}{\partial \theta_m} & \cdots & \frac{\partial \zeta_{m'}}{\partial \theta_m} \end{pmatrix}. \tag{1.94}$$

Let y be distributed with the density $p(y|\boldsymbol{\zeta})$ and the Fisher information matrix

$$\boldsymbol{\nu}(\boldsymbol{\zeta}) = \mathrm{Var}[R(y|\boldsymbol{\zeta})] = \mathrm{E}\left[\frac{\partial \ln p(y|\boldsymbol{\zeta})}{\partial \boldsymbol{\zeta}} \frac{\partial \ln p(y|\boldsymbol{\zeta})}{\partial \boldsymbol{\zeta}^T}\right]. \tag{1.95}$$

Since

$$\frac{\partial}{\partial \boldsymbol{\theta}} \ln p(y|\boldsymbol{\theta})) = \frac{\partial \boldsymbol{\zeta}}{\partial \boldsymbol{\theta}} \left[\frac{\partial}{\partial \boldsymbol{\zeta}} \ln p(y|\boldsymbol{\zeta})\right]_{\boldsymbol{\zeta}=\boldsymbol{\zeta}(\boldsymbol{\theta})} = \mathbf{F} R[\boldsymbol{\zeta}(\boldsymbol{\theta})],$$

it follows from the definition of the Fisher information matrix that

$$\boldsymbol{\mu}(\boldsymbol{\theta}) = \mathbf{F} \, \boldsymbol{\nu}(\boldsymbol{\zeta}) \, \mathbf{F}^T. \tag{1.96}$$

The transformation formula (1.96) is useful when a regression-type model for parameters $\boldsymbol{\zeta}$ is introduced,

$$\boldsymbol{\zeta} = \boldsymbol{\zeta}(\mathbf{x}, \boldsymbol{\theta}), \tag{1.97}$$

with the dependence on variables $\mathbf{x}$. In this case

$$\mathbf{F} = \mathbf{F}(\mathbf{x}, \boldsymbol{\theta}) = \frac{\partial \boldsymbol{\zeta}^T(\mathbf{x}, \boldsymbol{\theta})}{\partial \boldsymbol{\theta}}.$$

We refer to model (1.97) as generalized regression. The examples of generalized regression are

$$\boldsymbol{\zeta} = \mathbf{f}^T(\mathbf{x})\boldsymbol{\theta}, \tag{1.98}$$

as in the first example of Section 1.5.1, and

$$\zeta = \pi[\mathbf{f}^T(\mathbf{x})\boldsymbol{\theta}], \tag{1.99}$$

as in the second example. Note that $\mathbf{F} = \mathbf{f}$ for model (1.98), and $\mathbf{F} = \dot{\pi}\,\mathbf{f}$ for model (1.99).

Remark 1.2 In (1.97) – (1.99) we could have used the notation η instead of ζ to draw reader's attention to regression-type nature of the above transformations. Note, however, that in the beginning of this section we discuss transformation of *parameters*, $\boldsymbol{\theta} \to \zeta$. Because we reserve the symbol η for response functions throughout the book, we feel that if in this section we used η and called it a "parameter," this could have confused the reader. See also examples in Section 5.4.

As far as we know, in the experimental design literature only in the "normal" case have different types of components of ζ been parameterized, namely, the expectation(s) of the response(s) and its variance (variance-covariance matrix). See, for instance, Atkinson and Cook (1995) [17], Dette and Wong (1999) [98] or Fedorov and Leonov (2004) [143]. A rare exception is the beta regression considered by Wu et al. (2005) [415].

Recalling that the total information matrix is the weighted sum of information matrices of single observations,

$$\underline{\mathbf{M}}(\boldsymbol{\theta}, \xi_N) = \sum_{i=1}^n r_i \boldsymbol{\mu}(\mathbf{x}_i, \boldsymbol{\theta}) = \sum_{i=1}^n r_i \mathbf{F}(\mathbf{x}_i, \boldsymbol{\theta}) \boldsymbol{\nu}(\mathbf{x}_i, \zeta) \mathbf{F}^T(\mathbf{x}_i, \boldsymbol{\theta}), \tag{1.100}$$

one can immediately see a strong similarity of the latter formula and (1.62), i.e., a similarity between multiresponse linear regression and the generalized regression.

In what follows we provide a collection of Fisher information matrices $\boldsymbol{\nu} = \boldsymbol{\nu}(\zeta)$ for a number of popular single- and two-parameter distributions. These matrices play a central role in the design and analysis of experiments and are called *"elemental information matrices."* Almost all of the reported elemental information matrices and the corresponding references can be found in Bernardo and Smith (1994) [46]; Johnson et al. (1994, 1995) [218], [219]; Lehmann and Casella (1998) [252]; and Johnson et al. (2005) [217].

1.6.1   Univariate distributions

Table 1.1 contains elemental information expressions for single-parameter distributions. Elemental information matrices for two-parameter distributions are given in Table 1.3.

The distributions in Table 1.3 include the Weibull and Pareto, which are often used for modeling survival or lifetime data. Elaborations of the Laplace distribution are in Kotz et al. (2001) [236]. If one of the two parameters of the

TABLE 1.1: Elemental information for single-parameter distributions

Distribution	Density	Mean Variance	Information $\nu(\zeta)$
Bernoulli (p) $0 \le p \le 1$	$p^y(1-p)^{1-y}$	p $p(1-p)$	$1/[p(1-p)]$
Geometric (p) $0 \le p \le 1$	$(1-p)^y p$	$(1-p)/p$ $(1-p)/p^2$	$1/[p^2(1-p)]$
Binomial (p,n) $0 \le p \le 1$	$\binom{n}{y}p^y(1-p)^{n-y}$	np $np(1-p)$	$n/[p(1-p)]$
Neg. Bin. (p,m) $0 \le p \le 1$	$\binom{m+y-1}{m-1}p^m(1-p)^y$	$m(1-p)/p$ $m(1-p)/p^2$	$m/[p^2(1-p)]$
Hypergeometric (p,N,n) $0 \le p \le 1$	$\dfrac{\binom{n}{y}\binom{N-n}{Np-y}}{\binom{N}{Np}}$	np $\dfrac{np(1-p)(N-n)}{N-1}$	$\dfrac{(N-1)n}{p(1-p)(N-n)}$
Poisson (λ) $\lambda > 0$	$\dfrac{\lambda^y e^{-\lambda}}{y!}$	λ λ	$1/\lambda$

distributions in Table 1.3 is assumed to be known, then the elemental information for the other (unknown) parameter equals the corresponding diagonal element of the elemental information matrix. In many settings it is helpful to work with transformations of the original parameters ζ, such as log or logit functions of ζ, which can vary between $-\infty$ and ∞. We use the notation ϑ for such transformations, and notation $\nu(\vartheta)$ for elemental information matrix when the parameters ϑ, not ζ, are considered functions of controls $\mathbf{x}$ and regression parameters $\boldsymbol{\theta}$. Tables 1.2 and 1.4 contain information or information matrices for popular choices of those new parameters. The multivariate normal distribution and multinomial distribution are described in the next subsection. Many further references on multivariate distributions can be found in Johnson et al. (1997) [220] and Kotz et al. (2000) [235].

1.6.2 Two multivariate distributions

Normal distribution. Let $\mathbf{Y} \in R^l$ have a normal distribution, i.e.,

$$p(\mathbf{y}|\mathbf{a}, \boldsymbol{\Sigma}) = (2\pi)^{-l/2}|\boldsymbol{\Sigma}|^{-1/2}\exp\left\{-\frac{1}{2}(\mathbf{y}-\mathbf{a})\boldsymbol{\Sigma}^{-1}(\mathbf{y}-\mathbf{a})^T\right\}.$$

TABLE 1.2: Transformed elemental information for single-parameter distributions

Distribution	New Parameter ϑ	Information $\nu(\vartheta)$
Bernoulli (p)	$\vartheta = \ln \frac{p}{1-p}$	$e^{\vartheta}/(1+e^{\vartheta})^2$
Binomial (p, n)	$\vartheta = \ln \frac{p}{1-p}$	$n e^{\vartheta}/(1+e^{\vartheta})^2$
Poisson (λ)	$\vartheta = \ln \lambda$	e^{ϑ}
Geometric (p)	$\vartheta = \ln \frac{p}{1-p}$	$1/(1+e^{\vartheta})$
Neg. Bin. (p, m)	$\vartheta = \ln \frac{p}{1-p}$	$m/(1+e^{\vartheta})$

We let $\boldsymbol{\theta}$ represent the unknown parameters defining the mean $\mathbf{a}(\mathbf{x}, \boldsymbol{\theta})$ and the variance-covariance matrix $\boldsymbol{\Sigma}(\mathbf{x}, \boldsymbol{\theta})$. Then the (α, β) element of the information matrix for $\boldsymbol{\theta}$ is

$$\mu_{\alpha\beta} = \frac{\partial \mathbf{a}}{\partial \theta_{\alpha}} \boldsymbol{\Sigma}^{-1} \frac{\partial \mathbf{a}^T}{\partial \theta_{\beta}} + \frac{1}{2} \text{tr} \left(\boldsymbol{\Sigma}^{-1} \frac{\partial \boldsymbol{\Sigma}}{\partial \theta_{\alpha}} \boldsymbol{\Sigma}^{-1} \frac{\partial \boldsymbol{\Sigma}}{\partial \theta_{\beta}} \right); \qquad (1.101)$$

see Magnus and Neudecker (1988) [262], p. 325.

The information matrix for the $l + (l + 1)l/2$ parameters $\mathbf{a}$ and $\boldsymbol{\Sigma}$ appears complicated, so we introduce notation to express it in a more compact form; see Magnus and Neudecker (1988), Chapter 2.4, or Harville (1997) [195], Chapter 16.4. Let $\text{vec}\boldsymbol{\Sigma}$ be a vector that is constructed from $\boldsymbol{\Sigma}$ and consists of l^2 components. To build it, stack the columns of $\boldsymbol{\Sigma}$ beneath each other so that the first column of $\boldsymbol{\Sigma}$ is on top, followed by the second column of $\boldsymbol{\Sigma}$, etc.; the l-th column of $\boldsymbol{\Sigma}$ is therefore at the bottom of the stack. Because $\boldsymbol{\Sigma}$ is symmetric, this vector $\text{vec}\boldsymbol{\Sigma}$ contains considerable redundancy. To obtain a parsimonious column vector with the same information as is in $\boldsymbol{\Sigma}$, eliminate all elements that come from the super-diagonal elements of $\boldsymbol{\Sigma}$. The resulting vector, with only $l(l + 1)/2$ elements, is denoted $\text{vech}\boldsymbol{\Sigma}$.

The *duplication matrix* $\mathbf{D}_l$ (see Magnus and Neudecker (1988) [262], Chapter 3.8) is a linear transform that links $\text{vec}\boldsymbol{\Sigma}$ and $\text{vech}\boldsymbol{\Sigma}$:

$$\mathbf{D}_l \text{vech}\boldsymbol{\Sigma} = \text{vec}\boldsymbol{\Sigma}.$$

$\mathbf{D}_l$ is a unique matrix of dimension $l^2 \times l(l + 1)/2$. We use $\mathbf{D}_l$ to express an elemental information matrix with parameters $\boldsymbol{\vartheta} = [\mathbf{a}^T, (\text{vech}\boldsymbol{\Sigma})^T]^T$ in a relatively compact format:

$$\boldsymbol{\nu}(\boldsymbol{\vartheta}) = \begin{pmatrix} \boldsymbol{\Sigma}^{-1} & 0 \\ 0 & \frac{1}{2} \mathbf{D}_m^T \left(\boldsymbol{\Sigma}^{-1} \otimes \boldsymbol{\Sigma}^{-1} \right) \mathbf{D}_m \end{pmatrix}. \qquad (1.102)$$

TABLE 1.3: Elemental information matrices for two-parameter distributions

Distribution	Density	Mean Variance	Information Matrix $\nu(\zeta)$
Normal (a,σ^2)	$\dfrac{1}{\sqrt{2\pi\sigma^2}}\,e^{\frac{-(y-a)^2}{2\sigma^2}}$	a σ^2	$\sigma^{-2}\begin{pmatrix}1 & 0 \\ 0 & \frac{1}{2}\sigma^{-2}\end{pmatrix}$
Beta (α,β) $\alpha>0,\beta>0$	$B(\alpha,\beta)y^{\alpha-1}(1-y)^{\beta-1}$	$\alpha/(\alpha+\beta)$ $\dfrac{\alpha\beta}{(\alpha+\beta)^2(\alpha+\beta+1)}$	$\begin{pmatrix}\dot\psi(\alpha)-\dot\psi(\alpha+\beta) & -\dot\psi(\alpha+\beta) \\ -\dot\psi(\alpha+\beta) & \dot\psi(\beta)-\dot\psi(\alpha+\beta)\end{pmatrix}$
Gamma (α,β) $\alpha>0,\beta>0$	$\dfrac{1}{\Gamma(\alpha)\beta^\alpha}\,y^{\alpha-1}e^{-y/\beta}$	$\alpha\beta$ $\alpha\beta^2$	$\begin{pmatrix}\dot\psi(\alpha) & 1/\beta \\ 1/\beta & \alpha/\beta^2\end{pmatrix}$
Logistic (a,b) $-\infty<a<\infty$ $b>0$	$\dfrac{e^{-(y-a)/b}}{b[1+e^{-(y-a)/b}]^2}$	a $b^2\pi^2/3$	$\frac{1}{3}\begin{pmatrix}b^{-2} & 0 \\ 0 & 1+b^{-2}\end{pmatrix}$
Cauchy (a,b) $-\infty<a<\infty$ $b>0$	$\dfrac{b}{\pi[b^2+(y-a)^2]}$	Do not exist	$\frac{1}{2b^2}I$
Weibull (α,β) $\alpha>0,\beta>0$	$\dfrac{\alpha}{\beta}\left(\dfrac{y}{\beta}\right)^{\alpha-1}e^{-(y/\beta)^\alpha}$	$\beta\Gamma(1+\alpha^{-1})$ $\beta^2[\Gamma(1+2\alpha^{-1})-\Gamma^2(1+\alpha^{-1})]$	$\begin{pmatrix}\frac{\pi^2}{6}+\frac{(1-\gamma)^2}{\alpha^2} & \frac{\gamma-1}{\beta} \\ \frac{\gamma-1}{\beta} & \frac{\alpha^2}{\beta^2}\end{pmatrix}$
Pareto (α,σ) $\alpha>2$ (for variance) $\sigma>0$	$\dfrac{\alpha}{x}\left(\dfrac{y}{\sigma}\right)^{-\alpha}$	$\sigma\left(\dfrac{\alpha}{\alpha-1}\right)$ $\dfrac{\alpha\sigma^2}{(\alpha-1)^2(\alpha-2)}$	$\begin{pmatrix}\frac{\alpha}{\sigma^2(\alpha+2)} & -\frac{1}{\sigma(\alpha+1)} \\ -\frac{1}{\sigma(\alpha+1)} & \frac{1}{\alpha^2}\end{pmatrix}$

$\psi(\alpha)=\frac{\dot\Gamma(\alpha)}{\Gamma(\alpha)}$ and $\dot\psi(\alpha)=\frac{d\psi(\alpha)}{d\alpha}$ are the digamma and trigamma functions; $\gamma=0.5772$ is Euler's constant, see Abramovitz and Stegun (1972) [2]

TABLE 1.4: Transformed elemental information matrices for two-parameter distributions

Distribution	New Parameters $\boldsymbol{\vartheta}$	Information Matrix $\boldsymbol{\nu}(\boldsymbol{\vartheta})$
$\mathcal{N}(a, \sigma^2)$	$\vartheta_1 = a$ $\vartheta_2 = \ln \sigma^2$	$\begin{pmatrix} 1/e^{\vartheta_2} & 0 \\ 0 & 1/2 \end{pmatrix}$
$\mathcal{N}(a, a^2)$	$\vartheta = \ln a$	3
$\mathcal{N}(a, k^2 a^2)$	$\vartheta_1 = \ln a$ $\vartheta_2 = k^2$	$\begin{pmatrix} 2 + 1/\vartheta_2 & 1/\vartheta_2 \\ 1/\vartheta_2 & 1/(2\vartheta_2^2) \end{pmatrix}$
Beta (α, β)	$\vartheta_1 = \ln \alpha$ $\vartheta_2 = \ln \beta$	$\begin{pmatrix} e^{2\vartheta_1} \dot{\psi}(e^{\vartheta_1}) & 0 \\ 0 & e^{2\vartheta_2} \dot{\psi}(e^{\vartheta_2}) \end{pmatrix}$ $-\dot{\psi}(e^{\vartheta_1} + e^{\vartheta_2}) \begin{pmatrix} e^{2\vartheta_1} & 1 \\ 1 & e^{2\vartheta_2} \end{pmatrix}$
Gamma (α, β)	$\vartheta_1 = \ln \alpha$ $\vartheta_2 = \ln \beta$	$e^{\vartheta_1} \begin{pmatrix} e^{\vartheta_1} \dot{\psi}(e^{\vartheta_1}) & 1 \\ 1 & 1 \end{pmatrix}$
Logistic (a, b)	$\vartheta_1 = a$ $\vartheta_2 = \ln b$	$\frac{1}{3} \begin{pmatrix} e^{-2\vartheta_2} & 0 \\ 0 & 1 + e^{2\vartheta_2} \end{pmatrix}$
Cauchy (a, b)	$\vartheta_1 = a$ $\vartheta_2 = \ln b$	$\frac{1}{2} \begin{pmatrix} e^{-2\vartheta_2} & 0 \\ 0 & 1 \end{pmatrix}$
Weibull (α, β)	$\vartheta_1 = \ln \alpha$ $\vartheta_2 = \ln \beta$	$\begin{pmatrix} \frac{\pi^2}{6} + (1 - \gamma)^2 & \frac{\gamma - 1}{e^{\vartheta_2}} \\ \frac{\gamma - 1}{e^{\vartheta_2}} & e^{2\vartheta_1} \end{pmatrix}$

For example, for the bivariate normal distribution with parameters $\boldsymbol{\theta} = (a_1, a_2, \sigma_1^2, \rho\sigma_1\sigma_2, \sigma_2^2)^T$,

$$\mathbf{D}_2 = \begin{pmatrix} 1 & 0 & 0 \\ 0 & 1 & 0 \\ 0 & 1 & 0 \\ 0 & 0 & 1 \end{pmatrix},$$

which inserted in (1.102) yields the compact re-expression of the elemental information matrix:

$$\boldsymbol{\nu}(\boldsymbol{\vartheta}) = \frac{1}{1 - \rho^2} \begin{pmatrix} \boldsymbol{\Sigma}^{-1} & \mathbf{0} \\ \mathbf{0} & \mathbf{B} \end{pmatrix}, \qquad (1.103)$$

where

$$\Sigma^{-1} = \begin{pmatrix} \frac{1}{\sigma_1^2} & -\frac{\rho}{\sigma_1\sigma_2} \\ -\frac{\rho}{\sigma_1\sigma_2} & \frac{1}{\sigma_2^2} \end{pmatrix},$$

$$\mathbf{B} = \frac{1}{1-\rho^2} \begin{pmatrix} \frac{2-\rho^2}{4\sigma_1^4} & -\frac{\rho}{\sigma_1^3\sigma_2} & \frac{\rho^2}{2\sigma_1^2\sigma_2^2} \\ -\frac{\rho}{\sigma_1^3\sigma_2} & \frac{1+\rho^2}{\sigma_1^2\sigma_2^2} & -\frac{\rho}{\sigma_1\sigma_2^3} \\ \frac{\rho^2}{2\sigma_1^2\sigma_2^2} & -\frac{\rho}{\sigma_1\sigma_2^3} & \frac{2-\rho^2}{4\sigma_2^4} \end{pmatrix}.$$

Multinomial distribution. For multinomial observations $\mathbf{y} = (y_1, \ldots, y_l, y_{l+1})$,

$$p(\mathbf{y}|\boldsymbol{\vartheta}, n) = \frac{n!}{y_1! \cdots y_l! y_{l+1}!} \vartheta_1^{y_1} \cdots \vartheta_l^{y_l} \vartheta_{l+1}^{y_{l+1}},$$

where

$$\sum_{i=1}^{l+1} y_i = n \quad \text{and} \quad \sum_{i=1}^{l+1} \vartheta_i = 1,$$

see Bernardo and Smith (1994) [46], Chapter 5.4. There are actually only l independent parameters. The standard option is to take the elemental parameters as $\boldsymbol{\vartheta} = (\vartheta_1, \ldots, \vartheta_l)^T$, noting that $\vartheta_{l+1} = 1 - \sum_{i=1}^{l} \vartheta_i$.

The elemental information matrix for $\boldsymbol{\vartheta}$ is

$$\boldsymbol{\nu}(\boldsymbol{\vartheta}) = \frac{n}{\vartheta_{l+1}} \begin{pmatrix} \frac{\vartheta_1+\vartheta_{l+1}}{\vartheta_1} & 1 & \cdots & 1 \\ 1 & \frac{\vartheta_2+\vartheta_{l+1}}{\vartheta_2} & \cdots & 1 \\ \cdots & \cdots & \cdots & \cdots \\ 1 & 1 & \cdots & \frac{\theta_l+\vartheta_{l+1}}{\vartheta_1} \end{pmatrix}. \tag{1.104}$$

The latter can be rewritten as

$$\boldsymbol{\nu}(\boldsymbol{\vartheta}) = n \begin{pmatrix} \vartheta_1 & 0 & \cdots & 0 \\ 0 & \vartheta_2 & \cdots & 0 \\ \cdots & \cdots & \cdots & \cdots \\ 0 & 0 & \cdots & \vartheta_l \end{pmatrix}^{-1} + \frac{n}{\vartheta_{l+1}} \mathbf{ll}^T, \tag{1.105}$$

where $\mathbf{l}^T = (1, \ldots, 1)$. Now it follows from (1.105) and (10.13) with $\alpha = \vartheta_{l+1}^{-1}$ that

$$\boldsymbol{\nu}^{-1}(\boldsymbol{\vartheta}) = \frac{1}{n} \begin{pmatrix} \vartheta_1 & 0 & \cdots & 0 \\ 0 & \vartheta_2 & \cdots & 0 \\ \cdots & \cdots & \cdots & \cdots \\ 0 & 0 & \cdots & \vartheta_l \end{pmatrix} - \frac{1}{n} \boldsymbol{\vartheta}\boldsymbol{\vartheta}^T. \tag{1.106}$$

Examples of the use of the elemental information matrices are considered in Sections 5.4, 6.4, and 6.5.

1.7   Nonlinear Regression with Normally Distributed Observations

In this section we focus on parameter estimation for nonlinear normal models. In a sense, we bridge the results on estimation that are discussed in Sections 1.1 – 1.4, with those discussed in Section 1.6. We confine ourselves to the case of normally distributed measurements, but still consider a rather general regression framework that includes (a) nonlinear response functions, (b) multiresponse models and (c) models with unknown parameters in variance. An iterated estimator that is asymptotically equivalent to the MLE is introduced in Section 1.7.1 where the main results are formulated. This iterated estimator is a natural generalization of the traditional *iteratively reweighted least squares* (IRLS) algorithms. It includes not only the squared deviations of the predicted responses from the observations, but also the squared deviations of the predicted variance-covariance matrix from observed residual matrices. In this way, the combined iterated estimator (*combined iteratively reweighted least squares*, or CIRLS) allows us to bridge least squares estimation and the MLE. In Section 1.7.2 several examples are presented that admit closed-form formulae for iterated estimators. Results of simulation studies that illustrate the performance of various iterative procedures are discussed in Section 1.7.3. For more details, see Fedorov and Leonov (2004) [143].

As in Sections 1.1 and 1.5, suppose that r_i independent observations are taken at predictor levels $\mathbf{x}_i$, and $\sum_{i=1}^{n} r_i = N$. Let the observed $k \times$) vectors $\mathbf{y}_{ij}$ be normally distributed,

$$\mathbf{y}_{ij}|\mathbf{x}_i \sim \mathcal{N}\left[\boldsymbol{\eta}(\mathbf{x}_i, \boldsymbol{\theta}), \mathbf{S}(\mathbf{x}_i, \boldsymbol{\theta})\right], \quad j = 1, \ldots, r_i, \qquad (1.107)$$

where $\boldsymbol{\eta}(\mathbf{x}, \boldsymbol{\theta}) = [\eta_1(\mathbf{x}, \boldsymbol{\theta}), \ldots, \eta_k(\mathbf{x}, \boldsymbol{\theta})]^T$, $\mathbf{S}(\mathbf{x}, \boldsymbol{\theta})$ is a $k \times k$ matrix, and $\boldsymbol{\theta} \in \boldsymbol{\Theta} \subset R^m$ are unknown parameters. Throughout the rest of the chapter, we will use notation

$$\sum_{i,j} = \sum_{i=1}^{n}\sum_{j=1}^{r_i}, \quad \sum_{i} = \sum_{i=1}^{n},$$

and omit limits of summation unless stated otherwise.

For model (1.107), rewrite the formula (1.101) for the Fisher information matrix in more detail:

$$\boldsymbol{\mu}(\mathbf{x}, \boldsymbol{\theta}) = \boldsymbol{\mu}(\mathbf{x}, \boldsymbol{\theta}; \boldsymbol{\eta}, \mathbf{S}) = \{\mu_{\alpha\beta}(\mathbf{x}, \boldsymbol{\theta})\}_{\alpha,\beta=1}^{m}, \quad \text{where} \qquad (1.108)$$

$$\mu_{\alpha\beta}(\mathbf{x}, \boldsymbol{\theta}) = \frac{\partial \boldsymbol{\eta}^T(\mathbf{x}, \boldsymbol{\theta})}{\partial \theta_\alpha} \mathbf{S}^{-1}(\mathbf{x}, \boldsymbol{\theta}) \frac{\partial \boldsymbol{\eta}(\mathbf{x}, \boldsymbol{\theta})}{\partial \theta_\beta}$$

$$+ \frac{1}{2} \operatorname{tr} \left[\mathbf{S}^{-1}(\mathbf{x}, \boldsymbol{\theta}) \frac{\partial \mathbf{S}(\mathbf{x}, \boldsymbol{\theta})}{\partial \theta_\alpha} \mathbf{S}^{-1}(\mathbf{x}, \boldsymbol{\theta}) \frac{\partial \mathbf{S}(\mathbf{x}, \boldsymbol{\theta})}{\partial \theta_\beta}\right];$$

see also Muirhead (1982) [290], Chapter 1. In general, the dimension and structure of $\mathbf{y}, \boldsymbol{\eta}$, and $\mathbf{S}$ can vary for different $\mathbf{x}$. To indicate this, we could have introduced a subscript k_i for every $\mathbf{x}_i$, but for notational brevity we retain the traditional notation $\mathbf{y}_i$, $\boldsymbol{\eta}(\mathbf{x}_i, \boldsymbol{\theta})$ and $\mathbf{S}(\mathbf{x}_i, \boldsymbol{\theta})$ when it does not cause confusion. The log-likelihood function $\mathcal{L}_N(\boldsymbol{\theta})$ in (1.84) is

$$\mathcal{L}_N(\boldsymbol{\theta}) = -\frac{1}{2N} \sum_{i,j} \{\ln |\mathbf{S}(\mathbf{x}_i, \boldsymbol{\theta})|$$

$$+ [\mathbf{y}_{ij} - \boldsymbol{\eta}(\mathbf{x}_i, \boldsymbol{\theta})]^T \mathbf{S}^{-1}(\mathbf{x}_i, \boldsymbol{\theta}) [\mathbf{y}_{ij} - \boldsymbol{\eta}(\mathbf{x}_i, \boldsymbol{\theta})]\}. \tag{1.109}$$

Any vector $\boldsymbol{\theta}_N$ that maximizes the log-likelihood function $\mathcal{L}_N(\boldsymbol{\theta})$,

$$\boldsymbol{\theta}_N = \arg \max_{\boldsymbol{\theta} \in \Theta} \mathcal{L}_N(\boldsymbol{\theta}) \tag{1.110}$$

is called a maximum likelihood estimator (MLE). Introduce the following assumptions.

Assumption 1.1 *The set Θ is compact; $\mathbf{x}_i \in \mathfrak{X}$, where $\mathfrak{X}$ is compact and all components of $\boldsymbol{\eta}(\mathbf{x}, \boldsymbol{\theta})$ and $\mathbf{S}(\mathbf{x}, \boldsymbol{\theta})$ are continuous with respect to $\boldsymbol{\theta}$ uniformly in Θ, with $\mathbf{S}(\mathbf{x}, \boldsymbol{\theta}) \geq \mathbf{S}_0$, where $\mathbf{S}_0$ is a positive definite matrix. The true vector of unknown parameters $\boldsymbol{\theta}_t$ is an internal point of Θ.*

Let

$$l(\mathbf{x}, \boldsymbol{\theta}, \boldsymbol{\theta}_t) = \ln |\mathbf{S}(\mathbf{x}, \boldsymbol{\theta})| + \text{tr} \left[\mathbf{S}^{-1}(\mathbf{x}, \boldsymbol{\theta}) \, \mathbf{S}(\mathbf{x}, \boldsymbol{\theta}_t)\right]$$

$$+ [\boldsymbol{\eta}(\mathbf{x}, \boldsymbol{\theta}) - \boldsymbol{\eta}(\mathbf{x}, \boldsymbol{\theta}_t)]^T \mathbf{S}^{-1}(\mathbf{x}, \boldsymbol{\theta}) \, [\boldsymbol{\eta}(\mathbf{x}, \boldsymbol{\theta}) - \boldsymbol{\eta}(\mathbf{x}, \boldsymbol{\theta}_t)]. \tag{1.111}$$

Assumption 1.2 *The sum $\sum_i r_i \, l(\mathbf{x}_i, \boldsymbol{\theta}, \boldsymbol{\theta}_t)/N$ converges uniformly in Θ to a continuous function $\nu(\boldsymbol{\theta}, \boldsymbol{\theta}_t)$,*

$$\lim_{N \to \infty} N^{-1} \sum_i r_i \, l(\mathbf{x}_i, \boldsymbol{\theta}, \boldsymbol{\theta}_t) = \nu(\boldsymbol{\theta}, \boldsymbol{\theta}_t), \tag{1.112}$$

and the function $\nu(\boldsymbol{\theta}, \boldsymbol{\theta}_t)$ attains its unique minimum at $\boldsymbol{\theta} = \boldsymbol{\theta}_t$.

Following Jennrich (1969) [212], Theorem 6, it can be shown that under Assumptions 1.1 and 1.2, the MLE is a measurable function of observations and is strongly consistent; see also Fedorov (1974) [128]; Heyde (1997) [199], Chapter 12; Pázman (1993) [307]; Wu (1981) [410]. Condition (1.112) is based on the fact that

$$E\left\{[\mathbf{y} - \boldsymbol{\eta}(\mathbf{x}, \boldsymbol{\theta})]^T \mathbf{S}^{-1}(\mathbf{x}, \boldsymbol{\theta}) \, [\mathbf{y} - \boldsymbol{\eta}(\mathbf{x}, \boldsymbol{\theta})]\right\}$$

$$= [\boldsymbol{\eta}(\mathbf{x}, \boldsymbol{\theta}_t) - \boldsymbol{\eta}(\mathbf{x}, \boldsymbol{\theta})]^T \mathbf{S}^{-1}(\mathbf{x}, \boldsymbol{\theta}) \, [\boldsymbol{\eta}(\mathbf{x}, \boldsymbol{\theta}_t) - \boldsymbol{\eta}(\mathbf{x}, \boldsymbol{\theta})] + \text{tr} \left[\mathbf{S}^{-1}(\mathbf{x}, \boldsymbol{\theta}) \, \mathbf{S}(\mathbf{x}, \boldsymbol{\theta}_t)\right],$$

and the Kolmogorov law of large numbers; see Rao (1973) [334], Chapter 2c.3.

If in addition to Assumptions 1.1 and 1.2, all components of $\boldsymbol{\eta}(\mathbf{x}, \boldsymbol{\theta})$ and $\mathbf{S}(\mathbf{x}, \boldsymbol{\theta})$ are twice differentiable with respect to $\boldsymbol{\theta}$ for all $\boldsymbol{\theta} \in \boldsymbol{\Theta}$, and the limit matrix

$$\lim_{N \to \infty} \frac{1}{N} \sum_i r_i \, \boldsymbol{\mu}(\mathbf{x}_i, \boldsymbol{\theta}_t) \; = \; \mathbf{M}(\boldsymbol{\theta}_t) \tag{1.113}$$

exists and is regular, then $\boldsymbol{\theta}_N$ is asymptotically normally distributed,

$$\sqrt{N}(\boldsymbol{\theta}_N - \boldsymbol{\theta}_t) \; \sim \; \mathcal{N}\left[0, \mathbf{M}^{-1}(\boldsymbol{\theta}_t)\right]. \tag{1.114}$$

Note that the selection of the series $\{\mathbf{x}_i\}_1^n$ is crucial for the consistency and precision of $\boldsymbol{\theta}_N$.

Remark 1.3 Given N and $\{\mathbf{x}_i\}_1^n$, a design measure can be defined as

$$\xi_N(\mathbf{x}) \; = \; \frac{1}{N} \sum_i r_i \, \delta_{\mathbf{x}_i}(\mathbf{x}), \quad \delta_{\mathbf{x}}(\mathbf{z}) = \{1 \; \text{if} \; \mathbf{z} = \mathbf{x}, \text{ and } 0 \text{ otherwise}\}.$$

If the sequence $\{\xi_N(\mathbf{x})\}$ weakly converges to $\xi(\mathbf{x})$, then the limiting function $\nu(\boldsymbol{\theta}, \boldsymbol{\theta}_t)$ in the "identifiability" Assumption 1.2 takes the form

$$\nu(\boldsymbol{\theta}, \boldsymbol{\theta}_t) = \int l(\mathbf{x}, \boldsymbol{\theta}, \boldsymbol{\theta}_t) d\xi(\mathbf{x}),$$

cf. Malyutov (1988) [266]. Most often, within the optimal design paradigm, the limit design ξ is a discrete measure, i.e., a collection of support points $\{\mathbf{x}_i, \; i = 1, ..., n\}$ with weights p_i, such that $\sum_i p_i = 1$; see Chapter 2 for details.

1.7.1 Iterated estimators and combined least squares

If the variance-covariance matrices of the observations $\{\mathbf{y}_{ij}\}$ are known, i.e., $\mathbf{S}(\mathbf{x}_i, \boldsymbol{\theta}) = \mathbf{S}(\mathbf{x}_i)$, then (1.109) leads to the generalized least squares estimator (GLSE):

$$\tilde{\boldsymbol{\theta}}_N = \arg\min_{\boldsymbol{\theta}} \sum_{i,j} \left[\mathbf{y}_{ij} - \boldsymbol{\eta}(\mathbf{x}_i, \boldsymbol{\theta})\right]^T \mathbf{S}^{-1}(\mathbf{x}_i) \left[\mathbf{y}_{ij} - \boldsymbol{\eta}(\mathbf{x}_i, \boldsymbol{\theta})\right]; \tag{1.115}$$

cf. (1.46) and (1.60) for single and multiresponse cases, respectively. When the variance function $\mathbf{S}$ depends on $\boldsymbol{\theta}$, it is tempting to replace (1.115) by

$$\tilde{\boldsymbol{\theta}}_N = \arg\min_{\boldsymbol{\theta}} \sum_{i,j} \left[\mathbf{y}_{ij} - \boldsymbol{\eta}(\mathbf{x}_i, \boldsymbol{\theta})\right]^T \mathbf{S}^{-1}(\mathbf{x}_i, \boldsymbol{\theta}) \left[\mathbf{y}_{ij} - \boldsymbol{\eta}(\mathbf{x}_i, \boldsymbol{\theta})\right], \tag{1.116}$$

which, in general, is not consistent; cf. (1.56), see Fedorov (1974) [128]. In such circumstances, one has to resort to iterative procedures similar to (1.52), (1.53), which require an intermediate step of "freezing" parameter estimates in the variance function $\mathbf{S}(\mathbf{x}, \boldsymbol{\theta})$. See, for example, Jobson and Fuller (1980) [215]; Carroll and Ruppert (1982) [60]; Carroll and Ruppert (1988) [61], Chapter 2; Davidian and Giltinan (1995) [90], Chapter 2.3.3.

Let

$$
\begin{aligned}
\tilde{\boldsymbol{\theta}}_N &= \lim_{N \to \infty} \boldsymbol{\theta}_s, \text{ where} &\text{(1.117)} \\
\boldsymbol{\theta}_s &= \arg\min_{\boldsymbol{\theta}} \frac{1}{N} \sum_{i,j} [\mathbf{y}_{ij} - \boldsymbol{\eta}(\mathbf{x}_i, \boldsymbol{\theta})]^T \, \mathbf{S}^{-1}(\mathbf{x}_i, \boldsymbol{\theta}_{s-1}) \, [\mathbf{y}_{ij} - \boldsymbol{\eta}(\mathbf{x}_i, \boldsymbol{\theta})].
\end{aligned}
$$

(formally we have to write $\boldsymbol{\theta}_{s,N}$ instead of $\boldsymbol{\theta}_s$, but we drop subscript N to simplify notations). The estimator $\tilde{\boldsymbol{\theta}}_N$ is called *iteratively reweighted least squares* (IRLS) estimator. If $\boldsymbol{\eta}(\mathbf{x}, \boldsymbol{\theta})$ depends nontrivially on all components of vector $\boldsymbol{\theta}$, then the IRLS estimator is strongly consistent and asymptotically normal, $\sqrt{N}(\tilde{\boldsymbol{\theta}}_N - \boldsymbol{\theta}_t) \sim \mathcal{N}\left[0, \tilde{\mathbf{M}}^{-1}(\boldsymbol{\theta}_t)\right]$, with the asymptotic variance-covariance matrix

$$
\tilde{\mathbf{M}}^{-1}(\boldsymbol{\theta}_t) = \left\{ \lim_{N \to \infty} N^{-1} \left[\sum_i r_i \, \frac{\partial \boldsymbol{\eta}(\mathbf{x}_i, \boldsymbol{\theta})}{\partial \boldsymbol{\theta}} \mathbf{S}^{-1}(\mathbf{x}_i, \boldsymbol{\theta}) \frac{\partial \boldsymbol{\eta}(\mathbf{x}_i, \boldsymbol{\theta})}{\partial \boldsymbol{\theta}^T} \right]\Bigg|_{\boldsymbol{\theta} = \boldsymbol{\theta}_t} \right\}^{-1};
$$

see Beal and Sheiner (1988) [39]; Hardin and Hilbe (1997) [191], Chapter 4; Jobson and Fuller (1980) [215]; Malyutov (1982) [265]; or Vonesh and Chinchilli (1997) [388]. Note that $\tilde{\mathbf{M}}(\boldsymbol{\theta}_t) \le \mathbf{M}(\boldsymbol{\theta}_t)$, in terms of nonnegative definite matrix ordering, or Loewner ordering; cf. (1.18). Here the matrix $\mathbf{M}(\boldsymbol{\theta}_t)$ is the limiting matrix for the MLE; see (1.113). The reason for the "inferiority" of $\tilde{\mathbf{M}}(\boldsymbol{\theta}_t)$ is that the IRLS does not account for the information contained in the variance function $\mathbf{S}(\mathbf{x}, \boldsymbol{\theta})$.

A natural step after (1.117) is the introduction of the *combined iteratively reweighted least squares* estimator (CIRLS), which includes squared deviations of the predicted variance-covariance matrix $\mathbf{S}(\mathbf{x}, \boldsymbol{\theta})$ from observed residual matrices:

$$
\hat{\boldsymbol{\theta}}_N = \lim_{s \to \infty} \boldsymbol{\theta}_s, \qquad\qquad\qquad \text{(1.118)}
$$

where

$$
\boldsymbol{\theta}_s = \arg\min_{\boldsymbol{\theta} \in \boldsymbol{\Theta}} V_N(\boldsymbol{\theta}, \boldsymbol{\theta}_{s-1}),
$$

$$
\begin{aligned}
V_N(\boldsymbol{\theta}, \boldsymbol{\theta}') &= \frac{1}{N} \sum_{i,j} [\mathbf{y}_{ij} - \boldsymbol{\eta}(\mathbf{x}_i, \boldsymbol{\theta})]^T \, \mathbf{S}^{-1}(\mathbf{x}_i, \boldsymbol{\theta}') \, [\mathbf{y}_{ij} - \boldsymbol{\eta}(\mathbf{x}_i, \boldsymbol{\theta})] \\
&\quad + \frac{1}{2N} \sum_{i,j} \mathrm{tr} \left[\{ \Delta_{ij}(\boldsymbol{\theta}') - \Delta\boldsymbol{\eta}(\mathbf{x}_i; \boldsymbol{\theta}, \boldsymbol{\theta}') - \mathbf{S}(\mathbf{x}_i, \boldsymbol{\theta}) \} \, \mathbf{S}^{-1}(\mathbf{x}_i, \boldsymbol{\theta}') \right]^2 \quad \text{(1.119)}
\end{aligned}
$$

with

$$
\Delta_{ij}(\boldsymbol{\theta}') = [\mathbf{y}_{ij} - \boldsymbol{\eta}(\mathbf{x}_i, \boldsymbol{\theta}')] \, [\mathbf{y}_{ij} - \boldsymbol{\eta}(\mathbf{x}_i, \boldsymbol{\theta}')]^T \qquad \text{(1.120)}
$$

and

$$\Delta\boldsymbol{\eta}(\mathbf{x}_i; \boldsymbol{\theta}, \boldsymbol{\theta}') = [\boldsymbol{\eta}(\mathbf{x}_i, \boldsymbol{\theta}) - \boldsymbol{\eta}(\mathbf{x}_i, \boldsymbol{\theta}')] \, [\boldsymbol{\eta}(\mathbf{x}_i, \boldsymbol{\theta}) - \boldsymbol{\eta}(\mathbf{x}_i, \boldsymbol{\theta}')]^T. \qquad (1.121)$$

To prove the convergence of the combined iterated estimator, together with Assumption 1.1, we need an additional assumption. Let

$$\begin{aligned} \tilde{l}(\mathbf{x}, \boldsymbol{\theta}, \boldsymbol{\theta}_t) &= [\boldsymbol{\eta}(\mathbf{x}, \boldsymbol{\theta}) - \boldsymbol{\eta}(\mathbf{x}, \boldsymbol{\theta}_t)]^T \, \mathbf{S}_1^{-1} \, [\boldsymbol{\eta}(\mathbf{x}, \boldsymbol{\theta}) - \boldsymbol{\eta}(\mathbf{x}, \boldsymbol{\theta}_t)] \\ &+ \operatorname{tr}\left\{ [\mathbf{S}(\mathbf{x}, \boldsymbol{\theta}) - \mathbf{S}(\mathbf{x}, \boldsymbol{\theta}_t)] \, \mathbf{S}_1^{-1} \right\}^2. \end{aligned} \qquad (1.122)$$

Assumption 1.3 *The variance function satisfies* $\mathbf{S}(\mathbf{x}, \boldsymbol{\theta}) \le \mathbf{S}_1$ *for all* $\mathbf{x} \in \mathfrak{X}$ *and* $\boldsymbol{\theta} \in \Theta$, *where* $\mathbf{S}_1$ *is a positive definite matrix. Design measures* $\xi_N(\mathbf{x})$ *converge weakly to* $\xi(\mathbf{x})$, *and the function*

$$\tilde{\nu}(\boldsymbol{\theta}, \boldsymbol{\theta}_t) = \int \tilde{l}(\mathbf{x}, \boldsymbol{\theta}, \boldsymbol{\theta}_t) d\xi(\mathbf{x}) \qquad (1.123)$$

is continuous with respect to $\boldsymbol{\theta}$, *and attains its unique minimum at* $\boldsymbol{\theta} = \boldsymbol{\theta}_t$.

The following theorem establishes the asymptotic equivalence of the combined iterated estimator (1.118), (1.119) and the MLE (1.110). The introduction of stationary points of the log-likelihood function in the statement of the theorem is similar to the definition of the MLE in Cramèr (1946) [83].

Theorem 1.1 *Under the regularity Assumptions 1.1 and 1.3,*

$$\lim_{N \to \infty} P\{\hat{\boldsymbol{\theta}}_N \in \Theta_N\} = 1,$$

where Θ_N *is a set of stationary points of the log-likelihood function* $\mathcal{L}_N(\boldsymbol{\theta})$,

$$\Theta_N = \left\{ \boldsymbol{\theta} : \frac{\partial \mathcal{L}_N(\boldsymbol{\theta})}{\partial \theta_j} = 0, \ j = 1, \dots, m \right\}.$$

For the proof of Theorem 1.1, see the Appendix in Fedorov and Leonov (2004) [143].

Remark 1.4 The introduction of the term $\Delta\boldsymbol{\eta}(\mathbf{x}_i; \boldsymbol{\theta}, \boldsymbol{\theta}')$ in (1.121) together with Assumption 1.3 guarantees that for any $\boldsymbol{\theta}'$, the unique minimum of $\lim_{N \to \infty} E\left[V_N(\boldsymbol{\theta}, \boldsymbol{\theta}') \right] / N$ with respect to $\boldsymbol{\theta}$ is attained at $\boldsymbol{\theta} = \boldsymbol{\theta}_t$; for details, see Lemma 1 in Fedorov and Leonov (2004) [143]. Note that if the CIRLS (1.118), (1.119) converges, then $\Delta\boldsymbol{\eta}(\mathbf{x}_i; \boldsymbol{\theta}_s, \boldsymbol{\theta}_{s-1}) \to 0$ as $s \to \infty$. Therefore, this term may be omitted if a starting point $\boldsymbol{\theta}_0$ is close enough to the true value; see Section 1.7.2.1 for an example. In the simulation study of Section 1.7.3, we consider a modified CIRLS without the term $\Delta\boldsymbol{\eta}(\mathbf{x}_i; \boldsymbol{\theta}_s, \boldsymbol{\theta}_{s-1})$,

$$\bar{\boldsymbol{\theta}}_N = \lim_{s \to \infty} \boldsymbol{\theta}_s, \qquad (1.124)$$

where

$$\boldsymbol{\theta}_s = \arg\min_{\boldsymbol{\theta} \in \Theta} \bar{V}_N(\boldsymbol{\theta}, \boldsymbol{\theta}_{s-1}),$$

$$\bar{V}_N(\boldsymbol{\theta}, \boldsymbol{\theta}') = \frac{1}{N} \sum_{i,j} [\mathbf{y}_{ij} - \boldsymbol{\eta}(\mathbf{x}_i, \boldsymbol{\theta})]^T \mathbf{S}^{-1}(\mathbf{x}_i, \boldsymbol{\theta}') [\mathbf{y}_{ij} - \boldsymbol{\eta}(\mathbf{x}_i, \boldsymbol{\theta})]$$

$$+ \frac{1}{2N} \sum_{i,j} \mathrm{tr} \left[\{\Delta_{ij}(\boldsymbol{\theta}') - \mathbf{S}(\mathbf{x}_i, \boldsymbol{\theta})\} \mathbf{S}^{-1}(\mathbf{x}_i, \boldsymbol{\theta}') \right]^2, \tag{1.125}$$

where $\Delta_{ij}(\boldsymbol{\theta}')$ is introduced in (1.120). This method will be referred to as MIRLS in the sequel.

Remark 1.5 If function $\tilde{\nu}(\boldsymbol{\theta}, \boldsymbol{\theta}_t)$ defined in (1.123) attains its unique minimum at $\boldsymbol{\theta} = \boldsymbol{\theta}_t$, then so does function $\nu(\boldsymbol{\theta}, \boldsymbol{\theta}_t) = \int l(\mathbf{x}, \boldsymbol{\theta}, \boldsymbol{\theta}_t) \, d\xi(\mathbf{x})$, where $l(\mathbf{x}, \boldsymbol{\theta}, \boldsymbol{\theta}_t)$ is defined in (1.111); see Remark 1.3. To verify this, note that if $\mathbf{S}$ and $\mathbf{S}_*$ are positive definite matrices, then the matrix function

$$g(\mathbf{S}) = \ln |\mathbf{S}| + \mathrm{tr}[\mathbf{S}^{-1}\mathbf{S}_*]$$

attains its unique minimum at $\mathbf{S} = \mathbf{S}_*$; see Seber (1984) [355], Appendix A7.

Remark 1.6 If in (1.119) one chooses $\boldsymbol{\theta}' = \boldsymbol{\theta}$ and, similar to (1.116), considers

$$\hat{\hat{\boldsymbol{\theta}}}_N = \arg \min_{\boldsymbol{\theta} \in \boldsymbol{\Theta}} V_N(\boldsymbol{\theta}, \boldsymbol{\theta}),$$

then using the approach described in Fedorov (1974) [128], it can be verified that this "non-reweighted" estimator $\hat{\hat{\boldsymbol{\theta}}}_N$ is, in general, inconsistent.

Remark 1.7 If the normality assumption is replaced by the assumption that vectors $\mathbf{y}_{ij}$ have the finite fourth moment, then the estimator (1.118), (1.119) can be generalized to the latter case as well. For example, for a single-response model, $k = 1$, the second term on the right-hand side of (1.119) becomes

$$\frac{1}{N} \sum_{i,j} \frac{\left\{ [y_{ij} - \eta(\mathbf{x}_i, \boldsymbol{\theta}')]^2 - \Delta\eta(\mathbf{x}_i; \boldsymbol{\theta}, \boldsymbol{\theta}') - S(\mathbf{x}_i, \boldsymbol{\theta}) \right\}^2}{S_1(\mathbf{x}_i, \boldsymbol{\theta}')},$$

where $S_1(\mathbf{x}, \boldsymbol{\theta}) = E\{[y - \eta(\mathbf{x}, \boldsymbol{\theta})]^2 - S(\mathbf{x}, \boldsymbol{\theta})\}^2 = E[y - \eta(\mathbf{x}, \boldsymbol{\theta})]^4 - S^2(\mathbf{x}, \boldsymbol{\theta})$, and the expectation is taken under the assumption that $\boldsymbol{\theta} = \boldsymbol{\theta}_t$. Note that $E[y - \eta(\mathbf{x}, \boldsymbol{\theta})]^4 = 3S^2(\mathbf{x}, \boldsymbol{\theta})$ in the normal case, which leads to (1.119). Note also that the term $S^2(\mathbf{x}, \boldsymbol{\theta})$ appears in other estimation methods, for example, in least squares on squared residuals discussed in Davidian and Carroll (1987) [89], Section 3.1.2.

Remark 1.8 For the single-response case, the CIRLS is similar to the iterated estimator proposed by Davidian and Carroll (1987) [89]. However, they partition the parameter vector into two subvectors, with the second one appearing only in the variance function, and perform iterations on each term separately. Moreover, for cases where parameters in the expectation and variance functions coincide, the second term disappears completely from the iterations and hence their iterated estimator does not lead to the MLE. We emphasize that for finite sample size N, the CIRLS converges to the MLE only with probability $P_N \leq 1$, however $\lim_{N \to \infty} P_N = 1$.

1.7.2   Examples of iterated estimators

1.7.2.1   Multiresponse linear model with constant covariance matrix

To describe multiresponse linear models that are discussed in this and next sections, it is expedient to outline a practical problem where these models are routinely used. Consider a dose-response study where r_i patients are enrolled in a treatment group (cohort) i, and dose levels $\mathbf{x}_i = (x_{i1}, \ldots, x_{ik})$ are administered to each patient within the cohort; $i = 1, \ldots, n$. (Say, dose x_{il} is administered during patient's l-th visit to a clinic, $l = 1, \ldots, k$). Because patients within a given cohort get several doses and have several measurements taken, by a predictor "level" we mean a set (sequence) $\mathbf{x}_i$.

We assume that measurements $\mathbf{y}_{ij}$ for patient j in cohort i satisfy

$$\mathbf{y}_{ij} = \mathbf{F}^T(\mathbf{x}_i)\boldsymbol{\gamma} + \boldsymbol{\varepsilon}_{ij}, \quad \text{where} \quad \boldsymbol{\varepsilon}_{ij} \sim \mathcal{N}(\mathbf{0}, \mathbf{S}), \qquad (1.126)$$

where $\mathbf{y}_{ij} = (y_{ij,1}, \ldots, y_{ij,k})^T$; $\boldsymbol{\gamma} = (\gamma_1, \ldots, \gamma_{m_\gamma})^T$ is a vector of so-called "response" parameters; $\mathbf{F}(\mathbf{x}_i) = [\mathbf{f}(x_{i1}), \ldots, \mathbf{f}(x_{ik})]$; and $\mathbf{f}(x) = [f_1(x), \ldots, f_{m_\gamma}(x)]^T$ is a vector of basis functions; cf. (1.1), (1.2).

Remark 1.9 In general, individual levels x_{il} may be vector-valued. For example, if a patient receives a combination treatment with q drugs, then $\mathbf{x}_i = (\mathbf{x}_{i1}, \ldots, \mathbf{x}_{ik})$, where $\mathbf{x}_{il} = (x_{il}^1, \ldots, x_{il}^q)$, and x_{il}^u denotes the l-th dose level of drug u that is administered to patients from cohort i; $u = 1, \ldots, q$.

Let $\boldsymbol{\theta}$ be the combined vector of unknown parameters, i.e., $\boldsymbol{\theta} = (\boldsymbol{\gamma}, \mathbf{S})$, or more accurately,

$$\boldsymbol{\theta}^T = (\boldsymbol{\gamma}^T; S_{11}, S_{21}, \ldots, S_{k1}; \ S_{22}, S_{32}, \ldots, S_{k2}; \ \ldots; \ S_{kk}) = \left[\boldsymbol{\gamma}^T, \text{vech}^T(\mathbf{S})\right].$$

We follow Harville (1997) [195], Chapter 16.4, in using the notation vech for element-wise "vectorization" of a $k \times k$ symmetric matrix. The simplest estimator of the response parameter $\boldsymbol{\gamma}$ is given by

$$\tilde{\boldsymbol{\gamma}}_N = \left[\sum_i r_i \mathbf{F}(\mathbf{x}_i)\mathbf{F}^T(\mathbf{x}_i)\right]^{-1} \sum_{i,j} \mathbf{F}(\mathbf{x}_i)\mathbf{y}_{ij},$$

which is unbiased (though not efficient) and thus provides a choice of $\boldsymbol{\gamma}_0$, which allows for dropping the term $\Delta\boldsymbol{\eta}(\mathbf{x}_i; \boldsymbol{\theta}, \boldsymbol{\theta}')$ on the right-hand side of (1.119) and considering the modified algorithm MIRLS introduced in (1.124), (1.125); see Remark 1.4. In this case the modified function $\bar{V}_N(\boldsymbol{\theta}, \boldsymbol{\theta}')$ in (1.125) reduces to

$$\bar{V}_N(\boldsymbol{\theta}, \boldsymbol{\theta}') = \frac{1}{N} \sum_{i,j} \left[\mathbf{y}_{ij} - \mathbf{F}^T(\mathbf{x}_i)\boldsymbol{\gamma}\right]^T (\mathbf{S}')^{-1} \left[\mathbf{y}_{ij} - \mathbf{F}^T(\mathbf{x}_i)\boldsymbol{\gamma}\right]$$

$$+ \frac{1}{2N} \sum_{i,j} \text{tr} \left[\{[\mathbf{y}_{ij} - \mathbf{F}^T(\mathbf{x}_i)\boldsymbol{\gamma}'][\mathbf{y}_{ij} - \mathbf{F}^T(\mathbf{x}_i)\boldsymbol{\gamma}']^T - \mathbf{S}\} (\mathbf{S}')^{-1}\right]^2. \quad (1.127)$$

Parameters γ and $\mathbf{S}$ in (1.127) are nicely partitioned, and each step in the iterative procedure (1.124), (1.125) can be presented in closed form:

$$\gamma_s = \mathbf{M}_{s-1}^{-1}\mathbf{Y}_{s-1}, \quad \mathbf{S}_s = \frac{1}{N}\sum_{i,j}\left[\mathbf{y}_{ij} - \mathbf{F}^T(\mathbf{x}_i)\gamma_{s-1}\right]\left[\mathbf{y}_{ij} - \mathbf{F}^T(\mathbf{x}_i)\gamma_{s-1}\right]^T,$$

(1.128)

where

$$\mathbf{M}_s = \sum_i r_i\,\mathbf{F}(\mathbf{x}_i)\mathbf{S}_s^{-1}\mathbf{F}^T(\mathbf{x}_i), \quad \mathbf{Y}_s = \sum_{i,j}\mathbf{F}(\mathbf{x}_i)\mathbf{S}_s^{-1}\mathbf{y}_{ij};$$

cf. Fedorov (1977) [129]. Consequently,

$$\hat{\gamma}_N = \lim_{s\to\infty}\gamma_s \quad \text{and} \quad \hat{\mathbf{S}}_N = \lim_{s\to\infty}\mathbf{S}_s.$$

The information matrix $\mu(\mathbf{x}, \theta)$ is blockwise with respect to γ and vech($\mathbf{S}$),

$$\mu(\mathbf{x}, \theta) = \begin{bmatrix} \mu_{\gamma\gamma}(\mathbf{x}) & \mathbf{0} \\ \mathbf{0} & \mu_{SS} \end{bmatrix},$$

where $\mu_{\gamma\gamma}(x) = \mathbf{F}(x)\mathbf{S}^{-1}\mathbf{F}^T(x)$; $\mathbf{0}$'s are zero matrices of proper size and μ_{SS} does not depend on $\mathbf{x}$. Thus, the asymptotic variance-covariance matrices can be computed separately. For instance,

$$\text{Var}[\hat{\gamma}_N] \simeq \left[\sum_i r_i\,\mathbf{F}(\mathbf{x}_i)\hat{\mathbf{S}}_N^{-1}\mathbf{F}^T(\mathbf{x}_i)\right]^{-1}.$$

Note that the formula for $\mathbf{S}_s$ on the right-hand side of (1.128) is valid only if all k components are measured at all points $\mathbf{x}_i$. Otherwise, $\mathbf{S}_s$ cannot be presented in closed form for any nondiagonal case.

1.7.2.2 Multiresponse linear model with random coefficients

Compared to the example of Section 1.7.2.1, in this section there are several differences:

- Predictors $\mathbf{x}_i$ may have different length k_i. For example, in a dose-response study patients from different cohorts i may receive different numbers of doses.

- Measurement errors ε_{ij} are uncorrelated.

- Random variation of response parameters γ is allowed.

Let γ_{ij} be individual parameters of patient j in cohort i; $j = 1, \ldots, r_i$; $i = 1, \ldots, n$. Next, assume that parameters $\{\gamma_{ij}\}$ are independently sampled from the normal population with

$$\text{E}[\gamma_{ij}] = \gamma_0, \quad \text{Var}[\gamma_{ij}] = \Lambda,$$

(1.129)

where γ_0 and Λ are often referred to as population, or global parameters; cf. Section 2.11. Then the model of observations may be written as

$$\mathbf{y}_{ij} = \mathbf{F}^T(\mathbf{x}_i)\gamma_{ij} + \varepsilon_{ij}, \quad \text{where} \quad \varepsilon_{ij} \sim \mathcal{N}\left(\mathbf{0}, \sigma^2 \mathbf{I}_{k_i}\right), \tag{1.130}$$

so that $\mathbf{y}_{ij}$ and ε_{ij} are $k_i \times 1$ vectors, $\mathbf{F}(\mathbf{x}_i)$ is an $m_\gamma \times k_i$ matrix, and $\mathbf{I}_k$ denotes a $k \times k$ identity matrix. From (1.129) and (1.130) it follows that

$$\mathrm{E}[\mathbf{y}_{ij}] = \mathbf{F}^T(\mathbf{x}_i)\gamma_0; \quad \mathrm{Var}[\mathbf{y}_{ij}] = \mathbf{S}(\mathbf{x}_i, \Lambda, \sigma^2) = \mathbf{F}^T(\mathbf{x}_i)\Lambda\mathbf{F}(\mathbf{x}_i) + \sigma^2\mathbf{I}_{k_i}, \tag{1.131}$$

We first assume that Λ is diagonal, i.e., $\Lambda_{\alpha\beta} = \mathrm{diag}(\lambda_\alpha)$, $\alpha = 1, \ldots, m_\gamma$.

Straightforward exercises in matrix algebra lead from (1.108) to the following representation of the information matrix:

$$
\begin{aligned}
\boldsymbol{\mu}_N(\boldsymbol{\theta}) &= \sum_{i=1}^n r_i\, \boldsymbol{\mu}(\mathbf{x}_i, \boldsymbol{\theta}) = \begin{pmatrix} \boldsymbol{\mu}_{N,\gamma\gamma} & \mathbf{0}_{m,m} & \mathbf{0}_{m,1} \\ \mathbf{0}_{m,m} & \boldsymbol{\mu}_{N,\lambda\lambda} & \boldsymbol{\mu}_{N,\lambda\sigma} \\ \mathbf{0}_{1,m} & \boldsymbol{\mu}_{N,\lambda\sigma}^T & \boldsymbol{\mu}_{N,\sigma\sigma} \end{pmatrix} \\
&= \sum_{i=1}^n r_i \begin{pmatrix} \boldsymbol{\mu}_{\gamma\gamma,i} & \mathbf{0}_{m,m} & \mathbf{0}_{m,1} \\ \mathbf{0}_{m,m} & \boldsymbol{\mu}_{\lambda\lambda,i} & \boldsymbol{\mu}_{\lambda\sigma,i} \\ \mathbf{0}_{1,m} & \boldsymbol{\mu}_{\lambda\sigma,i}^T & \boldsymbol{\mu}_{\sigma\sigma,i} \end{pmatrix},
\end{aligned} \tag{1.132}
$$

where we drop subscript γ in m_γ to simplify notations, and

$$\boldsymbol{\mu}_{\gamma\gamma,i} = \mathbf{F}(\mathbf{x}_i)\mathbf{S}_i^{-1}\mathbf{F}^T(\mathbf{x}_i); \quad \mathbf{S}_i = \mathbf{S}(\mathbf{x}_i, \Lambda, \sigma^2),$$

$$\{\boldsymbol{\mu}_{\lambda\lambda,i}\}_{\alpha\beta} = \frac{1}{2}\left[\mathbf{F}_\alpha(\mathbf{x}_i)\mathbf{S}_i^{-1}\mathbf{F}_\beta^T(\mathbf{x}_i)\right]^2, \quad \alpha, \beta = 1, \ldots, m;$$

$$\{\boldsymbol{\mu}_{\lambda\sigma,i}\}_\alpha = \frac{1}{2}\mathbf{F}_\alpha(\mathbf{x}_i)\mathbf{S}_i^{-2}\mathbf{F}_\alpha^T(\mathbf{x}_i), \quad \alpha = 1, \ldots, m; \quad \mu_{\sigma\sigma,i} = \frac{1}{2}\,\mathrm{tr}\left[\mathbf{S}_i^{-2}\right];$$

$$\mathbf{F}_\alpha(\mathbf{x}_i) = [f_\alpha(x_{i1}), \ldots, f_\alpha(x_{ik_i})]; \quad \text{and} \quad \mathbf{0}_{a,b} \text{ is an } a \times b \text{ matrix of zeros.}$$

Thus sets of parameters γ and $\{\Lambda, \sigma\}$ are mutually orthogonal. This makes estimation problems computationally more affordable. Iterated estimators, similar to the example in Section 1.7.2.1, can be written as

$$\hat{\gamma}_N = \lim_{s\to\infty} \gamma_s, \quad \hat{\Lambda}_N = \lim_{s\to\infty} \Lambda_s, \quad \hat{\sigma}_N^2 = \lim_{s\to\infty} \sigma_s^2,$$

where

$$\gamma_{s+1} = \mathbf{M}_{\gamma,s}^{-1}\mathbf{Y}_s, \quad \mathbf{M}_{\gamma,s} = \sum_i r_i\, \mathbf{F}(\mathbf{x}_i)\mathbf{S}_{si}^{-1}\mathbf{F}^T(\mathbf{x}_i),$$

$$\mathbf{Y}_s = \sum_{i,j} \mathbf{F}(\mathbf{x}_i)\mathbf{S}_{si}^{-1}\mathbf{y}_{ij}, \quad \mathbf{S}_{si} = \mathbf{S}(\mathbf{x}_i, \Lambda_s, \sigma_s^2),$$

$$\begin{pmatrix} \Lambda_{s+1} \\ \sigma_{s+1}^2 \end{pmatrix} = \begin{pmatrix} \mathbf{M}_{s,\lambda\lambda} & \mathbf{M}_{s,\lambda\sigma} \\ \mathbf{M}_{s,\lambda\sigma}^T & M_{s,\sigma\sigma} \end{pmatrix}^{-1} \begin{pmatrix} \mathbf{y}_{s,1} \\ y_{s,2} \end{pmatrix}, \tag{1.133}$$

where $\mathbf{\Lambda}_s = (\Lambda_{s1}, \ldots, \Lambda_{sm})^T$; $\mathbf{M}_{s,\lambda\lambda}$ is an $m \times m$ matrix; $\mathbf{M}_{s,\lambda\sigma}$ and $\mathbf{y}_{s,1}$ are $m \times 1$ vectors; $\mathbf{M}_{s,\lambda\lambda}$, $\mathbf{M}_{s,\lambda\sigma}$, and $M_{s,\sigma\sigma}$ are the same as $\boldsymbol{\mu}_{N,\lambda\lambda}$, $\boldsymbol{\mu}_{N,\lambda\sigma}$, and $\boldsymbol{\mu}_{N,\sigma\sigma}$, respectively, except that $\mathbf{S}_{si}$ should be substituted for $\mathbf{S}_i$,

$$\{\mathbf{y}_{s,1}\}_\alpha = \frac{1}{2} \sum_{i,j} \left\{ \mathbf{F}_\alpha(\mathbf{x}_i) \mathbf{S}_{si}^{-1} \left[\mathbf{y}_{ij} - \mathbf{F}(\mathbf{x}_i)^T \boldsymbol{\gamma}_s \right] \right\}^2, \quad \alpha = 1, \ldots, m;$$

$$y_{s,2} = \frac{1}{2} \sum_{i,j} [\mathbf{y}_{ij} - \mathbf{F}(\mathbf{x}_i)^T \boldsymbol{\gamma}_s] \, \mathbf{S}_{si}^{-2} \, [\mathbf{y}_{ij} - \mathbf{F}(\mathbf{x}_i)^T \boldsymbol{\gamma}_s].$$

The proof of (1.133) is given in Fedorov and Leonov (2004) [143]. For a discussion on how to tackle the general case of nondiagonal matrix $\mathbf{\Lambda}$, see Remark 8 in Fedorov and Leonov (2004) [143].

Remark 1.10 In pharmacokinetic (PK) and pharmacodynamic (PD) studies, predictor x is the time of taking a blood sample. Thus in a PK/PD context, $\mathbf{x}_i$ is a sequence of k_i sampling times for patients in cohort i. Results developed for the linear model (1.129), (1.130) can be generalized to nonlinear models, as in

$$\mathrm{E}[\mathbf{y}|\boldsymbol{\gamma}, \mathbf{x}] = \boldsymbol{\eta}(\mathbf{x}, \boldsymbol{\gamma}), \quad \mathrm{Var}[\mathbf{y}|\boldsymbol{\gamma}, \mathbf{x}] = \mathbf{S}(\mathbf{x}, \boldsymbol{\gamma}; \sigma^2). \tag{1.134}$$

In the context of compartmental PK models, functions η_l are typically sums of exponential functions. For examples of PK models, see Sections 7.2 – 7.5.

1.7.2.3 Separation of response and variance parameters

Consider a simple two-parameter model (1.107) with a single response, $k = 1$:

$$\eta(x, \boldsymbol{\theta}) \equiv \theta_1, \quad S(x, \boldsymbol{\theta}) \equiv \theta_2, \quad \text{where} \quad \boldsymbol{\theta} = (\theta_1, \theta_2)^T, \tag{1.135}$$

for which the MLE is

$$\theta_{N1} = \bar{y} = \frac{1}{N} \sum_{ij} y_{ij}, \quad \theta_{N2} = \frac{1}{N} \sum_{i,j} (y_{ij} - \bar{y})^2. \tag{1.136}$$

For model (1.135):

(a) The CIRLS converges to the maximum likelihood estimate (1.136) after a single iteration from an arbitrary initial condition.

(b) For the MIRLS, it takes two iterations to converge to the MLE (1.136).

To verify (a), first note that the expression for the function $V_N(\boldsymbol{\theta}, \boldsymbol{\theta}')$ in (1.119) is reduced to

$$V_N(\boldsymbol{\theta}, \boldsymbol{\theta}') = \frac{1}{N\theta_2'} \sum_{i,j} (y_{ij} - \theta_1)^2$$

$$+ \frac{1}{2N(\theta_1')^2} \sum_{i,j} \left[(y_{ij} - \theta_1')^2 - (\theta_1 - \theta_1')^2 - \theta_2 \right]^2. \tag{1.137}$$

Next, let's find $\arg\min_{\boldsymbol{\theta}} V_N(\boldsymbol{\theta}, \boldsymbol{\theta}')$ by equating partial derivatives to zero:

$$\frac{\partial V_N(\boldsymbol{\theta}, \boldsymbol{\theta}')}{\partial \theta_1} = -\frac{2}{N\theta_2'} \sum_{i,j} (y_{ij} - \theta_1)$$

$$-\frac{2(\theta_1 - \theta_1')}{N(\theta_1')^2} \sum_{i,j} \left[(y_{ij} - \theta_1')^2 - (\theta_1 - \theta_1')^2 - \theta_2 \right] = 0, \tag{1.138}$$

$$\frac{\partial V_N(\boldsymbol{\theta}, \boldsymbol{\theta}')}{\partial \theta_2} = -\frac{1}{N(\theta_1')^2} \sum_{i,j} \left[(y_{ij} - \theta_1')^2 - (\theta_1 - \theta_1')^2 - \theta_2 \right] = 0. \tag{1.139}$$

It follows from (1.139) that the second term on the right-hand side of (1.138) is equal to zero and, therefore,

$$\arg\min_{\theta_1} V_N(\boldsymbol{\theta}, \boldsymbol{\theta}') = \frac{1}{N} \sum_{i,j} y_{ij} = \bar{y}.$$

Now using $\theta_1 = \bar{y}$ in (1.139) gives

$$\theta_2 = \frac{1}{N} \sum_{i,j} (y_{ij} - \theta_1')^2 - (\bar{y} - \theta_1')^2 = \frac{1}{N} \left(\sum_{i,j} y_{ij}^2 - N\bar{y}^2 \right) = \frac{1}{N} \sum_{i,j} (y_{ij} - \bar{y})^2,$$

which confirms that the CIRLS converges to the MLE (1.136) after a single iteration.

Similarly, the function $\bar{V}_N(\boldsymbol{\theta}, \boldsymbol{\theta}')$ in (1.125) may be written as

$$\bar{V}_N(\boldsymbol{\theta}, \boldsymbol{\theta}') = \frac{1}{N\theta_2'} \sum_{i,j} (y_{ij} - \theta_1)^2 + \frac{1}{2N(\theta_1')^2} \sum_{i,j} \left[(y_{ij} - \theta_1')^2 - \theta_2 \right]^2, \tag{1.140}$$

therefore

$$\frac{\partial \bar{V}_N(\boldsymbol{\theta}, \boldsymbol{\theta}')}{\partial \theta_1} = -\frac{2}{N\theta_2'} \sum_{i,j} (y_{ij} - \theta_1) \quad \text{and} \quad \arg\min_{\theta_1} \bar{V}_N(\boldsymbol{\theta}, \boldsymbol{\theta}') = \bar{y}.$$

Solving equation $\partial \bar{V}_N(\boldsymbol{\theta}, \boldsymbol{\theta}')/\partial \theta_2 = 0$ for θ_2 immediately leads to

$$\arg\min_{\theta_2} \bar{V}_N(\boldsymbol{\theta}, \boldsymbol{\theta}') = \frac{1}{N} \sum_{i,j} (y_{ij} - \theta_1')^2.$$

Thus, the first component of MIRLS converges to the MLE (1.136) after the single iteration, but the second component converges, in general, after two iterations.

Note also that for this simple model, the IRLS is not applicable at all because parameter θ_2 does not enter the response function $\eta(x, \boldsymbol{\theta})$, and thus this parameter cannot be estimated from (1.117).

1.7.3 Simulations

For the simulation study we selected simple one-parameter models to demonstrate the specifics of different iterative estimation procedures. The response function is either a linear function $\eta(x, \theta) = \theta x$, or an exponential function $\eta(x, \theta) = e^{\theta x}$, with the variance function $S(x, \theta) = e^{\theta x}$. Predictors x_i form a uniform grid in [0,1], $x_i = i/N$, $i = 1, \ldots, N$, where N is the number of data points (predictor levels) in each simulation run (simulated data set). For each example, we take $K_{sets} = 1000$ data sets.

Data points y_i are generated as

$$y_i = \eta(x_i, \theta_t) + \varepsilon_i, \quad \text{with} \quad \theta_t = 3, \quad \varepsilon_i \sim \mathcal{N}[0, S(x_i, \theta_t)].$$

So in the notation of Section 1.7, $N = n$ and $r_i \equiv 1$. For each data set, four methods of parameter estimation were used:

(1) CIRLS estimator $\hat{\theta}_N$, as introduced in (1.118), (1.119).

(2) Modified estimator MIRLS $\bar{\theta}_N$, as introduced in (1.124), (1.125).

(3) Traditional IRLS $\tilde{\theta}_N$ as introduced in (1.117).

(4) The maximum likelihood estimator (1.110).

The iterations for the first three methods were terminated when for two consecutive estimates θ_s and θ_{s+1} the convergence criterion was satisfied,

$$\left| \frac{\theta_{s+1} - \theta_s}{\theta_s} \right| < 0.001,$$

or the maximal number of iterations $N_{iter} = 20$ was reached. The initial condition θ_{0u} for the u-th data set, the same for all three iterative algorithms, was selected randomly,

$$\theta_{0u} = \theta_t + \sqrt{2\theta_t}\, \epsilon_u, \quad \text{where} \quad \epsilon_u \sim \mathcal{N}(0,1).$$

All computations were performed in MATLAB$^{\circledR}$. For the minimization, MATLAB function *fminbnd* was used, with boundaries $\Omega = [-5, 10]$ for the parameter values. This function exploits Golden Section search and parabolic interpolation; for details, see Forsythe et al. (1976) [163].

Example 1.1

For the first run, selected are exponential response and variance functions,

$$\eta(x, \theta) = S(x, \theta) = e^{\theta x}, \tag{1.141}$$

with $N = 20$ data points for each data set. Figure 1.2 exhibits the results for CIRLS, MIRLS, and IRLS algorithms. The histograms of parameter estimates are given on the left, while the histograms of the number of iterations to

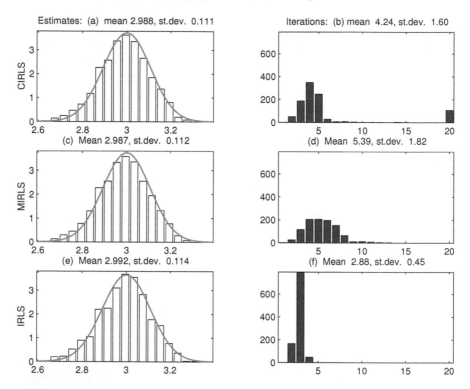

FIGURE 1.2: Example 1.1: $\eta(x,\theta) = S(x,\theta) = e^{\theta x}$, 20 points per set. Top – CIRLS, middle – MIRLS, bottom – IRLS.

converge are presented on the right. The parameter estimates for the maximum likelihood method are not presented since they coincide with the estimates of MIRLS.

The height of each bar in the left subplots (a), (c) and (e) is equal to

$$h_\alpha = \#\{\theta_u \in [A_\alpha, A_{\alpha+1}]\}\Delta/K_{sets}, \quad u = 1,\ldots,K_{sets},$$

where θ_u is the estimate of the corresponding iterative procedure for set u, and Δ is the bin width, $\Delta = A_\alpha - A_{\alpha-1}$. The solid lines in (a), (c) and (e) correspond to the normal density with mean $\theta_t = 3$ and standard deviation $\sigma(\theta_N) = 0.1072$ for the CIRLS and MIRLS, subplots (a) and (c), and $\sigma(\tilde{\theta}_N) = 0.1095$ for the IRLS, subplot (e). For the CIRLS, plotted are only the estimates for convergent sets: in this example there were 107 sets out of 1000 with no convergence of the CIRLS. This does not contradict Theorem 1.1 because of its asymptotic character, but requires us to take a closer look at the data sets for which the CIRLS did not converge.

The analysis of such nonconvergent data sets shows the following tendency. Independent of the initial condition θ_{0u}, after a single iteration the CIRLS estimate θ_1 is in a relatively small vicinity, on the order of $0.05 - 0.15$, of the

MLE θ_N. Then for nonconvergent data sets, estimates θ_s start to diverge from θ_N in the "oscillating" fashion,

$$(\theta_{s+1} - \theta_N)(\theta_s - \theta_N) < 0, \quad |\theta_{s+1} - \theta_N| \geq |\theta_s - \theta_N|, \qquad (1.142)$$

and, finally, there are two limiting points of the algorithm, θ' and θ'', such that

$$\theta'' = \arg\min_{\theta \in \Theta} V_N(\theta, \theta'), \quad \text{and} \quad \theta' = \arg\min_{\theta \in \Theta} V_N(\theta, \theta'').$$

The existence of such θ' and θ'' contradicts the convergence condition of the fixed-point method; see (1.143) and the inequality (A.8) in Fedorov and Leonov (2004) [143].

On the contrary, for the MIRLS algorithm (1.124), (1.125), it takes longer to converge to the vicinity of θ_N if $|\theta_{0u} - \theta_N|$ is large enough. Still, for all considered data sets, this modified algorithm always converged to the MLE θ_N though a theoretical proof of its convergence has yet to be established.

To clarify the behavior of the two algorithms, we took one of the data sets for which the CIRLS algorithm did not converge, and analyzed function $V_N(\theta, \theta')$ of CIRLS introduced in (1.119) and function $\bar{V}_N(\theta, \theta')$ of MIRLS introduced in (1.125). The observations are given by

$$\{y\}_1^{20} = \{1.24, \ -0.39, \ 1.04, \ 1.79, \ 2.45, \ 0.88, \ 1.73, \ 4.34, \ 1.52, \ 2.84,$$

$$5.82, \ 9.82, \ 4.24, \ 9.95, \ 7.03, \ 9.98, \ 10.65, \ 19.74, \ 20.86, \ 10.65\}.$$

The MLE for this set is $\theta_N = 2.93$. Starting from $\theta_0 = 2.93$, the CIRLS is diverging from θ_N as described in (1.142), and finally oscillates between the two limiting points $\theta' = 2.85$ and $\theta'' = 2.98$. Figure 1.3 shows contour plots of functions V_N and $\bar{V}_N$.

The left subplots, (a) and (c), present contour plots of functions $V_N(\theta, \theta')$ and $\bar{V}_N(\theta, \theta')$ in the small vicinity of θ_N: $\theta, \theta' \in [\theta_N - 0.12, \theta_N + 0.12]$. The right subplots, (b) and (d), demonstrate the behavior of these two functions in the larger area: $\theta, \theta' \in [\theta_N - 3, \theta_N + 3]$. The solid line shows function

$$A_N(\theta') = \arg\min_{\theta} V_N(\theta, \theta')$$

in top subplots ((a) and (b)) for the CIRLS, and function

$$\bar{A}_N(\theta') = \arg\min_{\theta} \bar{V}_N(\theta, \theta')$$

in bottom subplots ((c) and (d)) for the MIRLS. The diagonal dotted lines $\theta = \theta'$ and $\theta = 2\theta_N - \theta'$ intersect at the central point (θ_N, θ_N).

As seen in Figure 1.3(a), in a relatively small vicinity Ω_1 of the MLE θ_N, the derivative of the function $A_N(\theta')$ satisfies the inequality $A_N'(\theta') < -1$, which implies that

$$|A_N(\theta_1') - A_N(\theta_2')| > K_1|\theta_1' - \theta_2'| \text{ for some } K_1 > 1 \text{ and } \theta_1', \theta_2' \in \Omega_1. \ (1.143)$$

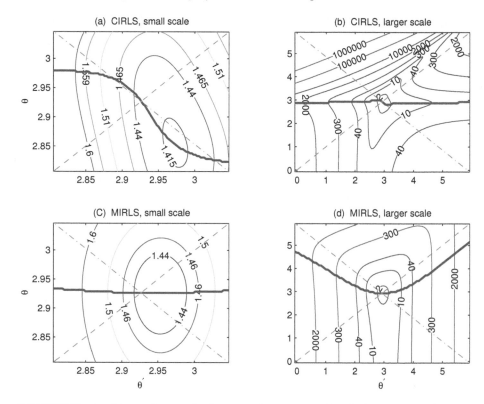

FIGURE 1.3: Example 1.1: Isolines of functions $V(\theta, \theta')$ (CIRLS, top) and $\bar{V}(\theta, \theta')$ (MIRLS, bottom), CIRLS-divergent set.

This means that the convergence condition of the fixed point theorem is violated; see inequality (A.8) in Fedorov and Leonov (2004) [143]. On the other hand, for values of θ' that are relatively far from θ_N, the curve $A_N(\theta')$ is close to θ_N and rather flat; see Figure 1.3(b). That is why the CIRLS converges quite quickly to a small vicinity of θ_N, even for "bad" initial conditions.

Vice versa, the function $\bar{A}_N(\theta')$ is close to θ_N and flat in the small vicinity of θ_N, see Figure 1.3(c), but it goes away from θ_N when the distance between θ' and θ_N increases; see Figure 1.3(d). Still, the derivative of the function $\bar{A}_N(\theta')$ satisfies $|\bar{A}'_N(\theta')| < 1$, which explains why the MIRLS converges, though slowly, to the MLE θ_N when the initial condition is quite far from θ_N.

For comparison purposes, we performed similar analysis for one of the data sets for which the CIRLS converges. The observations for this set are

$$\{y\}_1^{20} = \{1.76, \; -0.46, \; 1.31, \; 1.25, \; 2.83, \; 1.09, \; 2.99, \; 2.37, \; 1.08, \; 3.67,$$

$$4.16, \; 5.33, \; 6.23, \; 3.63, \; 12.86, \; 15.42, \; 12.35, \; 12.04, \; 18.18, \; 18.29\},$$

with $\theta_N = 2.92$. The behavior of the two algorithms for this set is illustrated in

Figure 1.4. Now both methods have similar performance in the small vicinity of θ_N. Still, as in the nonconvergent case, the function $A_N(\theta')$ is flat and close to θ_N when $\theta' - \theta_N$ is large enough, while the function $\bar{A}_N(\theta')$ exhibits some curvature when θ' goes away from θ_N.

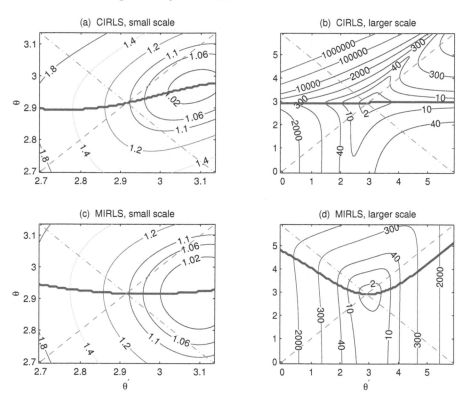

FIGURE 1.4: Example 1.1: Isolines of functions $V(\theta, \theta')$ (top, CIRLS) and $\bar{V}(\theta, \theta')$ (bottom, MIRLS), CIRLS-convergent set.

It is worthwhile noting that for model (1.141), the general formula (1.108) for the Fisher information at a point x is reduced to

$$\mu(x, \theta) = \frac{(\eta'_\theta)^2}{S} + \frac{(S'_\theta)^2}{2\,S^2} = x^2 e^{\theta x} + x^2/2. \qquad (1.144)$$

Therefore, for the selected θ_t and $\{x_i = i/N\}$, the second term on the right-hand side of (1.144) is negligible compared to the first one. In other words, for this model the information contained in the variance component is small compared to the information contained in the response function. Thus, in the iterative procedures CIRLS and MIRLS the additional terms do not contribute too much, and the traditional IRLS performs quite well; see Figure 1.2, bottom subplots (e) and (f). The sample estimates

$$\hat{\sigma}(\theta_N) = 0.112, \quad \hat{\sigma}(\tilde{\theta}_N) = 0.114,$$

are in a good accordance with the theoretical values

$$\sigma(\theta_N) = \left[\sum_i \mu(x_i, \theta_t)\right]^{-0.5} = 0.1072, \quad \sigma(\tilde{\theta}_N) = \left[\sum_i x_i^2 e^{\theta_t x_i}\right]^{-0.5} = 0.1095.$$

Note that if one includes those data sets for which the CIRLS does not converge and computes the sample statistics for all 1000 sets, then the mean estimate changes from 2.988 to 2.985, and its standard deviation from 0.111 to 0.118. This confirms that for the nonconvergent data sets, the CIRLS algorithm oscillates in a relatively small vicinity of θ_N.

Remark 1.11 Since the CIRLS algorithm converges to a relatively small vicinity of the MLE θ_N after a single iteration, it seems natural to try the following modification of the CIRLS, which we will refer to as CIRLS2:

- Use the CIRLS on the first iteration only;

- Then switch to the MIRLS algorithm starting from the second iteration.

It turned out that this modified algorithm always converged to the MLE, so the histogram of the parameter estimates is exactly the same as for the MIRLS. However, convergence properties of the modified algorithm CIRLS2 are much better: for 48 data sets, it converged after two iterations; for 884 sets it converged after three iterations; and for the remaining 68 sets the convergence was reached after four iterations. These numbers clearly demonstrate the superiority of the modified algorithm CIRLS2 for this example. Obviously, there are other possible modifications (run CIRLS for two or three iterations, then switch to MIRLS; use CIRLS as long as the distance between two consecutive estimates decreases, etc.).

Example 1.2

According to Theorem 1.1, it can be expected that if the number of data points N in the data sets increases, then the number of sets for which the CIRLS algorithm does not converge, would decrease. To verify this, for the second example we selected $N = 80$, without changing any other settings. Figure 1.5 presents histograms for parameter estimates and the number of iterations to converge for this example. The number of nonconvergent CIRLS sets drops to 44. The standard deviations of the MLE and the IRLS are equal to 0.0563 and 0.0576, respectively. Similar to Example 1.1, if one includes all the data sets, then the sample statistics for the parameter estimates essentially do not change.

Example 1.3

Now selected are linear response and exponential variance,

$$\eta(x, \theta) = \theta x, \quad S(x, \theta) = e^{\theta x}. \tag{1.145}$$

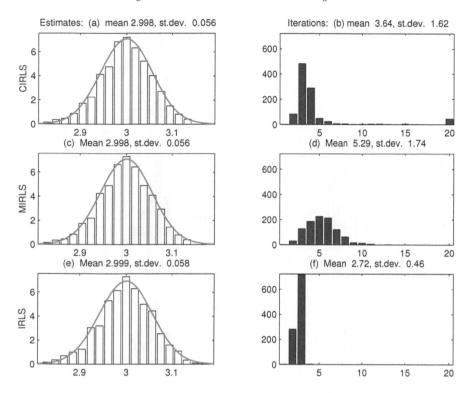

FIGURE 1.5: Example 1.2: $\eta(x,\theta) = S(x,\theta) = e^{\theta x}$, 80 points per set.

For this model, the Fisher information at a point x is equal to

$$\mu(x,\theta) = x^2 e^{-\theta x} + x^2/2. \qquad (1.146)$$

Therefore, for the selected θ_t and $\{x_i\}$ the information contained in the variance component is significant compared to the information in the response function. So it can be expected that the traditional IRLS for this model would be inferior to the CIRLS and MIRLS since the latter two methods take the second term on the right-hand side of (1.146) into account.

Figure 1.6 shows histograms of parameter estimates and the number of iterations to converge for model (1.145) with $N = 20$. As expected, the combined iteratively reweighted algorithms outperform the IRLS with respect to both precision of parameter estimates and the number of iterations to converge. The standard deviation of the MLE and the IRLS for model (1.145) equals

$$\sigma(\theta_N) = 0.473, \quad \sigma(\tilde{\theta}_N) = 1.065,$$

respectively, while the sample values are

$$\hat{\sigma}(\theta_N) = 0.520, \quad \hat{\sigma}(\tilde{\theta}_N) = 1.246.$$

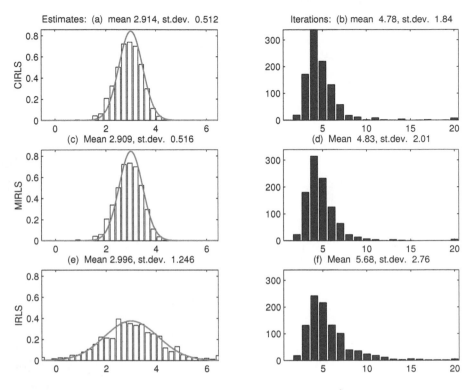

FIGURE 1.6: Example 1.3: $\eta(x,\theta) = \theta x$, $S(x,\theta) = e^{\theta x}$, 20 points per set.

As the reader may notice, there are a few cases for both MIRLS and IRLS when iterative algorithms did not converge after 20 iterations. It turned out that in all those cases the iterative procedures did converge, but it required more than 20 iterations.

To summarize, our simulation study demonstrated that when the information contained in the variance component is comparable to the information in the response function, our combined iterated estimator, is significantly superior to the traditional reweighted methods. We also found out that the "simplified" version of the proposed estimator, which we call MIRLS, while converging noticeably slower than CIRLS, does it more frequently. Therefore, if reasonable initial values of unknown parameters are available, this simplified estimator may be recommended.

Chapter 2

Convex Design Theory

2.1 From Optimal Estimators to Optimal Designs 49
2.2 Optimality Criteria 52
    2.2.1 Optimality criteria related to parameter space 52
    2.2.2 Criteria related to variance of predicted response 57
    2.2.3 Criteria that include unknown parameters 59
    2.2.4 Compound criteria 60
2.3 Properties of Optimality Criteria 61
2.4 Continuous Optimal Designs 62
    2.4.1 Information matrix and optimal designs 64
    2.4.2 Necessary and sufficient conditions for optimality 65
2.5 Sensitivity Function and Equivalence Theorems 67
2.6 Equivalence Theorem: Examples 71
2.7 Optimal Designs with Prior Information 77
2.8 Regularization 79
2.9 Optimality Criterion Depends on Estimated Parameters or Unknown
Constants 80
2.10 Response Function Contains Uncontrolled and Unknown Independent
Variables 84
2.11 Response Models with Random Parameters 85
    2.11.1 Known population mean and variance parameters 86
    2.11.2 Known variance parameters 89
    2.11.3 Estimation of population mean parameters 91

2.1 From Optimal Estimators to Optimal Designs

As pointed out in Section 1.1, for any design ξ_N the LSE $\hat{\boldsymbol{\theta}}_N$ is the best one in the sense that

$$\text{Var}[\hat{\boldsymbol{\theta}}_N] = \min_{\tilde{\boldsymbol{\theta}}} \text{Var}[\tilde{\boldsymbol{\theta}}_N], \tag{2.1}$$

where minimization is performed with respect to all linear unbiased estimators. In a more general nonlinear situation, as discussed in Section 1.5, the MLE $\boldsymbol{\theta}_N$ also possesses certain optimality properties in that asymptotically, as $N \to \infty$, the variance-covariance matrix $\text{Var}[\boldsymbol{\theta}_N]$ is inversely proportional to $\mathbf{M}^{-1}(\xi_N, \boldsymbol{\theta})$ and attains the lower bound in Cramèr-Rao inequality under certain regularity conditions on the distribution of $\{y_{ij}\}$; see references after (1.89). So the next rather natural question is whether it is possible to "minimize" $\text{Var}[\hat{\boldsymbol{\theta}}_N]$ or $\text{Var}[\boldsymbol{\theta}_N]$ among all possible designs.

As in Chapter 1, we start with the simpler linear model (1.1), (1.2) for which various optimization problems (criteria of optimality) are introduced. Then in Section 2.2.3 we extend the criteria to the more general setting.

The equality (1.14) suggests to address the following optimization problem: find the optimal design

$$\xi_N^* = \arg\max_{\xi_N} \mathbf{M}(\xi_N) = \arg\min_{\xi_N} \mathbf{D}(\xi_N), \tag{2.2}$$

where optimization is understood in terms of ordering of nonnegative definite matrices and is performed with respect to arbitrary designs ξ_N as defined in (1.3), i.e., collection of support points x_i and number of replications r_i such that x_i belong to a prespecified *design region* $\mathfrak{X}$ and $\sum_{i=1}^n r_i = N$. Note that our controls, i.e., variables entering the optimization problem, are n and $\{x_i, r_i\}_1^n$. It turns out that unlike (2.1), in general, it is not possible to solve the latter optimization problem, which is demonstrated by the following simple example; cf. Silvey (1980) [360], Chapter 1.3.

Example 2.1 *Consider the linear model (1.1), (1.2) with known variance σ^2, where*

$$\mathbf{f}(x) = (1, x)^T, \quad \boldsymbol{\theta} = (\theta_1, \theta_2)^T, \quad x \in [-1, 1], \tag{2.3}$$

so that the response function $\eta(x, \boldsymbol{\theta}) = \theta_1 + \theta_2 x$. Then for model (2.3) the solution of the optimization problem (2.2) does not exist.

To validate the statement of the example, first note that the information matrices $\boldsymbol{\mu}(x)$ and $\mathbf{M}(\xi_N)$ for model (2.3) are given, up to the constant σ^2, by

$$\boldsymbol{\mu}(x) = \begin{pmatrix} 1 & x \\ x & x^2 \end{pmatrix}, \quad \mathbf{M}(\xi_N) = \begin{pmatrix} N & \sum_i r_i x_i \\ \sum_i r_i x_i & \sum_i r_i x_i^2 \end{pmatrix}; \tag{2.4}$$

cf. (1.21), (1.90). Suppose that there exists a design $\xi_N^* = \{x_i^*, r_i^*\}$ such that for an arbitrary design ξ_N

$$\mathbf{z}^T \left[\mathbf{M}(\xi_N^*) - \mathbf{M}(\xi_N)\right] \mathbf{z} \geq 0 \quad \text{for any} \quad \mathbf{z} = (z_1, z_2)^T. \tag{2.5}$$

It follows from (2.4) that

$$\mathbf{M}(\xi_N^*) - \mathbf{M}(\xi_N) = \begin{pmatrix} 0 & \sum_i r_i^* x_i^* - \sum_i r_i x_i \\ \sum_i r_i^* x_i^* - \sum_i r_i x_i & \sum_i r_i^* x_i^{*2} - \sum_i r_i x_i^2 \end{pmatrix},$$

and

$$\mathbf{z}^T \left[\mathbf{M}(\xi_N^*) - \mathbf{M}(\xi_N)\right] \mathbf{z} = 2z_1 z_2 \left(\sum_i r_i^* x_i^* - \sum_i r_i x_i\right)$$

$$+ z_2^2 \left(\sum_i r_i^* x_i^{*2} - \sum_i r_i x_i^2\right). \tag{2.6}$$

It is obvious that for the design ξ_N^* to satisfy (2.5), it is necessary that

$$\xi_N^* = \{x_1^* = -1, x_2^* = 1; \quad r_1^* + r_2^* = N\}. \tag{2.7}$$

Indeed, if (2.7) is not true, then $\sum_i r_i^* x_i^{*2} < N$, and taking $z_1 = 0$, $z_2 = 1$ and a design ξ_N such that

$$\xi_N = \{x_1 = -1, x_2 = 1,\ r_1 + r_2 = N\},$$

leads to

$$\mathbf{z}^T \left[\underline{\mathbf{M}}(\xi_N^*) - \underline{\mathbf{M}}(\xi_N)\right] \mathbf{z} = \sum_i r_i^* x_i^{*2} - N < 0,$$

which contradicts (2.5). So let (2.7) be valid. We can confine ourselves to two-point designs $\xi_N = \{x_1 = -1, x_2 = 1; r_1 + r_2 = N\}$ and $z_2 = 1$. Then it follows from (2.6) that

$$\mathbf{z}^T \left[\underline{\mathbf{M}}(\xi_N^*) - \underline{\mathbf{M}}(\xi_N)\right] \mathbf{z} = 2z_1 \left[(r_2^* - r_1^*) - (r_2 - r_1)\right].$$

(a) If $r_1^* = r_2^* = N/2$, then take $z_1 = 1$ and a design ξ_N such that $r_2 - r_1 > 0$; for example, $r_1 = N/2 - 1$ and $r_2 = N/2 + 1$. Then $\mathbf{z}^T \left[\underline{\mathbf{M}}(\xi_N^*) - \underline{\mathbf{M}}(\xi_N)\right] \mathbf{z} = -4 < 0$, which contradicts (2.5).

(b) If $r_2^* - r_1^* \neq 0$, then take a design ξ_N such that $r_1 = r_2^*$, $r_2 = r_1^*$, and let $z_1 = -sign(r_2^* - r_1^*)$. Then

$$\mathbf{z}^T \left[\underline{\mathbf{M}}(\xi_N^*) - \underline{\mathbf{M}}(\xi_N)\right] \mathbf{z} = -4(r_2^* - r_1^*)\ sign(r_2^* - r_1^*) < 0,$$

which again contradicts (2.5). $\square$

Example 2.1 demonstrates that even for very simple models like (2.3) the solution of the optimization problem (2.2) does not exist, and therefore more modest objectives are in place. In particular, we will search for the solution of the following optimization problem:

$$\xi_N^* = \arg\min_{\xi_N} \Psi\left[\underline{\mathbf{M}}(\xi_N)\right], \tag{2.8}$$

where Ψ is a scalar functional that is usually called a criterion of optimality. As in the formulation of any optimization problem, it is necessary to accurately specify the set of admissible solutions, i.e., the set of admissible designs in our context. Given the number of observations N, these designs, as defined in (1.3), may be any combinations of n support points $\mathbf{x}_i \in \mathfrak{X}$ and number of replications r_i at $\mathbf{x}_i$, such that $\sum_i r_i = N$ and $n \leq N$. In the definition (1.3) it is important that $p_i = r_i/N$, i.e., p_i is a rational number of form a/N with integer a, and not an arbitrary positive number between zero and one. Jumping a few pages ahead, we remark that designs similar to ξ_N, but with weights p_i varying continuously between 0 and 1, will be the main subject of this book; see Section 2.4.

To summarize, the problem (2.8) is a discrete optimization problem with respect to frequencies r_i, or equivalently weights $p_i = r_i/N$. This combinatorial problem may be extremely difficult from both analytical and computational points of view. To emphasize this statement, rewrite (2.8) in a more explicit form,

$$\xi_N^* = \{x_i^*, p_i^*\}_1^{n^*} = \arg\min_{x_i, p_i, n} \Psi\left[\underline{\mathbf{M}}(\{x_i, p_i\}_1^n)\right], \tag{2.9}$$

where $x_i \in \mathfrak{X}$, $p_i = r_i/N$ and $\sum_i r_i = N$. Theoretical results are known only for symmetric design regions (cubes and spheres) and for simple basis functions such as first- or second-order polynomials.

In the next section we present some examples of popular optimality criteria. We distinguish criteria related to (a) the parameter space and to (b) the predicted response. The rest of the chapter is devoted to continuous designs that provide an approximate solution to the optimization problem (2.8).

2.2 Optimality Criteria

2.2.1 Optimality criteria related to parameter space

The equation

$$(\boldsymbol{\theta} - \hat{\boldsymbol{\theta}}_N)^T \, \mathbf{M}(\xi_N) \, (\boldsymbol{\theta} - \hat{\boldsymbol{\theta}}_N) = R^2 \tag{2.10}$$

defines an ellipsoid of concentration; see Cramèr (1946) [83], Chapter 21.10; Klepikov and Sokolov (1961) [234], Appendix 1; Fedorov (1972) [127], Chapter 1.8. The ellipsoid of concentration generates confidence regions for normal linear models; e.g., see Pukelsheim (1993) [328], Chapter 3. The "larger" the matrix $\mathbf{M}(\xi_N)$ (the "smaller" the variance-covariance matrix $\mathbf{D}(\xi_N)$), the "smaller" the ellipsoid of concentration. So it is intuitively clear that the "maximization" of the matrix $\mathbf{M}(\xi_N)$ ("minimization" of $\mathbf{D}(\xi_N)$) should lead to the improved precision of the estimator $\hat{\boldsymbol{\theta}}_N$.

To provide an explanation of how the information matrix comes into play in the construction of confidence regions, consider the case of a single parameter θ. Suppose that after N observations one can construct an estimator $\hat{\theta}_N$ that is (approximately) normally distributed with mean θ_t and variance V_N. Then the ratio $(\hat{\theta}_N - \theta_t)/\sqrt{V_N}$ is (approximately) normally distributed with zero mean and unit variance, and the (approximate) confidence interval with the coverage probability $1 - \alpha$ is

$$CI_{1-\alpha} = \left\{ \theta : \frac{|\theta - \hat{\theta}_N|}{\sqrt{V_N}} \leq z_{\alpha/2} \right\},$$

where $z_{\alpha/2}$ is the $100(1 - \alpha/2)$ percentile of the standard normal distribution. For example, in the location parameter model

$$y_i = \theta_t + \varepsilon_i, \ \varepsilon_i \sim \mathcal{N}(0, \sigma^2),$$

where σ^2 is known, one may take the sample mean $\hat{\theta}_N = \sum_{i=1}^N y_i/N \sim \mathcal{N}(\theta_t, \sigma^2/N)$, for which

$$CI_{1-\alpha, \ norm} = \left\{ \theta : \frac{|\theta - \hat{\theta}_N|}{\sigma/\sqrt{N}} \leq z_{\alpha/2} \right\}. \tag{2.11}$$

Note that the square of the standard normal random variable (r.v.) coincides with χ_1^2, the χ^2-distributed r.v. with one degree of freedom, and $z_{\alpha/2}^2 = \chi_{1,\alpha}^2$ where $\chi_{1,\alpha}^2$ is the $100(1-\alpha)$ percentile of χ_1^2 distribution. So

$$\frac{(\hat{\theta}-\theta_N)^2}{\sigma^2/N} = N\,M\,(\hat{\theta}-\theta_N)^2 \sim \chi_1^2,$$

where $M = \sigma^{-2}$ is the Fisher information of the r.v. y_i. Therefore, the confidence interval in (2.11) is equivalent to the confidence interval

$$CI_{1-\alpha,\,\chi^2} = \left\{\theta:\ NM\,(\theta-\hat{\theta}_N)^2 \le \chi_{1,\alpha}^2\right\}. \tag{2.12}$$

In the case of an m-dimensional parameter $\boldsymbol{\theta}$, we have the direct analog of (2.12) since the ellipsoidal confidence region with coverage probability $1-\alpha$ is defined as

$$CI_{1-\alpha,\,\chi^2} = \left\{\boldsymbol{\theta}:\ (\boldsymbol{\theta}-\hat{\boldsymbol{\theta}}_N)^T\,\underline{\mathbf{M}}(\xi_N)\,(\boldsymbol{\theta}-\hat{\boldsymbol{\theta}}_N) \le \chi_{m,\alpha}^2\right\}, \tag{2.13}$$

where $\chi_{m,\alpha}^2$ is the $100(1-\alpha)$ percentile of χ^2 distribution with m degrees of freedom.

In the rest of this section we simplify the notation and, if not stated otherwise, use $\underline{\mathbf{M}}$ and $\underline{\mathbf{D}}$ instead of $\underline{\mathbf{M}}(\xi_N)$ and $\underline{\mathbf{D}}(\xi_N)$, respectively.

Among the most popular optimality criteria are the following:

D-optimality:

$$\Psi = |\underline{\mathbf{D}}| = |\underline{\mathbf{M}}|^{-1}, \tag{2.14}$$

D-criterion seems a reasonable measure of the "size" of the ellipsoid (2.10) since its volume is proportional to $|\underline{\mathbf{D}}|^{1/2}$:

$$Volume = V(m)R^m\,|\underline{\mathbf{D}}|^{1/2}, \quad \text{where}\ \ V(m) = \frac{\pi^{m/2}}{\Gamma(m/2+1)},$$

where R is introduced in (2.10), and $\Gamma(u)$ is the Gamma function; see Bellman (1995) [43], Chapter 6, p. 101. Note that $V(2) = \pi$ (area in 2-D) and $V(3) = 4\pi/3$. D-criterion is often called a generalized variance criterion.

E-optimality:

$$\Psi = \lambda_{\min}^{-1}[\underline{\mathbf{M}}] = \lambda_{\max}[\underline{\mathbf{D}}], \tag{2.15}$$

where $\lambda_{\min}(\mathbf{B})$ and $\lambda_{\max}(\mathbf{B})$ are minimal and maximal eigenvalues of matrix $\mathbf{B}$, respectively. Note that the length of the largest principal axis of the confidence ellipsoid is $2\,\lambda_{\max}^{1/2}[\underline{\mathbf{D}}]$, and therefore minimization of E-criterion will also lead to the reduction of ellipsoid's linear "size."

A-, or linear optimality:

$$\Psi = \text{tr}[\mathbf{A}\underline{\mathbf{D}}], \tag{2.16}$$

where $\mathbf{A}$ is an $m \times m$ nonnegative definite matrix, often called a *utility matrix*. For example, if $\mathbf{A} = m^{-1}\mathbf{I}_m$, where $\mathbf{I}_m$ is an $m \times m$ identity matrix, the A-criterion is based on the average variance of the parameter estimates:

$$\Psi = m^{-1}\text{tr}[\underline{\mathbf{D}}] = m^{-1}\ \text{tr}[\underline{\mathbf{M}}^{-1}] = m^{-1}\sum_{i=1}^{m}\text{Var}(\widehat{\theta}_i). \tag{2.17}$$

It is worthwhile noting that D- and E-criteria are the limiting cases of a more general criterion:

$$\Psi_\gamma(\underline{\mathbf{M}}) = \left(m^{-1}\text{tr}[\underline{\mathbf{M}}^{-\gamma}]\right)^{1/\gamma} = (m^{-1}\text{tr}[\underline{\mathbf{D}}^\gamma])^{1/\gamma}; \tag{2.18}$$

see Kiefer (1974) [229]. If γ tends to 0, then (2.18) results in D-optimality (2.14). If $\gamma \to \infty$, then (2.18) results in E-optimality (2.15).

A useful relation exists between D-, A-, and E-optimality:

$$|\underline{\mathbf{D}}|^{1/m} \le m^{-1}\text{tr}[\underline{\mathbf{D}}] \le \lambda_{\max}(\underline{\mathbf{D}}), \tag{2.19}$$

which is a special case of a more general inequality

$$|\underline{\mathbf{D}}|^{1/m} \le \left(m^{-1}\text{tr}[\underline{\mathbf{D}}^\gamma]\right)^{1/\gamma} \le \lambda_{\max}(\underline{\mathbf{D}}) \text{ for any } \gamma > 0; \tag{2.20}$$

see Fedorov and Hackl (1997) [135], Chapter 2. To verify (2.20), first note that (10.8) implies that the matrix $\underline{\mathbf{D}}^\gamma$ may be defined for any $\gamma > 0$ as

$$\underline{\mathbf{D}}^\gamma = \mathbf{P}^T\mathbf{\Lambda}^\gamma\mathbf{P}, \text{ where } \mathbf{\Lambda}^\gamma = \text{Diag}[(\lambda_\alpha)^\gamma], \tag{2.21}$$

and $\mathbf{P}$ is the orthogonal matrix formed by eigenvectors of $\underline{\mathbf{D}}$. Next, it follows from (2.21), (10.9), and (10.10) that

$$|\underline{\mathbf{D}}| = |\mathbf{\Lambda}| = \prod_{\alpha=1}^{m}\lambda_\alpha, \quad \text{tr}[\underline{\mathbf{D}}^\gamma] = \sum_{\alpha=1}^{m}(\lambda_\alpha)^\gamma. \tag{2.22}$$

To prove the left inequality in (2.20), raise both sides to the power γ. Together with (2.22) this leads to the celebrated inequality between geometric and arithmetic means of nonnegative numbers:

$$\left[\prod_{\alpha=1}^{m}(\lambda_\alpha)^\gamma\right]^{1/m} \le m^{-1}\sum_{\alpha=1}^{m}(\lambda_\alpha)^\gamma, \tag{2.23}$$

which follows from Jensen's inequality for the logarithmic function; see Beckenbach and Bellman (1961) [41], Chapter 1.16. The right inequality in (2.20) is obvious since $m^{-1}\sum_\alpha \lambda_\alpha^\gamma \le [\lambda_{max}(\underline{\mathbf{D}})]^\gamma$.

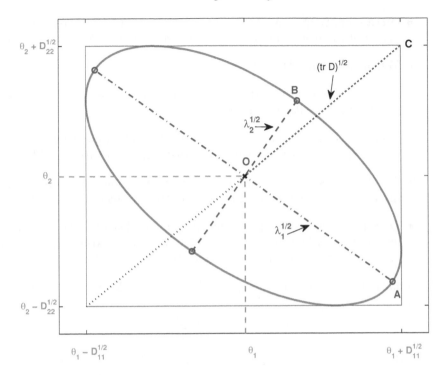

FIGURE 2.1: Ellipsoid of concentration (2.10) with $R = 1$; nondiagonal matrix. Dash-dotted and dashed lines correspond to the largest and the smallest principal axes, respectively.

Note also that it follows from (2.22) with $\gamma = 1$ that the minimization of A-criterion in (2.16) is equivalent to the minimization of the average of the eigenvalues of $\mathbf{D}$, and in that regard A-criterion is another measure of the "size" of the ellipsoid. Moreover, $\mathrm{tr}(\mathbf{D})$ is equal to the square of the half-length of the diagonal of a rectangle that is circumsribed around the ellipsoid.

Figure 2.1 illustrates different criteria of optimality in a two-dimensional case, $m = 2$, for a nondiagonal matrix $\underline{\mathbf{D}}$:

$$\underline{\mathbf{D}} = \begin{pmatrix} D_{11} & D_{12} \\ D_{12} & D_{22} \end{pmatrix}, \quad D_{12} \neq 0.$$

If λ_1 and λ_2 denote the maximal and minimal eigenvalues of $\underline{\mathbf{D}}$, respectively, then the values of different criteria are

- D-criterion: $|\underline{\mathbf{D}}| = \lambda_1\lambda_2 = (\overline{OA} \cdot \overline{OB})^2$, square of the product of the half-lengths of principal axes. .

- E-criterion: $\lambda_{\max}[\underline{\mathbf{D}}] = \lambda_1 = (\overline{OA})^2$, square of the half-length of the largest (major) principal axis.

- A-criterion: $\text{tr}[\underline{\mathbf{D}}] = \lambda_1 + \lambda_2 = D_{11} + D_{22} = (\overline{OC})^2$, square of the half-length of the rectangle's diagonal. For this example $\mathbf{A} = \mathbf{I}_2$ in (2.16).

- Volume (area in 2-D) $= \pi\sqrt{\lambda_1\lambda_2}$.

D-optimal designs are most popular among theoretical and applied researchers due to the following considerations:

- D-optimal designs minimize the volume of the ellipsoid of concentration. This property is easy to explain to practitioners in various fields.

- D-optimal designs are invariant with respect to nondegenerate transformations of parameters (e.g., changes in the parameter scale).

- D-optimal designs are attractive in practice because they often perform well according to other optimality criteria; see Atkinson and Donev (1992) [19], Chapter 11; Fedorov and Hackl (1997) [135].

To compare two different designs $\xi_{N,1}$ and $\xi_{N,2}$, a so-called relative D-efficiency is used:

$$\text{Eff}_D(\xi_{N,1}, \xi_{N,2}) = \left[\frac{|\mathbf{M}(\xi_{N,1})|}{|\mathbf{M}(\xi_{N,2})|}\right]^{1/m}, \qquad (2.24)$$

see Atkinson and Donev (1992) [19], Chapter 10. The rationale for the introduction of relative D-efficiency as in (2.24) is rather transparent: if $\mathbf{M}$ is a diagonal matrix and $\underline{\mathbf{D}} = \mathbf{M}^{-1}$, then

$$|\underline{\mathbf{M}}|^{-1/m} = \left(\prod_{i=1}^{m} m_{ii}\right)^{-1/m} = \left(\prod_{i=1}^{m} d_{ii}\right)^{1/m},$$

and thus $|\underline{\mathbf{M}}|^{-1/m}$ is the geometric mean of parameter variances.

A rather useful interpretation of the A-criterion appears in risk optimization problems. Indeed, let $g(\boldsymbol{\theta})$ be a smooth loss function that attains its minimum at $\boldsymbol{\theta} = \boldsymbol{\theta}_t$. Performing the Taylor expansion at $\boldsymbol{\theta}_t$, one has

$$g(\hat{\boldsymbol{\theta}}) \simeq g(\boldsymbol{\theta}_t) + \frac{1}{2}(\hat{\boldsymbol{\theta}} - \boldsymbol{\theta}_t)^T \left.\frac{\partial^2 g(\boldsymbol{\theta})}{\partial\boldsymbol{\theta}\,\partial\boldsymbol{\theta}^T}\right|_{\boldsymbol{\theta}=\boldsymbol{\theta}_t} (\hat{\boldsymbol{\theta}} - \boldsymbol{\theta}_t).$$

Taking expectation of both sides of the last expression leads to

$$\text{E}[g(\hat{\boldsymbol{\theta}})] - g(\boldsymbol{\theta}_t) \simeq \text{tr}(\mathbf{A}\mathbf{D}), \quad \text{where } \mathbf{A} = \frac{1}{2}\left.\frac{\partial^2 g(\boldsymbol{\theta})}{\partial\boldsymbol{\theta}\,\partial\boldsymbol{\theta}^T}\right|_{\boldsymbol{\theta}=\boldsymbol{\theta}_t}. \qquad (2.25)$$

The function $g(\boldsymbol{\theta})$ is often called a utility function. Note that with the matrix $\mathbf{A}$ as defined in (2.25), the A-criterion is invariant with respect to one-to-one transformation of parameters.

The three criteria, D-, E-, and A-, can be generalized if linear combinations

$\zeta = \mathbf{L}^T \boldsymbol{\theta}$ of the unknown parameters are of interest, where $\mathbf{L}$ is an $m \times s$ matrix of rank s. The variance-covariance matrix of ζ is given by

$$\text{Var}\{\hat{\zeta}\} = \mathcal{D} = \mathbf{L}^T \underline{\mathbf{M}}^{-1} \mathbf{L}, \tag{2.26}$$

and the above-mentioned criteria can be applied to find optimal designs for estimating ζ if $\underline{\mathbf{D}}$ is replaced with $\mathcal{D}$ in (2.14), (2.15), and (2.16).

If $\mathbf{L}$ is an $m \times 1$ vector, say $\mathbf{L} = \mathbf{c}$ and, therefore, $\zeta = \mathbf{c}^T \boldsymbol{\theta}$ consists of only one component, then a criterion

$$\Psi = \mathbf{c}^T \underline{\mathbf{M}}^{-1} \mathbf{c} \tag{2.27}$$

is called *c*-**criterion**. A *c*-optimal design minimizes the variance of a specific linear combination (or, in general, some scalar function) of the model parameters. The disadvantage of *c*-optimal designs is that they are often singular, i.e., the corresponding variance-covariance matrix is degenerate. Note that *c*-optimality is a special case of *A*-optimality since

$$\mathbf{c}^T \underline{\mathbf{M}}^{-1} \mathbf{c} = \text{tr}[\mathbf{A}_c \, \underline{\mathbf{M}}^{-1}], \quad \text{where} \quad \mathbf{A}_c = \mathbf{c}\mathbf{c}^T, \tag{2.28}$$

which follows from the identity (10.10). For examples, see (6.13), (8.10).

A useful relationship exists between (2.27) and the *E*-criterion (2.15). Suppose we are interested in a design that is good for any $\mathbf{c}$. Then it seems reasonable to consider

$$\Psi(\underline{\mathbf{M}}) = \max_{\mathbf{c}} \frac{\mathbf{c}^T \underline{\mathbf{M}}^{-1} \mathbf{c}}{\mathbf{c}^T \mathbf{c}}. \tag{2.29}$$

Taking into account that

$$\max_{\mathbf{c}} \frac{\mathbf{c}^T \underline{\mathbf{M}}^{-1} \mathbf{c}}{\mathbf{c}^T \mathbf{c}} = \lambda_{\min}^{-1}(\underline{\mathbf{M}}), \tag{2.30}$$

cf. (1.37), we find that (2.29) coincides with the *E*-criterion. It is worthwhile noting that (2.30) is a special case of the inequality

$$\prod_{\alpha=1}^{s} \lambda_{m-s+\alpha} \leq |\mathbf{L}^T \mathbf{D} \mathbf{L}| \leq \prod_{\alpha=1}^{s} \lambda_{\alpha}, \tag{2.31}$$

where λ_{α} are eigenvalues of $\mathbf{D}$, and $\mathbf{L}$ is an $m \times s$ matrix of rank s such that $\mathbf{L}^T \mathbf{L} = \mathbf{I}_s$; see Seber (2008) [356], Chapter 6.2.

2.2.2 Criteria related to variance of predicted response

For linear functions $\eta(\mathbf{x}, \boldsymbol{\theta}) = \boldsymbol{\theta}^T \mathbf{f}(\mathbf{x})$, the predicted response at a given point $\mathbf{x}$ is $\hat{\eta}(\mathbf{x}, \boldsymbol{\theta}) = \hat{\boldsymbol{\theta}}_N^T \mathbf{f}(\mathbf{x})$, and its variance is calculated as

$$\underline{d}(\mathbf{x}) = \mathbf{f}^T(\mathbf{x}) \underline{\mathbf{M}}^{-1} \mathbf{f}(\mathbf{x}); \tag{2.32}$$

cf. (2.26). Because of (10.10), the expression for $\underline{d}(\mathbf{x})$ in (2.32) may be written as

$$\underline{d}(\mathbf{x}) = \operatorname{tr}\left[\mathbf{f}(\mathbf{x})\mathbf{f}^T(\mathbf{x})\,\underline{\mathbf{M}}^{-1}\right].\tag{2.33}$$

If the goal is in the most precise prediction at a particular point $\mathbf{x}_0$, then the criterion

$$\Psi(\underline{\mathbf{M}}) = \underline{d}(\mathbf{x}_0)\tag{2.34}$$

provides a popular choice. If the goal is to know the response sufficiently well on some set $\mathcal{Z}$, then two popular criteria are

$$\Psi(\underline{\mathbf{M}}) = \int_{\mathcal{Z}} w(\mathbf{x})\underline{d}(\mathbf{x})d\mathbf{x}\tag{2.35}$$

and

$$\Psi(\underline{\mathbf{M}}) = \max_{\mathbf{x}\in\mathcal{Z}} w(\mathbf{x})\underline{d}(\mathbf{x}),\tag{2.36}$$

where $w(\mathbf{x})$ describes the relative importance of the response at $\mathbf{x}$. The criterion (2.35) is often called *I-criterion*, and (2.36) is the **minimax criterion**.

Most of criteria based on (2.32) are special cases of A-optimality; see (2.16). For instance, if the integral

$$\int_{\mathcal{Z}} w(\mathbf{x})\hat{\eta}(\mathbf{x},\boldsymbol{\theta})d\mathbf{x}$$

is to be estimated, then it follows from (10.10) that the corresponding optimality criterion is

$$
\begin{aligned}
\Psi(\underline{\mathbf{M}}) &= \int_{\mathcal{Z}} w(\mathbf{x})\mathbf{f}^T(\mathbf{x})\underline{\mathbf{M}}^{-1}\mathbf{f}(\mathbf{x})d\mathbf{x} = \operatorname{tr}\left[\underline{\mathbf{M}}^{-1}\int_{\mathcal{Z}} w(\mathbf{x})\mathbf{f}(\mathbf{x})\mathbf{f}^T(\mathbf{x})d\mathbf{x}\right]\\
&= \operatorname{tr}\left[\mathbf{A}\underline{\mathbf{M}}^{-1}\right],\quad \text{where}\quad \mathbf{A} = \int_{\mathcal{Z}} w(\mathbf{x})\mathbf{f}(\mathbf{x})\mathbf{f}^T(\mathbf{x})d\mathbf{x}.
\end{aligned}\tag{2.37}
$$

Similarly, (2.34) can be presented as

$$\Psi(\underline{\mathbf{M}}) = \mathbf{f}^T(\mathbf{x}_0)\underline{\mathbf{M}}^{-1}\mathbf{f}(\mathbf{x}_0) = \operatorname{tr}\left[\mathbf{A}_0\underline{\mathbf{M}}^{-1}\right],\quad \text{where}\quad \mathbf{A}_0 = \mathbf{f}(x_0)\mathbf{f}^T(\mathbf{x}_0)dx,$$

or as

$$\Psi(\underline{\mathbf{M}}) = \mathbf{c}_0^T\mathbf{M}^{-1}\mathbf{c}_0,\quad \text{where}\quad \mathbf{c}_0 = \mathbf{f}(\mathbf{x}_0);$$

cf. (2.27).

For other criteria, see Fedorov (1972) [127], Silvey (1980) [360], or Pukelsheim (1993) [328], including more examples of "alphabetical" optimality.

2.2.3 Criteria that include unknown parameters

We start this section by mentioning criteria that include unknown parameters in linear models. For instance, we may compare different estimates via

$$\sum_{\alpha=1}^{m} \frac{\text{Var}\{\hat{\theta}_\alpha\}}{\theta_\alpha^2}.$$

The corresponding criterion is

$$\Psi(\underline{\mathbf{M}}, \boldsymbol{\theta}) = \text{tr}[\mathbf{V}^2(\boldsymbol{\theta}) \, \underline{\mathbf{M}}^{-1}], \qquad (2.38)$$

where $\mathbf{V}(\boldsymbol{\theta}) = \text{Diag}[\theta_i^{-1}]$ is a diagonal matrix with elements θ_i^{-1} on the diagonal. The criterion (2.38) resembles (2.16); however, there exists an important difference between (2.38) and all other criteria introduced in Sections 2.2.1 and 2.2.2: now the criterion depends on unknown parameters. Obviously, in such circumstances the construction of optimal or even "good" designs becomes much more challenging than in situations when the criterion does not depend on $\boldsymbol{\theta}$. This brings us to the similar issue that arises in nonlinear models, namely the dependence of the information matrix $\underline{\mathbf{M}}(\xi_N, \boldsymbol{\theta})$ and the variance-covariance matrix $\underline{\mathbf{D}}(\xi_N, \boldsymbol{\theta})$ on unknown parameters $\boldsymbol{\theta}$. One of the potential approaches is to construct *locally optimal* designs: first specify a prior estimate (preliminary guess) of $\boldsymbol{\theta}$, e.g., $\tilde{\boldsymbol{\theta}}$, and then address the optimization problem for the given $\tilde{\boldsymbol{\theta}}$. Once the value $\tilde{\boldsymbol{\theta}}$ is fixed, the optimization problems (criteria of optimality) related to parameter space, as in Section 2.2.1, would be identical to that for linear models, with the addition of the prior estimate of $\boldsymbol{\theta}$. The concept of locally optimal designs will be considered in detail in Chapter 5 where we discuss the case of nonlinear regression models.

Here we just mention that the problem can be tackled by various techniques that help mitigate the dependence of optimal designs on estimated parameters and include:

- Minimax designs,

$$\xi_N^* = \arg\min_{\xi_N} \max_{\boldsymbol{\theta} \in \boldsymbol{\Theta}} \Psi[\underline{\mathbf{M}}(\xi_N), \boldsymbol{\theta}], \qquad (2.39)$$

  where $\boldsymbol{\Theta}$ is a given compact set in $\mathbf{R}^m$; cf. Atkinson and Fedorov (1988) [22];

- Designs that minimize the average criterion value,

$$\xi_N^* = \arg\min_{\xi_N} \int_{\boldsymbol{\Theta}} \Psi[\underline{\mathbf{M}}(\xi_N), \boldsymbol{\theta}] \, \mathcal{A}(d\boldsymbol{\theta}), \qquad (2.40)$$

  where $\mathcal{A}(d\boldsymbol{\theta})$ describes the "importance" of different values of $\boldsymbol{\theta}$ and may be interpreted as a prior "belief" in those parameter values. The criterion (2.40) brings us closer to the Bayesian setting; cf. Gladitz and Pilz (1982) [177]; Chaloner (1984) [64]; Pronzato and Walter (1985, 1988) [323], [324]; Chaloner and Verdinelli (1995) [65]); Pilz (1991) [309].

In both (2.39) and (2.40) we replace the original criterion with the secondary one by excluding dependence on $\boldsymbol{\theta}$, either by considering the worst-case scenario or by averaging over the given set $\boldsymbol{\Theta}$. While minimax and Bayesian approaches take into account prior uncertainties, they lead to optimization problems that are computationally more demanding than the construction of locally optimal designs. Instead of preliminary estimates of unknown parameters, one has to provide an uncertainty set for the minimax approach and a prior distribution for Bayesian designs. The latter task is often based on a subjective judgment. Locally optimal designs serve as a reference point for other candidate designs, and sensitivity analysis with respect to parameter values is always required to validate the properties of a particular optimal design.

Another alternative is based on adaptation:

1. Start with the "guesstimate" $\boldsymbol{\theta}_0$ and construct

$$\xi_{N_1}^* = \arg \min_{\xi_{N_1}} \ \Psi[\mathbf{M}(\xi_{N_1}), \boldsymbol{\theta}_0]$$

2. Perform N_1 experiments according to the design $\xi_{N_1}^*$, find $\hat{\boldsymbol{\theta}}_{N_1}$, then use the estimate $\hat{\boldsymbol{\theta}}_{N_1}$ to construct

$$\xi_{N_2}^* = \arg \min_{\xi_{N_2}} \ \Psi[\mathbf{M}(\xi_{N_1}^*) + \mathbf{M}(\xi_{N_2}), \hat{\boldsymbol{\theta}}_{N_1}].$$

3. Perform N_2 experiments according to the design $\xi_{N_2}^*$, find $\hat{\boldsymbol{\theta}}_{N_2}$ from $N_1 + N_2$ observations, then use the estimate $\hat{\boldsymbol{\theta}}_{N_2}$ to construct

$$\xi_{N_3}^* = \arg \min_{\xi_{N_3}} \ \Psi[\mathbf{M}(\xi_{N_1}^*) + \mathbf{M}(\xi_{N_2}^*) + \mathbf{M}(\xi_{N_3}), \hat{\boldsymbol{\theta}}_{N_2}], \ \text{etc.}$$

Because of the dependence of the criterion on parameter values, the described adaptive procedure uses estimates of unknown parameters. However, for linear models the information matrix itself does not depend on parameters. We discuss adaptive designs for nonlinear models in Chapters 5 and 8.

2.2.4   Compound criteria

There are situations when a practitioner may be interested in multiple objectives; for instance, in parameter estimation and in estimation of the response function at a given point $\mathbf{x}_0$. In the former case, D-optimality looks attractive, while in the latter case c-optimality may be a reasonable choice. It is rather natural to combine the two criteria and introduce

$$\Psi(\mathbf{M}) = w_1|\mathbf{M}| + w_2\mathbf{c}^T\mathbf{M}^{-1}\mathbf{c},$$

where $\mathbf{c} = \mathbf{f}(\mathbf{x}_0)$ and $w_1 + w_2 = 1$. Of course, other combinations may be considered and more than two criteria may be included; see Läuter (1974) [249]. More complicated ways of pursuing multiple objectives will be discussed in Section 4.3.

2.3 Properties of Optimality Criteria

Monotonicity. A property that is common for all optimality criteria introduced in the previous section is monotonicity:

$$\Psi(\underline{\mathbf{M}}) \leq \Psi(\underline{\mathbf{M}}') \quad \text{if} \quad \underline{\mathbf{M}} \geq \underline{\mathbf{M}}', \tag{2.41}$$

where $\underline{\mathbf{M}}$ and $\underline{\mathbf{M}}'$ are nonnegative definite matrices, so that Ψ is a monotonically nonincreasing function. The second inequality in (2.41) is understood in terms of Loewner ordering; see Section 1.1.1. Together with the additivity of the information matrix, cf. (1.21), inequality (2.41) means that extra observations cannot worsen the optimality criterion. More data can only help and never harm.

Homogeneity. The following relation holds for all considered criteria:

$$\Psi(\underline{\mathbf{M}}) = \Psi(N\mathbf{M}) = \gamma(N)\Psi(\mathbf{M}), \tag{2.42}$$

where γ is a nonincreasing function and

$$\mathbf{M} = N^{-1}\underline{\mathbf{M}} = \sum_{i=1}^{n} p_i \boldsymbol{\mu}(\mathbf{x}_i) \tag{2.43}$$

is the *normalized* information matrix, with $p_i = r_i/N$ and $\sum_{i=1}^{n} p_i = 1$. Thus, we can separate the dependence of the criterion on N and $\mathbf{M}$. However, matrix $\mathbf{M}$ still depends on N implicitly through p_i. Functions of type (2.42) are called homogeneous functions.

Convexity. The considered optimality criteria are convex functions or may be transformed into convex ones. A function $\Psi(\mathbf{M})$ defined on a convex set $\mathcal{M}$ is called convex if for any $\alpha \in [0, 1]$, and any $\mathbf{M}_1$, $\mathbf{M}_2 \in \mathcal{M}$

$$\Psi(\mathbf{M}) \leq (1 - \alpha)\Psi(\mathbf{M}_1) + \alpha\Psi(\mathbf{M}_2), \tag{2.44}$$

where $\mathbf{M}$ is a convex combination of $\mathbf{M}_1$ and $\mathbf{M}_2$, i.e.,

$$\mathbf{M} = (1 - \alpha)\mathbf{M}_1 + \alpha\mathbf{M}_2. \tag{2.45}$$

The function $\Psi(\mathbf{M}) = |\mathbf{M}|^{-1}$ is not convex, but the convexity of functions

$$\Psi(\mathbf{M}) = -\ln|\mathbf{M}| \tag{2.46}$$

and

$$\Psi(\mathbf{M}) = |\mathbf{M}|^{-1/m} \tag{2.47}$$

follows immediately from (10.14) and (10.15), respectively.

To proof the convexity of the other criteria, use the inequality (10.16).

2.4 Continuous Optimal Designs

As mentioned in Section 2.1, it is difficult to find a solution of the discrete optimization problem (2.9), in terms of both analytical and numerical analyses. Special efforts are required to find the optimal set $\{x_i^*, p_i^*\}_1^{n^*}$ for any given N. Some of these difficulties could be avoided if the discreteness of the weights p_i were ignored and the weights were assumed to be real numbers in the interval $[0, 1]$. Designs that allow weights to vary continuously in [0,1] will be called "continuous" designs. Such a modification allows us to extend the set of discrete designs and utilize a powerful theory of convex optimization.

From now on, if not stated otherwise, we will not use the number of observations N in reference to designs. By a continuous, or normalized design we mean an arbitrary combination of n support points $\mathbf{x}_i$ and weights p_i, such that

$$\xi = \{\mathbf{x}_i,\ p_i\}_1^n\ , \quad \text{where}\ \ \mathbf{x}_i \in \mathfrak{X},\ \ 0 \le p_i \le 1\ \text{and}\ \sum_{i=1}^n p_i = 1. \tag{2.48}$$

Continuous designs differ from exact designs defined in (1.3) in that there is no restriction in (2.48) on the number n of support points $\mathbf{x}_i$ and that weights p_i may vary continuously in [0,1].

Let $\xi_1 = \{\mathbf{x}_{1i}, p_{1i}\}_1^n$ and $\xi_2 = \{\mathbf{x}_{2i}, p_{2i}\}_1^n$ be two continuous designs with support points $\{\mathbf{x}_{1i}\}_1^{n_1}$ and $\{\mathbf{x}_{2i}\}_1^{n_2}$, respectively. Then for any $0 \le \alpha \le 1$ we may define a new design

$$\xi = (1 - \alpha)\xi_1 + \alpha\xi_2 \tag{2.49}$$

as follows. If a point $\mathbf{x}_{1i}$ belongs to ξ_1 only, then its weight in the design ξ is $(1 - \alpha)p_{1i}$. Similarly, if $\mathbf{x}_{2i}$ belongs to ξ_2 only, then its weight in ξ is αp_{2i}. Support points that are common to both designs have the weight $(1 - \alpha)p_{1i} + \alpha p_{2i}$ in the design ξ.

The set of points $\mathbf{x}_i$ in the design region $\mathfrak{X}$ for which the design ξ has nonzero weights p_i is called the support set of ξ and denoted by

$$\text{supp}\xi = \{\mathbf{x}_i \in \mathfrak{X}\ :\ p(\mathbf{x}_i) > 0\}.$$

From the definition of weights $\{p_i\}$ in (2.48) it is obvious that any probability measure defined on the design region $\mathfrak{X}$ can be a design; correspondingly, $\xi(d\mathbf{x})$ will be called a *design measure*. For a definition of probability measures and a compact description of the corresponding calculus, see Rao (1973) [334], Appendix 2A.

The extension of the design concept to probability measures allows us to replace the normalized information matrix in (2.43) with

$$\mathbf{M}(\xi) = \int_{\mathfrak{X}} \boldsymbol{\mu}(\mathbf{x})\xi(d\mathbf{x}), \tag{2.50}$$

where the integration is understood in the Stieltjes-Lebesgue sense. Combining (2.49) and (2.50) results in

$$\mathbf{M}(\xi) = (1 - \alpha)\mathbf{M}(\xi_1) + \alpha\mathbf{M}(\xi_2). \tag{2.51}$$

Of course, (2.43) is a special case of (2.50). There is a fundamental theoretical reason for the use of summation over a discrete set of support points as in (2.43) versus a more general integration as in (2.50); see Theorem 2.1.

Main optimization problem. Let $\Xi(\mathfrak{X})$ be the set of all probability measures on $\mathfrak{X}$. In the context of continuous designs we define an optimal design as a solution of the optimization problem

$$\xi^* = \arg \min_{\xi \in \Xi(\mathfrak{X})} \Psi\left[\mathbf{M}(\xi)\right]. \tag{2.52}$$

We omit "$\in \Xi(\mathfrak{X})$" whenever this is not misleading. Problem (2.52) and its various modifications are the main focus of the book. Note that for a mathematically rigorous formulation, one has to use "inf" in (2.52) instead of "min" since, in general, the minimum may not be attained over the set of admissible solutions in $\Xi(\mathfrak{X})$. To avoid such "nonexistence," we make the following assumptions:

(A1) $\mathfrak{X}$ is compact, and

(A2) The information matrix $\boldsymbol{\mu}(\mathbf{x})$ is continuous with respect to $\mathbf{x} \in \mathfrak{X}$.

In the case of linear model (1.1), (1.2), assumption (A2) is equivalent to the assumption of continuity of basis functions $\mathbf{f}(\mathbf{x})$. For nonlinear models discussed in Section 1.4, assumption (A2) should be replaced with the assumption of continuity of partial derivatives $\mathbf{f}(\mathbf{x}, \boldsymbol{\theta}) = \partial\eta(\mathbf{x}, \boldsymbol{\theta})/\partial\boldsymbol{\theta}$ for any $\boldsymbol{\theta} \in \boldsymbol{\Theta}$; see (1.72).

Many experimental design problems can be solved relatively easily if they are approximated by (2.52). The word "approximated" should draw the reader's attention to the fact that, in general, the solution of (2.52) does not provide the exact solution of (2.9). However, it is often acceptable as an approximate solution, in particular when the number of observations N is relatively large and one rounds $r_i = Np_i$ to the nearest integer while keeping $r_1 + \ldots + r_n = N$. For more details, see Section 3.3; see also Pukelsheim (1993) [328], Chapter 12.

Alternative optimization problem. Similar to the set $\Xi(\mathfrak{X})$ of all probability measures on $\mathfrak{X}$, one may define the set of information matrices

$$\mathcal{M}(\mathfrak{X}) = \{\mathbf{M}(\xi) \colon \xi \in \Xi(\mathfrak{X})\}. \tag{2.53}$$

The optimization problem (2.52) has the following analog:

$$\mathbf{M}(\xi^*) = \mathbf{M}^* = \arg \min_{\mathbf{M} \in \mathcal{M}(\mathfrak{X})} \Psi(\mathbf{M}). \tag{2.54}$$

In theory, the problem (2.54) is easier to solve than (2.52): to solve the former, one has to work not with probability measures but with information matrices that belong to the finite-dimensional space of order $m(m+1)/2$; see Wolkowicz et al. (2000) [407]. However, in some situations it is more difficult to construct $\mathcal{M}(\mathfrak{X})$ numerically than to solve (2.52). In addition, practitioners most often think in terms of predictors (or independent variables) that must be properly selected, but seldom in terms of the mapping of $\Xi(\mathfrak{X})$ to $\mathcal{M}(\mathfrak{X})$. Thus, in this book we focus on solving the problem (2.52).

2.4.1 Information matrix and optimal designs

We start this section by formulating the result that is usually referred to as Carathéodory's Theorem; see Fedorov (1972) [127], Chapter 2.1, or Pukelsheim (1993) [328], Chapter 8.2.

Let ν be a probability measure defined on $S_0 \subset R^k$, and let S be the set of all possible $s_\nu = \int_{S_0} s\, \nu(ds)$. Then any element of S may be represented as a convex combination

$$\sum_{i=1}^{n_0} \nu_i s_i, \quad \text{with} \quad \sum_{i=1}^{n_0} \nu_i = 1, \tag{2.55}$$

where $s_i \in S_0$ and $n_0 \leq k + 1$. If s_ν is a boundary point of S, then $n_0 \leq k$.

Theorem 2.1 *Let assumptions (A1) and (A2) hold. Then*

1. *For any design ξ the information matrix $\mathbf{M}(\xi)$ is symmetric and non-negative definite.*

2. *The set $\mathcal{M}(\mathfrak{X})$ is compact and convex.*

3. *For any matrix $\mathbf{M}$ from $\mathcal{M}(\mathfrak{X})$ there exists a design ξ that contains no more than $n_0 = m(m+1)/2 + 1$ points with nonzero weights, such that $\mathbf{M}(\xi) = \mathbf{M}$. If $\mathbf{M}$ is a boundary point of $\mathcal{M}(\mathfrak{X})$, then $n_0 = m(m+1)/2$.*

Proof.

1. The symmetry of the information matrix $\mathbf{M}(\xi)$ follows from the definition of the normalized information matrix (2.50) and the symmetry of the information matrix $\mu(\mathbf{x})$ in (1.21); cf. (1.86).

2. Compactness of $\mathcal{M}(\mathbf{X})$ is a direct consequence of assumptions (A1) and (A2). Convexity is stated in (2.51).

3. According to (2.50), the set $\mathcal{M}(\mathfrak{X})$ is a convex hull of the set $\{\mu(\mathbf{x}) : \mathbf{x} \in \mathfrak{X}\}$. Due to the symmetry of $\mu(\mathbf{x})$, the actual dimension of this set is $k = m(m+1)/2$. Consequently, Carathéodory's Theorem states that any element from $\mathcal{M}(\mathfrak{X})$ may be represented as a convex combination of no more than n_0 elements $\mu(\mathbf{x}_i)$:

$$\mathbf{M}(\xi) = \sum_{i=1}^{n_0} p_i \mu(\mathbf{x}_i), \quad \sum_{i=1}^{n_0} p_i = 1,$$

where $n_0 \leq k + 1$ in general, and $n_0 \leq k$ for boundary points. The choice of $\{\mathbf{x}_i, p_i\}_1^{n_0}$ for ξ completes the proof. $\square$

Part 3 of Theorem 2.1 is of great practical relevance. It allows us to restrict the search of optimal design to designs with no more than n_0 support points. Therefore, those who are reluctant to exercise with Stieltjes-Lebesgue integrals may think in terms of designs with a finite number of support points.

Whenever it is not explicitly stated otherwise, we assume that assumptions (A1) and (A2) are satisfied, so that the validity of Theorem 2.1 is assured.

2.4.2 Necessary and sufficient conditions for optimality

Suppose that the optimality criterion $\Psi(\mathbf{M})$ satisfies the following four "regularity" assumptions.

(B1) $\Psi(\mathbf{M})$ is a convex function; see (2.44), (2.45).

(B2) $\Psi(\mathbf{M})$ is a monotonically nonincreasing function; see (2.41).

(B3) Let $\Xi(q) = \{\xi \colon \Psi[\mathbf{M}(\xi)] \leq q < \infty\}$. Then there exists a real number q such that the set $\Xi(q)$ is non-empty.

(B4) For any $\xi \in \Xi(q)$ and $\overline{\xi} \in \Xi$,

$$\Psi\left[(1 - \alpha)\mathbf{M}(\xi) + \alpha\mathbf{M}(\overline{\xi})\right] = \Psi\left[\mathbf{M}(\xi)\right] \qquad (2.56)$$

$$+ \alpha \int_{\mathcal{X}} \psi(\mathbf{x}, \xi)\overline{\xi}(d\mathbf{x}) + o(\alpha|\xi, \overline{\xi}), \text{ where } \lim_{\alpha \to 0} \frac{o(\alpha|\xi, \overline{\xi})}{\alpha} = 0.$$

Assumptions (B1) and (B2) refer to convexity and monotonicity as discussed in Section 2.3, where it was shown that all popular criteria satisfy these assumptions. Assumption (B3) modestly assumes the existence of designs that have a finite value of the optimality criterion. The most restrictive assumption is (B4). It states the existence of the directional, or Gâteaux derivative

$$\frac{\partial\Psi(\xi; \overline{\xi})}{\partial\alpha} = \lim_{\alpha \to 0} \frac{\Psi\left[(1 - \alpha)\mathbf{M}(\xi) + \alpha\mathbf{M}(\overline{\xi})\right] - \Psi[\mathbf{M}(\xi)]}{\alpha} \qquad (2.57)$$

for any ξ and $\overline{\xi}$; see Pshenichnyi (1971) [327], p. 21; Avriel (2003) [26], Chapter 4.3. Moreover, this derivative must admit a rather specific form

$$\int_{\mathcal{X}} \psi(\mathbf{x}, \xi)\overline{\xi}(d\mathbf{x}). \qquad (2.58)$$

The meaning of $\psi(\mathbf{x}, \xi)$ will be discussed and interpreted in the next section.

Most of criteria discussed in Section 2.3 satisfy (B4). However, the E-criterion (2.15) and the criterion (2.36), which is related to the variance of the predicted response, in general, do not satisfy (B4). Assumption (B4) may be violated in cases when optimal designs are singular, in particular for the linear criterion (2.26) with rank$(\mathbf{L}) < m$; see Ermakov (1983) [115] and Pukelsheim (1993) [328] for details.

Theorem 2.2 *Suppose that assumptions (A1), (A2) and (B1) – (B4) hold. Then*

1. *There exists an optimal design ξ^* that contains no more than $m(m+1)/2$ support points.*

2. *The set of optimal designs is convex.*

3. *A necessary and sufficient condition for a design ξ^* to be optimal is the inequality*

$$\min_{\mathbf{x} \in \mathfrak{X}} \psi(\mathbf{x}, \xi^*) \geq 0. \tag{2.59}$$

4. *The function $\psi(\mathbf{x}, \xi^*)$ is equal to zero almost everywhere in $\mathrm{supp}\xi^*$.*

Proof.

1. The existence of an optimal design follows from the compactness of $\mathcal{M}$ (cf. Theorem 2.1) and assumption (B3). Because of the monotonicity of Ψ, $\mathbf{M}(\xi^*)$ must be a boundary point of $\mathcal{M}$. According to part 3 of Theorem 2.1, there exists an optimal design with no more than $m(m+1)/2$ support points.

2. Let ξ_1^* and ξ_2^* be optimal, i.e.,

$$\Psi[\mathbf{M}(\xi_1^*)] = \Psi[\mathbf{M}(\xi_2^*)] = \min_{\xi} \Psi[\mathbf{M}(\xi)]$$

and let $\xi^* = (1 - \alpha)\xi_1^* + \alpha\xi_2^*$. Then it follows from assumption (B1) that

$$\Psi[\mathbf{M}(\xi^*)] \leq (1 - \alpha)\Psi[\mathbf{M}(\xi_1^*)] + \alpha\Psi[\mathbf{M}(\xi_2^*)] = \min_{\xi} \Psi[\mathbf{M}(\xi)],$$

which proves the optimality of ξ^*.

3. If $\Psi[\mathbf{M}(\xi)]$ is a convex function of ξ, then the nonnegativity of the directional derivative at ξ^* is a necessary and sufficient condition for the optimality of ξ^*. Therefore, it follows from assumption (B4) that the inequality

$$\min_{\xi} \int_{\mathfrak{X}} \psi(\mathbf{x}, \xi^*)\, \xi(d\mathbf{x}) \geq 0 \tag{2.60}$$

is a necessary and sufficient condition for the optimality of ξ^*. The inequality (2.59) follows from (2.60) if one takes into account that

$$\min_{\xi} \int_{\mathfrak{X}} \psi(\mathbf{x}, \xi^*)\, \xi(d\mathbf{x}) = \min_{\mathbf{x} \in \mathfrak{X}} \psi(\mathbf{x}, \xi^*). \tag{2.61}$$

4. Let us assume that there exists a subset $\mathfrak{X}'$ such that

$$\mathfrak{X}' \subset \mathrm{supp}\xi^*, \quad \xi^*(\mathfrak{X}') \geq C > 0, \quad \text{and} \quad \psi(\mathbf{x}, \xi^*) \geq \gamma > 0 \text{ for } \mathbf{x} \in \mathfrak{X}.$$

Then it follows from (2.59) that

$$\int_{\mathfrak{X}} \psi(\mathbf{x}, \xi^*)\, \xi^*(d\mathbf{x}) \geq \gamma\, C. \tag{2.62}$$

However, (2.62) contradicts the equality

$$\int_{\mathfrak{X}} \psi(\mathbf{x}, \xi^*) \, \xi^*(d\mathbf{x}) = 0,$$

which is a direct consequence of assumption (B4) for $\xi = \bar{\xi} = \xi^*$. This contradiction finishes the proof. $\square$

It is useful to note that under the assumptions of Theorem 2.2 the following inequality holds for the optimal design ξ^* and any design ξ:

$$\min_{\mathbf{x} \in \mathfrak{X}} \psi(\mathbf{x}, \xi) \leq \Psi[\mathbf{M}(\xi^*)] - \Psi[\mathbf{M}(\xi)]. \tag{2.63}$$

To verify this inequality, take the design $\bar{\xi} = (1 - \alpha)\xi + \alpha\xi^*$ and use the convexity assumption (B1), from which it follows that

$$\frac{\Psi[\mathbf{M}(\bar{\xi})] - \Psi[\mathbf{M}(\xi)]}{\alpha} \leq \Psi[\mathbf{M}(\xi^*)] - \Psi[\mathbf{M}(\xi)].$$

Thus, when $\alpha \to 0$, then assumption (B4) implies

$$\Psi[\mathbf{M}(\xi^*)] - \Psi[\mathbf{M}(\xi)] \geq \int_{\mathfrak{X}} \psi(\mathbf{x}, \xi) \, \xi^*(d\mathbf{x}) \geq \min_{\mathbf{x} \in \mathfrak{X}} \psi(\mathbf{x}, \xi).$$

For a given design ξ, the inequality (2.63) provides a useful relation between the minimum of $\psi(\mathbf{x}, \xi)$ over the design region $\mathfrak{X}$ and the "criterion-wise closeness" of the design ξ to the optimal design ξ^*. This inequality will be used in the proof of the convergence of numerical procedures for the construction of optimal designs; see Sections 3.1.3, 3.2.

2.5 Sensitivity Function and Equivalence Theorems

The function $\psi(\mathbf{x}, \xi)$ plays a major role in convex design theory. In particular, as shown in Chapter 3, it is critical for the development of efficient iterative procedures for the construction of continuous optimal designs. It follows from part 4 of Theorem 2.2 that $\psi(\mathbf{x}, \xi^*)$ indicates the location of the support points of the optimal design ξ^*, i.e., points that provide the most information with respect to the chosen optimality criterion. Note also that moving some small measure from the support set of ξ to a point $\mathbf{x}$ decreases $\Psi[\mathbf{M}(\xi)]$ by approximately $\alpha\psi(\mathbf{x}, \xi)$.

To find a closed-form expression for $\psi(\mathbf{x}, \xi)$, introduce the following notations. For arbitrary fixed ξ and $\bar{\xi}$, let

$$\xi_\alpha = \xi_\alpha(\xi, \bar{\xi}) = (1 - \alpha)\xi + \alpha\bar{\xi} = \xi + \alpha(\bar{\xi} - \xi), \tag{2.64}$$

and

$$\mathbf{M}_\alpha = \mathbf{M}_\alpha(\xi,\bar{\xi}) = \mathbf{M}(\xi) + \alpha\left[\mathbf{M}(\bar{\xi}) - \mathbf{M}(\xi)\right]. \tag{2.65}$$

Obviously,

$$\lim_{\alpha\to 0}\mathbf{M}_\alpha = \mathbf{M}(\xi), \text{ and } \frac{\partial\mathbf{M}_\alpha}{\partial\alpha} = \mathbf{M}(\bar{\xi}) - \mathbf{M}(\xi). \tag{2.66}$$

For arbitrary fixed ξ and $\bar{\xi}$, the function $\Psi[\mathbf{M}_\alpha]$ is a function of the scalar argument α, which we denote by $G(\alpha)$:

$$G(\alpha) = G(\alpha;\xi;\bar{\xi}) = \Psi[\mathbf{M}_\alpha]. \tag{2.67}$$

If assumption (B4) holds, then it follows from (2.56) that the derivative $\lim_{\alpha\to 0} G'(\alpha)$ exists (Gâteaux, or directional derivative) and equals

$$\dot{G}(\xi,\bar{\xi}) = \lim_{\alpha\to 0} G'(\alpha) = \int\bar{\xi}(d\mathbf{x})\psi(\mathbf{x},\xi). \tag{2.68}$$

Moreover, if one uses an atomized measure $\bar{\xi} = \xi_\mathbf{x}$, i.e., a discrete design that is supported on a single point $\mathbf{x}$, then $\dot{G}(\xi,\bar{\xi}) = \psi(\mathbf{x},\xi)$.

We show below how to calculate the function $\psi(\mathbf{x},\xi)$ utilizing standard formulae of matrix differential calculus.

D-criterion: $\Psi = -\ln|\mathbf{M}|$. Use formula (10.3). Then (2.66) implies

$$G'(\alpha) = -\text{tr}\{\mathbf{M}_\alpha^{-1}[\mathbf{M}(\bar{\xi}) - \mathbf{M}(\xi)]\}, \tag{2.69}$$

and it follows from (2.50) that

$$\dot{G}(\xi,\bar{\xi}) = -\text{tr}\left\{\mathbf{M}^{-1}(\xi)\int\bar{\xi}(d\mathbf{x})\left[\boldsymbol{\mu}(\mathbf{x}) - \mathbf{M}(\xi)\right]\right\} =$$

$$= \int\bar{\xi}(d\mathbf{x})\left\{m - \text{tr}[\mathbf{M}^{-1}(\xi)\,\boldsymbol{\mu}(\mathbf{x})]\right\},$$

and, therefore, for D-criterion,

$$\psi(\mathbf{x},\xi) = m - \text{tr}[\mathbf{M}^{-1}(\xi)\,\boldsymbol{\mu}(\mathbf{x})]. \tag{2.70}$$

A-criterion: $\Psi = \text{tr}[\mathbf{A}\mathbf{M}^{-1}]$. Use formulae (10.4) and (10.5). Then

$$G'(\alpha) = -\text{tr}\left\{\mathbf{A}\mathbf{M}_\alpha^{-1}\left[\mathbf{M}(\bar{\xi}) - \mathbf{M}(\xi)\right]\mathbf{M}_\alpha^{-1}\right\}, \tag{2.71}$$

and

$$\dot{G}(\xi,\bar{\xi}) = \int\bar{\xi}(d\mathbf{x})\left\{\text{tr}[\mathbf{A}\mathbf{M}^{-1}(\xi)] - \text{tr}\left[\boldsymbol{\mu}(\mathbf{x})\mathbf{M}^{-1}(\xi)\mathbf{A}\mathbf{M}^{-1}(\xi)\right]\right\}.$$

Therefore, for A-criterion,

$$\psi(\mathbf{x}, \xi) = \text{tr}[\mathbf{A}\mathbf{M}^{-1}(\xi)] - \text{tr}[\boldsymbol{\mu}(\mathbf{x})\mathbf{M}^{-1}(\xi)\mathbf{A}\mathbf{M}^{-1}(\xi)]. \qquad (2.72)$$

The function

$$\varphi(\mathbf{x}, \xi) = -\psi(\mathbf{x}, \xi) + C \qquad (2.73)$$

is called the "sensitivity function" of the corresponding criterion; see Fedorov and Hackl (1997) [135], Chapter 2.4. The constant C is equal to the number m of estimated parameters for the D-criterion and to $\Psi(\xi)$ for all other criteria considered so far. Table 2.1 shows the sensitivity function for several popular optimality criteria, where we introduce a shorter notation $\Psi(\xi) = \Psi[\mathbf{M}(\xi)]$. For the sake of simplicity we assume that $\text{rank}[\mathbf{M}(\xi^*)] = m$, i.e., ξ^* is non-singular. There exist a number of design problems where this is not true; cf. Pukelsheim (1993) [328]. However, in many cases simple regularization procedures allow us to obtain practical solutions that approximate singular optimal designs with respect to the selected criteria; cf. (1.26).

TABLE 2.1: Sensitivity function $\varphi(\mathbf{x}, \xi)$ for various criteria Ψ; $\mathbf{D} = \mathbf{M}^{-1}$

$\Psi(\xi)$	$\varphi(\mathbf{x}, \xi)$	C
$\ln \|\mathbf{D}\|$	$d(\mathbf{x}, \xi) = \text{tr}[\boldsymbol{\mu}(\mathbf{x})\mathbf{D}]$	m
$\text{tr}[\mathbf{A}\mathbf{D}], \ A \geq 0$	$\text{tr}[\boldsymbol{\mu}(\mathbf{x})\mathbf{D}\mathbf{A}\mathbf{D}]$	$\text{tr}[\mathbf{A}\mathbf{D}]$
$\text{tr}[\mathbf{D}^\gamma]$	$\text{tr}[\boldsymbol{\mu}(\mathbf{x})\mathbf{D}^{\gamma+1}]$	$\text{tr}[\mathbf{D}^\gamma]$
$\text{tr}[\boldsymbol{\mu}(\mathbf{x}_0)]\mathbf{D}$	$\text{tr}[\boldsymbol{\mu}(\mathbf{x})\mathbf{D}\boldsymbol{\mu}(\mathbf{x}_0)\mathbf{D}]$	$\text{tr}[\boldsymbol{\mu}(\mathbf{x}_0)\mathbf{D}]$
$\int w(\tilde{\mathbf{x}})\text{tr}\,[\boldsymbol{\mu}(\tilde{\mathbf{x}})\mathbf{D}]\,d\tilde{\mathbf{x}}$	$\text{tr}\,[\boldsymbol{\mu}(\mathbf{x})\mathbf{D}\int w(\tilde{\mathbf{x}})\boldsymbol{\mu}(\tilde{\mathbf{x}})\mathbf{D}\,d\tilde{\mathbf{x}}]$	$\int w(\tilde{\mathbf{x}})\text{tr}\,[\boldsymbol{\mu}(\tilde{\mathbf{x}})\mathbf{D}]\,d\tilde{\mathbf{x}}$
$\lambda_{\min} = \lambda_{\min}(\mathbf{M})$ $= \lambda_{\max}^{-1}(\mathbf{D})$	$\sum_{i=1}^a \pi_i \mathbf{P}_i^T \boldsymbol{\mu}(\mathbf{x})\mathbf{P}_i$ $\lambda_{\min}\mathbf{P}_i = \mathbf{M}\mathbf{P}_i$, a is algebraic multiplicity of $\lambda_{\min}$, $\sum_{i=1}^a \pi_i = 1, \ 0 \leq \pi_i \leq 1$	$\lambda_{\min}$

It follows from (2.73) and Table 2.1 that for D-criterion the inequality (2.63) may be rewritten as

$$\ln \frac{|\mathbf{M}^{-1}(\xi)|}{|\mathbf{M}^{-1}(\xi^*)|} \ \leq \ \max_{\mathbf{x} \in \mathfrak{X}} d(\mathbf{x}, \xi) - m; \qquad (2.74)$$

see Kiefer (1961) [228], Wynn (1970) [416], and Section 3.1.3 for its use. Note also that for the linear response function $\eta(\mathbf{x}, \boldsymbol{\theta}) = \boldsymbol{\theta}^T \mathbf{f}(\mathbf{x})$, the sensitivity function of D-criterion may be presented as

$$d(\mathbf{x}, \xi) = \mathbf{f}^T(\mathbf{x})\mathbf{D}\mathbf{f}(\mathbf{x}); \qquad (2.75)$$

cf. (2.32), (2.33).

Equivalence Theorems. It has been a long tradition in experimental design theory to make use of so-called "equivalence theorems" that are obvious modifications of Theorem 2.2 for various optimality criteria. The most celebrated one is the Kiefer-Wolfowitz equivalence theorem for the D-criterion; e.g., see Kiefer and Wolfowitz (1960) [232], Karlin and Studden (1966) [225], Fedorov (1969, 1972) [125], [127], Whittle (1973) [405]. See also Fedorov (1971) [126], Fedorov and Malyutov (1972) [148].

Theorem 2.3 *The following design optimization problems are equivalent:*

1. $\min_\xi |\mathbf{D}(\xi)|$.

2. $\min_\xi \max_\mathbf{x} d(\mathbf{x}, \xi)$.

3. $\max_\mathbf{x} d(\mathbf{x}, \xi) = m$.

To see the relation between Theorem 2.3 and Theorem 2.2, take $\Psi = \ln|\mathbf{D}|$, $\psi(\mathbf{x}, \xi) = m - d(\mathbf{x}, \xi)$ and consider the linear model (1.1), (1.2). Note that

$$\begin{aligned}
\mathrm{Var}[\mathbf{f}^T(\mathbf{x})\hat{\boldsymbol{\theta}}] &= \mathbf{f}^T(\mathbf{x})\underline{\mathbf{M}}^{-1}(\xi)\mathbf{f}(\mathbf{x}) \\
&= N^{-1}\mathbf{f}^T(\mathbf{x})\mathbf{D}(\xi)\mathbf{f}(\mathbf{x}) = N^{-1}d(\mathbf{x}, \xi),
\end{aligned}$$

therefore, observations in the D-optimal design must be taken at points where the variance of the predicted response is the largest. This fact is in good agreement with intuition. For nonlinear models discussed in Section 1.4, the vector of basis functions $\mathbf{f}(\mathbf{x})$ must be replaced with the vector of partial derivatives $\mathbf{f}(\mathbf{x}, \boldsymbol{\theta}) = \partial\eta(\mathbf{x}, \boldsymbol{\theta})/\partial\boldsymbol{\theta}$; cf. (1.72).

Note that the optimization problem

$$\xi^* = \arg\min_\xi \max_\mathbf{x} \, d(\mathbf{x}, \xi) \qquad (2.76)$$

is of practical interest on its own because its solution gives the design that minimizes the maximum variance of the estimated response for all points in $\mathfrak{X}$. Two facts should be emphasized. First, the maximum is taken over the whole design region $\mathfrak{X}$; cf. (2.36). Second, it is assumed that all observations have constant variance σ^2 of measurement errors. Otherwise, (2.76) must be replaced by

$$\xi^* = \arg\min_\xi \max_\mathbf{x} \, [\lambda(\mathbf{x}) \, d(\mathbf{x}, \xi)], \qquad (2.77)$$

where $\lambda(\mathbf{x})$ is defined in (1.44).

A theorem similar to Theorem 2.3 may be formulated for other optimality criteria as follows.

Theorem 2.4 *The following design problems are equivalent:*

1. $\min_{\xi} \Psi(\xi)$.

2. $\min_{\xi} \max_{\mathbf{x}} \varphi(\mathbf{x}, \xi)$, *with* $\varphi(\mathbf{x}, \xi)$ *defined in (2.73).*

3. $\max_{\mathbf{x}} \varphi(\mathbf{x}, \xi) = \Psi(\xi)$.

2.6 Equivalence Theorem: Examples

In this section we show how to use the Equivalence Theorems 2.2 – 2.4 to validate the optimality of a specific design. In what follows we utilize the following lemma; see Silvey (1980) [360], Lemma 5.1.3; Fedorov (1972) [127], corollary 1 to Theorem 2.3.1.

Lemma 2.1 *Consider the regression model (1.1), (1.2). Suppose a D-optimal design is supported on m distinct points. Then the weights of all support points are equal:* $w_i = 1/m$, $i = 1, \ldots, m$.

Proof. The normalized information matrix $\mathbf{M}(\xi)$ may be written as $\mathbf{M}(\xi) = N^{-1}\sigma^{-2}\mathcal{F}\mathcal{F}^T$; see (1.5), (1.17). Thus for an arbitrary design ξ with n support points,

$$\mathcal{F}\mathcal{F}^T = \tilde{\mathcal{F}}\mathbf{W}\tilde{\mathcal{F}}^T, \quad \text{where } \tilde{\mathcal{F}}^T = \begin{bmatrix} f_1(x_1) & f_2(x_1) & \cdots & f_m(x_1) \\ f_1(x_2) & f_2(x_2) & \cdots & f_m(x_2) \\ f_1(x_n) & f_2(x_n) & \cdots & f_m(x_n) \end{bmatrix}, \quad (2.78)$$

and $\mathbf{W} = \mathrm{diag}(r_1, r_2, \ldots, r_n)$. When $n = m$, then the matrix $\tilde{\mathcal{F}}$ is a square $m \times m$ matrix and

$$|\mathcal{F}\mathcal{F}^T| = |\tilde{\mathcal{F}}|^2 \prod_{i=1}^{m} r_i.$$

Therefore, to find a D-optimal design when the matrix $\tilde{\mathcal{F}}$ is nonsingular, one has to solve the optimization problem

$$\prod_{i=1}^{m} w_i \to \max, \quad \text{subject to } w_i \geq 0, \quad \sum_{i=1}^{m} w_i = 1, \quad (2.79)$$

where $w_i = r_i / \sum_{i=1}^{m} r_i$. It follows from symmetry arguments that the solution of the optimization problem (2.79) is $w_i = 1/m$, $i = 1, \ldots, m$. $\square$

Example 2.2 Linear regression: Consider a linear regression model (1.1), (1.2) with

$$\mathbf{f}(x) = (1, x)^T, \quad \boldsymbol{\theta} = (\theta_1, \theta_2)^T, \quad \mathfrak{X} = [-1, 1]. \tag{2.80}$$

Direct calculations lead to the following presentation of the normalized information matrix $\mathbf{M}(\xi)$:

$$\mathbf{M}(\xi) = \begin{pmatrix} 1 & \sum_i w_i x_i \\ \sum_i w_i x_i & \sum_i w_i x_i^2 \end{pmatrix},$$

so that $|\mathbf{M}(\xi)| = \sum_i w_i x_i^2 - \left(\sum_i w_i x_i\right)^2 = \sum_i w_i (x_i - \bar{x})^2$,

$$\mathbf{M}^{-1}(\xi) = \frac{1}{|\mathbf{M}(\xi)|} \begin{pmatrix} \sum_i w_i x_i^2 & \sum_i w_i x_i \\ \sum_i w_i x_i & 1 \end{pmatrix},$$

and

$$d(x, \xi) = \mathbf{f}^T(x)\mathbf{M}^{-1}(\xi)\mathbf{f}(x) = \frac{\sum_i w_i x_i^2 - 2x \sum_i w_i x_i + x^2}{|\mathbf{M}(\xi)|^2}. \tag{2.81}$$

For the information matrix $\mathbf{M}(\xi)$ to be nonsingular, the optimal design ξ must have at least two support points. If there are two support points, then Lemma 2.1 implies that $w_1 = w_2 = 1/2$. Let $x_1 = 1$, $x_2 = -1$, i.e.,

$$\xi^* = \{x_1 = 1, \ x_2 = -1, \ w_1 = w_2 = 1/2\}. \tag{2.82}$$

Then

$$|\mathbf{M}(\xi)| = 1, \quad \sum_i w_i x_i = 0, \quad \sum_i w_i x_i^2 = 1,$$

and it follows from (2.81) that $d(x, \xi) = 1 + x^2$. Therefore, according to Theorem 2.3, design ξ^* in (2.82) is indeed *D*-optimal.

The optimality of the design ξ^* in (2.82) for the linear model (2.80) may be obtained as a corollary of the more general result for polynomial models: we follow Silvey (1980) [360], Section 5.1.4; de la Garza (1954) [91]; and Guest (1958) [184]. For more details on optimal design for polynomial models, see Hoel (1958, 1961, 1965b) [201], [202], [204]; Karlin and Studden (1966) [225]; Fedorov (1972) [127], Chapter 2.3; Pukelsheim (1993) [328], Chapter 9.5. For some recent references on the application of the "de la Garza phenomenon" for nonlinear models, see Yang (2010) [419], Dette and Melas (2011) [95].

Example 2.3 Polynomial regression: consider a regression model (1.1), (1.2) with

$$\mathbf{f}(x) = (1, x, \ldots, x^{m-1})^T, \quad \boldsymbol{\theta} = (\theta_1, \theta_2, \ldots, \theta_m)^T, \quad \mathfrak{X} = [-1, 1], \tag{2.83}$$

for which the variance of prediction $d(x, \xi)$ is a polynomial of degree $2m - 2$, i.e., $d(x, \xi) = a_1 + a_2 x_1 + a_{2m-1} x^{2m-2}$. There are at most $2m - 3$ stationary points of $d(x, \xi)$. Since $\mathbf{M}(\xi)$ is a positive definite matrix and the coefficient a_{2m-1} is positive, there are at most $m - 1$ local minima and $m - 2$ local maxima. For the information matrix $\mathbf{M}(\xi)$ to be nonsingular, there must be two more maxima at the boundary points $x = \pm 1$, and, therefore, the number of support points of D-optimal design must be exactly m. Lemma 2.1 implies now that weights of all support points are equal to $1/m$, and that the problem of finding points of maxima of $d(x, \xi)$ is equivalent to the problem of finding points $\{x_1, \ldots, x_{m-2}\}$ of maxima of the Vandermonde determinant $|\mathbf{V}|$, where

$$\mathbf{V} = \begin{pmatrix} 1 & 1 & \cdots & 1 \\ 1 & -1 & \cdots & (-1)^{m-1} \\ 1 & x_1 & \cdots & x_1^{m-1} \\ \cdots & \cdots & \cdots & \cdots \\ 1 & x_{m-2} & \cdots & x_{m-2}^{m-1} \end{pmatrix}.$$

Note now that the response $\eta(x) = \mathbf{f}^T(x)\boldsymbol{\theta}$ may be presented via the Lagrange interpolation formula:

$$\eta(x) = \sum_{j=1}^{m} \eta(x_j) L_j(x), \text{ where } L_j(x) = \prod_{i \neq j, \, i=1}^{m} \frac{x - x_i}{x_j - x_i},$$

where $L_j(x)$ are Lagrange interpolation polynomials over m distinct points $x_1, \ldots, x_m$. Polynomials $L_j(x)$ may be presented as

$$L_j(x) = \frac{F(x)}{(x - x_j)F'(x_j)}, \text{ with } F(x) = \prod_{j=1}^{m}(x - x_j) \qquad (2.84)$$

(indeed, $F'(x) = \sum_{j=1}^{m} \prod_{i \neq j, \, i=1}^{m}(x - x_i)$, so $F'(x_j) = \prod_{i \neq j}(x_j - x_i)$). The variance of prediction $d(x, \xi)$ is, therefore, proportional to $\sum_{j=1}^{m} L_j^2(x)$, and to find $m - 2$ internal points of D-optimal design, one needs to find $m - 2$ solutions x_j of the equation

$$L_j'(x_j) = 0, \ x_j \in (-1, 1), \ j = 1, \ldots, m - 2. \qquad (2.85)$$

It follows from (2.84) that

$$F'(x) = \left[L_j'(x)(x - x_j) + L_j(x) \right] F'(x_j),$$

$$F''(x) = \left[L_j''(x)(x - x_j) + 2L_j'(x) \right] F'(x_j).$$

Thus, equations (2.85) and $F''(x) = 0$ have identical roots. Since the two D-optimal points are $+1$ and -1, one may search for $F(x)$ as

$$F(x) = A(x^2 - 1)F_{m-2}(x),$$

where $F_{m-2}(x)$ is a polynomial of degree $m - 2$. It follows now from the theory of orthogonal polynomials that $F_{m-2}(x)$ is the derivative of the Legendre polynomial $P_{m-1}(x)$. Indeed, in this case the definition of Legendre polynomials implies that

$$F'(x) = A\frac{d}{dx}\left[(x^2 - 1)P'_{m-1}x)\right] = A(m-1)mP_{m-1}(x)$$

and

$$F''(x) = A(m-1)mP'_{m-1}(x).$$

Therefore, the D-optimal design for the polynomial regression model (2.83) is supported on two boundary points $x = \pm 1$ and $m - 2$ roots of the derivative of the Legendre polynomial $P_{m-1}(x)$.

Example 2.4 Trigonometric regression: consider *trigonometric regression* with the set of basis functions

$$\mathbf{f}(x) = (1, \ \sin x, \ \cos x, \dots, \ \sin kx, \ \cos kx)^T, \ \ 0 \le x < 2\pi, \qquad (2.86)$$

so that the number of parameters $m = 2k + 1$; cf. Hoel (1965a) [203]; Fedorov (1972) [127], Chapter 2.4; Ermakov and Zhigljavsky (1987) [116]; Pukelsheim (1993) [328], Chapter 9.16; Fedorov and Hackl (1997) [135], Chapter 2.5. Due to symmetry arguments and invariance with respect to rotation, it seems reasonable to consider the uniform design (measure) on $[0, 2\pi)$ as a candidate, i.e., $\xi^u(dx) = 1/(2\pi)$. To demonstrate that this design is indeed D-optimal, first note that for any integer α

$$\int_0^{2\pi} \sin \alpha x \, dx = \int_0^{2\pi} \cos \alpha x \, dx = 0, \qquad (2.87)$$

because of periodicity of sine and cosine, and that

$$\int_0^{2\pi} \sin \alpha x \sin \beta x \, dx = \int_0^{2\pi} \cos \alpha x \sin \beta x \, dx = \int_0^{2\pi} \cos \alpha x \cos \beta x \, dx = 0, \qquad (2.88)$$

for any integer $\alpha \ne \beta$ because the integrals in (2.88) may be reduced to the integrals of type (2.87) by so-called "product-to-sum" trigonometric identities, as in

$$2 \sin x \sin y = [\cos(x - y) - \cos(x + y)],$$
$$2 \cos x \cos y = [\cos(x - y) + \cos(x + y)],$$
$$2 \sin x \cos y = [\sin(x + y) + \sin(x - y)]. \qquad (2.89)$$

Next,

$$\int_0^{2\pi} \sin^2 \alpha x \, dx = \int_0^{2\pi} \cos^2 \alpha x \, dx = \pi \qquad (2.90)$$

because of the first two identities in (2.89). Therefore, (2.87), (2.88) and (2.90) imply that

$$\mathbf{M}(\xi^u) = \int_0^{2\pi} \mathbf{f}(x)\mathbf{f}^T(x)\xi^u(dx) = \begin{pmatrix} 1 & 0 & \cdots & 0 \\ 0 & 1/2 & \cdots & 0 \\ \vdots & \vdots & \ddots & \vdots \\ 0 & 0 & \cdots & 1/2 \end{pmatrix}, \quad (2.91)$$

$$\mathbf{D}(\xi^u) = \begin{pmatrix} 1 & 0 & \cdots & 0 \\ 0 & 2 & \cdots & 0 \\ \vdots & \vdots & \ddots & \vdots \\ 0 & 0 & \cdots & 2 \end{pmatrix}, \quad (2.92)$$

from which it follows that for any $x \in [0, 2\pi]$

$$d(x, \xi^u) = \mathbf{f}^T(x)\mathbf{D}(\xi^u)\mathbf{f}(x) = 1 + \sum_{\alpha=1}^{k} 2(\sin^2 \alpha x + \cos^2 \alpha x) \equiv$$

$$\equiv 2k + 1 = m. \quad (2.93)$$

From Theorem 2.3 it follows now that the design ξ^u is D-optimal.

For the criterion $\Psi = \mathrm{tr}[\mathbf{D}^\gamma]$, according to Table 2.1,

$$\varphi(x, \xi^u) = \mathbf{f}^T(x)\mathbf{D}^{\gamma+1}\mathbf{f}(x) = 1 + 2^{\gamma+1}\sum_{\alpha=1}^{k} 2(\sin^2 \alpha x + \cos^2 \alpha x)$$

$$= 1 + 2^{\gamma+1}k ,$$

and

$$\mathrm{tr}[\mathbf{D}^\gamma] = 1 + 2^\gamma 2k = 1 + 2^{\gamma+1}k,$$

which proves that the design ξ^u is optimal in the sense of (2.18) for any $\gamma > 0$.

From a practical viewpoint, the design ξ^u with infinitely many support points is hardly useful. A more practical alternative is a design ξ_n with $n \geq m$ support points such that

$$\xi_n = \left\{ x_i = \varphi + 2\pi\frac{i-1}{n}, \ w_i = \frac{1}{n}, \ i = 1, \ldots, n \right\}. \quad (2.94)$$

To prove the optimality of the design ξ_n for any $n \geq m$, it is sufficient to show that the information matrix $\mathbf{M}(\xi_n)$ coincides with the information matrix $\mathbf{M}(\xi^u)$ in (2.91). Note that $\mathbf{M}(\xi_n) = \sum_{i=1}^{n} \boldsymbol{\mu}(x_i)/n$, where

$$\boldsymbol{\mu}(x_i) = \begin{pmatrix} 1 & \sin x_i & \cdots & \cos kx_i \\ \sin x_i & \sin^2 x_i & \cdots & \sin x_i \cos kx_i \\ \vdots & \vdots & \ddots & \vdots \\ \cos kx_i & \cos kx_i \sin x_i & \cdots & \cos^2 kx_i \end{pmatrix}. \quad (2.95)$$

Use the following trigonometric identities:

$$\sum_{i=0}^{n-1} \sin(\varphi + iy) = \sin\left[\varphi + \frac{(n-1)y}{2}\right] \sin\frac{ny}{2} \, cosec\frac{y}{2} \, ,$$

$$\sum_{i=0}^{n-1} \cos(\varphi + iy) = \cos\left[\varphi + \frac{(n-1)y}{2}\right] \sin\frac{ny}{2} \, cosec\frac{y}{2} \, , \qquad (2.96)$$

see Gradshteyn and Ryzhik (1994) [181], Chapter 1.341. For the elements of the first row/column of $\mathbf{M}(\xi_n)$, use (2.96) with $y = 2\pi\alpha/n$, $\alpha = 1, \ldots, k$. Then $\sin(ny/2) = \sin(\pi\alpha) = 0$, and therefore all nondiagonal elements in the first row/column are equal to zero.

For nondiagonal elements of other rows/columns use formula (2.89), which will reduce the sum of products of trigonometric functions to the sums similar to those on the left-hand side of (2.96). For example,

$$M_{23}(\xi_n) = \frac{1}{n}\sum_{i=1}^{n} \sin x_i \cos x_i = \frac{1}{2n}\sum_{i=1}^{n} \sin 2x_i = 0$$

by the same argument as for the elements of the first row/column.

For the diagonal elements of the matrix $\mathbf{M}(\xi_n)$, use the following identities

$$\sum_{i=0}^{n-1} \sin^2 iy = \frac{n-1}{2} - \frac{\cos ny \, \sin[(n-1)y]}{2\sin y},$$

$$\sum_{i=0}^{n-1} \cos^2 iy = \frac{n+1}{2} + \frac{\cos ny \, \sin[(n-1)y]}{2\sin y}; \qquad (2.97)$$

see Gradshteyn and Ryzhik (1994) [181], Chapter 1.351. For $y = 2\pi/n$,

$$\sum_{i=0}^{n-1} \sin^2 iy = \frac{n-1}{2} - \frac{\cos(2\pi) \sin(2\pi - y)}{2\sin y} = \frac{n-1}{2} + \frac{1}{2} = \frac{n}{2},$$

$$\sum_{i=0}^{n-1} \cos^2 iy = \frac{n+1}{2} - \frac{1}{2} = \frac{n}{2}.$$

Finally, we have to show that functions $F_1(\varphi) = \sum_{i=0}^{n-1} \sin^2(\varphi + iy)$ and $F_2(\varphi) = \sum_{i=0}^{n-1} \cos^2(\varphi + iy)$ are invariant with respect to φ. For this, take derivatives of these functions:

$$F_1'(\varphi) = -F_2'(\varphi) = 2\sum_{i=0}^{n-1} \sin(\varphi + iy)\cos(\varphi + iy) = \sum_{i=0}^{n-1} \sin[2(\varphi + iy)] = 0$$

because of the first identity in (2.96). Thus all diagonal elements of the matrix $\mathbf{M}(\xi_n)$, except the first one, are equal to $1/2$, which proves that $\mathbf{M}(\xi_n) = \mathbf{M}(\xi^u)$ and that ξ_n is indeed D-optimal.

2.7 Optimal Designs with Prior Information

Consider the linear regression model as in (1.1) or (1.4), where σ^2 is known. Suppose that the prior information about the parameter $\boldsymbol{\theta}$ is available and that the prior unbiased estimator is $\hat{\boldsymbol{\theta}}_0$ with the variance-covariance matrix $\mathbf{D}_0$. As discussed at the end of Section 1.1, the best linear unbiased estimator (BLUE) is

$$\boldsymbol{\theta}^* = \left[\mathbf{D}_0^{-1} + \underline{\mathbf{M}}(\xi_N)\right]^{-1} \left[\mathbf{D}_0^{-1}\hat{\boldsymbol{\theta}}_0 + \underline{\mathbf{M}}(\xi_N)\,\hat{\boldsymbol{\theta}}_N\right],$$

with the variance-covariance matrix $\mathbf{D}_B$ as in (1.34),

$$\mathbf{D}_B = \left[\mathbf{D}_0^{-1} + \underline{\mathbf{M}}(\xi_N)\right]^{-1}.$$

Therefore, it is natural to optimize various functionals depending on the matrix $\mathbf{D}_B$ or its normalized version

$$\mathbf{D}_B(\xi) = N \cdot \mathbf{D}_B = \mathbf{M}_B^{-1}(\xi), \tag{2.98}$$

where

$$\mathbf{M}_B(\xi) = \mathbf{M}_0 + \mathbf{M}(\xi), \;\; \mathbf{M}_0 = \frac{1}{N}\,\mathbf{D}_0^{-1}, \;\; \mathbf{M}(\xi) = \frac{1}{N}\,\underline{\mathbf{M}}(\xi_N). \tag{2.99}$$

If D-criterion is considered, then one will address the following optimization problem:

$$\xi^* = \arg\max_{\xi} |\mathbf{M}_0 + \mathbf{M}(\xi)|. \tag{2.100}$$

The criterion in (2.100) is called Bayesian D-optimality; cf. Chaloner (1984) [64], Section 1; Pilz (1991) [309]; Chaloner and Verdinelli (1995) [65], Section 2.1. Unlike standard non-Bayesian design criteria, it is obvious from the definition of the matrix $\mathbf{M}_B(\xi)$ in (2.99) that Bayesian optimal designs do depend on the variance σ^2 and the number of observations N.

Note also that for normal linear regression models, the optimization problem (2.100) is equivalent to maximization of the Shannon information of the posterior distribution; see Lindley (1956) [258], Bernardo (1979) [45].

In general, if the optimality criterion $\Psi[\mathbf{M}]$ satisfies the regularity conditions of Sections 2.3 and 2.4, then so does the criterion $\Psi[\mathbf{M}_0 + \mathbf{M}(\xi)]$ as a function of $\mathbf{M}(\xi)$. To find out expressions for directional derivatives and sensitivity functions of Bayesian designs, note that the analog of the matrix $\mathbf{M}_\alpha$ in (2.65) is now

$$\mathbf{M}_{B,\alpha} = \mathbf{M}_B(\xi) + \alpha\left[\mathbf{M}_B(\bar{\xi}) - \mathbf{M}_B(\xi)\right] = \mathbf{M}_B(\xi) + \alpha\left[\mathbf{M}(\bar{\xi}) - \mathbf{M}(\xi)\right]; \tag{2.101}$$

therefore,

$$\lim_{\alpha \to \alpha} \mathbf{M}_{B,\alpha} = \mathbf{M}_B(\xi), \quad \text{and} \quad \frac{\partial \mathbf{M}_{B,\alpha}}{\partial \alpha} = \mathbf{M}(\bar{\xi}) - \mathbf{M}(\xi). \tag{2.102}$$

It follows from (10.3) that for Bayesian D-criterion

$$G'(\alpha) = -\mathrm{tr}\{\mathbf{M}_{B,\alpha}^{-1}[\mathbf{M}(\bar\xi) - \mathbf{M}(\xi)]\} \tag{2.103}$$

and

$$\dot G(\xi, \bar\xi) = \int \bar\xi(d\mathbf{x}) \left\{\mathrm{tr}[\mathbf{M}_B^{-1}(\xi)\,\mathbf{M}(\xi)] - \mathrm{tr}[\mathbf{M}_B^{-1}(\xi)\,\boldsymbol\mu(\mathbf{x})]\right\}.$$

So the integrand in the expression for the directional derivative for Bayesian D-criterion (2.100) is

$$\psi(\mathbf{x}, \xi) = \mathrm{tr}[\mathbf{M}_B^{-1}(\xi)\mathbf{M}(\xi)] - \mathrm{tr}[\mathbf{M}_B^{-1}(\xi)\,\boldsymbol\mu(\mathbf{x})]; \tag{2.104}$$

see condition (B4) in Section 2.4.2. The corresponding sensitivity function is

$$d_B(\mathbf{x}, \xi) = \mathrm{tr}[\mathbf{M}_B^{-1}(\xi)\,\boldsymbol\mu(\mathbf{x})]. \tag{2.105}$$

It is worthwhile noting that if a preliminary experiment is performed and the matrix $\mathbf{D}_0^{-1}$ is its information matrix, then the problem similar to that of maximization of the determinant $|\mathbf{D}_0^{-1} + \mathbf{M}(\xi_N)|$ was considered in a number of papers that addressed iterative construction of D-optimal designs; see Dykstra (1971) [113], Evans (1979) [120], Johnson and Nachtsheim (1983) [216], among others. Such settings may be viewed as two-stage design problems: one starts with the initial experiment and then attempts to complement the existing design with the most "informative" second-stage design. The algorithms discussed in these papers are conceptually very close to those discussed in Chapters 3.1, 3.2, 5.3, while the normalized version of the optimization problem (2.100) is algebraically identical to finding optimal two-stage design.

To make the link between the two problems transparent, let us assume that the total number of observations in the two-stage design is N, the first experimental stage has N_0 observations, the second stage has $N - N_0$ observations and is stochastically independent of the first stage (i.e., the decision to continue with the second stage is not conditioned on the observed responses of the first stage). Let the nonnormalized information matrices of the individual stages be $\underline{\mathbf{M}}(\xi_{N_0})$ and $\underline{\mathbf{M}}(\xi_{N-N_0})$. Then the total (two-stage) nonnormalized information matrix is

$$\underline{\mathbf{M}}(\xi_N) = \underline{\mathbf{M}}(\xi_{N_0}) + \underline{\mathbf{M}}(\xi_{N-N_0}),$$

and the combined BLUE is

$$\hat{\boldsymbol\theta}_{tot} = \underline{\mathbf{M}}^{-1}(\xi_N) \left[\underline{\mathbf{M}}^{-1}(\xi_{N_0})\hat{\boldsymbol\theta}_{N_0} + \underline{\mathbf{M}}^{-1}(\xi_{N-N_0})\hat{\boldsymbol\theta}_{N-N_0}\right];$$

cf. (1.31). The normalized information matrix of the two-stage design is

$$\mathbf{M}(\xi_{tot}) = \frac{1}{N}\underline{\mathbf{M}}(\xi_N) = \frac{1}{N}\left[N_0\frac{\mathbf{M}(\xi_{N_0})}{N_0} + (N - N_0)\frac{\mathbf{M}(\xi_{N_0})}{N - N_0}\right],$$

so

$$\mathbf{M}(\xi_{tot}) = \delta\mathbf{M}(\xi_0) + (1 - \delta)\mathbf{M}(\xi), \tag{2.106}$$

where $\delta = N_0/N$ is the fraction of observations in the first stage; $\{\xi_0, \mathbf{M}(\xi_0)\}$ and $\{\xi, \mathbf{M}(\xi)\}$ are the normalized design and normalized information matrix of the first and second stages, respectively. Therefore, the terms $\mathbf{M}(\xi_{tot})$, $\delta\mathbf{M}(\xi_0)$, $(1-\delta)\mathbf{M}(\xi)$ in (2.106) correspond to $\mathbf{M}_B(\xi)$, $\mathbf{M}_0$, $\mathbf{M}(\xi)$ in (2.99). The design ξ_{N_0}, or its normalized version ξ_0, may be viewed as a forced-in portion of the total experiment, when a practitioner wants to perform N_0 observations at preselected levels of the control variable $\mathbf{x}$.

The optimization problem of finding a two-stage D-optimal design that is analogous to the optimization problem (2.100) is

$$\xi^* = \arg\max_\xi |\delta\mathbf{M}(\xi_0) + (1-\delta)\mathbf{M}(\xi)|. \tag{2.107}$$

Using the same arguments as in the proof of (2.104), one can show that the function $\psi(\mathbf{x}, \xi)$ that corresponds to two-stage D-optimality is

$$\psi(\mathbf{x}, \xi) = (1-\delta)\left\{\text{tr}[\mathbf{M}^{-1}(\xi_{tot})\mathbf{M}(\xi)] - \text{tr}[\mathbf{M}^{-1}(\xi_{tot})\,\boldsymbol{\mu}(\mathbf{x})]\right\}, \tag{2.108}$$

and the sensitivity function is

$$d(\mathbf{x}, \xi_{tot}) = \text{tr}[\mathbf{M}^{-1}(\xi_{tot})\,\boldsymbol{\mu}(\mathbf{x})]. \tag{2.109}$$

Two-stage optimal designs as in (2.107) are often called composite optimal designs; see Fedorov and Hackl (1997) [135], Chapter 2.6. It is obvious that, in general, the solution of the optimization problem (2.107) depends on the initial design ξ_0 and its relative weight δ.

For examples of the application of two-stage, or composite designs, see Chapters 8.1.4 and 8.3.

2.8 Regularization

When optimal designs are singular, i.e., the rank of the information matrix is less than m, one has to replace the inverse $\mathbf{M}^{-1}$ by the generalized inverse $\mathbf{M}^-$ as in (1.24). The estimator $\hat{\boldsymbol{\gamma}}$ in (1.24) is unique, i.e., it does not depend on the type of generalized inverse, and the limit transition technique (1.25) and (1.26) work fine. The optimal design problem is much more difficult since the singularity of $\mathbf{M}$ causes problems for differentiating $\Psi(\mathbf{M})$. In general, the singular case needs a more sophisticated technique and is beyond the scope of this book. Here we outline a possible modification of the original optimization problem that may be helpful.

Recall that assumption (B4) states the existence of the directional derivative of $\Psi(\mathbf{M})$; see Section 2.4. In the case of singular optimal designs, introduce

$$\Psi_\delta(\xi) = \Psi_\delta[\mathbf{M}(\xi)] = \Psi\left[(1-\delta)\mathbf{M}(\xi) + \delta\mathbf{M}(\xi_0)\right], \tag{2.110}$$

where $0 < \delta < 1$ and $\mathrm{rank}[\mathbf{M}(\xi_0)] = m$. If assumption (B4) is fulfilled for $\Psi(\mathbf{M})$ when $\mathbf{M}$ is regular, then it is valid for $\Psi_\delta(\xi)$ whatever the design ξ is. Indeed, it follows from (2.110) that for arbitrary designs ξ_1 and ξ_2,

$$\Psi_\delta\left[(1 - \alpha)\mathbf{M}(\xi_1) + \alpha\mathbf{M}(\xi_2)\right] = \Psi\{(1 - \delta)[(1 - \alpha)\mathbf{M}(\xi_1) + \alpha\mathbf{M}(\xi_2)] + \delta\mathbf{M}(\xi_0)\}$$

$$= \Psi\left\{(1 - \alpha)[(1 - \delta)\mathbf{M}(\xi_1) + \delta\mathbf{M}(\xi_0)] + \alpha[(1 - \delta)\mathbf{M}(\xi_2) + \delta\mathbf{M}(\xi_0)]\right\}.$$

The validity of assumption (B4) for the criterion Ψ_δ now follows from the last expression if in (2.56) one takes $\xi = (1 - \delta)\xi_1 + \delta\xi_0$ and $\bar\xi = (1 - \delta)\xi_2 + \delta\xi_0$. If

$$\xi_\delta^* = \arg\min_\xi \Psi_\delta(\xi), \tag{2.111}$$

then it follows from the convexity of $\Psi_\delta(\xi)$ that

$$\Psi(\xi_\delta^*) - \Psi(\xi^*) \leq \delta\left[\Psi(\xi_0) - \Psi(\xi^*)\right]. \tag{2.112}$$

The proper choice of δ and ξ_0 may ensure the "practical" optimality of ξ_δ^*.

The optimization problem (2.111) is a special case of (2.52) where all necessary assumptions including assumption (B4) hold. Therefore, Theorems 2.2 and 2.4 work. For example, the sensitivity function of the D-criterion is

$$\varphi(\mathbf{x}, \bar\xi) = \mathrm{tr}[\boldsymbol{\mu}(\mathbf{x})\mathbf{M}^{-1}(\bar\xi)], \quad \text{and} \quad C = \mathrm{tr}[\mathbf{M}^{-1}(\bar\xi)\mathbf{M}(\xi)],$$

where $\bar\xi = (1 - \delta)\xi + \delta\xi_0$; see (2.73). For the linear criterion $\mathrm{tr}[\mathbf{A}\mathbf{M}^{-1}(\bar\xi)]$,

$$\varphi(\mathbf{x}, \bar\xi) = \mathrm{tr}[\boldsymbol{\mu}(\mathbf{x})\mathbf{M}^{-1}(\bar\xi)\mathbf{A}\mathbf{M}^{-1}(\bar\xi)],$$

and

$$C = \mathrm{tr}[\mathbf{A}\mathbf{M}^{-1}(\bar\xi)\mathbf{M}(\xi)\mathbf{M}^{-1}(\bar\xi)].$$

Note that the inverse of the matrix $\mathbf{M}(\bar\xi)$ exists because of the regularity of $\mathbf{M}(\xi_0)$ and the definition of $\bar\xi$.

2.9 Optimality Criterion Depends on Estimated Parameters or Unknown Constants

Consider a design problem where the optimality criterion $\Psi(\mathbf{M}, \mathbf{u})$ depends on variables or parameters $\mathbf{u} \in \mathbf{U}$ that cannot be controlled by the experimenter. See, for example, criterion (2.38), which depends on values θ_α, $\alpha = 1, \ldots, m$; cf. Section 2.2. To a large extent, the dependence of the optimality criterion on unknown parameters discussed in this section is similar to the dependence of locally optimal designs on unknown parameters in nonlinear regression models, which we address in Chapter 5. The difference, however, is that for linear regression models the information matrix itself does not depend on unknown parameters while for nonlinear models it does.

We assume that the optimality criterion $\Psi(\mathbf{M}, \mathbf{u})$ satisfies assumptions (A1), (A2) and (B1) – (B4) for every $\mathbf{u} \in \mathbf{U}$. In general, it is impossible to find the design that is best for all $\mathbf{u}$. Therefore, we will discuss optimal designs "on average" and "minimax designs"; cf. Section 2.2.3. A design that is optimal on average is defined as

$$\xi_{\mathcal{A}}^* = \arg\min_\xi \int_{\mathbf{U}} \Psi[\mathbf{M}(\xi), \mathbf{u}] \, \mathcal{A}(d\mathbf{u}) = \arg\min_\xi \Psi_{\mathcal{A}}[\mathbf{M}(\xi)], \qquad (2.113)$$

where $\int_{\mathbf{U}} \mathcal{A}(d\mathbf{u}) = 1$, and $\mathcal{A}(d\mathbf{u})$ may be interpreted as a measure of our trust in a particular value of $\mathbf{u}$. In the Bayesian approach, such a measure is considered an *a priori* distribution of $\mathbf{u}$. Parameters $\mathbf{u}$ may coincide with the estimated parameters $\boldsymbol{\theta}$ as in (2.38), but, in general, they may be different from $\boldsymbol{\theta}$.

The minimax criterion defines the optimal design as

$$\xi_M^* = \arg\min_\xi \max_{\mathbf{u}} \Psi[\mathbf{M}(\xi), \mathbf{u}]. \qquad (2.114)$$

To discuss optimality on average and minimax optimality, we need an analog of assumption (B4) where the dependence of the criterion on $\mathbf{u}$ is introduced explicitly.

($\tilde{B}4'$) For any $\xi \in \Xi(q)$ and $\bar{\xi} \in \Xi$

$$\Psi\left[(1 - \alpha)\mathbf{M}(\xi) + \alpha\mathbf{M}(\bar{\xi}), \mathbf{u}\right] = \Psi[\mathbf{M}(\xi), \mathbf{u}]$$
$$+ \alpha \int \psi(\mathbf{x}, \xi; \mathbf{u})\bar{\xi}(d\mathbf{x}) + o(\alpha|\xi, \bar{\xi}), \qquad (2.115)$$

where $\lim_{\alpha \to 0} \alpha^{-1} o(\alpha|\xi, \bar{\xi}) = 0$ uniformly in $\mathbf{U}$.

Optimality on average. We assume that the set $\mathbf{U}$ is compact. The design $\xi_{\mathcal{A}}^*$ is often called Bayesian in the literature. We prefer to refer to the design $\xi_{\mathcal{A}}^*$ as "optimal design on average" and not Bayesian design in order to avoid a mix-up with the solution of the optimization problem (2.100) for which we reserve the label "Bayesian."

The optimization problem (2.113) is relatively simple. As integration is a linear operation, we can reformulate Theorems 2.2 and 2.4 for $\Psi_{\mathcal{A}}(\mathbf{M})$ by introducing

$$\psi(\mathbf{x}, \xi) = \int_{\mathbf{U}} \psi(\mathbf{x}, \xi; \mathbf{u})\mathcal{A}(d\mathbf{u}) \qquad (2.116)$$

and

$$\varphi(\mathbf{x}, \xi) = \int_{\mathbf{U}} \varphi(\mathbf{x}, \xi; \mathbf{u})\mathcal{A}(d\mathbf{u}), \qquad (2.117)$$

where $\psi(\mathbf{x}, \xi; \mathbf{u})$ is introduced in (2.115), and $\varphi(\mathbf{x}, \xi; \mathbf{u})$ is defined via the analog of (2.73) where analogs of constant C on the right-hand side of (2.73) are obtained by integrating the corresponding values of C with respect to the measure $\mathcal{A}(d\mathbf{u})$.

If the optimality criterion is of type (2.38) and if $\mathbf{u}$ coincides with $\boldsymbol{\theta}$, then

$$\int \text{tr}\left[\mathbf{V}^2(\boldsymbol{\theta})\,\mathbf{M}^{-1}(\xi)\right]\,\mathcal{A}(d\boldsymbol{\theta}) = \text{tr}\left[\overline{\mathbf{V}}^2\,\mathbf{M}^{-1}(\xi)\right], \tag{2.118}$$

where $\overline{\mathbf{V}}^2 = \int \mathbf{V}^2(\boldsymbol{\theta})\mathcal{A}(d\boldsymbol{\theta})$, and therefore the criterion (2.118) is a special case of the A-criterion. For the D-optimality the analog of the criterion (2.38) corresponds to minimization of the determinant $|\mathbf{V}(\boldsymbol{\theta})\,\mathbf{M}^{-1}(\xi)\,\mathbf{V}(\boldsymbol{\theta})|$. Since $|\mathbf{V}(\boldsymbol{\theta})\,\mathbf{M}^{-1}(\xi)\,\mathbf{V}(\boldsymbol{\theta})| = |\mathbf{V}(\boldsymbol{\theta})|^2\,|\mathbf{M}(\xi)|^{-1}$, then

$$\arg\min_{\xi}|\mathbf{V}(\boldsymbol{\theta})\,\mathbf{M}^{-1}(\xi)\,\mathbf{V}(\boldsymbol{\theta})| = \arg\min_{\xi}|\mathbf{M}^{-1}(\xi)|;$$

therefore, D-optimal designs based on relative errors do not depend on parameter values.

Minimax design. We make use of the relation

$$\frac{\partial}{\partial\alpha}\max_{\mathbf{u}\in\mathbf{U}}g(\alpha,\mathbf{u}) = \max_{\mathbf{u}\in\mathbf{U}^*}\frac{\partial g(\alpha,\mathbf{u})}{\partial\alpha}, \tag{2.119}$$

which is true if $\mathbf{U}$ is compact and if the corresponding derivative exists everywhere in $\mathbf{U}$. The set $\mathbf{U}^*$ is defined as

$$\mathbf{U}^* = \{\mathbf{u}|\ \mathbf{u} = \mathbf{u}(\alpha) = \arg\max_{\mathbf{u}\in\mathbf{U}}g(\alpha,\mathbf{u})\},$$

cf. Pshenichnyi (1971) [327], Chapter 3. We get

$$\frac{\partial}{\partial\alpha}\max_{\mathbf{u}\in\mathbf{U}}\Psi\left[(1-\alpha)\mathbf{M}(\xi) + \alpha\mathbf{M}(\bar{\xi}),\mathbf{u}\right]_{\alpha=0}$$

$$= \max_{\mathbf{u}\in\mathbf{U}(\xi)}\frac{\partial}{\partial\alpha}\Psi\left[(1-\alpha)\mathbf{M}(\xi) + \alpha\mathbf{M}(\bar{\xi}),\mathbf{u}\right]_{\alpha=0}$$

$$= \max_{\mathbf{u}\in\mathbf{U}(\xi)}\int\psi(\mathbf{x},\xi;\mathbf{u})\bar{\xi}(d\mathbf{x}), \tag{2.120}$$

where

$$\mathbf{U}(\xi) = \{\mathbf{u}|\ \mathbf{u} = \mathbf{u}(\xi) = \arg\max_{\mathbf{u}\in\mathbf{U}}\Psi[\mathbf{M}(\xi),\mathbf{u}]\}.$$

Nonlinearity of the maximization procedure leads to the necessary and sufficient condition of optimality, which is more complicated than that in Theorems 2.2 and 2.4.

Theorem 2.5 *A necessary and sufficient condition for ξ_M^* to be optimal is the existence of a measure ζ^* such that*

$$\min_{\mathbf{x}}\tilde{\psi}(\mathbf{x},\xi_M^*;\zeta^*) \geq 0, \tag{2.121}$$

where

$$\tilde{\psi}(\mathbf{x}, \xi; \zeta) = \int_{\mathbf{U}(\xi)} \psi(\mathbf{x}, \xi; \mathbf{u})\, \zeta(d\mathbf{u}). \tag{2.122}$$

Proof. The proof is analogous to the corresponding part of the proof of Theorem 2.2. The difference is that we use (2.120) and the fact that

$$\min_{\overline{\xi}} \max_{\zeta} \int_{\mathbf{x}} \int_{\mathbf{U}(\xi)} \psi(\mathbf{x}, \xi; \mathbf{u})\overline{\xi}(dx)\, \zeta(d\mathbf{u})$$

$$= \min_{\overline{\xi}} \max_{\mathbf{u} \in \mathbf{U}(\xi)} \int_{\mathbf{x}} \psi(\mathbf{x}, \xi; \mathbf{u})\, \overline{\xi}(dx)$$

$$= \max_{\zeta} \min_{\mathbf{x}} \int_{\mathbf{U}(\xi)} \psi(\mathbf{x}, \xi; \mathbf{u})\, \zeta(d\mathbf{u})$$

$$= \max_{\zeta} \min_{\overline{\xi}} \int_{\mathbf{x}} \int_{\mathbf{U}(\xi)} \psi(\mathbf{x}, \xi; \mathbf{u})\, \overline{\xi}(dx)\zeta(d\mathbf{u}). \tag{2.123}$$

Condition (2.121) is obviously more difficult to verify than the corresponding conditions in Theorems 2.2 and 2.4. However, in a number of special cases it has a relatively simple form. For instance, consider a criterion $\Psi(\mathbf{M}, \mathbf{u}) = \mathbf{u}^T \mathbf{M}^{-1} \mathbf{u}$. If $\mathbf{U} = \{\mathbf{u}\colon \mathbf{u}^T \mathbf{u} = 1\}$, then we have a direct analog of the E-criterion since

$$\max_{\mathbf{u} \in \mathbf{U}} \Psi(\mathbf{M}, \mathbf{u}) = \max_{\mathbf{u} \in \mathbf{U}} \mathbf{u}^T \mathbf{M}^{-1} \mathbf{u} = \lambda_{\max}, \tag{2.124}$$

where $\lambda_{\max}$ is the largest eigenvalue of the matrix $\mathbf{M}^{-1}(\xi) = \mathbf{D}(\xi)$; cf. (2.15), (2.29). Some algebra shows that

$$\psi(\mathbf{x}, \mathbf{u}, \xi) = \mathbf{u}^T \mathbf{M}^{-1}(\xi)\mathbf{u} - \left[\mathbf{u}^T \mathbf{M}^{-1}(\xi)\mathbf{f}(\mathbf{x})\right]^2. \tag{2.125}$$

If the maximum in (2.124) is attained at the unique $\mathbf{u} = \mathbf{u}_{\max}$, then (2.121) is equivalent to the inequality

$$\left[\mathbf{f}^T(\mathbf{x})\mathbf{u}_{\max}\right]^2 \leq \lambda_{\max}^{-1}(\xi^*), \tag{2.126}$$

where $\mathbf{u}_{\max}$ is the corresponding eigenvector. If (2.124) has more than one solution, then (2.126) must be replaced by the inequality

$$\sum_{\ell=1}^{\alpha'} \zeta_\ell \left[\mathbf{f}^T(\mathbf{x})\mathbf{u}_\ell\right]^2 \leq \lambda_{\max}^{-1}(\xi^*), \tag{2.127}$$

where α' is the multiplicity of $\lambda_{\max}(\xi^*)$, and $\{\mathbf{u}_\ell\}_1^{\alpha'}$ is the set of the corresponding eigenvectors.

Intuitively, optimizing the minimax criterion provides the experimenter with a design that guarantees reasonably good results even in the case of worst values of $\mathbf{u}$. Unfortunately, sometimes the worst $\mathbf{u}$ occurs more than once. Then we have to treat all these worst $\mathbf{u}$'s appropriately, and that explains the integration with respect to the measure ζ. In most cases, this integration is a weighted sum similar to (2.127).

2.10   Response Function Contains Uncontrolled and Unknown Independent Variables

So far the independent variables $\mathbf{x} \in \mathfrak{X}$ were assumed to be controlled by the experimenter. Weather conditions in agricultural experiments, or temperature, atmospheric pressure, and wind direction in environmental studies are examples of variables $\mathbf{z} \in \mathbf{Z}$ that are beyond the experimenter's control. In the following, we split the independent variables into two groups and use notation $\mathbf{f}(\mathbf{x}, \mathbf{z})$ instead of $\mathbf{f}(\mathbf{x})$,

$$y = \mathbf{f}^T(\mathbf{x}, \mathbf{z})\, \boldsymbol{\theta} + \varepsilon, \tag{2.128}$$

where variables $\mathbf{x} \in \mathfrak{X} \subset R^k$ are assumed to be controlled and the variables $\mathbf{z} \in \mathbf{Z}$ are assumed to be uncontrolled. Usually the value of $\mathbf{z}$ becomes known after the completion of the experiment. The nonnormalized information matrix is

$$\underline{\mathbf{M}}(\xi_N) = \sum_{i=1}^{n} \sum_{j=1}^{r_i} \mathbf{f}(\mathbf{x}_i, \mathbf{z}_{ij})\mathbf{f}^T(\mathbf{x}_i, \mathbf{z}_{ij}). \tag{2.129}$$

In (2.129) we assume that $\mathbf{x}_i$ can be selected and fixed prior to the experiment. For instance, in a dose-response study $\{\mathbf{x}_i\}$ are doses that are tested. On the other hand, values $\{\mathbf{z}_{ij}\}$ are specific for each observation: each patient has his/her values of certain factors such as age, gender, etc. It is reasonable to assume that $\{\mathbf{z}_{ij}\}$ are sampled from a population that is described by the probability distribution $\zeta(d\mathbf{z})$. Then for sufficiently large $N = \sum_{i=1}^{n} r_i$,

$$N^{-1}\underline{\mathbf{M}}(\xi_N) \simeq \sum_{i=1}^{n} p_i \int \mathbf{f}(\mathbf{x}_i, \mathbf{z})\mathbf{f}^T(\mathbf{x}_i, \mathbf{z})\zeta(d\mathbf{z}), \quad p_i = r_i/N,$$

or

$$N^{-1}\underline{\mathbf{M}}(\xi_N) \simeq \mathbf{M}(\xi, \zeta) = \int_{\mathfrak{X}} \int_{\mathbf{Z}} \mathbf{f}(\mathbf{x}, \mathbf{z})\mathbf{f}^T(\mathbf{x}, \mathbf{z})\zeta(d\mathbf{z})\xi(d\mathbf{x})$$

$$= \int_{\mathfrak{X}} \boldsymbol{\mu}(\mathbf{x}, \zeta)\xi(d\mathbf{x}), \quad \text{where } \boldsymbol{\mu}(\mathbf{x}, \zeta) = \int_{\mathbf{Z}} \mathbf{f}(\mathbf{x}, \mathbf{z})\mathbf{f}^T(\mathbf{x}, \mathbf{z})\zeta(d\mathbf{z}). \tag{2.130}$$

For the sake of simplicity, we assume in (2.130) that $\mathbf{f}(\mathbf{x}, \mathbf{z})$ is continuous with respect to $\mathbf{x}$ and $\mathbf{z}$. The optimal design is defined as

$$\xi^* = \arg \min_{\xi} \Psi\left[\mathbf{M}(\xi, \zeta)\right]. \tag{2.131}$$

Following the exposition of Sections 2.4 and 2.5, one can verify that Theorems 2.2 and 2.3 remain valid if $\boldsymbol{\mu}(\mathbf{x})$ is replaced by $\boldsymbol{\mu}(\mathbf{x}, \zeta)$. For instance, the necessary and sufficient conditions for the D-criterion is

$$\text{tr}\left[\boldsymbol{\mu}(\mathbf{x}, \zeta)\mathbf{M}^{-1}(\xi, \zeta)\right] \leq m. \tag{2.132}$$

Note that this condition is different from the necessary and sufficient condition for the D-optimality on average, which follows from (2.116) and is formulated as

$$\int_{\mathbf{U}} \text{tr} \left[\boldsymbol{\mu}(\mathbf{x}, \mathbf{u}) \mathbf{M}^{-1}(\xi, \mathbf{u}) \right] \mathcal{A}(d\mathbf{u}) \leq m. \qquad (2.133)$$

Generalization to the case when the distribution of $\mathbf{z}$ depends on $\mathbf{x}$, i.e., when one has to consider measures $\zeta(d\mathbf{z}|\mathbf{x})$, is straightforward.

In conclusion, we want to emphasize that the results of this section are quite different from what we will discuss in chapters on nonlinear models. Here we integrate out *a priori* unknown variables from the information matrix of a single observation. On the contrary, in the nonlinear case we will integrate out unknown (estimated) parameters from the optimality criterion. Moreover, at the end of the experiment variables $\mathbf{z}_{ij}$ become known exactly while unknown parameters must be estimated.

2.11 Response Models with Random Parameters

We consider experiments where observations $\mathbf{y}_{ij}$ are taken from an i-th object, $i = 1, \ldots, n$, under conditions $\mathbf{x}_{ij}$, $j = 1, \ldots, k_i$. We associate index i with individuals in medico-biological studies, with a date in meteorology, or with a tested item in engineering. Let us assume that the response function has the same functional form for all objects, cf. (1.57):

$$\mathbf{y}_{ij} = \mathbf{F}^T(\mathbf{x}_{ij})\boldsymbol{\gamma}_i + \boldsymbol{\varepsilon}_{ij}, \qquad (2.134)$$

where the vector $\boldsymbol{\gamma}_i = (\gamma_{i1}, \ldots, \gamma_{i,n_i})^T$ of individual parameters reflects specific features of the i-th object. Let the variability of $\boldsymbol{\gamma}_i$ be described by a probability distribution with mean $\boldsymbol{\gamma}^0$ and the variance-covariance matrix $\boldsymbol{\Omega}$ (global, or population parameters). We further assume that the observational errors are uncorrelated, have zero mean and variance σ^2, and are independent of $\boldsymbol{\gamma}_i$.

If repeated observations are possible for object i at the experimental condition $\mathbf{x}_{ij}$, we use notation r_{ij} for the number of repetitions at $\mathbf{x}_{ij}$ and $r_i = \sum_{j=1}^{k_i} r_{ij}$ for the total number of observations performed on object i.

Estimation Problem. The model (2.134) is usually called a regression model with random coefficients or a mixed effects model; see Spjotvoll (1977) [367], Demidenko (2004) [93], Pinheiro and Bates (2002) [311], Verbeke and Molenberghs (2000) [386]. Statistical analyses of such models may address various goals, for example,

(a) estimation of the individual parameters $\boldsymbol{\gamma}_i$,

(b) estimation of the population (global) parameters $\boldsymbol{\gamma}^0 = \text{E}\{\boldsymbol{\gamma}_i\}$,

(c) estimation of variance parameters σ^2 and $\mathbf{\Omega}$,

(d) various combinations of the above.

In general, for data collection one may use different designs for different objects i. We use the notation $\boldsymbol{\theta} = \{\boldsymbol{\gamma}^0, \ \mathbf{\Omega}, \ \sigma^2\}$ for the combined vector of unknown parameters, to emphasize that, unlike many previous sections, in the mixed models setting we have to estimate more parameters; cf. Chapter 7 and Section 7.1, in particular.

2.11.1   Known population mean and variance parameters

In this section we assume that parameters $\boldsymbol{\gamma}^0$, σ^2 and $\mathbf{\Omega}$ are known. Introduce the following notations; cf. (1.11), (1.12), (1.62), (1.63):

$$\underline{\mathbf{M}}_i \ = \ \sigma^{-2} r_i \mathbf{M}(\xi_i) = \sigma^{-2} r_i \sum_{j=1}^{r_i} p_{ij} \ \mathbf{F}(\mathbf{x}_{ij}) \mathbf{F}^T(\mathbf{x}_{ij}), \qquad (2.135)$$

$$\underline{\mathbf{Y}}_i \ = \ \sigma^{-2} r_i \mathbf{Y}_i = \sigma^{-2} r_i \sum_{j=1}^{r_i} p_{ij} \ \mathbf{F}(\mathbf{x}_{ij}) \mathbf{y}_{ij}, \qquad (2.136)$$

$$\mathbf{S}_i \ = \ \sum_{j=1}^{r_i} \left[\mathbf{y}_{ij} - \mathbf{F}^T(\mathbf{x}_{ij}) \widehat{\boldsymbol{\gamma}}_i \right] \left[\mathbf{y}_{ij} - \mathbf{F}^T(x_{ij}) \widehat{\boldsymbol{\gamma}}_i \right]^T, \qquad (2.137)$$

$$\widehat{\boldsymbol{\gamma}}_i \ = \ \underline{\mathbf{M}}_i^{-1} \underline{\mathbf{Y}}_i, \qquad (2.138)$$

$$\breve{\boldsymbol{\gamma}}_i \ = \ \left(\underline{\mathbf{M}}_i + \mathbf{\Omega}^{-1} \right)^{-1} \left(\underline{\mathbf{M}}_i \widehat{\boldsymbol{\gamma}}_i + \mathbf{\Omega}^{-1} \boldsymbol{\gamma}^0 \right), \qquad (2.139)$$

$$\xi_i \ = \ \{\mathbf{x}_{ij}, \ p_{ij}\}, \quad p_{ij} = r_{ij}/r_i. \qquad (2.140)$$

For the sake of simplicity, we assume the regularity of all matrices that are inverted.

Estimators $\{\widehat{\boldsymbol{\gamma}}_i\}$ and $\{\breve{\boldsymbol{\gamma}}_i\}$ are the usual least squares estimators (LSEs) of individual parameters and its shrinkage versions, respectively; cf. Rao (1965) [333]. From the results presented in Section 1.3.3 it follows that the estimator $\widehat{\boldsymbol{\gamma}}_i$ minimizes, in the Loewner sense, the variance-covariance matrix of linear conditionally unbiased estimators: $\mathrm{E}(\widehat{\boldsymbol{\gamma}}_i | \boldsymbol{\gamma}_i) = \boldsymbol{\gamma}_i$ and

$$\mathbf{D}(\widehat{\boldsymbol{\gamma}}_i) = \mathrm{E}_\varepsilon \left[(\widehat{\boldsymbol{\gamma}}_i - \boldsymbol{\gamma}_i) (\widehat{\boldsymbol{\gamma}}_i - \boldsymbol{\gamma}_i)^T | \boldsymbol{\gamma}_i \right] = \underline{\mathbf{M}}_i. \qquad (2.141)$$

Thus the estimator $\widehat{\boldsymbol{\gamma}}_i$ is the best individual estimator of the i-th object among conditionally unbiased estimators. However, if one is interested in the "goodness" of parameter estimation "on average" across the whole population $\{\boldsymbol{\gamma}_i\}$, then it is reasonable to consider an estimator that minimizes the mean squared error matrix,

$$\boldsymbol{\gamma}_i^* = \arg \min_{\tilde{\boldsymbol{\gamma}}_i} \mathrm{E} \left[(\tilde{\boldsymbol{\gamma}}_i - \boldsymbol{\gamma}_i)(\tilde{\boldsymbol{\gamma}}_i - \boldsymbol{\gamma}_i)^T \right], \qquad (2.142)$$

where $\mathrm{E}\tilde{\boldsymbol{\gamma}}_i = \mathrm{E}_{\boldsymbol{\gamma}}[\mathrm{E}_\varepsilon(\tilde{\boldsymbol{\gamma}}_i)] = \boldsymbol{\gamma}^0$. Direct calculations show that $\boldsymbol{\gamma}_i^* = \breve{\boldsymbol{\gamma}}_i$; see

Rao (1965) [333]. The mean squared error matrix of $\breve{\gamma}_i$ is

$$\mathbf{D}(\breve{\gamma}_i) = \mathrm{E}_{\gamma}\mathrm{E}_{\varepsilon}\left[(\breve{\gamma}_i - \gamma_i)(\breve{\gamma}_i - \gamma_i)^T\right] = \left(\underline{\mathbf{M}}_i + \mathbf{\Omega}^{-1}\right)^{-1}. \tag{2.143}$$

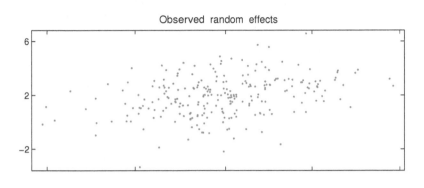

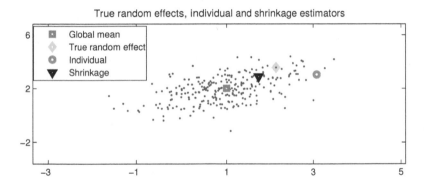

FIGURE 2.2: Individual and global (shrinkage) estimators. Top panel: observed random effects $\mathbf{y}_i$. Bottom panel: true random effects γ_i.

Figure 2.2 illuminates the difference between $\widehat{\gamma}_i$ and $\breve{\gamma}_i$ for the simplest random effects model

$$\mathbf{y}_i = \gamma_i + \varepsilon_i, \text{ where } \gamma_i \sim \mathcal{N}(\gamma^0, \mathbf{\Omega}), \; \varepsilon_i \sim \mathcal{N}(\mathbf{0}, \mathbf{I}_2), \tag{2.144}$$

$$\gamma^0 = \begin{pmatrix} 1 \\ 2 \end{pmatrix}, \; \mathbf{\Omega} = \begin{pmatrix} 1 & 0.5 \\ 0.5 & 2 \end{pmatrix},$$

and $\mathbf{I}_2$ is a 2×2 identity matrix. In the notations of the model (2.134), $r_i \equiv 1$ for all objects i (thus, we drop index j), and $\mathbf{F}(\mathbf{x}_i) \equiv \mathbf{I}_2$. For the model (2.144), formulae (2.135) – (2.139) reduce to

$$\underline{\mathbf{M}}_i = \sigma^{-2}\mathbf{I}_2; \; \underline{\mathbf{Y}}_i = \sigma^{-2}\mathbf{y}_i; \; \widehat{\gamma}_i = \mathbf{y}_i; \; \breve{\gamma}_i = (\mathbf{I}_2 + \mathbf{\Omega}^{-1})^{-1}(\mathbf{y}_i + \mathbf{\Omega}^{-1}\gamma^0). \tag{2.145}$$

The top panel of Figure 2.2 displays observations $\{y_i\}$; the bottom panel shows "true" random effects $\{\gamma_i\}$, together with the individual estimator $\widehat{\gamma}_{i*}$ (circle), shrinkage estimator $\breve{\gamma}_{i*}$ (triangle) and γ_{i*} (diamond) for one particular object $i*$.

The estimator (2.139) can be viewed as the one that uses prior information about the population from which the individual parameters are sampled, and the estimator $\breve{\gamma}_i$ is "better" than $\widehat{\gamma}_i$ if one cares about the "common" (population) good.

Unlike $\widehat{\gamma}_i$, the estimator $\breve{\gamma}_i$ is a conditionally biased estimator of γ_i. Indeed, it follows from (2.139) that

$$
\begin{aligned}
\mathrm{E}(\breve{\gamma}_i|\gamma_i) &= \left(\underline{\mathbf{M}}_i + \mathbf{\Omega}^{-1}\right)^{-1}\left(\underline{\mathbf{M}}_i\gamma_i + \mathbf{\Omega}^{-1}\gamma^0\right) \\
&= \gamma_i + \left(\underline{\mathbf{M}}_i + \mathbf{\Omega}^{-1}\right)^{-1}\mathbf{\Omega}^{-1}(\gamma^0 - \gamma_i).
\end{aligned}
$$

Direct calculations show that the mean squared error matrix of $\breve{\gamma}_i$ conditional on γ_i is

$$
\mathrm{E}_\varepsilon\left[(\widehat{\gamma}_i - \gamma_i)(\widehat{\gamma}_i - \gamma_i)^T|\gamma_i\right] \tag{2.146}
$$

$$
= \left(\underline{\mathbf{M}}_i + \mathbf{\Omega}^{-1}\right)^{-1}\left[\underline{\mathbf{M}}_i + \mathbf{\Omega}^{-1}(\gamma^0 - \gamma_i)(\gamma^0 - \gamma_i)^T\mathbf{\Omega}^{-1}\right]\left(\underline{\mathbf{M}}_i + \mathbf{\Omega}^{-1}\right)^{-1}.
$$

Therefore, it follows from (2.141) and (2.146) that for small $\|\gamma^0 - \gamma_i\|$ the estimator $\breve{\gamma}_i$ is still better than $\widehat{\gamma}_i$ with respect to the conditional mean squared error matrix. However, for larger $\|\gamma^0 - \gamma_i\|$ the estimator $\breve{\gamma}_i$ is inferior to $\widehat{\gamma}_i$ in the above sense.

If repeated observations can be performed on the i-th object, then one can apply the machinery of continuous designs. The design problems for estimators $\widehat{\gamma}_i$ and $\breve{\gamma}_i$ are

$$
\xi^* = \arg\min_\xi \Psi\left[\mathbf{M}(\xi)\right], \text{ where } \mathbf{M}(\xi) = \int_{\mathcal{X}} \mathbf{F}(\mathbf{x})\mathbf{F}^T(\mathbf{x})\xi(d\mathbf{x}), \tag{2.147}
$$

and

$$
\xi^* = \arg\min_\xi \Psi\left[\mathbf{M}_{tot}(\xi)\right], \text{ where } \mathbf{M}_{tot}(\xi) = \mathbf{M}(\xi) + r_i^{-1}\mathbf{\Omega}^{-1}, \tag{2.148}
$$

respectively. In (2.148), r_i is the number of observations available for object i. Optimization problems (2.147) and (2.148) were considered in Sections 2.4 and 2.7, respectively. A generalization to cases where the matrix $\mathbf{F}(\mathbf{x})$ differs between objects is straightforward.

While examples exist where repeated observations are possible, e.g., in multicenter clinical trials, they are not numerous; see Fedorov and Jones (2005) [139]. More often, the repeated observation setting looks artificial, for example when repeated blood samples in pharmacokinetic studies are taken at the same time points; see Pronzato and Pázman (2001) [321], Retout et al. (2001) [339].

We would like to emphasize that, in general, designs that are optimal for individuals, i.e., defined by (2.147), are different from those that are optimal for "common good", i.e., defined by (2.148).

2.11.2 Known variance parameters

In this section we assume that parameters σ^2 and $\boldsymbol{\Omega}$ are known while global mean $\boldsymbol{\gamma}^0$ and individual parameters $\boldsymbol{\gamma}_i$ are to be estimated. One can verify that the total sum of squares can be presented as follows (cf. Spjotvoll (1977) [367]):

$$
\begin{aligned}
SS &= \sum_{i=1}^{n} \sum_{j=1}^{r_i} \left[\mathbf{y}_{ij} - \mathbf{F}^T(\mathbf{x}_{ij}) \boldsymbol{\gamma}_i \right]^T \left[\mathbf{y}_{ij} - \mathbf{F}^T(\mathbf{x}_{ij}) \boldsymbol{\gamma}_i \right] \\
&= \sum_{i=1}^{n} \left[\mathbf{S}_i + (\breve{\boldsymbol{\gamma}}_i - \boldsymbol{\gamma}_i)^T (\underline{\mathbf{M}}_i + \boldsymbol{\Omega}^{-1})(\breve{\boldsymbol{\gamma}}_i - \boldsymbol{\gamma}_i) \right] \\
&\quad + \sum_{i=1}^{n} (\widehat{\boldsymbol{\gamma}}_i - \boldsymbol{\gamma}^0)^T (\underline{\mathbf{M}}_i^{-1} + \boldsymbol{\Omega})^{-1} (\widehat{\boldsymbol{\gamma}}_i - \boldsymbol{\gamma}^0).
\end{aligned}
\tag{2.149}
$$

It immediately follows from (2.149) that the least squares estimator for $\boldsymbol{\gamma}^0$ (also a BLUE) is

$$
\widehat{\boldsymbol{\gamma}}^0 = \left[\sum_{i=1}^{n} (\underline{\mathbf{M}}_i^{-1} + \boldsymbol{\Omega})^{-1} \right]^{-1} \sum_{i=1}^{n} (\underline{\mathbf{M}}_i^{-1} + \boldsymbol{\Omega})^{-1} \widehat{\boldsymbol{\gamma}}_i = \sum_{i=1}^{n} W_i \widehat{\boldsymbol{\gamma}}_i,
\tag{2.150}
$$

where $W_i \sim (\underline{\mathbf{M}}_i^{-1} + \boldsymbol{\Omega})^{-1}$, $\sum_i W_i = 1$, and

$$
\mathrm{Var}(\widehat{\boldsymbol{\gamma}}^0) = \left[\sum_{i=1}^{n} (\underline{\mathbf{M}}_i^{-1} + \boldsymbol{\Omega})^{-1} \right]^{-1}.
\tag{2.151}
$$

In a special case when $\xi_i \equiv \xi$ and $\underline{\mathbf{M}}_i \equiv \underline{\mathbf{M}}$, $i = 1, \ldots, n$, i.e., all objects are observed under the same design setting, one gets

$$
\widehat{\boldsymbol{\gamma}}^0 = \frac{1}{n} \sum_{i=1}^{n} \widehat{\boldsymbol{\gamma}}_i, \quad \text{and} \quad \mathrm{Var}(\widehat{\boldsymbol{\gamma}}^0) = \frac{1}{n} \left(\underline{\mathbf{M}}^{-1} + \boldsymbol{\Omega} \right).
\tag{2.152}
$$

Thus, the corresponding continuous design problem is

$$
\xi^* = \arg \min_{\xi} \ \Psi \left\{ \frac{1}{n} \left[r^{-1} \mathbf{M}^{-1}(\xi) + \boldsymbol{\Omega} \right] \right\}.
\tag{2.153}
$$

From a computational point of view, the problem of finding the optimal design in (2.153) requires a minor modification in finding the directional derivative.

To illustrate a practical situation with different designs ξ_i for different objects, consider a multicenter clinical trial where patients are enrolled in n centers. By $\mathbf{x}_{ij}$ we denote the j-th dose (combination of doses) that can be administered in center i, and by r_{ij} the number of patients on dose $\mathbf{x}_{ij}$. In general, doses in different centers can be different, and therefore one can consider different designs $\xi_i = \{\mathbf{x}_{ij}, p_{ij}\}_{j=1}^{k_i}$ for different centers i, $i = 1, \ldots, n$.

If r and n are given, the calculation of the directional derivative for D-criterion leads to the following necessary and sufficient condition of D-optimality, cf. Section 2.5 and formula (10.3):

$$\text{tr}[\mathbf{M}(\xi^*) + r\mathbf{M}(\xi^*)\mathbf{\Omega}\mathbf{M}(\xi^*)]^{-1}\boldsymbol{\mu}(\mathbf{x}) \leq \text{tr}[\mathbf{I} + r\mathbf{\Omega}\mathbf{M}(\xi^*)]^{-1}, \qquad (2.154)$$

where $\boldsymbol{\mu}(\mathbf{x}) = \sigma^{-2}\,\mathbf{F}(\mathbf{x})\mathbf{F}^T(\mathbf{x})$.

The optimization problem (2.153) is relatively simple for the linear criterion. Indeed,

$$\xi^* = \arg\min_{\xi}\ \text{tr}\left\{\frac{\mathbf{A}}{n}\left[r^{-1}\mathbf{M}^{-1}(\xi) + \mathbf{\Omega}\right]\right\} = \arg\min_{\xi}\ \text{tr}[\mathbf{A}\mathbf{M}^{-1}(\xi)]. \quad (2.155)$$

Therefore, given n and r, the linear optimal designs for the considered random effects model coincide with the linear optimal designs for the linear regression with deterministic $\boldsymbol{\gamma}$.

In practice the number of observations r_i for object i is either small or moderate. Thus, the continuous optimization problem (2.153) is of limited value. However, there is one area of application where solving the problem (2.153) may be useful, namely, the design of multicenter clinical trials where the number of patients enrolled in each given center i may be large enough and thus, the continuous optimization problem makes practical sense; see Fedorov and Jones (2005) [139].

Staying with discrete designs, one can make a rather useful observation in the case of $\underline{\mathbf{M}}_i \equiv r\mathbf{M}(\xi)$. Introducing the total number of observations $Q = nr$, we can rewrite the variance of $\boldsymbol{\gamma}^0$ in (2.152) as

$$\text{Var}(\widehat{\boldsymbol{\gamma}}^0) = \frac{\mathbf{M}^{-1}(\xi)}{Q} + \frac{\mathbf{\Omega}}{n}. \qquad (2.156)$$

If Q is fixed, then the first term on the right-hand side of (2.156) is constant, and one has to select n as large as possible to "minimize" the variance-covariance matrix $\text{Var}(\widehat{\boldsymbol{\gamma}}^0)$. Therefore, saturated designs with $r = dim(\boldsymbol{\gamma})$ will be beneficial for this case. Note also that in this case only the first term depends on the allocation of observations, and for linear criteria of optimality, for given Q, the linear optimal design will coincide with the one for a standard regression problem where $\boldsymbol{\gamma}_i = \boldsymbol{\gamma}$; cf. (2.155).

The design problem becomes more complicated if one introduces costs of observations, e.g., costs of initiation of a new center in multicenter clinical trials, or enrolling a new patient in PK/PD studies, etc. Let

$$Q = nr + nq, \qquad (2.157)$$

where q is the cost of "observing" any single object, and it is assumed that any single observation "costs" one unit. If Q in (2.157) is fixed, then $n = Q/(r+q)$, and for the linear optimality criterion,

$$\Psi = \text{tr}\left\{\mathbf{A}\left[\frac{\mathbf{M}^{-1}(\xi)}{nr} + \frac{\mathbf{\Omega}}{n}\right]\right\} = \left\{\frac{\text{tr}[\mathbf{A}\mathbf{M}^{-1}(\xi)]}{r} + \text{tr}(\mathbf{A}\mathbf{\Omega})\right\}\frac{r+q}{Q}. \quad (2.158)$$

The direct minimization of the expression on the right-hand side of (2.158) with respect to r leads to

$$r^* = \sqrt{q \, \frac{\text{tr}[\mathbf{A}\mathbf{M}^{-1}(\xi)]}{\text{tr}(\mathbf{A}\boldsymbol{\Omega})}}.$$

One can verify that $\Psi = \Psi(\xi, n, r) = \Psi(\xi, Q, q)$ is the increasing function of $\text{tr}[\mathbf{A}\mathbf{M}^{-1}(\xi)]$, and once again the "standard" linear optimal designs provide the solution. Note that for other optimality criteria, in particular for D-optimality, this is not true.

2.11.3   Estimation of population mean parameters

Often in clinical trials very few observations per patient are available. Moreover, repeated observations may be impossible. For instance, in PK/PD studies a standard design variable is time, and $\mathbf{x}_i$ indicates a sequence of times when blood samples are taken for patient i; see Chapter 7. In this case, the concept of continuous design performed on a given subject is not applicable. However, the proper selection of $\{\mathbf{x}_{ij}\}$ may significantly increase information about the model parameters. In this setting, it is expedient to view $\boldsymbol{\mu}(\mathbf{x}_i) = \left[\mathbf{M}^{-1}(\mathbf{x}_i) + \boldsymbol{\Omega}\right]^{-1}$ as the information matrix of a "single independent observation" (single individual) that corresponds to multiple measurements $\{\mathbf{y}_{ij}\}$ for patient i at times $\{x_{ij}\}$. If r_i is the number of patients observed at times $\mathbf{x}_i$, then the information matrix of the experiment can be written as

$$\underline{\mathbf{M}}(\xi_N) = \sum_{i=1}^{n} r_i \left[\mathbf{M}^{-1}(\mathbf{x}_i) + \boldsymbol{\Omega}\right]^{-1}, \tag{2.159}$$

where $\xi_N = \{\mathbf{x}_i, \ p_i = r_i/N\}$; cf. (2.150), (2.151). If r_i are moderately large, then a transition to continuous designs becomes reasonable, and we may introduce

$$\mathbf{M}(\xi) = N^{-1}\underline{\mathbf{M}}(\xi_N) = \sum_{i=1}^{n} p_i \boldsymbol{\mu}(\mathbf{x}_i), \tag{2.160}$$

where $\boldsymbol{\mu}(\mathbf{x}_i) = \left[\mathbf{M}^{-1}(\mathbf{x}_i) + \boldsymbol{\Omega}\right]^{-1}$. The design problem can be introduced as

$$\xi^* = \arg\min_{\xi} \Psi[\mathbf{M}(\xi)], \tag{2.161}$$

where $\mathbf{M}(\xi)$ is defined in (2.160). The optimization problem (2.161) is identical to the problem (2.52), and the Equivalence Theorem 2.2 can be applied.

Optimal designs defined by (2.161) have a tendency to include those candidate points $\mathbf{x}_i \in \mathfrak{X}$ that contain more observations. For instance, if $\mathbf{x}_i = (x_{i1}, x_{i2})$ and $\mathbf{x}_{i'} = (x_{i1}, x_{i2}, x_{i3})$, then the point $\mathbf{x}_{i'}$ will be always selected over $\mathbf{x}_i$ because

$$\mathbf{M}(\mathbf{x}_{i'}) \geq \mathbf{M}(\mathbf{x}_i)$$

where the inequality is understood in the Loewner sense. However, once the costs of observations are introduced, points with smaller number of observations may be selected in the optimal designs. For more details on cost-based designs, see Chapter 4. For examples of cost-based designs, see Sections 6.4.2, 6.5.1, 6.5.2, 7.2.3, 7.2.4, 7.4.2, 9.2.

More details on linear random effects models can be found in

- Estimation: Kiefer and Wolfowitz (1956) [231], Rao (1965) [333], Spjotvoll (1977) [367], Mallet (1986) [263], Verbeke and Molenberghs (2000) [386], Pinheiro and Bates (2002) [311]. Littell et al. (2006) [260].

- Numerical procedures: Jennrich and Schluchter (1986) [213].

- Design: Fedorov et al. (1993) [136], Fedorov and Leonov (2004) [142], Schmelter (2007) [350], Schmelter (2007) [351], Schmelter et al. (2007) [352].

Chapter 3

Algorithms and Numerical Techniques

3.1 First-Order Algorithm: D-Criterion 93
    3.1.1 Forward iterative procedure 94
    3.1.2 Some useful recursive formulae 95
    3.1.3 Convergence of algorithms 96
    3.1.4 Practical numerical procedures 100
3.2 First-Order Algorithm: General Case 101
3.3 Finite Sample Size 105
3.4 Other Algorithms 108

In this chapter we focus on iterative procedures for the construction of optimal continuous (normalized) designs. In Section 3.1 we introduce first-order iterative procedures for the D-criterion. Then in Section 3.2 we describe first-order procedures for the general case of convex criteria. The major developments of the numerical procedures were undertaken by Fedorov (1969, 1972) [125], [127]; Wynn (1970, 1972) [416], [417]; Atwood (1973) [25]; Tsay (1976) [385]; Wu and Wynn (1978) [409]; Wu (1978) [408]. The case of finite sample size is discussed in Section 3.3. A short survey of publications on other classes of numerical procedures for the construction of optimal designs is provided in Section 3.4.

3.1 First-Order Algorithm: D-Criterion

Let us start with an heuristic outline of an iterative procedure. Let ξ_s be the design that was obtained after s iteration steps; see (2.48) for the formal definition of the normalized design. At each iteration step we aim to improve the characteristics of the design with respect to some selected optimality criterion. For instance, the updated design may be obtained according to the following formula:

$$\xi_{s+1} = (1 - \alpha_s)\xi_s + \alpha_s\xi \ , \ \alpha_s > 0; \tag{3.1}$$

see (2.49) for a definition of the convex sum of two designs. In essence, we reduce weights of observations that are taken according to design ξ_s and instead add observations at points that correspond to design ξ. The question arises as to how to choose points in ξ.

First let us consider D-optimality. Recall that

$$d(\mathbf{x}, \xi_s) = \text{tr}[\mathbf{D}(\xi_s)\boldsymbol{\mu}(\mathbf{x})]$$

is the sensitivity function for the D-criterion (cf. Table 2.1) and that all support points of a D-optimal design coincide with maxima of the sensitivity function over the design region $\mathfrak{X}$; see Theorem 2.3. Thus, it may be expected that the design ξ_s will improve when one adds observations at points where the function $d(\mathbf{x}, \xi_s)$ attains its maximum. Recall that the function $d(\mathbf{x}, \xi_s)$ is the normalized variance of the estimated response at point $\mathbf{x}$; cf. (2.32). Thus, in order to obtain the improved design ξ_{s+1}, it makes sense to make observations at those points where the variance of the predicted response is the largest.

More formally, we describe this idea as follows:

(a) Given ξ_s, find

$$\mathbf{x}_{s+1} = \arg\max_{\mathbf{x} \in \mathfrak{X}} d(\mathbf{x}, \xi_s). \qquad (3.2)$$

(b) Add point $\mathbf{x}_{s+1}$ to the current design, i.e., construct

$$\xi_{s+1} = (1 - \alpha_s)\xi_s + \alpha_s \xi(\mathbf{x}_{s+1}), \qquad (3.3)$$

where $\xi(\mathbf{x})$ is a unit measure atomized at $\mathbf{x}$, i.e., $\xi(\mathbf{x}) = \{\mathbf{x},\ w_1 = 1\}$.

Steps (3.2) and (3.3) are repeated until a particular stopping rule is satisfied: for example, the maximal number of steps is reached or the difference in criteria values on consecutive steps is less than a preselected threshold.

3.1.1   Forward iterative procedure

To explore the theoretical reasons of a meaningful behavior of the iterative procedure (3.2), (3.3), let us compare values of determinants $|\mathbf{D}(\xi_s)|$ and $|\mathbf{D}(\xi_{s+1})|$ on two consecutive steps. If ξ_{s+1} satisfies (3.1), then it follows from (2.51) that

$$\ln|\mathbf{D}(\xi_{s+1})| = \ln|\mathbf{M}^{-1}(\xi_{s+1})| = \ln|[(1 - \alpha)\mathbf{M}(\xi_s) + \alpha\mathbf{M}(\xi)]^{-1}|.$$

Thus assumption (B4) of Section 2.4.2 and (2.73) imply that

$$\ln|\mathbf{D}(\xi_{s+1})| = \ln|\mathbf{D}(\xi_s)| + \alpha\left[m - \int d(\mathbf{x}, \xi_s)\, \xi(d\mathbf{x})\right] + o(\alpha, \xi_s, \xi). \qquad (3.4)$$

For sufficiently small α, the minimization of the function $\ln|\mathbf{D}(\xi_{s+1})|$ with respect to the added measure $\alpha\xi(d\mathbf{x})$ leads to

$$\min_{\xi} \ln|\mathbf{D}(\xi_{s+1})| \cong \ln|\mathbf{D}(\xi_s)| + \alpha\min_{\xi}\left[m - \int d(\mathbf{x}, \xi_s)\, \xi(d\mathbf{x})\right]$$

$$= \ln |\mathbf{D}(\xi_s)| + \alpha \left[m - \max_{\xi} \int d(\mathbf{x}, \xi_s) \, \xi(d\mathbf{x}) \right]. \qquad (3.5)$$

Observing that

$$\max_{\xi} \int d(\mathbf{x}, \xi_s) \, \xi(d\mathbf{x}) = \max_{\mathbf{x} \in \mathfrak{X}} \, d(\mathbf{x}, \xi_s), \qquad (3.6)$$

we conclude that for small α the one-point design defined in (3.2) is the best choice. Note that (3.5) implies that the iterative procedure (3.2), (3.3) improves the design by moving along the smallest directional derivative. In spite of its simplicity, equality (3.6) plays an important role in the numerical construction of optimal designs: it replaces the maximization problem $\max_\xi \int d(\mathbf{x}, \xi_s) \, \xi(d\mathbf{x})$ in the space of probability measures with the maximization problem $\max_{\mathbf{x}} \, d(\mathbf{x}, \xi_s)$ over the design region $\mathfrak{X}$ that most often belongs to a finite-dimensional Euclidean space.

To apply steps (3.2), (3.3), we need to specify both the direction and the "step length" α_s. The following three choices for $\{\alpha_s\}$ are among the most popular ones:

$$\lim_{s \to \infty} \alpha_s = 0, \quad \sum_{s=0}^{\infty} \alpha_s = \infty; \qquad (3.7)$$

$$\alpha_s = \arg \min_{\alpha} \Psi[(1 - \alpha)\xi_s + \alpha\xi(\mathbf{x}_{s+1})]; \qquad (3.8)$$

$$\alpha_s = \begin{cases} \alpha_{s-1}, & \text{if } \Psi[(1 - \alpha_{s-1})\xi_s + \alpha_{s-1}\xi(\mathbf{x}_{s+1})] < \Psi(\xi_s), \\ \gamma\alpha_{s-1}, & \text{otherwise, with a suitable choice of } \gamma < 1. \end{cases} \qquad (3.9)$$

The condition of divergence of the sum $\sum_s \alpha_s$ in (3.7) allows for the convergence of the iterative procedure (3.2), (3.3) even for rather "poor" initial designs; it is analogous to the condition for step lengths in various stochastic approximation procedures; cf. Robbins and Monro (1951) [341]. A generalized geometric sequence provides an example of the sequence satisfying (3.7):

$$\alpha_s = \frac{a_1}{n_0 + a_2 s},$$

where n_0 is the number of points in the initial design, and a_1, a_2 are positive constants.

For obvious reasons, rule (3.8) is called the steepest descent rule.

3.1.2 Some useful recursive formulae

Suppose that the individual information matrix can be factorized as

$$\boldsymbol{\mu}(\mathbf{x}) = \mathbf{g}(\mathbf{x})\mathbf{g}^T(\mathbf{x}). \qquad (3.10)$$

For example, such factorization is valid for

- Linear model $\eta(\mathbf{x}, \boldsymbol{\theta}) = \mathbf{f}^T(\mathbf{x})\boldsymbol{\theta}$ with known constant variance σ^2, for which $\mathbf{g}(\mathbf{x}) = \mathbf{f}(\mathbf{x})/\sigma$; cf. (1.90);

- Binary model (1.92) for which

$$\mathbf{g}(\mathbf{x}) = \mathbf{g}(\mathbf{x}, \boldsymbol{\theta}) = \frac{\dot{\pi}}{\sqrt{\pi(1 - \pi)}} \mathbf{f}(\mathbf{x});$$

see (1.93); see also examples in Section 5.4;

- Nonlinear model (1.107) with a single response, $k = 1$, when variance S does not depend on unknown parameters, i.e., $S(\mathbf{x}, \boldsymbol{\theta}) \equiv \sigma^2(\mathbf{x})$. In this case, according to (1.108),

$$\mathbf{g}(\mathbf{x}) = \mathbf{g}(\mathbf{x}, \boldsymbol{\theta}) = \frac{1}{\sigma(\mathbf{x})} \frac{\partial \eta(\mathbf{x}, \boldsymbol{\theta})}{\partial \boldsymbol{\theta}};$$

cf. (6.15).

Let $d(\mathbf{x}, \xi) = \mathbf{g}^T(\mathbf{x})\mathbf{M}^{-1}(\xi)\mathbf{g}(\mathbf{x})$. Then formula (10.11) implies

$$
\begin{aligned}
|\mathbf{D}^{-1}(\xi_{s+1})| &= |\mathbf{M}(\xi_{s+1})| = |(1 - \alpha)\mathbf{M}(\xi_s) + \alpha \mathbf{g}(\mathbf{x}_{s+1})\mathbf{g}^T(\mathbf{x}_{s+1})| \\
&= (1 - \alpha)^m \left(1 + \frac{\alpha d(\mathbf{x}_{s+1}, \xi_s)}{1 - \alpha}\right)|\mathbf{M}(\xi_s)|. \quad (3.11)
\end{aligned}
$$

Taking a derivative of the right-hand side of (3.11) with respect to α and equating it to zero, one may find that for the steepest descent rule (3.8)

$$\alpha_s = \arg\min_\alpha |\mathbf{D}(\xi_{s+1})| = \frac{d(\mathbf{x}_{s+1}, \xi_s) - m}{[d(\mathbf{x}_{s+1}, \xi_s) - 1]m}. \quad (3.12)$$

The following recursion may be derived from formula (10.12). It allows us to avoid the matrix inversion on each step of the iterative procedure:

$$
\begin{aligned}
\mathbf{D}(\xi_{s+1}) &= \frac{1}{1 - \alpha}\left[\mathbf{M}(\xi_s) + \frac{\alpha}{1 - \alpha}\mathbf{g}(\mathbf{x}_{s+1})\mathbf{g}^T(\mathbf{x}_{s+1})\right]^{-1} \\
&= \frac{\mathbf{D}(\xi_s)}{1 - \alpha}\left[\mathbf{I}_m - \frac{\alpha \mathbf{g}(\mathbf{x}_{s+1})\mathbf{g}^T(\mathbf{x}_{s+1})\mathbf{D}(\xi_s)}{1 - \alpha + \alpha d(\mathbf{x}_{s+1}, \xi_s)}\right]. \quad (3.13)
\end{aligned}
$$

3.1.3   Convergence of algorithms

In this section we assume that assumptions (A1) and (A2) of Section 2.4 are satisfied, and that the individual information matrix $\boldsymbol{\mu}(\mathbf{x})$ may be factorized as in (3.10). As discussed in Section 2.4, assumption (A2) may be replaced with the assumption of continuity of functions $\mathbf{g}(\mathbf{x})$ in (3.10).

Does the repeated application of steps (3.2), (3.3) lead to an optimal design when $s \to \infty$? The answer to this question is positive: we prove the following theorem for the steepest descent rule (3.8).

Theorem 3.1 *If sequence* $\{\xi_s\}$ *is defined in (3.2), (3.3) and the initial design* ξ_0 *is regular, then for the steepest descent rule (3.8)*

$$\lim_{s \to \infty} |\mathbf{D}(\xi_s)| = \min_{\xi \in \Xi(\mathfrak{X})} |\mathbf{D}(\xi)|, \qquad (3.14)$$

where $\Xi(\mathfrak{X})$ *is the set of all probability measures on the design region* $\mathfrak{X}$; *see* *(2.52).*

Proof.   Let $\Psi_s = |\mathbf{D}(\xi_s)|$ and $\delta_s = d(\mathbf{x}_{s+1}, \xi_s) - m$. It follows from (3.11) that

$$\frac{\Psi_s}{\Psi_{s+1}} = \frac{|\mathbf{M}(\xi_{s+1})|}{|\mathbf{M}(\xi_s)|} = (1 - \alpha_s)^{m-1} \left[1 - \alpha_s + \alpha_s(\delta_s + m)\right], \qquad (3.15)$$

and (3.12) implies that

$$r_{s+1} = \frac{\Psi_s}{\Psi_{s+1}} = \left(\frac{m + \delta_s}{m}\right)^m \left(\frac{m-1}{m-1+\delta_s}\right)^{m-1}. \qquad (3.16)$$

It follows from the definition of α_s in (3.12) that the sequence $\{\Psi_s\}$ is nonincreasing and bounded from below by zero ($\{\Psi_s\}$ are determinants of nonnegative definite matrices). Therefore this sequence converges, i.e.,

$$\lim_{s \to \infty} \Psi_s = \Psi. \qquad (3.17)$$

Let us assume that Ψ exceeds $\min_\xi |\mathbf{D}(\xi)| = \Psi^*$, i.e.,

$$\frac{\Psi}{\Psi^*} = 1 + \gamma, \quad \text{where } \gamma > 0. \qquad (3.18)$$

The inequality (2.74) may be rewritten as

$$d(\mathbf{x}_{s+1}, \xi_s) - m \geq \ln \frac{|\mathbf{D}(\xi_s)|}{\Psi^*}, \qquad (3.19)$$

and provides a useful relation between the closeness of $|\mathbf{D}(\xi_s)|$ to Ψ^* and closeness of $d(\mathbf{x}_{s+1}, \xi_s)$ to m. It follows from (3.19) that for all s

$$\delta_s \geq \gamma_1 > 0, \quad \text{where } \gamma_1 = \ln(1 + \gamma) > 0. \qquad (3.20)$$

Next, introduce function $r(\delta)$,

$$r(\delta) = \left(\frac{m + \delta}{m}\right)^m \left(\frac{m-1}{m-1+\delta}\right)^{m-1}.$$

Note that $r(0) = 1$ and $r(\delta)$ is monotonically increasing for positive δ since

$$\frac{dr}{d\delta} = \frac{(m-1)^{m-1}}{m^m} \frac{\delta(m+\delta)^{m-1}}{(m-1+\delta)^m} > 0 \text{ for } \delta > 0.$$

Thus, (3.20) implies that $r_{s+1} \geq 1 + \beta$, where $\beta = r(\gamma_1) - 1 > 0$, from which it follows that $\Psi_s / \Psi_{s+k+1} > (1 + \beta)^k$ for any integer k, and thus

$$\lim_{s \to \infty} \Psi_s = 0,$$

which contradicts (3.18). This proves the theorem. $\square$

Analogs of Theorem 3.1 are valid for sequences $\{\alpha_s\}$ that satisfy (3.7) or (3.9). Using the ideas from the proofs of Theorem 3.1 and Theorem 1 of Wynn (1970) [416], we establish the following result; cf. Theorem 3 of Tsay (1976) [385].

Theorem 3.2 *If sequence $\{\xi_s\}$ is defined in (3.2), (3.3) and the initial design ξ_0 is regular, then for the step length rule (3.7)*

$$\lim_{s \to \infty} |\mathbf{D}(\xi_s)| = \min_{\xi} |\mathbf{D}(\xi)|. \tag{3.21}$$

Proof. Let $\Psi_s = |\mathbf{D}(\xi_s)|$ and let us assume that the sequence $\{\Psi_s\}$ does not converge to $\Psi^* = \min_\xi |\mathbf{D}(\xi)|$. Let $\varepsilon > 0$ be an arbitrary fixed number. Introduce two complementary sets of indices, S_1 and S_2:

$$S_1 = S_1(\varepsilon) = \left\{ s : \frac{\Psi_s}{\Psi^*} \geq 1 + \frac{\varepsilon}{2} \right\}, \tag{3.22}$$

$$S_2 = S_2(\varepsilon) = \left\{ s : \frac{\Psi_s}{\Psi^*} < 1 + \frac{\varepsilon}{2} \right\}. \tag{3.23}$$

Note that S_1 is a "bad" set in that designs ξ_s, $s \in S_1$, are relatively "far" from the optimum in terms of the closeness of Ψ_s and Ψ^*. On the contrary, S_2 is a "good" set because designs ξ_s, $s \in S_2$, are in a "small" vicinity of the optimal design. The idea of the proof is as follows: we show that

(A) If $s \in S_1$, then designs ξ_s tend to improve and values Ψ_s tend to get closer to Ψ^* because the sum $\sum_s \alpha_s$ diverges.

(B) If $s \in S_2$, then for all sufficiently large indices s designs ξ_s cannot "leave" a small vicinity of the optimum because $\alpha_s \to 0$.

Let us first show that the set S_2 contains infinitely many indices s, i.e., that there exists a subsequence of design $\{\xi_{s'}\}$ such that

$$\lim_{s' \to \infty} \Psi_{s'} = \Psi^*.$$

Suppose that this is not true, i.e., all sufficiently large indices s belong to S_1. Let $\gamma_1 = \ln(1 + \varepsilon/2)$. Then it follows from (3.15) and (3.19) that

$$\frac{\Psi_s}{\Psi_{s+1}} \geq (1 - \alpha_s)^{m-1} [1 - \alpha_s + \alpha_s(\gamma_1 + m)],$$

and

$$\ln \frac{\Psi_s}{\Psi_{s+1}} \geq (m-1)\ln(1-\alpha_s) + \ln[1+\alpha_s(\gamma_1+m-1)]$$

$$= -\alpha_s(m-1) + \alpha_s(\gamma_1+m-1) + O(\alpha_s^2) \geq \frac{\alpha_s\gamma_1}{2} \quad (3.24)$$

for all sufficiently large $s > s_1^*$ because $\alpha_s \to 0$. Therefore,

$$\ln \frac{\Psi_s}{\Psi_{s+k+1}} \geq \frac{\gamma_1}{2} \sum_{i=s}^{s+k} \alpha_i,$$

and $\lim_{s\to\infty} \Psi_s = 0$ because the sum $\sum_i \alpha_i$ diverges. This contradicts the definition of the set S_1 in (3.22) because $\Psi^* > 0$, and proves that the set S_2 contains infinitely many indices s.

Note that because $\Psi_s \geq \Psi^*$ for any s, relations (3.15) and (3.19) imply that

$$\frac{\Psi_s}{\Psi_{s+1}} \geq (1-\alpha)^{m-1}(1-\alpha_s+\alpha_s m).$$

Now since $\alpha_s \to 0$, then

$$\ln \frac{\Psi_s}{\Psi_{s+1}} \geq (m-1)\ln(1-\alpha_s) + \ln[1+\alpha_s(m-1)] \geq -C\alpha_s^2$$

for all sufficiently large $s > s_2^*$, where the constant C depends on m only, and consequently

$$\frac{\Psi_s}{\Psi_{s+1}} \geq 1 - \varepsilon/4 \quad (3.25)$$

for all $s > s_2^*$.

Suppose now that $s \in S_2$ and $(s+1) \in S_1$. Then (3.23) and (3.25) lead to

$$\frac{\Psi_{s+1}}{\Psi^*} = \frac{\Psi_{s+1}}{\Psi_s}\frac{\Psi_s}{\Psi^*} \leq \frac{1+\varepsilon/2}{1-\varepsilon/4} \leq 1+\varepsilon \quad (3.26)$$

for all $\varepsilon < 1$. Next, note that (3.24) implies that if $(s+1) \in S_1$ for $s > s_1^*$, then $\Psi_{s+1} > \Psi_{s+2}$, and, therefore Ψ_{s+2} must satisfy the inequality

$$\frac{\Psi_{s+2}}{\Psi^*} \leq 1+\varepsilon.$$

Repeating this argument, we establish that

$$\Psi_s \leq (1+\varepsilon)\Psi^*$$

for any $s > \max\{s_1^*, s_2^*\}$. Since ε is arbitrary, this proves the theorem. $\square$

3.1.4   Practical numerical procedures

The numerical procedure (3.2), (3.3) provides a good starting point for understanding the theoretical background of the optimal design algorithms. In practice, various "tricks" that complement the standard iterative procedure are used in algorithms. Some of these useful complements are described below.

(1) The convergence rate is significantly improved if, in parallel to adding "good" points to the current design as in (3.2), we delete "bad" points from ξ_s. Such modification is often called a "backward" step; cf. Atwood (1973) [25]. Let $\xi_s = \{\mathbf{x}_{sj}, p_{sj}, \ j = 1, \ldots, n_s\}$ be the current design on step s. To accomplish the backward step, find

$$\mathbf{x}_{s+1}^- = \arg\min_{\mathbf{x} \in X_s} d(\mathbf{x}, \xi_s) = \arg\min_{j \in [1, n_s]} d(\mathbf{x}_{sj}, \xi_s), \qquad (3.27)$$

where $X_s = \operatorname{supp} \xi_s$, and either delete $\mathbf{x}_{s+1}^-$ from X_s completely, or reduce its weight. We may, for instance, replace (3.2) by

$$\mathbf{x}_{s+1} = \arg\max[d(\mathbf{x}_{s+1}^+, \xi_s) - m, \ m - d(\mathbf{x}_{s+1}^-, \xi_s)], \qquad (3.28)$$

where $\mathbf{x}_{s+1}^+$ is defined in (3.2), and use

$$\alpha_s = \begin{cases} \alpha_s', & \text{if } \mathbf{x}_{s+1} = \mathbf{x}_{s+1}^+, \\ -\min\left(\alpha_s', \dfrac{p_s}{1-p_s}\right), & \text{if } \mathbf{x}_{s+1} = \mathbf{x}_{s+1}^-; \end{cases} \qquad (3.29)$$

α_s' is given by one of the rules (3.7) – (3.9), and p_s is the weight of point $\mathbf{x}_{s+1}^-$ in the design ξ_s.

The explanation of the formula in the second line in (3.29) is as follows. If in the updated design one uses the step length α_s, then the weight of the "worst" point $\mathbf{x}_{s+1}^-$ becomes $p_{s,new} = (1 + \alpha_s)p_s - \alpha_s \geq 0$, from which it follows that α_s must be less than or equal to $p_s/(1 - p_s)$. When $\alpha_s = p_s/(1 - p_s)$, this means that the worst point $\mathbf{x}_{s+1}^-$ is completely removed from the current design.

(2) One may use both forward and backward steps in a single "combined" step of the iterative procedure: first, use (3.2) to find the best "new" point, and construct the updated design ξ_s^+ according to

$$\xi_s^+ = (1 - \alpha_s)\xi_s + \alpha_s \xi(\mathbf{x}_{s+1}), \qquad (3.30)$$

with $\alpha_s = \alpha_s'$. Then find the worst point in the current design according to

$$\mathbf{x}_{s+1}^- = \arg\min_{\mathbf{x} \in X_s^+} d(\mathbf{x}, \xi_s^+), \qquad (3.31)$$

where X_s^+ is the support set of the design ξ_s^+, and find

$$\xi_{s+1} = (1 - \alpha_s)\xi_s^+ + \alpha_s \xi(\mathbf{x}_{s+1}^-), \ \ \alpha_s = -\min\left(\alpha_s', \frac{p_s}{1 - p_s}\right), \qquad (3.32)$$

where p_s is the weight of point $\mathbf{x}_{s+1}^-$ in the design ξ_s^+.

(3) Sometimes it is more convenient to first make n^+ forward steps with $\mathbf{x}_{s+1}$ obtained from (3.2), and then to proceed with n^- backward steps based on (3.27). The number n^+ is called the length of the forward excursion, and n^- is called the length of the backward excursion.

(4) Points $\{\mathbf{x}_s\}$ have the tendency to cluster around support points of the optimal design. We can avoid this by using a simple "merging" procedure: check whether $\mathbf{x}_{s+1}$ satisfies the inequality

$$\max_{\mathbf{x}_{sj} \in X_s} (\mathbf{x}_{sj} - \mathbf{x}_{s+1})^T (\mathbf{x}_{sj} - \mathbf{x}_{s+1}) \leq r, \tag{3.33}$$

where the constant r is chosen on practical grounds. If a support point $\mathbf{x}_{sj}$ is close enough to $\mathbf{x}_{s+1}$ to satisfy (3.33), then $\mathbf{x}_{sj}$ is deleted from the design and its weight is added to that of $\mathbf{x}_{s+1}$. Alternatively, in some older publications it has been recommended to use the weighted average of $\mathbf{x}_{s+1}$ and $\mathbf{x}_{sj}$. Our experience demonstrates that the former rule works better and is, in addition, in better agreement with the theory. Indeed, observations must be taken at points where the function $d(\mathbf{x}, \xi^*)$ attains its maximum. Obviously, for a "reasonable" numerical procedure $d(\mathbf{x}, \xi_s)$ becomes "closer" to $d(\mathbf{x}, \xi^*)$ when $s \to \infty$. Therefore, for large s the point $\mathbf{x}_{s+1}$ is closer to the corresponding support point of the optimal design than neighboring points that were found in previous steps.

(5) Sometimes it may be computationally cumbersome to solve the maximization problem (3.2) precisely. Instead, it is sufficient to determine $\mathbf{x}_{s+1}$ such that $d(\mathbf{x}_{s+1}, \xi_s) - m \geq \delta_s > 0$.

(6) The iterative procedure is completed when some stopping rule is satisfied. At every iteration, we compute $\max_{\mathbf{x}} d(\mathbf{x}, \xi_s)$ and, therefore, from (3.19) it is straightforward to find out how close $|\mathbf{D}(\xi_s)|$ is to $|\mathbf{D}(\xi^*)|$ and to formulate an appropriate stopping rule. For example, one can check whether the expression on the left-hand side of (3.19) is less than a preselected "small" positive ε.

3.2 First-Order Algorithm: General Case

In what follows we suppose that assumptions (A1), (A2) and (B1) – (B4) hold and, therefore, we can use Theorem 2.2. However, we modify assumption (B4):
(B4′) For any $\xi \in \Xi(q)$ and $\bar{\xi} \in \Xi$,

$$\Psi[(1 - \alpha)\mathbf{M}(\xi) + \alpha\mathbf{M}(\bar{\xi})]$$
$$= \Psi[\mathbf{M}(\xi)] + \alpha \int \psi(\mathbf{x}, \xi) \bar{\xi}(d\mathbf{x}) + O(\alpha^2 | \xi, \bar{\xi}), \tag{3.34}$$

where $O(\alpha^2|\xi, \overline{\xi}) \le \alpha^2 K_q$ for some $K_q > 0$ uniformly with respect to ξ and $\overline{\xi}$.

To justify the use of the iterative procedure as in (3.1), we use exactly the same arguments as for the D-criterion in Section 3.1.1. It follows from assumption (B4') that

$$\Psi[\mathbf{M}(\xi_{s+1}] \cong \Psi[\mathbf{M}(\xi_s)] + \alpha \int \psi(\mathbf{x}, \xi_s)\, \xi(d\mathbf{x}), \tag{3.35}$$

and the minimum of the right-hand side of (3.35) with respect to $\xi(d\mathbf{x})$ is attained at the atomized measure $\xi(\mathbf{x}_s)$, where

$$\mathbf{x}_{s+1} = \arg\min_{\mathbf{x}} \psi(\mathbf{x}, \xi_s) = \arg\max_{\mathbf{x}} \varphi(\mathbf{x}, \xi_s); \tag{3.36}$$

see (2.73) and Table 2.1 for the definition of the sensitivity function $\varphi(\mathbf{x}, \xi)$. Therefore, the following iterative procedure may be considered:

(a) Given $\xi_s \in \Xi_q$, find $\mathbf{x}_{s+1}$ from (3.36).

(b) Construct

$$\xi_{s+1} = (1 - \alpha_s)\xi_s + \alpha_s\xi(\mathbf{x}_{s+1}), \tag{3.37}$$

where the sequence $\{\alpha_s\}$ may be chosen according to (3.7), (3.8), or (3.9).

It is worthwhile noting that the atomized design $\xi(\mathbf{x}_{s+1})$ at which the minimum of the expression on the right-hand side of (3.35) is attained, does not depend on the step length α_s. This explains the simplicity and popularity of first-order algorithms.

Theorems 3.3 and 3.4 are direct analogs of Theorems 3.1 and 3.2, respectively.

Theorem 3.3 *Let the assumptions of Theorem 2.2 and (B4') hold. If sequence $\{\xi_s\}$ is defined in (3.36), (3.37) and the initial design ξ_0 is regular, then for the steepest descent rule (3.8)*

$$\lim_{s\to\infty} \Psi[\mathbf{M}(\xi_s)] = \Psi^* = \min_{\xi} \Psi[\mathbf{M}(\xi_s)]. \tag{3.38}$$

Proof. Let $\Psi_s = \Psi[\mathbf{M}(\xi_s)]$. By definition, the sequence $\{\Psi_s\}$ is nonincreasing and, therefore, it converges:

$$\lim_{s\to\infty} \Psi_s = \Psi_\infty. \tag{3.39}$$

Assume that Ψ_∞ exceeds the optimal value Ψ^*:

$$\Psi_\infty - \Psi^* = \gamma_1 > 0. \tag{3.40}$$

Let γ be an arbitrary fixed positive number such that $\gamma < \gamma_1$. Then it follows from (2.63) and (3.40) that

$$\min_{\mathbf{x}} \psi(\mathbf{x}, \xi_s) \le \Psi^* - \Psi_s \le -\gamma_1 < -\gamma. \tag{3.41}$$

If $\mathbf{x}_{s+1}$ is selected according to (3.36) and

$$\xi_\alpha = (1 - \alpha)\xi_s + \alpha\xi(\mathbf{x}_{s+1}),$$

then assumption (B4′) implies for all sufficiently small α that

$$\Psi[\mathbf{M}(\xi_\alpha)] = \Psi_s + \alpha \min_{\mathbf{x}} \psi(\mathbf{x}, \xi_s) + O(\alpha^2), \tag{3.42}$$

and (3.41) entails

$$\Psi_s - \Psi[\mathbf{M}(\xi_\alpha)] \geq \alpha\gamma - K_q\alpha^2 = -K_q\left(\alpha - \frac{\gamma}{2K_q}\right)^2 + \frac{\gamma^2}{4K_q}. \tag{3.43}$$

If $\alpha = \frac{\gamma}{2K_q}$, then the definition of the step length rule (3.8) leads to the inequality

$$\Psi_s - \Psi_{s+1} \geq \Psi_s - \Psi[\mathbf{M}(\xi_\alpha)] = \frac{\gamma^2}{4K_q},$$

from which it follows that $\lim_{s\to\infty} \Psi_s = -\infty$. This contradicts (3.40) and proves the theorem. $\square$

Theorem 3.4 *If the assumptions of Theorem 3.3 are satisfied, then for the step length rule (3.7)*

$$\lim_{s\to\infty} \Psi[\mathbf{M}(\xi_s)] = \Psi^* = \min_{\xi} \Psi[\mathbf{M}(\xi_s)].$$

Proof. Let $\Psi_s = \Psi[\mathbf{M}(\xi_s)]$ and let us assume that the sequence $\{\Psi_s\}$ does not converge to Ψ^*. For an arbitrary fixed number $\varepsilon > 0$ introduce two complementary sets,

$$S_1 = S_1(\varepsilon) = \{s : \Psi_s - \Psi^* \geq \varepsilon/2\}, \tag{3.44}$$

$$S_2 = S_2(\varepsilon) = \{s : \Psi_s - \Psi^* < \varepsilon/2\}. \tag{3.45}$$

To show that the set S_2 contains infinitely many indices s, suppose that this is not true. Then (2.63), (3.42) and (3.44) lead to the inequality

$$\Psi_s - \Psi_{s+1} \geq \frac{\alpha_s\varepsilon}{2} - K_q\alpha_s^2 \geq \frac{\alpha_s\varepsilon}{4} \tag{3.46}$$

for all sufficiently large s and, consequently, since the sum $\sum_i \alpha_i$ diverges,

$$\lim_{s\to\infty} \Psi_s = -\infty,$$

which contradicts the definition of the set S_1 in (3.44).

Similar to the second part of the proof of Theorem 3.2, note that because $\Psi_s \geq \Psi^*$ for any s, then (3.42) implies that

$$\Psi_s - \Psi_{s+1} \geq -K_q\alpha_s^2 \geq -\varepsilon/2 \tag{3.47}$$

for all sufficiently large s. If $s \in S_2$ and $(s+1) \in S_1$, then (3.45) and (3.47) lead to

$$\Psi_{s+1} - \Psi^* = (\Psi_{s+1} - \Psi_s) + (\Psi_s - \Psi^*) < \varepsilon.$$

Finally, if $(s+1) \in S_1$, then $\Psi_{s+1} > \Psi_{s+2}$ because of (3.46), and, consequently,

$$\Psi_{s+2} - \Psi^* < \varepsilon$$

for all sufficiently large s. $\square$

Remark 3.1   To verify assumption (B4′), it is sufficient to prove that the function $G(\alpha) = G(\alpha; \xi; \bar{\xi})$, introduced in (2.67), has the second derivative $G''(\alpha)$ at $\alpha = 0$ and that $G''(0)$ is uniformly bounded with respect to $\xi \in \Xi(q)$ and $\bar{\xi}$. Let us show that this is true for D- and A-criteria. Indeed, it follows from (2.69), (10.4) and (10.5) that for the D-criterion

$$
\begin{aligned}
G''(\alpha) &= -\mathrm{tr}\left\{ \left[\mathbf{M}(\bar{\xi}) - \mathbf{M}(\xi)\right] \frac{d\mathbf{M}_\alpha^{-1}}{d\alpha} \right\} \\
&= \mathrm{tr}\left\{ \left[\mathbf{M}(\bar{\xi}) - \mathbf{M}(\xi)\right] \mathbf{M}_\alpha^{-1} \frac{d\mathbf{M}_\alpha}{d\alpha} \mathbf{M}_\alpha^{-1} \right\},
\end{aligned}
$$

and

$$\lim_{\alpha \to 0} G''(\alpha) = \mathrm{tr}\left\{ \left[\mathbf{M}(\bar{\xi}) - \mathbf{M}(\xi)\right] \mathbf{M}^{-1}(\xi) \right\}^2 = \mathrm{tr}\{\mathbf{M}(\bar{\xi})\mathbf{M}^{-1}(\xi) - \mathbf{I}_m\}^2.$$

For the A-criterion, assume that $\mathbf{A} = \mathbf{I}_m$. Then it follows from (2.71), (10.4) and (10.5) that

$$G''(\alpha) = \mathrm{tr}\left\{ \left[\mathbf{M}(\bar{\xi}) - \mathbf{M}(\xi)\right] \mathbf{M}_\alpha^{-2} \frac{d\mathbf{M}_\alpha^2}{d\alpha} \mathbf{M}_\alpha^{-2} \right\}.$$

Since

$$\frac{d\mathbf{M}_\alpha^2}{d\alpha} = 2\frac{d\mathbf{M}_\alpha}{d\alpha} \mathbf{M}_\alpha,$$

then it follows from (2.66) that

$$\lim_{\alpha \to 0} G''(\alpha) = 2\mathrm{tr}\{\left[\mathbf{M}(\bar{\xi}) - \mathbf{M}(\xi)\right] \mathbf{M}^{-2}(\xi) \left[\mathbf{M}(\bar{\xi}) - \mathbf{M}(\xi)\right] \mathbf{M}^{-1}(\xi)\}.$$

For more details on the convergence of iterative procedures with the general step length rule (3.7), see Wu and Wynn (1978) [409], in particular the discussion in Sections 3 and 4 that follows the proof of Dichotomous Theorem in Section 2.

Remark 3.2   In the proof of Theorems 3.3 and 3.4, we did not use the factorization assumption (3.10) for the information matrix of a single observation. Therefore, these theorems hold for the general case (1.101) where the information matrix is presented as the sum of two terms.

The rate of convergence can be improved if weights are reallocated within the design ξ_s, i.e., if

$$\mathbf{x}_s = \arg\min[\psi(\mathbf{x}_s^+, \xi_s), -\psi(\mathbf{x}_s^-, \xi_s)], \qquad (3.48)$$

where $\mathbf{x}_s^+ = \arg\min_{\mathbf{x}\in\mathfrak{x}} \psi(\mathbf{x}, \xi_s)$ and $\mathbf{x}^- = \arg\max_{\mathbf{x}\in X_s} \psi(\mathbf{x}, \xi_s)$. All modifications discussed in Section 3.1.4 are valid here and may help make the proposed algorithm more practical.

Regularization of numerical procedures. If assumption (B4$'$) does not hold, the convergence of sequences $\Psi[\mathbf{M}(\xi_s)]$ is not guaranteed. In particular, the numerical procedure may not converge when the optimal design is singular. One of the most reliable and relatively simple approaches is based on the concept of regularization as introduced in Section 2.8: we replace the minimization of $\Psi[\mathbf{M}(\xi)]$ by the minimization of $\Psi_\delta(\xi) = \Psi\left[(1-\delta)\mathbf{M}(\xi) + \delta\mathbf{M}(\xi_0)\right]$, where ξ_0 is some regular design; cf. (2.110), and the functions $\psi(\mathbf{x}, \xi)$ and $\varphi(\mathbf{x}, \xi)$ must be modified accordingly. For instance, for the D-criterion,

$$\begin{aligned}
\psi(\mathbf{x}, \xi) &= (1-\delta)\left\{\operatorname{tr}\left[\mathbf{M}^{-1}(\bar{\xi})\mathbf{M}(\xi)\right] - d(\mathbf{x}, \bar{\xi})\right\} \\
&= (1-\delta)\left[\int d(\mathbf{x}, \bar{\xi})\xi(d\mathbf{x}) - d(\mathbf{x}, \bar{\xi})\right], \qquad (3.49)
\end{aligned}$$

where $\bar{\xi} = (1-\delta)\xi + \delta\xi_0$. For the A-criterion,

$$\begin{aligned}
\psi(\mathbf{x}, \xi) &= (1-\delta)\left\{\operatorname{tr}\left[\mathbf{A}\mathbf{M}^{-1}(\bar{\xi})\mathbf{M}(\xi)\mathbf{M}^{-1}(\bar{\xi})\right]\right. \\
&\quad \left. - \mathbf{f}^T(\mathbf{x})\mathbf{M}^{-1}(\bar{\xi})\mathbf{A}\mathbf{M}^{-1}(\bar{\xi})\mathbf{f}(\mathbf{x})\right\} \\
&= (1-\delta)\left[\int \varphi(\mathbf{x}, \bar{\xi})\xi(d\mathbf{x}) - \varphi(\mathbf{x}, \bar{\xi})\right]. \qquad (3.50)
\end{aligned}$$

The expression on the last line of (3.50) is valid for any criterion that satisfies assumption (B4$'$).

From a theoretical point of view, it makes sense to decrease the regularization constant δ on later iterations. However, the rate of decrease of δ must be significantly less than that of α_s. We can expect that for an appropriate choice of the sequence $\delta = \delta(s)$, with $\delta(s) \to 0$,

$$\lim_{s\to\infty} \Psi[\mathbf{M}(\xi_{\delta(s),s})] = \min_\xi \Psi[\mathbf{M}(\xi)]. \qquad (3.51)$$

3.3 Finite Sample Size

Rounding procedures. Since the introduction of the design measure concept in Section 2.3, we have neglected the fact that for real experiments the number of observations r_i at each support point $\mathbf{x}_i$ is an integer. Consequently, for a fixed sample size N the weights $p_i = r_i/N$ do not vary continuously and belong to a finite discrete set $\{j/N, \ j = 0, 1, \ldots, N\}$. When it is necessary to emphasize the discrete character of weights, we call the corresponding designs "discrete"; other standard terms are "exact" and "finite sample size" design. More details can be found in Pukelsheim (1993) [328], Chapter 12.

Let n be the number of support points of the continuous (approximate) optimal design ξ^*. Suppose that the number of observations N is much greater than n. Then one can use standard numerical rounding:

$$r_i^* = \left\{ \begin{array}{ll} \lceil p_i N \rceil, & \text{if } \lceil p_i N \rceil - p_i N \leq 0.5, \\ \lceil p_i N \rceil - 1, & \text{otherwise}, \end{array} \right. \tag{3.52}$$

where $\lceil u \rceil$ is the smallest integer not less than u. Occasionally, (3.52) must be adjusted to keep the sum of rounded weights equal to N: $\sum_{i=1}^{n} r_i^* = N$.

Let ξ_N^* be the discrete optimal design, i.e., the solution of the optimization problem (2.9). Let $\tilde{\xi}_N$ be a rounded version of ξ^*. Obviously, in practice it is important to know how close values $\Psi[\mathbf{M}(\tilde{\xi}_N)]$ and $\Psi[\mathbf{M}(\xi_N^*)]$ are.

Theorem 3.5 *Let n be the number of support points of the design ξ^* and let function $\Psi(\mathbf{M})$ be monotonic and homogeneous; see (2.41) and (2.42). Then*

$$\Psi[\mathbf{M}(\xi^*)] \leq \Psi[\mathbf{M}(\xi_N^*)] \leq \frac{\gamma(N-n)}{\gamma(N)} \ \Psi[\mathbf{M}(\xi^*)]. \tag{3.53}$$

Proof. It follows from (2.41) and (2.42) that

$$\gamma(N-n)\Psi[\mathbf{M}(\xi^*)] = \Psi[(N-n)\mathbf{M}(\xi^*)] \geq \Psi\left[\sum_{i=1}^{n} (\lceil p_i N \rceil - 1) \ \boldsymbol{\mu}(\mathbf{x}_i^*)\right]$$

$$\geq \Psi[N\mathbf{M}(\xi_N^*)] \ \geq \ \Psi[N\mathbf{M}(\xi^*)] = \gamma(N)\Psi[\mathbf{M}(\xi^*)],$$

which proves (3.53). $\square$

For the D-criterion, Theorem 3.5 leads to the following inequality:

$$\frac{|\mathbf{D}(\xi_N^*)|}{|\mathbf{D}(\xi^*)|} \leq \left(\frac{N}{N-n}\right)^m.$$

There exist special cases where rounding procedures can be skipped. For instance, it was mentioned in Section 2.6 that for the trigonometric regression on the interval $[0, 2\pi]$, any design with equidistant support points ($n \geq m$) and equal weights is D-optimal. Therefore, for any $N > m$ one can easily construct the exact D-optimal design by allocating a single observation at each of N equidistant points. A similar situation occurs for the first-order polynomial regression on the sphere: allocation of observations at N "equidistant" points gives the exact D-optimal design.

Necessary Conditions. Most necessary conditions are based on the following simple idea: a distortion of the optimal design cannot lead to an improvement. Let ξ be a regular design. Suppose that a design ξ' is obtained from ξ by replacing a single observation at a point $\mathbf{x}$ with a single observation at a point $\mathbf{x}'$. Introduce

$$d_2(\mathbf{x}, \mathbf{x}', \xi) = \mathbf{f}(\mathbf{x}) \, \mathbf{D}(\xi) \, \mathbf{f}(\mathbf{x}'). \tag{3.54}$$

A simple exercise in matrix algebra together with (10.12) leads to the following formula for the D-criterion:

$$\frac{|\mathbf{D}(\xi)|}{|\mathbf{D}(\xi')|} = 1 - \frac{1}{N} \left[d(\mathbf{x}', \xi) - d(\mathbf{x}, \xi) \right] - \frac{1}{N^2} \left[d(\mathbf{x}, \xi) d(\mathbf{x}', \xi) - d_2(\mathbf{x}, \mathbf{x}', \xi) \right]. \tag{3.55}$$

It follows from (3.55) that for any support point $\mathbf{x}_i^* \in \mathrm{supp}\xi_N^*$ and any $\mathbf{x} \in \mathfrak{X}$,

$$d(\mathbf{x}_i^*, \xi_N^*) \geq d(\mathbf{x}, \xi_N^*) - \frac{1}{N}[d(\mathbf{x}_i^*, \xi_N^*) d(\mathbf{x}, \xi_N^*) - d_2(\mathbf{x}_i^*, \mathbf{x}, \xi_N^*)]. \tag{3.56}$$

Note that for any design ξ,

$$\sum_{i=1}^{n} p_i d(\mathbf{x}_i, \xi) = \sum_{i=1}^{n} p_i \mathbf{f}^T(\mathbf{x}_i) \mathbf{D}(\xi) \mathbf{f}(\mathbf{x}_i)$$

$$= \mathrm{tr} \left[\mathbf{D}(\xi) \sum_{i=1}^{n} p_i \mathbf{f}^T(\mathbf{x}_i) \mathbf{f}(\mathbf{x}_i) \right] = \mathrm{tr} \left[\mathbf{D}(\xi) \mathbf{M}(\xi) \right] = m. \tag{3.57}$$

Next, it follows from (3.54) that

$$\sum_{i=1}^{n} p_i d_2(\mathbf{x}_i, \mathbf{x}, \xi) = \sum_{i=1}^{n} p_i \mathbf{f}^T(\mathbf{x}) \mathbf{D}(\xi) \mathbf{f}(\mathbf{x}_i) \mathbf{f}^T(\mathbf{x}_i) \mathbf{D}(\xi) \mathbf{f}(\mathbf{x})$$

$$= \mathbf{f}^T(\mathbf{x}) \mathbf{D}(\xi) \left[\sum_{i=1}^{n} p_i \mathbf{f}^T(\mathbf{x}_i) \mathbf{f}^T(\mathbf{x}_i) \right] \mathbf{D}(\xi) \mathbf{f}(\mathbf{x})$$

$$= \mathbf{f}^T(\mathbf{x}) \mathbf{D}(\xi) \mathbf{f}(\mathbf{x}) = d(\mathbf{x}, \xi). \tag{3.58}$$

Therefore, the summation of both sides of (3.56) together with (3.57) and (3.58) lead to the inequality

$$d(\mathbf{x}, \xi_n^*) \leq m \, \frac{N}{N + 1 - m}; \tag{3.59}$$

cf. the last part of Theorem 2.3 for $N \to \infty$. Similar results may be derived for other optimality criteria.

Numerical Search. Almost all existing and widely used algorithms for discrete designs are modifications of algorithms discussed in Section 3.2. In particular, a family of first-order algorithms for the construction of optimal discrete designs can be obtained as follows. Let ξ_0 be an initial design with weights $p_i = r_i/N$. Then use a procedure based on the iteration steps (a, b) described at the beginning of Section 3.2 and set $\alpha_s \equiv N^{-1}$ for all s.

In general, such iterative procedures lead to an improvement in the initial design, but do not guarantee the convergence to the optimal design. To improve the algorithm, it is recommended to make several attempts starting with different initial designs. In practice, if iterations with $\alpha_s \equiv N^{-1}$ do not lead to further improvement after some step s, one can use the algorithm with diminishing step length as a benchmark, in order to evaluate by how much the optimal discrete design deviates from the continuous optimal design ξ^*.

Another family of algorithms can be constructed using formulae similar to (3.56). For example, for the D-criterion, an iterative procedure can be constructed where pairs of points $(\mathbf{x}_s^+, \mathbf{x}_s^-)$ are determined according to

$$
\begin{aligned}
(\mathbf{x}_s^+, \mathbf{x}_s^-) \;=\; \arg \max_{\mathbf{x}^+ \in \mathfrak{X},\ \mathbf{x}^- \in X_s} \{ & d(\mathbf{x}, \xi_s) - d(\mathbf{x}^-, \xi_s) \\
& - N^{-1}[d(\mathbf{x}^+, \xi_s)d(\mathbf{x}^-, \xi_s) - d_2(\mathbf{x}^+, \mathbf{x}^-, \xi_s)]\}.
\end{aligned} \quad (3.60)
$$

On each iteration step, the design is improved by deleting $\mathbf{x}_s^-$ and adding $\mathbf{x}_s^+$. This algorithm is computationally more demanding than the first-order algorithms but, in general, leads to better results. It is worthwhile to remark that removing the term of order $1/N$ on the right-hand side of (3.60) converts the algorithm to the relatively simple first-order exchange algorithm; cf. Atwood (1973) [25].

3.4   Other Algorithms

In this chapter we focused on the first-order optimization algorithm, with references provided in the beginning of the chapter. It is worthwhile to mention other classes of numerical procedures for the construction of optimal designs:

- Multiplicative algorithms: the earlier publications include Fellman (1974) [154]; Titterington (1976, 1978) [375]; [376]; Torsney (1977) [379]; Silvey et al. (1978) [362]. A very interesting historical account of the developments can be found in Torsney (2009) [381]. See also Torsney (1983) [380]; Pázman (1986) [306]; Pukelsheim and Torsney (1991) [329]; Pronzato et al. (2000) [325]; Torsney and Mandal (2006) [382]; Harman and Pronzato (2007) [194]; Dette et al. (2008) [97]; Torsney and Martín-Martín (2009) [383]; Yu (2010) [423]; Holland-Letz et al. (2012) [205]; Martín-Martín et al. (2012) [269].

- Haycroft et al. (2009) [196] discuss multiplicative algorithms in the context of general gradient methods.

- Various stochastic search algorithms which include, among other methods,

- Simulated annealing; see Bohachevsky et al. (1986) [48]; Haines (1987) [186]; Meyer and Nachtsheim (1988) [281]; Atkinson (1992) [14]; Duffull et al. (2002) [107];

- Genetic algorithm; see Hamada et al. (2001) [188];

- Stochastic evolutionary algorithm; see Jin et al. (2005) [214].

- Methods based on semidefinite programming; see Wolkowicz et al. (2000) [407].

See also a discussion in Berger and Wong (2009) [44], Chapters 11.3, 11.4.

Chapter 4

Optimal Design under Constraints

4.1 Single Constraint 111
    4.1.1 One-stage designs 111
    4.1.2 Two-stage designs 116
4.2 Multiple Constraints 117
4.3 Constraints for Auxiliary Criteria 120
4.4 Directly Constrained Design Measures 122

In this chapter we discuss optimal designs under constraints. The idea of incorporating constraints (costs, or penalties) in optimal design goes back to the seminal paper by Elfving (1952) [114] on the geometrical construction of c-optimal designs: at the very end of the paper, Elfving introduced a constraint on the total costs instead of the constraint on the number of observations. In the notation of this chapter, the former corresponds to (4.6) while the latter corresponds, as usual, to (4.5). Elfving introduced the optimal design problem with the single constraint, and as we show in Section 4.1, for normalized designs that problem can be rather easily reduced to the standard setting. The problem with multiple constraints is much more challenging; see a survey paper by Cook and Fedorov (1995) [79] for the relevant discussion. For other references, see Cook and Wong (1994) [80], Mentré et al. (1997) [277], Fedorov et al. (2002) [134].

We use the terms "cost-based designs," "cost-normalized," and "penalized designs" interchangeably and hope that this does not lead to confusion.

4.1 Single Constraint

4.1.1 One-stage designs

In Section 2.4, an optimal design ξ^* is defined as

$$\xi^* = \arg \min_{\xi} \Psi[\mathbf{M}(\xi)]; \tag{4.1}$$

it is assumed and extensively used that

$$\int \xi(d\mathbf{x}) = 1. \tag{4.2}$$

The constraint (4.2) may be considered a continuous analog of the constraint that is imposed on the number of observations N,

$$\sum_{i=1}^{n} r_i = N, \tag{4.3}$$

see (1.1). In fact, the problem (4.1), (4.2) can be viewed as an approximation of the following optimization problem:

$$\xi_N^* = \arg \min_{\xi_N} \Psi[N\mathbf{M}(\xi_N)], \tag{4.4}$$

subject to

$$\sum_{i=1}^{n} r_i = N \leq N^*, \tag{4.5}$$

if conditions of Section 2.4 hold. When measurements at a point $\mathbf{x}$ are associated with some cost, or penalty, $\phi(\mathbf{x})$, one can replace the constraint (4.5) with

$$\underline{\Phi}(\xi_N) = \sum_{i=1}^{n} r_i \phi(\mathbf{x}_i) \leq \Phi^*, \tag{4.6}$$

where Φ^* is the constraint on the total cost (penalty), or, equivalently, in the continuous design setting,

$$N\Phi(\xi_N) \leq \Phi^*, \quad \text{where } \Phi(\xi_N) = \sum_{i=1}^{n} p_i \phi(\mathbf{x}_i). \tag{4.7}$$

More generally, $\Phi(\xi) = \int_{\mathfrak{X}} \phi(\mathbf{x})\xi(d\mathbf{x})$. To simplify notations, we omit $\boldsymbol{\theta}$ from the arguments of the cost function, but a reader should keep in mind that costs (penalties) may depend on parameters. For instance, the penalty may depend on the response $\eta(\mathbf{x}, \boldsymbol{\theta})$.

Using the continuous approximation of (4.4) and (4.7), we arrive at the following optimization problem:

$$\xi^* = \arg \min_{\xi} \Psi[N\mathbf{M}(\xi)], \quad \text{subject to} \quad N\,\Phi(\xi) = \Phi^*. \tag{4.8}$$

It follows from the monotonicity and homogeneity of criteria Ψ (cf. Section 2.3), that the optimization problem (4.8) can be written as

$$\xi^* = \arg \min_{\xi} \Psi \left[\frac{\Phi^*}{\Phi(\xi)} \mathbf{M}(\xi) \right] = \arg \min_{\xi} \Psi \left[\frac{\mathbf{M}(\xi)}{\Phi(\xi)} \right]. \tag{4.9}$$

Obviously, the solution ξ^* of the optimization problem (4.9) does not depend either on N or Φ^*. However, to satisfy the constraint in (4.8), one needs to adjust the sample size:

$$N^* = \Phi^*/\Phi(\xi^*). \tag{4.10}$$

Note that in the "continuous" setting, the optimization problem (4.8) is equivalent to

$$\xi^* = \arg\min_{\xi} N\Phi(\xi), \quad \text{subject to } \Psi[N\mathbf{M}(\xi)] = \Psi^*. \tag{4.11}$$

In general, the criterion in (4.9) is not a convex function of $\xi \in \Xi(\mathfrak{X})$. However, this criterion is quasiconvex: a real-valued function g, defined on a convex set $X \subset R^n$, is said to be quasiconvex if

$$g[\alpha\mathbf{x}_1 + (1-\alpha)\mathbf{x}_2] \leq \max\{g(\mathbf{x}_1), g(\mathbf{x}_2)\}, \ 0 \leq \alpha \leq 1; \tag{4.12}$$

see Avriel (2003) [26], Chapter 6.1. For quasiconvex functions, most results used in convex optimization stay valid; see also the discussion of the criterion (4.34) later in this section.

To solve the optimization problem (4.9) for penalized designs, the expressions for directional derivatives as in (2.69) – (2.72) must be modified accordingly. For example, for the D-criterion,

$$\xi^* = \arg\min_{\xi} \left[-\ln \left| \frac{\mathbf{M}(\xi)}{\Phi(\xi)} \right| \right] = \arg\min_{\xi}[-\ln |\mathbf{M}(\xi)| + m \ln \Phi(\xi)].$$

If $\mathbf{M}_\alpha$ and $G(\alpha)$ are introduced as in (2.65) and (2.67), respectively, then the analog of (2.69) is

$$G'(\alpha) = -\text{tr}\{\mathbf{M}_\alpha^{-1}[\mathbf{M}(\bar{\xi}) - \mathbf{M}(\xi)]\} + \frac{m[\Phi(\bar{\xi}) - \Phi(\xi)]}{\Phi(\xi_\alpha)}, \tag{4.13}$$

so letting $\alpha \to 0$, we conclude that the analog of the function $\dot{G}(\xi, \bar{\xi})$ in (2.68) is

$$
\begin{aligned}
\dot{G}(\xi, \bar{\xi}) &= m - \int \bar{\xi}(d\mathbf{x})\text{tr}\left[\mathbf{M}^{-1}(\xi)\boldsymbol{\mu}(\mathbf{x})\right] + m \int \bar{\xi}(d\mathbf{x})\frac{\phi(\mathbf{x})}{\Phi(\xi)} - m \\
&= \int \bar{\xi}(d\mathbf{x})\left\{\frac{m\phi(\mathbf{x})}{\Phi(\xi)} - \text{tr}\left[\mathbf{M}^{-1}(\xi)\boldsymbol{\mu}(\mathbf{x})\right]\right\}. \tag{4.14}
\end{aligned}
$$

For the penalized D-criterion, the analog of function $\psi(\mathbf{x}, \xi)$ in (2.70) is

$$\psi_c(\mathbf{x}, \xi) = \frac{m\phi(\mathbf{x})}{\Phi(\xi)} - \text{tr}[\mathbf{M}^{-1}(\xi) \, \boldsymbol{\mu}(\mathbf{x})]. \tag{4.15}$$

Therefore, a necessary and sufficient condition of D-optimality of the design ξ is

$$\text{tr}\left[\mathbf{M}^{-1}(\xi) \, \boldsymbol{\mu}(\mathbf{x})\right] \leq \frac{m\phi(\mathbf{x})}{\Phi(\xi)}, \quad \forall \, \mathbf{x} \in \mathfrak{X}, \tag{4.16}$$

and on each forward step of the first-order optimization algorithm, one has to maximize the function

$$d_c(\mathbf{x}, \xi) = \text{tr}\left[\mathbf{M}^{-1}(\xi) \, \boldsymbol{\mu}(\mathbf{x})\right] - \frac{m\phi(\mathbf{x})}{\Phi(\xi)} \tag{4.17}$$

over $\mathfrak{X}$. On backward steps one has to minimize this function over the support set of the current design.

An alternative way of analyzing penalized designs can be obtained via the direct normalization of information matrices by the total cost $\underline{\Phi}(\xi_N)$. Indeed, let

$$\mathbf{M}_c(\xi_N) = \underline{\mathbf{M}}(\xi_N)/\underline{\Phi}(\xi_N) \;=\; \mathbf{M}(\xi_N)/\Phi(\xi_N). \qquad (4.18)$$

It follows from the definition of $\underline{\mathbf{M}}(\xi_N)$ and $\underline{\Phi}(\xi_N)$ that

$$\mathbf{M}_c(\xi_N) \;=\; \frac{\sum_i r_i \boldsymbol{\mu}(\mathbf{x}_i)}{\sum_i r_i \phi(\mathbf{x}_i)} \;=\; \sum_i \tilde{p}_i \,\boldsymbol{\mu}_c(\mathbf{x}_i), \qquad (4.19)$$

where

$$\tilde{p}_i = \frac{r_i \phi(\mathbf{x}_i)}{\underline{\Phi}(\xi_N)}, \quad \boldsymbol{\mu}_c(\mathbf{x}_i) = \frac{\boldsymbol{\mu}(\mathbf{x}_i)}{\phi(\mathbf{x}_i)}, \qquad (4.20)$$

and a cost-normalized design ξ_c is defined as $\xi_c = \{\mathbf{x}_i, \tilde{p}_i, \ \sum_i \tilde{p}_i = 1\}$. In the continuous setting cost-normalized designs can be introduced via

$$\mathbf{M}_c(\xi) = \mathbf{M}(\xi_c) = \int_{\mathfrak{X}} \boldsymbol{\mu}_c(\mathbf{x})\xi_c(d\mathbf{x}) = \mathbf{M}(\xi)/\Phi(\xi), \qquad (4.21)$$

where

$$\xi_c(d\mathbf{x}) = \xi(d\mathbf{x})\frac{\phi(\mathbf{x})}{\Phi(\xi)}, \quad \boldsymbol{\mu}_c(\mathbf{x}) = \frac{\boldsymbol{\mu}(\mathbf{x})}{\phi(\mathbf{x})}.$$

The results of Section 2.5 can be applied directly to cost-normalized designs (measures) ξ_c and cost-normalized information matrices $\mathbf{M}(\xi_c)$. For example, for D-optimality the function $\psi(\mathbf{x}, \xi)$ in (2.70) must be replaced with

$$\tilde{\psi}_c(\mathbf{x}, \xi_c) = m - \mathrm{tr}[\mathbf{M}^{-1}(\xi_c)\,\boldsymbol{\mu}_c(\mathbf{x})]. \qquad (4.22)$$

Therefore, a necessary and sufficient condition of D-optimality of the design ξ_c is

$$\mathrm{tr}\left[\mathbf{M}^{-1}(\xi_c)\,\boldsymbol{\mu}_c(\mathbf{x})\right] \;\leq\; m, \quad \forall\, \mathbf{x} \in \mathfrak{X}. \qquad (4.23)$$

In the iterative procedure based on cost-based designs, one has to maximize the sensitivity function

$$\tilde{d}_c(\mathbf{x}, \xi_c) = \mathrm{tr}[\mathbf{M}^{-1}(\xi_c)\,\boldsymbol{\mu}_c(\mathbf{x})]. \qquad (4.24)$$

The directional derivatives (4.15) and (4.22) are different, which is natural because they correspond to two different sets of probability measures, $\Xi(\mathfrak{X})$ and $\Xi(\mathfrak{X}_c)$. However, both (4.15) and (4.22) lead to the same necessary and sufficient condition of D-optimality. Indeed, it follows from (4.21) that the necessary and sufficient condition (4.23) is equivalent to (4.16). Therefore, the numerical procedures based on (4.17) and (4.24) lead to the same optimal designs.

Remark 4.1 It follows from (4.21) that the sensitivity function in (4.24) can be presented as

$$\tilde{d}_c(\mathbf{x}, \xi_c) = \text{tr} \left[\mathbf{M}^{-1}(\xi) \, \frac{\mu(\mathbf{x})}{\phi(\mathbf{x})} \right] \Phi(\xi). \qquad (4.25)$$

Let

$$\hat{d}_c(\mathbf{x}, \xi) = \text{tr} \left[\mathbf{M}^{-1}(\xi) \, \frac{\mu(\mathbf{x})}{\phi(\mathbf{x})} \right]. \qquad (4.26)$$

Then the maximization, with respect to $\mathbf{x}$, of $\hat{d}_c(\mathbf{x}, \xi^*)$ in (4.26) is equivalent to the maximization of $\tilde{d}_c(\mathbf{x}, \xi_c^*)$ in (4.25). This provides an explanation of using (4.26) as an analog of the sensitivity function in the first-order optimization algorithm for penalized designs; see (6.6) and (8.2). Note also that (4.21) implies that the directional derivative in (4.22) can be presented as

$$\tilde{\psi}_c(\mathbf{x}, \xi_c) = \left\{ \frac{m\phi(\mathbf{x})}{\Phi(\xi)} - \text{tr} \left[\mathbf{M}^{-1}(\xi) \, \mu(\mathbf{x}) \right] \right\} \frac{\Phi(\xi)}{\phi(\mathbf{x})}. \qquad (4.27)$$

Since $\Phi(\xi)$ and $\phi(\mathbf{x})$ are both positive, it follows from (4.27) that the numerical procedures based on (4.17) and (4.24) select new design points in the same direction. For further discussion of the use of (4.26), see Section 5.3.

Recall that when standard normalized designs $\xi = \{p_i, \mathbf{x}_i\}$ of Section 2.4 are constructed, the optimal weights p_i are multiplied by N, and values $r_i' = N p_i$ are rounded to the nearest integer r_i while preserving the equality $\sum_i r_i = N$; see Section 3.3. For penalized designs, if one uses the numerical procedure based on the sensitivity function $d_c(\mathbf{x}, \xi)$ in (4.17), the above algorithm of calculating the actual r_i will not change. On the other hand, if the numerical procedure for penalized designs is based on the sensitivity function $\tilde{d}_c(\mathbf{x}, \xi)$ in (4.24), then because of the change of measures $\xi \to \xi_c$, the optimal weights $\tilde{p}_i$ must be adjusted by costs $\phi(\mathbf{x}_i)$ to obtain $r_i' = \tilde{p}_i \Phi^* / \phi(\mathbf{x}_i)$. Unlike the case of standard normalization, for cost-based designs the allocation ratios r_{i2}/r_{i1} are, in general, not equal to the ratios of weights $\tilde{p}_{i2}/\tilde{p}_{i1}$ because

$$\frac{r_{i2}}{r_{i1}} = \frac{\tilde{p}_{i2}}{\tilde{p}_{i1}} \times \frac{\phi(\mathbf{x}_{i1})}{\phi(\mathbf{x}_{i2})}. \qquad (4.28)$$

For an illustration of (4.28), see examples in Sections 7.2.4 and 7.4.2.

In the examples of Sections 6.4.2, 6.5.1, 6.5.2 we use the first-order optimization procedure based on (4.26). In the examples of Sections 7.2.3, 7.2.4, 7.4.2 we utilize the first-order optimization procedure based on (4.24). In the examples of Section 9.2 we use the numerical procedure based on (4.17). Experimenting with different approaches did not reveal any preferences. However, only the approach based on (4.17) can be easily generalized for two-stage (composite) or Bayesian designs; see Section 4.1.2.

4.1.2   Two-stage designs

For two-stage designs, we assume that the design for the first stage ξ_0 is available and fixed, with sample size N_0. The total sample size is N, so that the sample size of the second stage is $N - N_0$; cf. Section 2.7.

When the total penalty for the two stages is limited by Φ^*, the optimal design can be defined as

$$\xi^* = \arg\min_{\xi} \Psi[N_0 \mathbf{M}(\xi_0) + (N - N_0)\mathbf{M}(\xi)] \qquad (4.29)$$

subject to

$$N_0 \Phi(\xi_0) + (N - N_0)\Phi(\xi) \leq \Phi^*, \qquad (4.30)$$

where the criterion Ψ is convex and homogeneous. Denoting $\delta = N_0/N$, rewrite (4.29), (4.30) as

$$\xi^* = \arg\min_{\xi} \Psi\{N[\delta \mathbf{M}(\xi_0) + (1 - \delta)\mathbf{M}(\xi)]\} \qquad (4.31)$$

subject to

$$N[\delta \Phi(\xi_0) + (1 - \delta)\Phi(\xi)] \leq \Phi^*. \qquad (4.32)$$

Assume that δ is fixed. The constraint in (4.32) implies $N(\xi) = \Phi^*/[\delta\Phi(\xi_0) + (1 - \delta)\Phi(\xi)]$, and thus

$$
\begin{aligned}
\xi^* &= \arg\min_{\xi} \Psi\{[\delta \mathbf{M}(\xi_0) + (1 - \delta)\mathbf{M}(\xi)]\ \Phi^*/[\delta\Phi(\xi_0) + (1 - \delta)\Phi(\xi)]\} \\
&= \arg\min_{\xi} \gamma(\Phi^*)\Psi\left[\frac{\delta \mathbf{M}(\xi_0) + (1 - \delta)\mathbf{M}(\xi)}{\delta\Phi(\xi_0) + (1 - \delta)\Phi(\xi)}\right],
\end{aligned} \qquad (4.33)
$$

where γ is a nonincreasing function; see (2.42). Thus the optimization problem for the second stage in the two-stage design is equivalent to

$$\xi^* = \arg\min_{\xi} \Psi\left[\frac{\mathbf{A} + \mathbf{M}(\xi)}{a + \Phi(\xi)}\right], \qquad (4.34)$$

where $\mathbf{A} = \frac{\delta}{1-\delta}\mathbf{M}(\xi_0)$ and $a = \frac{\delta}{1-\delta}\Phi(\xi_0)$. Both $\mathbf{A}$ and a are fixed given the fixed initial design ξ_0.

Similar to the criterion in (4.9), the criterion in (4.34) is quasiconvex; see (4.12). Consider the design $\bar{\xi} = (1 - \alpha)\xi^* + \alpha\xi$, where ξ^* is the optimal design and ξ is an arbitrary design. For D-optimality, the directional derivative of Ψ in the direction of $\bar{\xi}$ is

$$
\begin{aligned}
\frac{\partial}{\partial\alpha} &\log \left|\frac{\mathbf{A} + \mathbf{M}(\xi)}{a + \Phi(\xi)}\right|^{-1}_{\alpha=0} \\
&= m\,\frac{\Phi(\xi) - \Phi(\xi^*)}{a + \Phi(\xi^*)} - \mathrm{tr}\,\{[\mathbf{A} + \mathbf{M}(\xi^*)]^{-1}[\mathbf{M}(\xi) - \mathbf{M}(\xi^*)]\}, \quad (4.35)
\end{aligned}
$$

where m is the number of unknown parameters. For quasiconvex criteria, the necessary and sufficient condition of the optimality of ξ^* is nonnegativeness of the directional derivative (4.35),

$$\text{tr}\{[\mathbf{A} + \mathbf{M}(\xi^*)]^{-1}\mathbf{M}(\xi)\} - \frac{m\Phi(\xi)}{a + \Phi(\xi^*)}$$

$$\leq \quad \text{tr}\{[\mathbf{A} + \mathbf{M}(\xi^*)]^{-1}\mathbf{M}(\xi^*)\} - \frac{m\Phi(\xi^*)}{a + \Phi(\xi^*)} \,. \tag{4.36}$$

The inequality (4.36) is of little help because it should be verified for all possible ξ. However, instead of examining all possible designs, one can verify (4.36) only for designs atomized at a single point; see Section 2.5. Indeed, with $\mathbf{M}(\xi) = \int_{\mathfrak{X}} \boldsymbol{\mu}(\mathbf{x})\xi(d\mathbf{x})$ and $\Phi(\xi) = \int_{\mathfrak{X}} \phi(\mathbf{x})\xi(d\mathbf{x})$, one can verify that for any design ξ,

$$\max_{\xi} \left[\text{tr}\{[\mathbf{A} + \mathbf{M}(\xi^*)]^{-1}\mathbf{M}(\xi)\} - \frac{m\Phi(\xi)}{a + \Phi(\xi^*)} \right]$$

$$= \quad \max_{\xi} \left\{ \int_{\mathfrak{X}} \left[\text{tr}\{[\mathbf{A} + \mathbf{M}(\xi^*)]^{-1}\boldsymbol{\mu}(\mathbf{x})\} - \frac{m\phi(\mathbf{x})}{a + \Phi(\xi^*)} \right] \xi(d\mathbf{x}) \right\}$$

$$= \quad \max_{\mathbf{x} \in \mathfrak{X}} \left\{ \text{tr}\{[\mathbf{A} + \mathbf{M}(\xi^*)]^{-1}\boldsymbol{\mu}(\mathbf{x})\} - \frac{m\phi(\mathbf{x})}{a + \Phi(\xi^*)} \right\}. \tag{4.37}$$

Therefore, the inequality

$$\text{tr}\{[\mathbf{A} + \mathbf{M}(\xi^*)]^{-1}\boldsymbol{\mu}(\mathbf{x})\} - \frac{m\phi(\mathbf{x})}{a + \Phi(\xi^*)}$$

$$\leq \quad \text{tr}\{[\mathbf{A} + \mathbf{M}(\xi^*)]^{-1}\mathbf{M}(\xi^*)\} - \frac{m\Phi(\xi^*)}{a + \Phi(\xi^*)}, \ \forall \, \mathbf{x} \in \mathfrak{X}, \tag{4.38}$$

is the necessary and sufficient condition of optimality of ξ^*. The equality in (4.38) holds for all support points of ξ^*. The analog of the sensitivity function for the second stage in the two-stage design is

$$\varphi(\mathbf{x}, \xi) = \text{tr}\{[\mathbf{A} + \mathbf{M}(\xi)]^{-1}\boldsymbol{\mu}(\mathbf{x}) - \frac{m\phi(\mathbf{x})}{a + \Phi(\xi)}; \tag{4.39}$$

cf. (4.17) and Table 2.1. If $\mathbf{A} = \mathbf{0}$, $a = 0$, $\boldsymbol{\mu}(\mathbf{x}) = \mathbf{f}(\mathbf{x})\mathbf{f}^T(\mathbf{x})$, and $\phi(\mathbf{x}) \equiv$ *const*, then (4.39) coincides, up to the sign, with (2.70). The results of this section will be used in the examples of Chapters 6 and 8.

4.2 Multiple Constraints

It is clear from the previous section of this chapter that a single constraint does not cause too much difficulty and can be reduced to the standard case where the assumption (4.2) is valid. The construction of optimal designs with multiple constraints is a more challenging task. For the sake of simplicity we assume that the first constraint is as in (4.2), or $N \leq N^*$ in the nonnormalized case. Other type of constraints can be reduced to (4.2) using (4.18) and (4.19).

Let us start with the optimization problem (4.4) in the nonnormalized setting, with constraints (4.5) and additional constraints

$$\sum_{i=1}^{n} r_i \phi'(\mathbf{x}_i) \leq \mathbf{\Phi}^*, \tag{4.40}$$

where ϕ' and $\mathbf{\Phi}$ are $\ell \times 1$ vectors. After the normalization and the standard transition to normalized designs we face the optimization problem (4.1) subject to (4.2) and

$$\int_{\mathcal{X}} \phi'(\mathbf{x}) \xi(d\mathbf{x}) \leq \mathbf{C}, \quad \text{where} \quad \mathbf{C} = \mathbf{\Phi}^*/N. \tag{4.41}$$

We will use transformed functions

$$\phi(\mathbf{x}) = \phi'(\mathbf{x}) - \mathbf{C}, \tag{4.42}$$

which allows us to rewrite (4.41) as

$$\int_{\mathcal{X}} \phi(\mathbf{x}) \xi(d\mathbf{x}) \leq \mathbf{0}. \tag{4.43}$$

Theorem 4.1 *Let assumptions (A1), (A2) and (B1) – (B4) from Section 2.4 hold. Let designs from $\Xi(q)$ satisfy (4.43) and let the function $\phi(\mathbf{x})$ be continuous for all $\mathbf{x} \in \mathcal{X}$. Then the following statements hold:*

1. *For any optimal design there exists a design with the same information matrix that contains no more than $m(m+1)/2 + \ell$ support points.*

2. *A necessary and sufficient condition for a design ξ^* to be optimal is the inequality*
$$\min_{\mathbf{x}} q(\mathbf{x}, \mathbf{u}^*, \xi^*) \geq 0,$$
where $q(\mathbf{x}, \mathbf{u}, \xi) = \psi(\mathbf{x}, \xi) + \mathbf{u}^T \phi(\mathbf{x})$, $\mathbf{u}^* = \arg\max_{\mathbf{u} \in \mathbf{U}} \min_{\mathbf{x}} q(\mathbf{x}, \mathbf{u}, \xi^*)$, and $\mathbf{U} = \{\mathbf{u} : \mathbf{u} \in R^\ell, u_i \geq 0, i = 1, \ldots, \ell\}$.

3. *The set of optimal designs is convex.*

4. *The function $q(\mathbf{x}, \mathbf{u}^*, \xi^*)$ attains zero almost everywhere in $\mathrm{supp}\xi^*$.*

Proof.
1. Note that any pair $\{\mathbf{M}(\xi), \Phi(\xi)\}$ belongs to the convex hull of
$$\{\mu(\mathbf{x}), \phi(\mathbf{x})\} \in R^{m(m+1)/2+\ell}$$

and apply Carathéodory's Theorem; cf. Theorem 2.1.

2. The inequality

$$\min_{\xi} \int \psi(\mathbf{x}, \xi^*) \, \xi(d\mathbf{x}) \geq \mathbf{0}, \tag{4.44}$$

together with the inequality (4.43), constitutes a necessary and sufficient condition of optimality of ξ^*. In general, no single-point design exists that satisfies both (4.43) and (4.44), unlike some previously considered cases; see (2.60), (2.61) and (4.36), (4.37).

The Lagrangian theory indicates the duality of the optimization problem (4.43), (4.44) and the maximin problem

$$\max_{\mathbf{u} \in U} \min_{\xi} \int q(\mathbf{x}, \mathbf{u}, \xi^*) \, \xi(d\mathbf{x}); \tag{4.45}$$

see Laurent (1972) [248], Chapter 7. Since

$$\min_{\xi} \int q(\mathbf{x}, \mathbf{u}, \xi^*) \, \xi(d\mathbf{x}) = \min_{\mathbf{x} \in \mathfrak{X}} q(\mathbf{x}, \mathbf{u}, \xi^*),$$

the optimization problem (4.45) is equivalent to

$$\max_{\mathbf{u} \in U} \min_{\mathbf{x}} q(\mathbf{x}, \mathbf{u}, \xi^*),$$

which confirms the second assertion of the theorem. The proofs of the other two parts of the theorem coincide with that of the corresponding results for the unconstrained case. □

Numerical procedures. The numerical procedures discussed in Chapter 3 must be modified in order to handle the optimization problem defined in (4.1), (4.2), (4.43). The simplest version of an iterative procedure is based on the first-order algorithm and comprises the following steps:

(a) Given $\xi_s \in \Xi(q)$, find

$$\xi^s = \arg\min_{\xi} \int \psi(\mathbf{x}, \xi_s) \xi(d\mathbf{x}), \quad \text{subject to} \quad \int \phi(\mathbf{x}) \xi(d\mathbf{x}) \leq \mathbf{0}. \tag{4.46}$$

(b) Choose $0 \leq \alpha_s \leq 1$ and construct

$$\xi_{s+1} = (1 - \alpha_s)\xi_s + \alpha_s \xi^s. \tag{4.47}$$

Unlike the standard case, the optimization problem (4.46) cannot be reduced to the minimization of the function $\psi(\mathbf{x}, \xi_s)$, which is a relatively simple problem. The minimization can be simplified by applying Carathéodory's Theorem: one can verify the existence of a design ξ^s that has no more than $\ell + 1$ support points. Thus, (4.46) can be reduced to a finite-dimensional problem:

$$\xi^s = \left\{ \begin{array}{ccc} \mathbf{x}_1^s & \cdots & \mathbf{x}_{\ell+1}^s \\ p_1^s & \cdots & p_{\ell+1}^s \end{array} \right\} = \arg\min_{\{p_j, \mathbf{x}_j\}} \sum_{j=1}^{\ell+1} p_j \, \psi(\mathbf{x}_j, \xi_s) \tag{4.48}$$

subject to

$$p_j \geq 0, \quad \sum_{j=1}^{\ell+1} p_j \, \phi(\mathbf{x}_j) \leq \mathbf{0}, \quad \sum_{j=1}^{\ell+1} p_j = 1. \tag{4.49}$$

The proof of convergence of this iterative procedure is identical to that for the standard case; see Theorem 3.3. The optimization problem (4.48), (4.49) is practically solvable if the number of constraints ℓ and the dimension of $\mathfrak{X}$ is reasonably small.

As an example of the optimization problem (4.48), (4.49), consider the case of the single constraint $\ell = 1$, which is additional to the constraint (4.2). Assume that the constraint is active, i.e.,

$$p_1\phi(\mathbf{x}_1) + (1 - p_1)\phi(\mathbf{x}_2) = p_1[\phi(\mathbf{x}_1) - \phi(\mathbf{x}_2)] + \phi(\mathbf{x}_2) = 0.$$

Note that $\phi(\mathbf{x}_1)$ and $\phi(\mathbf{x}_2)$ must be of opposite signs, otherwise the design ξ^s is atomized on the single point. Let

$$p^* = p^*(\mathbf{x}_1, \mathbf{x}_2) = \frac{\phi(\mathbf{x}_2)}{\phi(\mathbf{x}_2) - \phi(\mathbf{x}_1)},$$

and

$$p_1^*(\mathbf{x}_1, \mathbf{x}_2) = \begin{cases} 1, & \text{if } p^* \geq 1, \\ p^*, & \text{if } 0 < p^* < 1, \\ 0, & \text{if } p^* \leq 0. \end{cases} \tag{4.50}$$

Combining (4.48) and (4.50) when $0 < p_1^*(\mathbf{x}_1, \mathbf{x}_2) < 1$, one gets the following optimization problem on step s:

$$\xi^s = \arg \min_{\mathbf{x}_1, \mathbf{x}_2} \{p_1^*(\mathbf{x}_1, \mathbf{x}_2)\psi(\mathbf{x}_1, \xi_s) + [1 - p_1^*(\mathbf{x}_1, \mathbf{x}_2)] \, \psi(\mathbf{x}_2, \xi_s)\}.$$

4.3 Constraints for Auxiliary Criteria

The approach developed in Section 4.1 can be applied with some modifications to a more general design problem:

$$\xi^* = \arg \min_{\xi} \Psi(\xi) \quad \text{subject to} \quad \Phi(\xi) \leq 0, \tag{4.51}$$

where the components of $\Phi^T = (\Phi_1, \ldots, \Phi_\ell)$ can be from a very general class of functions of ξ. All constraints are assumed to be active for ξ^*. In addition to assumptions (A1), (A2) and (B1) – (B4) from Section 2.4, let us assume that

(C1) All components of $\Phi(\xi)$ are convex;

(C2) There exists a real number q such that the set

$$\{\xi \colon \Psi(\xi) \le q < \infty, \ \Phi(\xi) \le 0\} = \Xi(q) \qquad (4.52)$$

is not empty;

(C3) For any $\xi \in \Xi(q)$ and $\overline{\xi} \in \Xi$,

$$\Phi\left[(1-\alpha)\xi + \alpha\overline{\xi}\right] = \Phi(\xi) + \alpha \int \phi(\mathbf{x}, \xi)\,\overline{\xi}(d\mathbf{x}) + o(\alpha|\xi, \overline{\xi}). \qquad (4.53)$$

Assumptions (C1), (C2), and (C3) are almost identical to assumptions (B1), (B3), and (B4) of Section 2.4, respectively, but deal with $\Phi(\xi)$ instead of $\Psi(\xi)$.

Extended version of Theorem 4.1. The analysis of (4.51) is based on ideas of Section 4.1 and makes use of the linearization of $\Phi(\xi)$ at ξ^*. A necessary and sufficient condition of optimality of the design ξ^* is identical to the one stated in part 2 of Theorem 4.1 with the obvious replacement of $\phi(\mathbf{x})$ with $\phi(\mathbf{x}, \xi^*)$. In this case we will speak of the "extended version" of Theorem 4.1.

To give a feeling of how the extended version of Theorem 4.1 works, below we provide two examples that can be embedded in the design problem (4.51).

Uncertainty of the model. Consider the problem of finding a D-optimal design for the response $\boldsymbol{\theta}_0^T \mathbf{f}_0(\mathbf{x})$ while ensuring that this design is reasonably "good" for the alternative responses $\boldsymbol{\theta}_j^T \mathbf{f}_j(\mathbf{x})$, $j = 1, \ldots, \ell$:

$$\begin{aligned}
\Psi(\xi) &= -\log|\mathbf{M}_0(\xi)|, \\
\Phi_j(\xi) &= -\log|\mathbf{M}_j(\xi)| - c_j , \quad j = 0, \ldots, \ell,
\end{aligned}$$

where $\mathbf{M}_j(\xi) = \int \mathbf{f}_j(\mathbf{x})\mathbf{f}_j^T(\mathbf{x})\,\xi(d\mathbf{x})$. Recall that for the D-criterion

$$\begin{aligned}
\psi(\mathbf{x}, \xi) &= m_0 - d_0(\mathbf{x}, \xi), \\
\phi_j(\mathbf{x}, \xi) &= m_j - d_j(\mathbf{x}, \xi),
\end{aligned}$$

where m_j is the number of unknown parameters in the j-th response function and $d_j(\mathbf{x}, \xi) = \mathbf{f}_j^T(\mathbf{x})\mathbf{M}_j^{-1}(\xi)\mathbf{f}_j(\mathbf{x})$. Assume further that all basis functions are continuous in $\mathcal{X}$ and that assumption (C2) holds. Then all assumptions of the extended version of Theorem 4.1 hold, and a necessary and sufficient condition of optimality of ξ^* is the existence of vector $\mathbf{u}^*$ such that

$$d(\mathbf{x}, \xi^*) + \sum_{j=1}^{\ell} u_j^* d_j(\mathbf{x}, \xi^*) \le m_0 + \sum_{j=1}^{\ell} u_j^* m_j, \qquad (4.54)$$

while $\Phi(\xi^*) = 0$. The equality in (4.54) holds at all support points of ξ^*.

Uncertainty with respect to the optimality criterion. Consider the problem of minimization of a particular criterion while having "acceptable" values of some auxiliary criteria. Let $\boldsymbol{\theta}^T \mathbf{f}(\mathbf{x})$ be the model of interest, and let the goal of the experiment be to find a design that minimizes $\Psi(\xi) = -\log|\mathbf{M}(\xi)|$, while keeping $\text{tr}[\mathbf{M}^{-1}(\xi)]$ at a relatively low level. This means that

$$\Phi(\xi) = \text{tr}[\mathbf{M}^{-1}(\xi)] - c.$$

The extended version of Theorem 4.1 states that a necessary and sufficient condition of optimality of ξ^* is the existence of $u^* \geq 0$ such that

$$d(\mathbf{x}, \xi^*) + u^* \mathbf{f}^T(\mathbf{x})\mathbf{M}^{-2}(\xi^*)\mathbf{f}(\mathbf{x}) \;\leq\; m + u^* \text{tr}[\mathbf{M}^{-1}(\xi^*)]. \qquad (4.55)$$

4.4   Directly Constrained Design Measures

In many spatial experiments, several closely located sensors do not contribute much more information than each individual sensor separately. In pharmacokinetic studies, with blood samples taken over time, it makes little sense to take consecutive samples too close in time because of limited added information and ethical concerns. In both examples the "density" of sensor/time allocation should be lower than some reasonable level. For a design measure ξ this means that

$$\xi(d\mathbf{x}) \leq \omega(d\mathbf{x}), \qquad (4.56)$$

where $\omega(d\mathbf{x})$ describes the maximal "number" of sensors per unit space $d\mathbf{x}$ (number of samples per unit time). It is assumed that $\int \omega(d\mathbf{x}) \geq 1$; if the equality holds, then we cannot do anything better than take $\xi(d\mathbf{x}) = \omega(d\mathbf{x})$. Let us consider the following optimization problem:

$$\xi^* = \arg\min \Psi(\xi) \;\; \text{subject to} \;\; \xi(d\mathbf{x}) \leq \omega(d\mathbf{x}). \qquad (4.57)$$

The solution of (4.57) is called a (Ψ, ω)-optimal design. Whenever this is not ambiguous we will skip (Ψ, ω).

Let us assume in addition to assumptions (B1) – (B4) from Section 2.4 that

(D)   The measure ω is atomless, i.e., for any ΔX there exists a subset $\Delta X' \subset \Delta X$ such that

$$\int_{\Delta X'} \omega(d\mathbf{x}) < \int_{\Delta X} \omega(d\mathbf{x}),$$

cf. Karlin and Studden (1966) [225], Chapter VIII.12. The sets Ξ and $\Xi(q)$ in (B4) have to satisfy the constraint (4.56). Let $\overline{\Xi}$ be a set of design measures such that $\xi(\Delta X) = \omega(\Delta X)$ for any $\Delta X \subset \text{supp}\xi$ and $\xi(\Delta X) = 0$ otherwise.

A function $\psi(\mathbf{x}, \xi)$ is said to separate sets X_1 and X_2 with respect to the measure $\omega(dx)$ if for any two sets $\Delta X_1 \subset X_1$ and $\Delta X_2 \subset X_2$ with equal nonzero measures

$$\int_{\Delta X_1} \psi(\mathbf{x}, \xi) \, \omega(dx) \le \int_{\Delta X_2} \psi(\mathbf{x}, \xi) \, \omega(dx). \tag{4.58}$$

Theorem 4.2 *If assumptions (B1) – (B4) and (D) hold, then*

1. $\xi^* \in \overline{\overline{\Xi}}$ *exists;*

2. *A necessary and sufficient condition of* (Ψ, ω)-*optimality for* $\xi^* \in \overline{\overline{\Xi}}$ *is that* $\psi(\mathbf{x}, \xi^*)$ *separates* $X^* = \mathrm{supp}\xi^*$ *and* $\mathfrak{X} \setminus X^*$.

Proof. The results of the theorem are based on the moment spaces theory.
1. The existence of an optimal design follows from the compactness of the set of information matrices. The fact that at least one optimal design belongs to $\overline{\overline{\Xi}}$ is a corollary of Liapunov's Theorem on the range of vector measures; cf. Karlin and Studden (1966) [225], Chapter VIII.12. This theorem states that for any design measure ξ satisfying (4.56), such that $\int_{\mathfrak{X}} \xi(dx) = \int_{\mathfrak{X}} q(\mathbf{x}) \, \omega(dx) = 1$ and $0 \le q(x) \le 1$, there exists a subset $X' \subset \mathfrak{X}$ such that

$$\int_{X'} \mathbf{f}(\mathbf{x})\mathbf{f}^T(\mathbf{x}) \, \omega(dx) = \mathbf{M}(\xi) \quad \text{and} \quad \int_{X'} \omega(dx) = 1,$$

where

$$\mathbf{M}(\xi) = \int_{\mathfrak{X}} \mathbf{f}(\mathbf{x})\mathbf{f}^T(\mathbf{x}) \, \xi(dx) = \int_{\mathfrak{X}} \mathbf{f}(\mathbf{x})\mathbf{f}^T(\mathbf{x}) q(\mathbf{x}) \omega(dx).$$

A measure $\xi'(dx)$ that satisfies $\xi'(dx) = \omega(dx)$ if $\mathbf{x} \in X'$ and $\xi'(dx) \equiv 0$ otherwise, can be considered a design from $\overline{\overline{\Xi}}$.
2. The necessity follows from the fact that if there exist subsets $\Delta X_1 \subset X^*$ and $\Delta X_2 \subset \mathfrak{X} \setminus X^*$ with nonzero measures such that

$$\int_{\Delta X_1} \psi(\mathbf{x}, \xi^*) \, \omega(dx) > \int_{\Delta X_2} \psi(\mathbf{x}, \xi^*) \, \omega(dx),$$

then deletion of ΔX_1 from the support set and subsequent inclusion of ΔX_2 causes a decrease of Ψ; cf. (2.63). This contradicts the optimality of ξ^*.
   To prove the sufficiency we assume that $\xi^* \in \overline{\overline{\Xi}}$ is non-optimal and $\xi \in \overline{\overline{\Xi}}$ is optimal, i.e.,

$$\Psi[\mathbf{M}(\xi^*)] > \Psi[\mathbf{M}(\xi)] + \delta \tag{4.59}$$

for some $\delta > 0$. Let $\overline{\xi} = (1 - \alpha)\xi^* + \alpha\xi$; then the convexity of Ψ implies that

$$\begin{aligned}
\Psi[\mathbf{M}(\overline{\xi})] &\le (1 - \alpha)\Psi[\mathbf{M}(\xi^*)] + \alpha\Psi[\mathbf{M}(\xi)] \\
&\le (1 - \alpha)\Psi[\mathbf{M}(\xi^*)] + \alpha\{\Psi[\mathbf{M}(\xi^*)] - \delta\} \\
&= \Psi[\mathbf{M}(\xi^*)] - \alpha\delta. \tag{4.60}
\end{aligned}$$

On the other hand, assumption (B4) states that

$$\Psi[\mathbf{M}(\overline{\xi})] = \Psi[\mathbf{M}(\xi^*)] + \alpha \int_{\mathfrak{X}} \psi(\mathbf{x}, \xi^*)\, \xi(d\mathbf{x}) + o(\alpha).$$

Let
$$\text{supp}\xi = (X^* \setminus D) \cup E$$

for $D \subset X^*$, $E \subset (\mathfrak{X} \setminus X^*)$, and $E \cap D = \emptyset$, where $\int_E \omega(d\mathbf{x}) = \int_D \omega(d\mathbf{x})$ to assure that $\int_{\mathfrak{X}} \xi(d\mathbf{x}) = \int_{\mathfrak{X}} \xi^*(d\mathbf{x}) = 1$. Then

$$\int_{\mathfrak{X}} \psi(\mathbf{x}, \xi^*)\, \xi(d\mathbf{x}) \tag{4.61}$$
$$= \int_{X^*} \psi(\mathbf{x}, \xi^*)\, \omega(d\mathbf{x}) + \int_E \psi(\mathbf{x}, \xi^*)\, \omega(d\mathbf{x}) - \int_D \psi(\mathbf{x}, \xi^*)\, \omega(d\mathbf{x}).$$

If $\overline{\xi} = \xi$ and $\alpha \to 0$ in assumption (B4), then

$$\int_{\mathfrak{X}} \psi(\mathbf{x}, \xi)\, \xi(d\mathbf{x}) = 0.$$

As a consequence,

$$\int_{X^*} \psi(\mathbf{x}, \xi^*)\, \omega(d\mathbf{x}) = \int_{\mathfrak{X}} \psi(\mathbf{x}, \xi^*)\, \xi^*(d\mathbf{x}) = 0.$$

The assumption of separation (4.58) implies

$$\int_E \psi(\mathbf{x}, \xi^*)\, \omega(d\mathbf{x}) \geq \int_D \psi(\mathbf{x}, \xi^*)\, \omega(d\mathbf{x}),$$

so
$$\int_{\mathfrak{X}} \psi(\mathbf{x}, \xi^*)\, \xi(d\mathbf{x}) \geq 0$$

and
$$\Psi[\mathbf{M}(\overline{\xi})] \geq \Psi[\mathbf{M}(\xi^*)] + o(\alpha). \tag{4.62}$$

The contradiction of (4.59) and (4.62) completes the proof. $\square$

To summarize, let us note that in spite of its seemingly abstract form, Theorem 4.2 contains the following, rather simple message. For the D-criterion, the sensitivity function $d(\mathbf{x}, \xi^*)$ must be the largest at support points of the optimal design ξ^*. The same statement is true for any sensitivity function $\varphi(\mathbf{x}, \xi^*)$ from Table 2.1: similar to the standard case, observations must be allocated at points where we know least about the response. Recall also that $\xi^*(d\mathbf{x}) = \omega(d\mathbf{x})$ at all support points.

How to use Theorem 4.2 in practice? In the example of sensor allocation, for a given spatial area ΔX, one can take the number of sensors $N^*(\Delta X)$ as

$$N^*(\Delta X) = \left[N \int_{\Delta X} \xi^*(d\mathbf{x}) \right]^+$$

and allocate them uniformly, e.g., at the nodes of some uniform grid.

Iterative procedure. Theorem 4.2 suggests that $\xi^*(d\mathbf{x})$ should be different from 0 in areas where the function $\psi(\mathbf{x}, \xi^*)$ is small. Therefore, relocating some measure from areas with higher values of this function to those with smaller values should improve ξ. This simple idea can be implemented in various numerical procedures. We consider one particular procedure that is similar to the iterative procedure based on the first-order algorithm.

(a) For a design $\xi_s \in \overline{\Xi}$, let $X_{1s} = \mathrm{supp}\xi_s$ and $X_{2s} = \mathfrak{X} \setminus X_{1s}$; find

$$\mathbf{x}_{1s} = \arg\max_{\mathbf{x} \in X_{1s}} \psi(\mathbf{x}, \xi_s) , \quad \mathbf{x}_{2s} = \arg\min_{\mathbf{x} \in X_{2s}} \psi(\mathbf{x}, \xi_s),$$

and two sets $D_s \subset X_{1s}$ and $E_s \subset X_{2s}$ such that $\mathbf{x}_{1s} \in D_s$, $\mathbf{x}_{2s} \in E_s$, and

$$\int_{D_s} \omega(d\mathbf{x}) = \int_{E_s} \omega(d\mathbf{x}) = \alpha_s$$

for some $\alpha_s > 0$.

(b) Construct ξ_{s+1} such that

$$\mathrm{supp}\xi_{s+1} = X_{1,s+1} = (X_{1s} \setminus D_s) \cup E_s.$$

If sequence $\{\alpha_s\}$ satisfies (3.7) and if the conditions of Theorem 4.2 and assumption (B4′) from Section 3.2 hold, then $\{\Psi(\xi_s)\}$ converges to the optimal design ξ^* defined by (4.57). The proof of this statement is almost identical to the proof of Theorem 3.3.

In most problems, $\omega(d\mathbf{x}) = q(\mathbf{x})d\mathbf{x}$. These cases may be reduced to the case where $q(\mathbf{x}) \equiv c$ for some real c by an appropriate transformation of the coordinates. For $q(\mathbf{x}) \equiv c$, all integrals may be replaced by sums over some regular grid elements in the computerized version of the iterative procedure. If these elements are fixed and D_s and E_s coincide with the grid elements, then the above iterative procedure may be considered a special version of the exchange algorithm with one simple constraint: no grid element can have more than one support point, and the weights of all support points are the same and equal to N^{-1}.

Chapter 5

Nonlinear Response Models

5.1 Bridging Linear and Nonlinear Cases 128
5.2 Mitigating Dependence on Unknown Parameters 129
5.3 Box and Hunter Adaptive Design 131
5.4 Generalized Nonlinear Regression: Use of Elemental Information Matrices 136
5.5 Model Discrimination 141

The main ideas that are used to construct optimal designs for nonlinear models are fundamentally similar to those in the linear case. This was the main reason for us spending so many pages exploring the latter. To bridge the two cases, let us start with the simple example of a single response with additive errors as in Section 1.4,

$$y_i = \eta(\mathbf{x}_i, \boldsymbol{\theta}) + \varepsilon_i, \tag{5.1}$$

where $\eta(\mathbf{x}, \boldsymbol{\theta})$ is a given nonlinear function, and $\{\varepsilon_i\}$ are independent random variables with zero mean and constant variance σ^2.

Recall that in the estimation problem we linearize the model, i.e., use the Taylor expansion up to the first-order term, cf. (1.72):

$$\eta(\mathbf{x}, \boldsymbol{\theta}) \simeq \eta(\mathbf{x}, \boldsymbol{\theta}_t) + (\boldsymbol{\theta} - \boldsymbol{\theta}_t)^T \mathbf{f}(\mathbf{x}, \boldsymbol{\theta}_t), \quad \mathbf{f}(\mathbf{x}, \boldsymbol{\theta}) = \frac{\partial \eta(\mathbf{x}, \boldsymbol{\theta})}{\partial \boldsymbol{\theta}}, \tag{5.2}$$

where $\boldsymbol{\theta}_t$ is the point of "immediate" interest. Depending on the problem at hand, $\boldsymbol{\theta}_t$ may correspond to the true value, the "guesstimate," the prior value of the parameter, etc. There exists a steady stream of publications where the second-order approximation of the response function is used; see Pázman (1986, 1993) [306] [307]; Pázman and Pronzato (1992, 1994, 2013) [319], [320], [322]. However, the methods advocated in these publications are substantially more complicated, and a question arises whether it is worthwhile to use very "precise" techniques while working with models that are just another approximation of the reality. For instance, the assumption about homogeneous variance can be easily viewed as an oversimplified description of observational errors. Likewise, the assumptions about the specific shape of $\eta(\mathbf{x}, \boldsymbol{\theta})$ (e.g., the response being described by the solution of a simple system of linear differential equations as in the examples of pharmacokinetic (PK) studies considered in Chapter 7) are related only to the basic features of the underlying phenomenon (drug absorption, disposition, metabolism and elimination in PK examples). Such assumptions often neglect many real-life factors that, when incorporated in the model, can make the underlying problem much more challenging than the addition of the higher-order terms in (5.2). From our point of view, the approximation (5.2) and what follows from it is a reasonable compromise between the complexity of the design problem and potential benefits that one may get by applying the corresponding designs.

Having said that, we nevertheless encourage an "evaluation" of the accuracy of the first-order approximation if it does not lead to unreasonable efforts. For instance, if the response $\eta(\mathbf{x}, \boldsymbol{\theta})$ is given in closed form (and not as an output of the numerical solution of the system of differential equations, as it often happens in PK studies with higher-order elimination, see (7.81)), then one can easily calculate the second-order correction to $\eta(\mathbf{x}, \boldsymbol{\theta}_t)$; see Remark 7.1 in Section 7.2.2 and examples in Section 7.5.6.

Similar to Chapter 2, we start the exposition in this chapter utilizing only the first two moments of the errors $\{\varepsilon_i\}$. The exploration of cases based on the explicit use of the distribution of observed responses is postponed to Section 5.4.

5.1   Bridging Linear and Nonlinear Cases

Consider the information matrix as presented in (1.75), (1.77) and (1.78). Recall that the variance of the LSE can be approximated by

$$\text{Var}[\hat{\boldsymbol{\theta}}_N] \cong \underline{\mathbf{M}}^{-1}(\xi_N, \boldsymbol{\theta}_t), \tag{5.3}$$

where $\boldsymbol{\theta}_t$ is the true parameter value. Similar to the linear case, it is expedient to introduce the normalized information matrix

$$\mathbf{M}(\xi, \boldsymbol{\theta}_t) = \frac{1}{N} \, \underline{\mathbf{M}}(\xi_N, \boldsymbol{\theta}_t), \tag{5.4}$$

or, in the continuous design setting,

$$\mathbf{M}(\xi, \boldsymbol{\theta}_t) = \int_{\mathfrak{X}} \boldsymbol{\mu}(\mathbf{x}, \boldsymbol{\theta}_t)\xi(d\mathbf{x}), \quad \boldsymbol{\mu}(\mathbf{x}, \boldsymbol{\theta}_t) = \sigma^{-2} \, \mathbf{f}(\mathbf{x}, \boldsymbol{\theta}_t)\mathbf{f}^T(\mathbf{x}, \boldsymbol{\theta}_t), \tag{5.5}$$

where $\mathbf{f}(\mathbf{x}, \boldsymbol{\theta}_t)$ is introduced in (5.2). We can exploit the ideas considered in Chapter 2, repeating everything, almost word for word, that led us to (2.52). Compared to the design problem in the linear case, there is one essential difference: the information matrix $\mathbf{M}(\xi, \boldsymbol{\theta}_t)$ depends on unknown parameters $\boldsymbol{\theta}_t$. Consequently, the solution of the optimization problem

$$\xi^*(\boldsymbol{\theta}_t) = \arg \min_{\xi \in \Xi} \, \Psi\left[\mathbf{M}(\xi, \boldsymbol{\theta}_t)\right] \tag{5.6}$$

does depend on $\boldsymbol{\theta}_t$ too. Chernoff (1953) [70] coined the term "locally optimal design" to emphasize that $\xi^*(\boldsymbol{\theta}_t)$ is optimal only for the specific parameter value. However, once we assume that $\boldsymbol{\theta}_t$ is given (for example, a "perfect guess"), then the full machinery presented in Chapters 2 and 3 can be applied. Let us emphasize two main distinctions between optimal designs for linear models and locally optimal designs for nonlinear models: in the latter case, the formulae (5.3) – (5.6) are only approximations (which can be questionable for moderate sample size N and rather large variance σ^2), and the parameter value θ_t is unknown. A rather extensive literature exists that is devoted to the construction of locally optimal designs. To name a few references, see Box and Lucas (1959) [54]; Fedorov (1969, 1972) [125], [127]; Cochran (1973) [77]; Silvey (1980) [360], Chapter 6; Kitsos et al. (1988) [233]; Ford et al. (1992) [162]; Atkinson and Donev (1992) [19], Chapter 18; Atkinson et al. (1993) [16].

It is clear that the direct applicability of locally optimal designs is much less obvious than the applicability of optimal designs in the linear case. Still, locally optimal designs are widely accepted as benchmarks that help to evaluate efficiency of more "practical" designs; see examples in Chapters 6 and 7. Moreover, the concept of locally optimal design can be extended in various directions, of which the most popular extensions are "averaged" criteria (often referred to as a Bayesian approach), minimax criteria, and adaptive (multi-stage) designs; see, for instance, Fedorov and Pázman (1968) [150]; Fedorov (1969, 1972) [125], [127]; Fedorov and Malyutov (1972) [148]; White (1973, 1975) [399], [398]; Chaloner and Verdinelli (1995) [65].

5.2 Mitigating Dependence on Unknown Parameters

Averaging. The idea of integrating out unknown parameters was partially explored in Section 2.9. Similar to (2.113), we can introduce the secondary criterion

$$\Psi_{\mathcal{F}}(\xi) = \int_{\Theta} \Psi[\mathbf{M}(\xi, \boldsymbol{\theta})]\, \mathcal{F}(d\boldsymbol{\theta}), \tag{5.7}$$

and replace the optimization problem (5.6) with

$$\xi_{\mathcal{F}}^* = \arg\min_{\xi}\ \Psi_{\mathcal{F}}(\xi). \tag{5.8}$$

The criterion (5.7) is associated with the Bayesian approach, and the corresponding optimal designs are often called Bayesian optimal designs; cf. Chaloner and Verdinelli (1995) [65]. We prefer to call these designs "conservative Bayesian designs" to emphasize that no prior information is used to improve the estimation of parameters $\boldsymbol{\theta}$ explicitly as it is traditionally done in the Bayesian setting. The analog of the optimization problem (2.100) of Section 2.7 is now

$$\Psi_{\mathcal{F}}(\xi) = \int_{\Theta} \ln|\mathbf{M}(\xi, \boldsymbol{\theta}) + \mathbf{D}_0^{-1}|\, \mathcal{F}(d\boldsymbol{\theta}), \tag{5.9}$$

where $\mathbf{D}_0$ is the variance-covariance matrix of the distribution $\mathcal{F}$.

Under mild regularity conditions integration and differentiation (i.e., calculation of directional derivatives in the design case) are interchangeable. Therefore, all results like Equivalence Theorems or numerical procedures can be readily derived from the results of Chapters 2 and 3 by adding integration in all corresponding formulae. For instance, for the A-criterion, the sensitivity function $\varphi(\mathbf{x}, \xi) = \operatorname{tr}[\boldsymbol{\mu}(\mathbf{x})\mathbf{M}^{-1}(\xi)\mathbf{A}\mathbf{M}^{-1}(\xi)]$ should be replaced with

$$\varphi(\mathbf{x}, \xi) = \int_{\Theta} \operatorname{tr}\left[\boldsymbol{\mu}(\mathbf{x}, \boldsymbol{\theta})\mathbf{M}^{-1}(\xi, \boldsymbol{\theta})\mathbf{A}\mathbf{M}^{-1}(\xi, \boldsymbol{\theta})\right] \mathcal{F}(d\boldsymbol{\theta}), \qquad (5.10)$$

with $\boldsymbol{\mu}(\mathbf{x}, \boldsymbol{\theta})$ defined in (5.5).

Some caution is required with criteria like the D-criterion; see (2.14), (2.46), (2.47), or Kiefer's criterion (2.18). In the former case we can introduce secondary criteria:

$$\int |\mathbf{M}(\xi, \boldsymbol{\theta})|^{-1}\mathcal{F}(d\boldsymbol{\theta}), \quad \int \ln |\mathbf{M}(\xi, \boldsymbol{\theta})|^{-1}\mathcal{F}(d\boldsymbol{\theta}), \quad \int |\mathbf{M}(\xi, \boldsymbol{\theta})|^{-1/m}\mathcal{F}(d\boldsymbol{\theta});$$
$$(5.11)$$

see Pronzato and Walter (1985, 1988) [323], [324]; Ermakov (1983) [115]; Chaloner and Verdinelli (1995) [65]. Each of the criteria in (5.11) leads, in general, to different optimal designs while locally optimal designs for the criteria $|\mathbf{M}(\xi, \boldsymbol{\theta})|^{-1}$, $\ln |\mathbf{M}(\xi, \boldsymbol{\theta})|^{-1}$ and $|\mathbf{M}(\xi, \boldsymbol{\theta})|^{-1/m}$ are obviously identical. Similarly, locally optimal designs for the linear criteria $\operatorname{tr}\left[\|\mathbf{M}^{-\gamma}(\xi, \boldsymbol{\theta})\|\right]^{1/\gamma}$ and $\operatorname{tr}\left[\|\mathbf{M}^{-\gamma}(\xi, \boldsymbol{\theta})\|\right]$ are the same, while optimal designs for criteria

$$\int \operatorname{tr}\left[\|\mathbf{M}^{-\gamma}(\xi, \boldsymbol{\theta})\|\right]^{1/\gamma} \mathcal{F}(d\boldsymbol{\theta}) \,, \quad \int \operatorname{tr}\left[\|\mathbf{M}^{-\gamma}(\xi, \boldsymbol{\theta})\|\right] \mathcal{F}(d\boldsymbol{\theta})$$

are, in general, different.

Note that in Section 2.9 the information matrix itself does not depend on model parameters, while in the problems in this section its dependence on $\boldsymbol{\theta}$ makes the integration formidably more difficult, and all computations are often discouragingly computer intensive.

Minimax approach. Similar to Section 2.9, we can replace (5.6) with the secondary optimization problem that corresponds to another, more cautious way of eliminating unknown parameters from the original criterion:

$$\xi^* = \arg\min_{\xi} \ \max_{\boldsymbol{\theta}\in\Theta} \ \Psi\left[\mathbf{M}(\xi, \boldsymbol{\theta})\right]. \qquad (5.12)$$

From an analytical viewpoint, there is nothing new in (5.12) compared to the optimization problem (2.114): indeed, $\boldsymbol{\theta}$ in (5.12) is the direct analog of $\mathbf{u}$ in (2.114). In particular, Theorem 2.5 holds, and the discussion of minimax designs in Section 2.9 can be repeated here. To make the optimization problem (5.12) computationally affordable, it is recommended to confine the parameter set Θ to a discrete set; cf. Atkinson and Fedorov (1988) [22]. See also examples in Section 6.5.

Other extensions of the locally optimal design concept can be made, in particular for optimal design under constraints: the results of Chapter 4 are applicable if one replaces $\boldsymbol{\mu}(\mathbf{x}), \mathbf{M}(\xi)$ with $\boldsymbol{\mu}(\mathbf{x}, \boldsymbol{\theta}), \mathbf{M}(\xi, \boldsymbol{\theta})$, and $\phi(\mathbf{x}), \Phi(\xi)$ with $\phi(\mathbf{x}, \boldsymbol{\theta}), \Phi(\xi, \boldsymbol{\theta})$. Obviously, the sensitivity functions will depend on $\boldsymbol{\theta}$ as well.

For a practitioner, an adaptive design is likely the most promising alternative to the locally optimal designs. However, one has to continue to use locally optimal designs as benchmarks. In particular, from a methodological perspective it is important to prove the convergence of the adaptive design to the locally optimal design with $\boldsymbol{\theta} = \boldsymbol{\theta}_t$. The adaptive approach is outlined in the next section.

5.3 Box and Hunter Adaptive Design

Let us recall the first-order optimization algorithm for the D-criterion; see Section 3.1. Rewrite the forward step in the nonlinear case by introducing an additional argument $\boldsymbol{\theta}_t$, cf. (3.2), (3.3):

$$\mathbf{x}_{s+1} = \arg\max_{\mathbf{x}} \; d(\mathbf{x}, \xi_s, \boldsymbol{\theta}_t), \tag{5.13}$$

where

$$d(\mathbf{x}, \xi_s, \boldsymbol{\theta}_t) = \mathbf{f}^T(\mathbf{x}, \boldsymbol{\theta}_t)\mathbf{M}^{-1}(\xi_s, \boldsymbol{\theta}_t)\mathbf{f}(\mathbf{x}, \boldsymbol{\theta}_t)$$

and

$$\mathbf{M}(\xi_{s+1}, \boldsymbol{\theta}_t) = (1 - \alpha_s)\mathbf{M}(\xi_s, \boldsymbol{\theta}_t) + \alpha_s \sigma^{-2}\mathbf{f}(\mathbf{x}_{s+1}, \boldsymbol{\theta}_t)\mathbf{f}^T(\mathbf{x}_{s+1}, \boldsymbol{\theta}_t). \tag{5.14}$$

Now let us associate the step index s with the number of observations N, and let $s = N$. Then the matrix $\mathbf{M}(\xi_N, \boldsymbol{\theta}_t)$ can be interpreted as the normalized information matrix while the nonnormalized matrix is presented as

$$\underline{\mathbf{M}}(\xi_N, \boldsymbol{\theta}_t) = \sum_{i=1}^{N} \sigma^{-2}\mathbf{f}(\mathbf{x}_i, \boldsymbol{\theta}_t)\mathbf{f}(\mathbf{x}_i, \boldsymbol{\theta}_t). \tag{5.15}$$

Note that in (5.15) some of the design points $\{\mathbf{x}_i\}$ may coincide; cf. (1.11). In nonnormalized notations, when $\alpha_N = 1/(N+1)$, the iterative procedure (5.13), (5.14) takes the form

$$\mathbf{x}_{N+1} = \arg\max_{\mathbf{x}} \; \underline{d}(\mathbf{x}, \xi_N, \boldsymbol{\theta}_t), \tag{5.16}$$

where

$$\underline{d}(\mathbf{x}, \xi_N, \boldsymbol{\theta}_t) = \mathbf{f}^T(\mathbf{x}, \boldsymbol{\theta}_t)\underline{\mathbf{M}}^{-1}(\xi_N, \boldsymbol{\theta}_t)\mathbf{f}(\mathbf{x}, \boldsymbol{\theta}_t)$$

and

$$\underline{\mathbf{M}}(\xi_{N+1}, \boldsymbol{\theta}_t) = \underline{\mathbf{M}}(\xi_N, \boldsymbol{\theta}_t) + \sigma^{-2}\mathbf{f}(\mathbf{x}_{N+1}, \boldsymbol{\theta}_t)\mathbf{f}^T(\mathbf{x}_{N+1}, \boldsymbol{\theta}_t). \tag{5.17}$$

The procedure (5.16), (5.17) can be viewed as a one-step-forward adaptive design. Indeed, (5.16) suggests to take the $(N+1)$-th observation at a point where the prediction of the response is the worst, i.e., $\mathrm{Var}[\eta(\mathbf{x}, \boldsymbol{\theta}_t)]$ is the largest. Step (5.17) provides a correction of the information matrix after the $(N+1)$-th observation has been taken. The procedure looks rather simple except for the fact that $\boldsymbol{\theta}_t$ is unknown. In real-life applications, parameter $\boldsymbol{\theta}_t$ should be estimated, which requires the modification of (5.16) and (5.17). Specifically, the unknown parameter $\boldsymbol{\theta}_t$ should be replaced with its current estimate $\boldsymbol{\theta}_N$ ("plug-in" approach), which leads to the following adaptive design:

$$\mathbf{x}_{N+1} = \arg\max_{\mathbf{x}\in\mathfrak{X}} \underline{d}(\mathbf{x}, \xi_N, \hat{\boldsymbol{\theta}}_N), \tag{5.18}$$

$$\hat{\boldsymbol{\theta}}_{N+1} = \arg\min_{\boldsymbol{\theta}\in\Theta} \sum_{j=1}^{N+1} [y_j - \eta(\mathbf{x}_j, \boldsymbol{\theta})]^2, \tag{5.19}$$

$$\underline{\mathbf{M}}(\xi_{N+1}, \hat{\boldsymbol{\theta}}_{N+1}) = \underline{\mathbf{M}}(\xi_N, \hat{\boldsymbol{\theta}}_{N+1}) + \sigma^{-2}\mathbf{f}(\mathbf{x}_{N+1}, \hat{\boldsymbol{\theta}}_{N+1})\mathbf{f}^T(\mathbf{x}_{N+1}, \hat{\boldsymbol{\theta}}_{N+1}). \tag{5.20}$$

The extension of the results to other optimality criteria is straightforward: one has to replace $\underline{d}(\mathbf{x}, \xi_N, \hat{\boldsymbol{\theta}}_N)$ on the right-hand side of (5.18) by the non-normalized version of the function $\varphi(\mathbf{x}, \xi)$ from Table 2.1. For example, for the A-criterion $\mathrm{tr}(\mathbf{AD})$, one has to use

$$\underline{\varphi}(\mathbf{x}, \xi_N, \hat{\boldsymbol{\theta}}_N) = \mathrm{tr}[\boldsymbol{\mu}(\mathbf{x}, \hat{\boldsymbol{\theta}}_N)\underline{\mathbf{M}}^{-1}(\xi_N, \hat{\boldsymbol{\theta}}_N)\mathbf{A}\underline{\mathbf{M}}^{-1}(\xi_N, \hat{\boldsymbol{\theta}}_N)],$$

where $\boldsymbol{\mu}(\mathbf{x}, \hat{\boldsymbol{\theta}}_N) = \mathbf{f}(\mathbf{x}, \hat{\boldsymbol{\theta}}_N)\mathbf{f}^T(\mathbf{x}, \hat{\boldsymbol{\theta}}_N)$.

The adaptive design in (5.18) – (5.20) was proposed in the Bayesian setting by Box and Hunter (1965) [53], who did not discuss the asymptotic properties of the procedure. It follows from (5.20) and (10.11) that

$$|\underline{\mathbf{M}}(\xi_{N+1}, \boldsymbol{\theta})| = |\underline{\mathbf{M}}(\xi_N, \boldsymbol{\theta})| \ [1 + \sigma^{-2}\mathbf{f}^T(\mathbf{x}_{N+1}, \boldsymbol{\theta})\underline{\mathbf{M}}^{-1}(\xi_N, \boldsymbol{\theta}) \ \mathbf{f}(\mathbf{x}_{N+1}, \boldsymbol{\theta})]. \tag{5.21}$$

Obviously, the maximization of the expression on the right-hand side of (5.21) is equivalent to the maximization problem

$$\max_{\mathbf{x}_{N+1}} \ \mathbf{f}(\mathbf{x}_{N+1}, \boldsymbol{\theta})\underline{\mathbf{M}}^{-1}(\xi_N, \boldsymbol{\theta}) \ \mathbf{f}^T(\mathbf{x}_{N+1}, \boldsymbol{\theta}). \tag{5.22}$$

In the linear case, the information matrix $\underline{\mathbf{M}}$ and basis functions $\mathbf{f}(\mathbf{x})$ do not depend on $\boldsymbol{\theta}$, and therefore the solution of (5.18) provides the largest increment of the determinant of the information matrix. In the nonlinear case, the solution of (5.18) assures the largest determinant of the matrix $\underline{\mathbf{M}}^{-1}(\xi_{N+1}, \hat{\boldsymbol{\theta}}_N)$ and not of the matrix $\underline{\mathbf{M}}^{-1}(\xi_{N+1}, \hat{\boldsymbol{\theta}}_{N+1})$. Still, one may expect that consecutive parameter estimates do not differ much, which would justify the use of the adaptive procedure (5.18) – (5.20). In the linear case, the procedure (5.18) – (5.20) can be viewed as the simplest first-order algorithm.

A similar idea (search for the largest increment/decrement of the criterion of interest) can be applied to other criteria of optimality that are discussed in the book. One can verify that the (approximately) largest decrement of the criterion is attained at the point

$$\mathbf{x}_{N+1} = \arg\max_{\mathbf{x} \in \mathfrak{X}} \varphi(\mathbf{x}, \xi_N, \hat{\boldsymbol{\theta}}_N); \tag{5.23}$$

see Fedorov (1969, 1972) [125], [127].

The adaptive designs based on (5.18) or, more generally, on (5.23) are driven by the idea of collecting maximal information per single observation. If a practitioner faces a restriction Φ^* on the total cost, instead of the restriction on the total number of observations, then one needs to adjust the selection of $\mathbf{x}_{N+1}$. The following route seems reasonable: if the cost of a single observation at $\mathbf{x}$ is $\phi(\mathbf{x})$, then spending of one "cost unit" provides an opportunity to make $1/\phi(\mathbf{x})$ observations at point $\mathbf{x}$. This suggests rewriting the expression in (5.20) as

$$\underline{\mathbf{M}}(\xi_{N+1}, \hat{\boldsymbol{\theta}}_{N+1}) \simeq \underline{\mathbf{M}}(\xi_N, \hat{\boldsymbol{\theta}}_{N+1}) + \frac{\sigma^{-2}}{\phi(\mathbf{x})} \mathbf{f}(\mathbf{x}_{N+1}, \hat{\boldsymbol{\theta}}_{N+1}) \mathbf{f}^T(\mathbf{x}_{N+1}, \hat{\boldsymbol{\theta}}_{N+1}). \tag{5.24}$$

Now it follows from (5.21) and (5.24) that for the D-criterion the next point $\mathbf{x}_{N+1}$ in the adaptive cost-based procedure may be selected as

$$\mathbf{x}_{N+1} = \arg\max_{\mathbf{x} \in \mathfrak{X}} \phi^{-1}(\mathbf{x})\, \underline{d}(\mathbf{x}, \xi_N, \hat{\boldsymbol{\theta}}_N). \tag{5.25}$$

The formula (5.25) provides a heuristic justification of the use of the formula (4.26) in the adaptive penalized designs; see Remark 4.1 in Section 4.1.1. In general, the cost function $\phi(\mathbf{x})$ may depend on model parameters as in the examples of Sections 6.4, 6.5, 8.2 and 8.3.

The discussion of the convergence of the adaptive procedure started with Fedorov (1969, 1972) [125], [127], and then other authors; see Lai (2001, 2003) [242], [243]. On an intuitive level, one can expect that when the estimate $\hat{\boldsymbol{\theta}}_N$ is "close" to the true value $\boldsymbol{\theta}_t$, then design points selected according to (5.18) will "cluster" around the optimal points of the locally optimal design (5.6). However, the formal proof of the strong consistency of the estimator $\hat{\boldsymbol{\theta}}_N$ and the convergence of the adaptive design $\{\xi_N\}$ to the locally optimal design in the weak sense, i.e.,

$$\Psi\left[\frac{1}{N}\, \underline{\mathbf{M}}(\xi_N, \boldsymbol{\theta}_t)\right] \;\to\; \Psi[\mathbf{M}(\xi^*, \boldsymbol{\theta}_t)], \tag{5.26}$$

is a formidable technical problem. The design points in the adaptive procedure are selected via the optimization of a function that involves the collected data. So observations become dependent, and therefore matrix $\underline{\mathbf{M}}(\xi_N, \hat{\boldsymbol{\theta}}_N)$ is no longer the information matrix in the traditional sense. For a discussion of the theoretical properties of this approach, see Ford and Silvey (1980) [161], Malyutov (1982) [264], Wu (1985) [411], Chaudhuri and Mykland (1993) [68], Ying and Wu (1997) [421], Hu (1998) [207], Rosenberger and Hughes-Oliver (1999) [343]. See also Wu (1985a,b) [411], [412]; McLeish and Tosh (1990) [273]; Atkinson and Donev (1992) [19], Chapter 11; Zacks (1996) [424]; Flournoy et al. (1998) [159]. For examples of adaptive model-based designs in biopharmaceutical applications, see Chapter 8.

It is worthwhile noting that unlike our current presentation in which the procedure (5.18) – (5.20) is derived from (5.13), (5.14), the historical path was just the opposite: first the adaptive procedure (5.18) – (5.20) was proposed by Box and Hunter, and only after that were numerical methods of optimal design construction developed, in particular by Wynn (1970, 1972) [416], [417], and Fedorov (1969, 1972) [125], [127].

On an intuitive level, the convergence of the adaptive procedure (5.18) – (5.20) to the locally optimal design seems plausible once the strong consistency of the estimator $\boldsymbol{\theta}_N$ is established, i.e., $\boldsymbol{\theta}_N \to \boldsymbol{\theta}_t$ a.s. as $N \to \infty$. Indeed, in this case the adaptive procedure becomes very "close" to the numerical procedure (5.16), (5.17), which converges to the locally optimal design. The proof of the strong consistency of $\hat{\boldsymbol{\theta}}_N$ requires a number of strong assumptions, and the corresponding discussion is beyond the scope of this book; see references after formula (5.26). However, the situation simplifies substantially if one considers the following modification of the procedure (5.18) – (5.20); cf. Fedorov and Uspensky (1975) [151].

(a) Select a design ξ_0 that consists of m support points, $\xi_0 = \{\mathbf{x}_{01}, \ldots, \mathbf{x}_{0m}\}$, where $m = dim(\boldsymbol{\theta})$ and $|\mathbf{M}(\xi_0, \boldsymbol{\theta})| > 0$ for all $\boldsymbol{\theta} \in \boldsymbol{\Theta}$.

(b) At step N, assign the $(N+1)$-th observation to the point

$$\mathbf{x}_{N+1} = \begin{cases} \arg\max_{\mathbf{x}} \ \underline{d}(\mathbf{x}, \xi_N, \hat{\boldsymbol{\theta}}_N), & \text{with probability } 1 - \delta, \\ \mathbf{x}_j \in \xi_0, & \text{with probability } \delta, \end{cases} \quad (5.27)$$

where points $\mathbf{x}_j$ may be selected either in the systematic way (each point from ξ_0 is selected once on m consecutive steps), or randomly sampled without replacement.

(c) Find $\hat{\boldsymbol{\theta}}_{N+1}$ from (5.19).

(d) Update the information matrix as in (5.20).

Note that with the fixed $\hat{\boldsymbol{\theta}}_N \equiv \boldsymbol{\theta}$, we do not need step (c) in the above procedure, and in this case the described iterative procedure becomes a minor modification of the regularized numerical procedure of Section 3.2; see formulae (3.49) – (3.51).

When the design region $\mathfrak{X}$ has a finite number of support points, then mixing adaptation with the regular initial design ξ_0 assures the strong consistency of $\hat{\boldsymbol{\theta}}_N$. In this case it is not difficult to show that

$$\lim_{N \to \infty} \frac{1}{N} \left[|\underline{\mathbf{M}}(\xi_N, \hat{\boldsymbol{\theta}}_N)| \right]^{1/m} = \arg\min_{\xi} \; [|(1 - \delta)\mathbf{M}(\xi, \boldsymbol{\theta}_t) + \delta\mathbf{M}(\xi_0, \boldsymbol{\theta}_t)|]^{1/m}.$$

Indeed, if $\bar{y}_{jN}$ denotes the average of observations performed at a point $\mathbf{x}_{0j}$ of the initial design ξ_0 during the first N steps, then

$$\bar{y}_{jN} = \eta(\mathbf{x}_{0j}, \boldsymbol{\theta}_t) + \tilde{\varepsilon}_j,$$

where $E(\tilde{\varepsilon}_j) = 0$ and $\mathrm{Var}(\tilde{\varepsilon}_j) \approx \sigma^2/(\delta N) \to 0$ as $N \to \infty$. Thus, the portion of observations performed at the points of the initial design will suffice for the consistent estimation of $\boldsymbol{\theta}$.

The adaptive procedure described in (5.18) – (5.20) is fully adaptive, i.e., it updates parameter estimates and allocates the next design point after each observation. In practice, this is not always feasible because of the logistics of the study, i.e., when the experiment is carried out in stages. In such situations parameter estimation and/or design are performed not after every individual observation, but after data from groups of observations are collected. Several modifications of the procedure (5.18) – (5.20) are possible. To describe such procedures, introduce the following notation.

Let n_k be the number of observations on stage k, let $N_j = \sum_{k=1}^{j} n_k$ be the total number of observations up to stage j, and let the estimation be performed after collecting N_1, N_2, ... observations,

$$\hat{\boldsymbol{\theta}}_{N_j} = \arg\min_{\boldsymbol{\theta}} \sum_{i=1}^{N_j} [y_i - \eta(\mathbf{x}_i, \boldsymbol{\theta})]^2. \tag{5.28}$$

There are two options of finding new design points on stage $j + 1$. For the sake of simplicity, we resort to the D-optimality and single-response case.

Option (a). New points can be added after each measurement, in which case

$$\mathbf{x}_{N+1} = \arg\max_{\mathbf{x}} \; \underline{d}(\mathbf{x}, \xi_N, \hat{\boldsymbol{\theta}}_{N_j}) \,, \quad N_j \leq N < N_{j+1}, \tag{5.29}$$

$$\underline{\mathbf{M}}(\xi_{N+1}) = \underline{\mathbf{M}}(\xi_N) + \sigma^{-2}\mathbf{f}(\mathbf{x}_{N+1}, \hat{\boldsymbol{\theta}}_{N_j})\mathbf{f}^T(\mathbf{x}_{N+1}, \hat{\boldsymbol{\theta}}_{N_j}). \tag{5.30}$$

Option (b). All design points of stage $j + 1$ can be allocated simultaneously, after the end of stage j. This option is analogous to the construction of two-stage, or composite design as described in Section 2.7; see (2.107). The design ξ_{N_j}, i.e., all design points of the first j stages, provides an analog of the first-stage design in the notations of Section 2.7, while the design $\Xi_{j+1} = \{\mathbf{x}_{N_j+1}, \mathbf{x}_{N_j+2}, \ldots, \mathbf{x}_{N_{j+1}}\}$ corresponds to the second stage of the composite design, and $\delta = N_j/N_{j+1}$.

First we find the solution $\xi = \xi_{j+1}$ of the normalized optimization problem (2.107) via the iterative algorithm (3.1), with forward and backward steps as in (3.30) – (3.32), where the sensitivity function $d(\mathbf{x}, \xi)$ must be replaced with the function $d(\mathbf{x}, \xi_{tot})$ defined in (2.109). If $\xi_{j+1} = \{(\mathbf{x}_{j+1,l}, \ w_{j+1,l}), \ l = 1, \ldots, k_{j+1}\}$ is the constructed normalized optimal design of the "second" stage, then one computes frequencies $\tilde{p}_{j+1,l} = w_{j+1,l} \ n_{j+1}$ and rounds them to the nearest integer $p_{j+1,l}$, to keep the equality $\sum_l p_{j+1,l} = n_{j+1}$ satisfied. So, design points $\mathbf{x}_{j+1,l}$ on stage $j + 1$ will be replicated $p_{j+1,l}$ times to obtain the design Ξ_{j+1}.

In the examples discussed above we focused on the D-criterion and single-response models. The extension of our discussion to other convex optimality criteria and multiresponse models is straightforward: one has to replace $\boldsymbol{\mu}(\mathbf{x}, \boldsymbol{\theta}) = \mathbf{f}(\mathbf{x}, \boldsymbol{\theta})\mathbf{f}^T(\mathbf{x}, \boldsymbol{\theta})$ with the general expression for the information matrix as in (1.108) and use the sensitivity functions from Table 2.1 for the corresponding adaptive procedures.

5.4   Generalized Nonlinear Regression: Use of Elemental Information Matrices

In this section we provide a set of tools that makes the optimal design of experiments as routine as possible for many popular distributions where parameters depend on controllable, and perhaps uncontrollable, variables. Once a model is selected, i.e., the response function and the distribution of responses, the design procedure consists of almost identical steps for all examples enumerated and discussed in this section. We hope that this collection of results will streamline the practical aspects of experimental design, and also may lead to the development of rather simple software that can incorporate all the cases we have considered. For more details, see Atkinson et al. (2012) [23].

So far in this chapter the only assumption on the distribution of observed responses was about the existence of the first two moments. Obviously, additional information, namely, a complete knowledge of distribution of observations may help in obtaining more precise inference about unknown parameters. In what follows, we use the concept of the elemental Fisher information matrix, which was introduced in Section 1.6. Similar to Section 1.6, we assume that the distribution $y \sim p(y|\boldsymbol{\zeta})$ is known together with its elemental information matrix; see Tables 1.1 – 1.4 in Section 1.6. If parameters $\boldsymbol{\zeta}$ are functions of control variables $\mathbf{x}$ and unknown parameters $\boldsymbol{\theta}$, i.e., $\boldsymbol{\zeta} = \boldsymbol{\zeta}(\mathbf{x}, \boldsymbol{\theta})$, then the information matrix of a single observation can be presented as

$$\boldsymbol{\mu}(\mathbf{x}, \boldsymbol{\theta}) \ = \ \mathbf{F}(\mathbf{x}, \boldsymbol{\theta}) \ \nu(\boldsymbol{\zeta}, \mathbf{x}, \boldsymbol{\theta}) \ \mathbf{F}^T(\mathbf{x}, \boldsymbol{\theta}), \quad \text{where } \mathbf{F}(\mathbf{x}, \boldsymbol{\theta}) = \frac{\partial \boldsymbol{\zeta}(\mathbf{x}, \boldsymbol{\theta})}{\partial \boldsymbol{\theta}}; \quad (5.31)$$

see (1.96) and Remark 1.2 about the choice of notations. Using (5.31) and

Theorem 2.2, we can modify Table 2.1 and arrive at Table 5.1, where $\mathbf{F} = \mathbf{F}(\mathbf{x}, \boldsymbol{\theta})$ and $\boldsymbol{\nu} = \boldsymbol{\nu}(\boldsymbol{\zeta}, \mathbf{x}, \boldsymbol{\theta})$ enter the sensitivity function explicitly.

TABLE 5.1: Sensitivity function for transformations; $\mathbf{D} = \mathbf{M}^{-1}$; λ_i are eigenvalues of the matrix $\mathbf{M}$

$\Psi(\xi)$	$\varphi(\mathbf{x}, \xi, \boldsymbol{\theta})$	C
$\ln|\mathbf{D}|, \;\; |\mathbf{D}|^{1/m}, \;\; \prod_{\alpha=1}^{m} \lambda_\alpha(\mathbf{D})$	$\mathrm{tr}[\boldsymbol{\nu}\; \mathbf{F}^T \mathbf{D} \mathbf{F}]$	m
$\ln|\mathbf{A}^T \mathbf{D} \mathbf{A}|, \; dim(\mathbf{A}) = k \times m,$ $\mathrm{rank}(\mathbf{A}) = k < m$	$\mathrm{tr}[\boldsymbol{\nu}\; \mathbf{B}^T (\mathbf{A}^T \mathbf{D} \mathbf{A})^{-1} \mathbf{B}]$ $\mathbf{B} = \mathbf{F}^T \mathbf{D} \mathbf{A}$	k
$\mathrm{tr}(\mathbf{D}), \;\; \sum_{\alpha=1}^{m} \lambda_\alpha(\mathbf{D})$	$\mathrm{tr}[\boldsymbol{\nu} \mathbf{F}^T \mathbf{D}^2 \mathbf{F}]$	$\mathrm{tr}(\mathbf{D})$
$\mathrm{tr}(\mathbf{A}^T \mathbf{D} \mathbf{A}), \;\; \mathbf{A} \geq 0$	$\mathrm{tr}\{\boldsymbol{\nu}\, [\mathbf{F}^T \mathbf{D} \mathbf{A}]^2\}$	$\mathrm{tr}(\mathbf{A}^T \mathbf{D} \mathbf{A})$
$\mathrm{tr}(\mathbf{D}^\gamma), \;\; \sum_{\alpha=1}^{m} \lambda_\alpha^\gamma(\mathbf{D})$	$\mathrm{tr}[\boldsymbol{\nu} \mathbf{F}^T \mathbf{D}^{\gamma+1} \mathbf{F}]$	$\mathrm{tr}(\mathbf{D}^\gamma)$

Now the adaptive procedure (5.18) – (5.20) should be replaced with

$$\mathbf{x}_{N+1} = \arg\max_{\mathbf{x}} \; \varphi(\mathbf{x}, \xi_N, \hat{\boldsymbol{\theta}}_N), \tag{5.32}$$

$$\hat{\boldsymbol{\theta}}_{N+1} = \arg\max_{\boldsymbol{\theta} \in \Theta} \; \mathcal{L}_N \left(\boldsymbol{\theta}, \{\mathbf{x}_i\}_1^N, \; \{\mathbf{y}_i\}_1^N \right), \tag{5.33}$$

$$\underline{\mathbf{M}}(\xi_{N+1}, \hat{\boldsymbol{\theta}}_{N+1}) = \underline{\mathbf{M}}(\xi_N, \hat{\boldsymbol{\theta}}_{N+1}) + \boldsymbol{\mu}(\mathbf{x}_{N+1}, \hat{\boldsymbol{\theta}}_{N+1}), \tag{5.34}$$

where the log-likelihood function $\mathcal{L}_N$ in (5.33) is the special case of (1.84) with $r_i \equiv 1$. The sensitivity function φ in (5.32) is obtained from the second column of Table 5.1, and the information matrix $\boldsymbol{\mu}(\mathbf{x}, \boldsymbol{\theta})$ in (5.34) is defined in (5.31).

Example 5.1 *Linear regression with normal errors and constant variance*

For normally distributed observations there are two elemental parameters, the mean a and the variance σ^2; see Table 1.3. Let the variance be constant and

$$\boldsymbol{\zeta}(\mathbf{x}, \boldsymbol{\theta}) = \begin{bmatrix} a(\mathbf{x}, \vartheta) \\ \sigma^2 \end{bmatrix} = \begin{bmatrix} \mathbf{f}^T(\mathbf{x}) & 0 \\ 0 & 1 \end{bmatrix} \begin{pmatrix} \vartheta \\ \sigma^2 \end{pmatrix}. \tag{5.35}$$

Often it is assumed that σ^2 does not depend on $\mathbf{x}$. Then it follows from (5.31) and Table 5.1 that

$$\boldsymbol{\mu}(\mathbf{x}, \boldsymbol{\theta}) = \frac{1}{\sigma^2} \begin{bmatrix} \mathbf{f}(\mathbf{x})\mathbf{f}^T(\mathbf{x}) & 0 \\ 0 & \sigma^{-2}/2 \end{bmatrix}, \tag{5.36}$$

where $\boldsymbol{\theta}^T = (\vartheta^T, \sigma^2)$. Note that the information matrix of the MLE $\hat{\boldsymbol{\theta}}$ is block diagonal, i.e., the first m components $\hat{\boldsymbol{\vartheta}}$ of $\hat{\boldsymbol{\theta}}$ are independent of the last one, $\hat{\sigma}^2$.

The information matrix for the design ξ is

$$\mathbf{M}(\xi,\boldsymbol{\theta}) = \begin{bmatrix} \sigma^{-2}\,\mathbf{M}_r(\xi) & 0 \\ 0 & \sigma^{-4}/2 \end{bmatrix}, \tag{5.37}$$

where $\mathbf{M}_r(\xi) = \int \mathbf{f}(\mathbf{x})\,\mathbf{f}^T(\mathbf{x})\,\xi(d\mathbf{x})$, i.e., it does not depend on $\boldsymbol{\theta}$. It follows from Table 5.1 that the sensitivity function of the D-criterion is

$$\varphi(\mathbf{x},\xi,\boldsymbol{\theta}) = \mathbf{f}(\mathbf{x})\,\mathbf{M}_r^{-1}(\xi)\,\mathbf{f}^T(\mathbf{x}) - m_r, \quad m_r = dim(\boldsymbol{\vartheta}),$$

and a necessary and sufficient condition for ξ to be optimal is the inequality

$$\mathbf{f}^T(\mathbf{x})\,\mathbf{M}_r^{-1}(\xi)\,\mathbf{f}(\mathbf{x}) \le m_r.$$

The latter inequality is, of course, the major part of the Kiefer-Wolfowitz equivalence theorem. Note that this inequality does not contain any unknown parameters.

Example 5.2 *Normal linear regression with independently parameterized variance*

Let us assume that $\boldsymbol{\theta}^T = (\boldsymbol{\vartheta}_r^T, \boldsymbol{\vartheta}_v^T)$ and

$$\zeta(\mathbf{x},\boldsymbol{\theta}) = \begin{bmatrix} a(\mathbf{x},\boldsymbol{\vartheta}_r) \\ \ln\sigma^2(\mathbf{x},\boldsymbol{\vartheta}_v) \end{bmatrix} = \begin{bmatrix} \mathbf{f}^T(\mathbf{x}) & 0 \\ 0 & \mathbf{g}^T(\mathbf{x}) \end{bmatrix}\begin{pmatrix} \boldsymbol{\vartheta}_r \\ \boldsymbol{\vartheta}_v \end{pmatrix}. \tag{5.38}$$

It follows from (5.31) and the first line of Table 1.4 that

$$\mathbf{M}(\xi) = \begin{bmatrix} \mathbf{M}_r(\xi) & 0 \\ 0 & \mathbf{M}_v(\xi)/2 \end{bmatrix}, \tag{5.39}$$

where $\mathbf{M}_r(\xi) = \int \mathbf{f}(\mathbf{x})\mathbf{f}^T(\mathbf{x})\xi(d\mathbf{x})$ and $\mathbf{M}_v(\xi) = \int \mathbf{g}(\mathbf{x})\mathbf{g}^T(\mathbf{x})\xi(d\mathbf{x})$. From Table 5.1 we obtain

$$e^{-\boldsymbol{\vartheta}_v^T\mathbf{g}(\mathbf{x})}\,\mathbf{f}^T(\mathbf{x})\mathbf{M}_r^{-1}(\xi)\mathbf{f}(\mathbf{x}) + \frac{1}{2}\,\mathbf{g}(\mathbf{x})\mathbf{M}_v^{-1}(\xi)\mathbf{g}^T(\mathbf{x}) \le m_r + m_v,$$

where $m_r = dim(\boldsymbol{\vartheta}_r)$ and $m_v = dim(\boldsymbol{\vartheta}_v)$; cf. Atkinson and Cook (1995) [17].

Example 5.3 *One-parameter families, linear predictor function and D-optimality*

Let $\zeta(\mathbf{x},\boldsymbol{\theta}) = h[\boldsymbol{\theta}^T\,\mathbf{f}(\mathbf{x})]$, where the range of the inverse link function h coincides with the domain of the corresponding parameter (e.g., between 0 and 1 for p from Table 1.1). From (5.31) and Table 5.1 it can be immediately seen that a necessary and sufficient condition for ξ to be optimal is the inequality

$$\lambda[\boldsymbol{\theta}^T\,\mathbf{f}(\mathbf{x})]\,\mathbf{f}^T(\mathbf{x})\,\mathbf{M}^{-1}(\xi)\,\mathbf{f}(\mathbf{x}) \le m,$$

where $\lambda(u) = \nu(u)g^2(u)$, $g(u) = \partial h(u)/\partial u$ and $\mathbf{M}(\xi) = \int \mathbf{f}(\mathbf{x})\mathbf{f}^T(\mathbf{x})\xi(d\mathbf{x})$; cf. Wu (1985) [411] and Ford et al. (1992) [162].

Example 5.4 *Binary response model*

This is a special case of Example 5.3. Start with the Bernoulli distribution with parameter p; see the first entry in Table 1.1. Then consider the transformation $p = \pi[\boldsymbol{\theta}^T \mathbf{f}(\mathbf{x})]$ as in (1.92) or (1.99). In this example,

$$m' = 1 \quad \text{and} \quad \frac{\partial p}{\partial \boldsymbol{\theta}} = \dot{\pi} \mathbf{f}(\mathbf{x}).$$

Therefore, it follows from (1.96) that

$$\boldsymbol{\mu}(\mathbf{x}, \boldsymbol{\theta}) = \frac{\dot{\pi}^2 \, \mathbf{f}(\mathbf{x})\mathbf{f}^T(\mathbf{x})}{\pi(1-\pi)},$$

which obviously coincides with (1.93).

For the logistic (logit) model,

$$\pi(z) = \pi_L(z) = e^z/(1+e^z) \quad \text{and} \quad \dot{\pi} = \pi(1-\pi); \tag{5.40}$$

therefore

$$\boldsymbol{\mu}(\mathbf{x}, \boldsymbol{\theta}) = \pi(z)[1 - \pi(z)]\mathbf{f}(\mathbf{x})\mathbf{f}(\mathbf{x}) = \frac{e^z}{(1+e^z)^2} \, \mathbf{f}(\mathbf{x})\mathbf{f}^T(\mathbf{x}), \tag{5.41}$$

where $z = \mathbf{f}^T(\mathbf{x})\boldsymbol{\theta}$.

Another popular example is the probit model

$$\pi_P(z) = \mathcal{N}(z) = \int_{-\infty}^z \psi_1(u)du, \quad \text{where} \quad \psi_1(z) = \dot{\pi}_P(z) = \frac{1}{\sqrt{2\pi}}e^{-z^2/2}; \tag{5.42}$$

i.e., $\mathcal{N}$ and ψ_1 denote the probability distribution function and density function of the standard normal distribution, respectively. For the probit binary model,

$$\boldsymbol{\mu}(\mathbf{x}, \boldsymbol{\theta}) = \frac{\psi_1^2(z)}{\mathcal{N}(z)\,[1 - \mathcal{N}(z)]} \, \mathbf{f}(\mathbf{x})\mathbf{f}^T(\mathbf{x}). \tag{5.43}$$

For many distributions, parameters satisfy certain constraints. For example, parameter λ must be positive for Poisson distribution, or parameter p must belong to the interval [0,1] for Bernoulli distribution; see Table 1.1. The direct use of linear parameterization as in (1.98) may violate these constraints. Therefore, the introduction of new parameters such as $\ln \lambda$ or $\ln[p/(1-p)]$ may be expedient.

Example 5.5 *Poisson regression*

Let $\ln \lambda(\mathbf{x}, \boldsymbol{\theta}) = \mathbf{f}^T(\mathbf{x})\boldsymbol{\theta}$. Then $\mathbf{F} = \exp[\mathbf{f}^T(\mathbf{x})\boldsymbol{\theta}] \, \mathbf{f}(\mathbf{x})$, and according to the last entry in Table 1.1,

$$\boldsymbol{\mu}(\mathbf{x}, \boldsymbol{\theta}) = \exp[\mathbf{f}^T(\mathbf{x})\boldsymbol{\theta}] \, \mathbf{f}(\mathbf{x})\mathbf{f}^T(\mathbf{x}).$$

Example 5.6 *Bivariate binary response model*

Consider two binary outcomes, efficacy and toxicity, from a clinical trial. The possible combinations are $y = (y_{11}, y_{10}, y_{01}, y_{00})$ with probabilities $\boldsymbol{\vartheta}^T = (\vartheta_1, \ldots, \vartheta_4)$. It is more intuitive to denote these probabilities as p_{11}, p_{10}, p_{01} and p_{00}, respectively. The interpretation of these probabilities is "probability of efficacy and toxicity", "probability of efficacy, no toxicity," etc. Let a "single" observation be an observation performed on a cohort of size n. Then

$$P(y|p, n) = \frac{n!}{y_{11}! y_{10}! y_{01}, ! y_{00}!} p_{11}^{y_{11}} p_{10}^{y_{10}} p_{01}^{y_{01}} p_{00}^{y_{00}}, \tag{5.44}$$

where $\sum_{i=1}^{2} \sum_{j=1}^{2} y_{ij} = n$ and $\sum_{i=1}^{2} \sum_{j=1}^{2} p_{ij} = 1$. Define $\boldsymbol{\zeta} = \mathbf{p} = (p_{11}, p_{10}, p_{01})$. It follows from (1.105) that the elemental information matrix for a bivariate binary random variable and a cohort of size n is

$$\boldsymbol{\nu}(\boldsymbol{\vartheta}) = n \begin{pmatrix} p_{11} & 0 & 0 \\ 0 & p_{10} & 0 \\ 0 & 0 & p_{01} \end{pmatrix}^{-1} + \frac{n \, \mathbf{1} \mathbf{1}^T}{1 - p_{11} - p_{10} - p_{01}}, \tag{5.45}$$

where $\mathbf{1}^T = (1, 1, 1)$. The formula (5.45) will be used in the examples in Sections 6.4 and 6.5.

Example 5.7 *Gamma regression*

In the case of gamma distributed observations there are several intuitively attractive ways to define the link function. One of these is to model the parameters α and β directly:

$$\ln \alpha = \mathbf{f}^T(\mathbf{x}) \boldsymbol{\vartheta}_\alpha$$
$$\ln \beta = \mathbf{g}^T(\mathbf{x}) \boldsymbol{\vartheta}_\beta$$

Direct differentiation gives

$$\mathbf{F}(\mathbf{x}, \boldsymbol{\theta}) = \begin{bmatrix} \alpha \mathbf{f}(\mathbf{x}) & 0 \\ 0 & \beta \mathbf{f}(\mathbf{x}) \end{bmatrix}, \tag{5.46}$$

where $\boldsymbol{\theta}^T = (\boldsymbol{\vartheta}_\alpha^T, \boldsymbol{\vartheta}_\beta^T)$, and the information matrix of a single observation at $\mathbf{x}$, according to Table 1.4, is

$$\boldsymbol{\mu}(\mathbf{x}, \boldsymbol{\theta}) = \alpha \begin{bmatrix} \alpha \psi'(\alpha) \mathbf{f}(\mathbf{x}) \mathbf{f}^T(\mathbf{x}) & \mathbf{f}(\mathbf{x}) \mathbf{g}^T(\mathbf{x}) \\ \mathbf{g}(\mathbf{x}) \mathbf{f}^T(\mathbf{x}) & \mathbf{g}(\mathbf{x}) \mathbf{g}^T(\mathbf{x}) \end{bmatrix}, \tag{5.47}$$

where $\alpha = e^{\mathbf{f}^T(\mathbf{x}) \boldsymbol{\vartheta}_\alpha}$. A necessary and sufficient condition for D-optimality follows immediately from (5.46) and Table 5.1:

$$\psi'(\alpha) \mathbf{f}^T(\mathbf{x}) \left(\mathbf{M}^{-1} \right)_{\alpha\alpha} \mathbf{f}(\mathbf{x}) + \frac{2}{\beta} \mathbf{f}^T(\mathbf{x}) \left(\mathbf{M}^{-1} \right)_{\alpha\beta} \mathbf{g}(\mathbf{x})$$

$$+ \frac{\alpha}{\beta^2} \mathbf{g}^T(\mathbf{x}) \left(\mathbf{M}^{-1}\right)_{\beta\beta} \mathbf{g}(\mathbf{x}) \leq m_\alpha + m_\beta,$$

where the matrices $\left(\mathbf{M}^{-1}\right)_{\alpha\alpha}$, $\left(\mathbf{M}^{-1}\right)_{\alpha\beta}$, $\left(\mathbf{M}^{-1}\right)_{\beta\beta}$ are the blocks of the inverse information matrix corresponding to parameters $\boldsymbol{\vartheta}_\alpha$ and $\boldsymbol{\vartheta}_\beta$, respectively. Of course, one has to remember that α and β are functions of $\mathbf{x}$ and of unknown parameters.

Example 5.8 *Reparameterization of normal model*

As another example of the application of formula (1.96), let's validate the first entry in Table 1.4 where $\boldsymbol{\zeta} = (a, \sigma^2)^T$ and $\boldsymbol{\vartheta} = (a, \ln \sigma^2)^T$. Since $\vartheta_2 = \ln \zeta_2$, then $\zeta_2 = e^{\vartheta_2}$,

$$\mathbf{F} = \left(\frac{\partial \boldsymbol{\zeta}}{\partial \boldsymbol{\vartheta}}\right) = \begin{pmatrix} 1 & 0 \\ 0 & \sigma^2 \end{pmatrix},$$

and according to (1.96),

$$\boldsymbol{\nu}(\boldsymbol{\vartheta}) = \mathbf{F}\, \boldsymbol{\nu}(\boldsymbol{\zeta})\, \mathbf{F}^T = \begin{pmatrix} 1 & 0 \\ 0 & \sigma^2 \end{pmatrix} \begin{pmatrix} \frac{1}{\sigma^2} & 0 \\ 0 & \frac{1}{2\sigma^4} \end{pmatrix} \begin{pmatrix} 1 & 0 \\ 0 & \sigma^2 \end{pmatrix}$$

$$= \begin{pmatrix} \frac{1}{\sigma^2} & 0 \\ 0 & 1/2 \end{pmatrix} = \begin{pmatrix} e^{-\theta_2} & 0 \\ 0 & 1/2 \end{pmatrix}.$$

5.5 Model Discrimination

In practice there may exist several candidate models that describe a given phenomenon or process reasonably well. In such situations it is beneficial to develop designs that discriminate between models, i.e., find the most adequate one. In what follows we will assume that there are two candidate models, both of which depend on the same set of independent variables and have the structure

$$y = \eta(\mathbf{x}) + \varepsilon; \tag{5.48}$$

cf. (1.1). We assume that random errors $\{\varepsilon\}$ satisfy (1.2) where, without loss of generality, $\sigma^2 = 1$. The response function $\eta(\mathbf{x})$ is one of two known functions $\eta_1(\mathbf{x}, \boldsymbol{\theta}_1)$ or $\eta_2(\mathbf{x}, \boldsymbol{\theta}_2)$, where $\boldsymbol{\theta}_1 \in \boldsymbol{\Theta}_1 \subset R^{m_1}$, $\boldsymbol{\theta}_2 \in \boldsymbol{\Theta}_2 \subset R^{m_2}$. An experiment is performed in order to decide which one of the two models is adequate.

The results of this section will be based on the least squares estimators. Let

$$v_j(\boldsymbol{\theta}_j) = \sum_{i=1}^{n} p_i [\bar{y}_i - \eta_j(x, \boldsymbol{\theta}_j)]^2,$$

with $p_i = r_i/N$; cf. the notation of Section 1.1, in particular equation (1.9). Define the least squares estimators of θ_j as

$$\hat{\theta}_j = \arg \min_{\theta_j \in \Theta_j} v_j(\theta_j). \tag{5.49}$$

Statistical methods of model discrimination are, in general, based on a comparison of the sum of squares $v_1(\hat{\theta}_1)$ and $v_2(\hat{\theta}_2)$. In what follows we consider differences

$$d_{21} = v_2(\hat{\theta}_2) - v_1(\hat{\theta}_1). \tag{5.50}$$

Basic optimality criterion. Optimal designs for discriminating between the models will depend upon which model is the true one and, in general, will depend on the parameters of the true model. Let us assume that the first model is true, i.e., $\eta(\mathbf{x}) = \eta_1(\mathbf{x}, \theta_1)$. Obviously, the larger the difference d_{21}, the greater our inclination of accepting η_1 as the true model. The behavior of d_{21} is primarily determined by the sum of squared deviations

$$\Delta_{21}(\xi) = \sum_{i=1}^{n} p_i[\eta(\mathbf{x}_i) - \eta_2(\mathbf{x}_i, \theta_2')]^2, \tag{5.51}$$

where

$$\theta_2' = \theta_2'(\xi) = \arg \min_{\theta_2 \in \Theta_2} \sum_{i=1}^{n} p_i[\eta(\mathbf{x}_i) - \eta_2(\mathbf{x}_i, \theta_2)]^2, \tag{5.52}$$

so that the solution of the optimization problem (5.52) depends on the design ξ. The quantity $\Delta_{21}(\xi)$ is a measure of the lack of fit when $\eta_2(\mathbf{x}_i, \theta_2')$ is substituted for $\eta(\mathbf{x})$. If η_1 is the true model, then the design ξ^* that maximizes $\Delta_{21}(\xi)$, i.e.,

$$\xi^* = \arg \max_{\xi} \Delta_{21}(\xi), \tag{5.53}$$

will provide the strongest evidence of the lack of fit of the second model.

Note that if Θ_2 coincides with R^{m_2}, $\eta_2(\mathbf{x}, \theta_2) = \theta_2^T \mathbf{f}_2(\mathbf{x})$, and the errors are independently and normally distributed, then $\Delta_{21}(\xi)$ is proportional to the noncentrality parameter of the χ^2 distribution of $v_2(\theta_2')$; see Rao (1973) [334], Chapter 3b. If $N \to \infty$, then the difference d_{21} converges almost surely to $\Delta_{21}(\xi)$ under rather mild assumptions.

Locally optimal designs. The optimization problem (5.53) is a special case of the optimization problem (2.114) based on the criterion

$$\min_{\theta_2 \in \Theta_2} \Delta_{21}(\xi, \theta_2), \quad \text{where} \quad \Delta_{21}(\xi, \theta_2) = -\int [\eta(\mathbf{x}) - \eta_2(\mathbf{x}, \theta_2)]^2 \xi(d\mathbf{x}), \tag{5.54}$$

and the integral with respect to $\xi(d\mathbf{x})$ replaces the weighted sum in (5.51). We can reformulate the optimization problem (2.114) as

$$\xi^* = \arg \max_{\xi} \min_{\theta_2 \in \Theta_2} \Delta_{21}(\xi, \theta_2), \tag{5.55}$$

with

$$\Delta_{21}(\xi, \theta_2) = \int [\eta(\mathbf{x}) - \eta_2(\mathbf{x}, \theta_2)]^2 \xi(d\mathbf{x}). \tag{5.56}$$

Results similar to those of Theorem 2.5 can be proved for the criterion (5.56), which is linear with respect to ξ. Indeed, to assure that all assumptions of Theorem 2.5 hold, it is sufficient to assume that $\eta(\mathbf{x})$ and $\eta_2(\mathbf{x}, \theta_2)$ are continuous functions of $\mathbf{x} \in \mathfrak{X}$ for all $\theta_2 \in \Theta_2$; cf. Atkinson and Fedorov (1974) [21], Fedorov (1981) [130]. The analog of the function $\psi(\mathbf{x}, \xi; \mathbf{u})$ in (2.115) is

$$\Delta_{21}(\xi, \theta_2) - \varphi_{21}(\mathbf{x}, \theta_2),$$

where $\varphi_{21}(\mathbf{x}, \theta_2) = [\eta(\mathbf{x}) - \eta_2(\mathbf{x}, \theta_2)]^2$.

Theorem 5.1 *The following statements hold:*

1. *A necessary and sufficient condition for a design ξ^* to be optimal is the existence of a measure ζ^* such that*

$$\varphi'_{21}(\mathbf{x}, \xi^*) \leq \Delta'_{21}(\xi^*), \tag{5.57}$$

   where

$$\varphi'_{21}(\mathbf{x}, \xi) = \varphi'_{21}(\mathbf{x}, \xi; \zeta) = \int_{\Theta_2(\xi)} \varphi_{21}(\mathbf{x}, \theta_2) \zeta(d\theta_2), \tag{5.58}$$

$$\Theta_2(\xi) = \{\theta_2 : \theta_2 = \theta_2(\xi) = \arg \min_{\theta_2 \in \Theta_2} \Delta_{21}(\xi, \theta_2)\}, \tag{5.59}$$

   $\int_{\Theta_2(\xi)} \zeta(d\theta_2) = 1$, *and* $\Delta'_{21}(\xi) = \min_{\theta_2 \in \Theta_2} \Delta_{21}(\xi, \theta_2)\}$.

2. *The function $\varphi'_{21}(\mathbf{x}, \xi^*)$ is equal to $\Delta'_{21}(\xi^*)$ at all support points of the design ξ^*.*

3. *The set of optimal designs is convex.*

Designs for discriminating between models are called T-optimal, where T stands for testing. If the set $\Theta_2(\xi)$ in (5.59) consists of the single point, then

$$\varphi'_{21}(\mathbf{x}, \xi^*) = [\eta(\mathbf{x}) - \eta_2(\mathbf{x}, \theta'_2)]^2,$$

with $\theta'_2 = \theta'_2(\xi^*)$. This makes (5.57) rather simple for verification. In particular, we note that all observations must be made at points where the function $\eta_2(\mathbf{x}, \theta'_2)$ deviates the most from $\eta(\mathbf{x})$.

Numerical procedures. Since T-optimal designs depend on parameters of the true model $\eta(\mathbf{x}) = \eta(\mathbf{x}, \theta_1)$, it is necessary to perform sensitivity analyses for several distinct values of θ_1. To construct optimal designs, one can use analogs of numerical procedures described in Chapter 3. For instance, a first-order algorithm may be based on the following iteration on step s:

(a) Given ξ_s, find

$$
\begin{aligned}
\boldsymbol{\theta}_{2s} &= \arg \min_{\boldsymbol{\theta}_2 \in \boldsymbol{\Theta}_2} \int [\eta(\mathbf{x}) - \eta_2(\mathbf{x}, \boldsymbol{\theta}_2)]^2 \xi_s(dx), \\
\mathbf{x}_s &= \arg \max_{\mathbf{x} \in \mathfrak{X}} [\eta(\mathbf{x}) - \eta_2(\mathbf{x}, \boldsymbol{\theta}_{2s})]^2.
\end{aligned}
$$

(b) Choose α_s with $0 \leq \alpha_s \leq 1$ and construct

$$
\xi_{s+1} = (1 - \alpha_s)\xi_s + \alpha_s \xi(\mathbf{x}_s).
$$

The corresponding forward iterative procedure converges to the optimal design under mild conditions. For instance, the assumptions that $\eta_2(\mathbf{x}, \boldsymbol{\theta}_{2s})$ is continuous for all $\boldsymbol{\theta}_{2s} \in \boldsymbol{\Theta}_2$ and that the optimization problem in (5.57) has a unique solution for ξ^* are sufficient to use the results from Chapter 3. Similar to the iterative procedure (3.27) – (3.29), one can alternate between forward and backward steps to accelerate convergence. If (5.57) does not have a unique solution, then the iterative procedure may not converge to the optimal design.

To assure the convergence of the iterative procedure to a "nearly" optimal design, one can use a regularization procedure that is similar to that of Section 2.8: replace ξ_s by $\overline{\xi}_s = (1 - \delta)\xi_s + \delta\overline{\xi}$, where $\overline{\xi}$ is a regular design, i.e., the least squares estimation problem

$$
\hat{\boldsymbol{\theta}}_2(\overline{\xi}) = \arg \min_{\boldsymbol{\theta}_2 \in \boldsymbol{\Theta}_2} \int [\eta(\mathbf{x}) - \eta_2(\mathbf{x}, \boldsymbol{\theta}_2)]^2 \, \overline{\xi}(dx)
$$

has a unique solution.

Example 5.9 Two linear models: consider a constant versus a quadratic model. The two response functions are

$$
\begin{aligned}
\eta_1(x, \theta_1) &= \theta_{11}, \\
\eta_2(x, \theta_2) &= \theta_{21} + \theta_{22}x + \theta_{23}x^2,
\end{aligned}
$$

with $|x| \leq 1$. Suppose that the first model is true.

Without any restrictions on the parameters, the adequacy of the constant model implies that of the quadratic model (for the special case of $\theta_{22} = \theta_{23} = 0$). This situation is typical for so-called "nested" models where one model is a special case of the other model.

To make the models distinct, we add the constraint $\theta_{22}^2 + \theta_{23}^2 \geq 1$. If the first model is true, then the noncentrality parameter is

$$
\Delta_{21}(\xi) = \min_{\theta_{22}^2 + \theta_{23}^2 \geq 1} \int \left(\theta_{11} - \theta_{21} - \theta_{22}x - \theta_{23}x^2\right)^2 \xi(dx). \tag{5.60}
$$

The minimum will evidently occur on the set $\theta_{22}^2 + \theta_{23}^2 = 1$.

To find the optimal design, we use the same approach as for the examples of Section 2.6: first, we select some design that is intuitively reasonable and then check the optimality utilizing Theorem 5.1.

The symmetry of the design space and the constrained model η_2 imply the symmetry of the optimal design with respect to the origin. Thus, we can try the design

$$\xi^* = \left\{ \begin{array}{ccc} -1 & 0 & 1 \\ \frac{1}{4} & \frac{1}{2} & \frac{1}{4} \end{array} \right\}.$$

Note that there exist two solutions of (5.60) for this design, specifically

$$\theta_{21}^{(1)} = \theta_{11} - \frac{1}{2}, \ \theta_{22}^{(1)} = 0, \ \theta_{23}^{(1)} = 1$$

and

$$\theta_{21}^{(2)} = \theta_{11} + \frac{1}{2}, \ \theta_{22}^{(2)} = 0, \ \theta_{23}^{(2)} = -1.$$

Therefore, the sensitivity function is

$$\varphi'_{21}(x, \xi^*) = \sum_{\ell=1}^{2} \zeta_\ell \left(\theta_{11} - \theta_{21}^{(\ell)} - \theta_{22}^{(\ell)} x - \theta_{23}^{(\ell)} x^2 \right)^2.$$

For any ζ_1 and ζ_2 such that $\zeta_1 + \zeta_2 = 1$, the sensitivity function turns out to be $\phi_{21}(x, \xi^*) = (\frac{1}{2} - x^2)^2$ and has maximal values of $1/4$ at the support points of the design ξ^*. Thus, ξ^* is T-optimal. Note that the design ξ^* does not depend on θ_{11}.

However, if the second model is true, then optimal designs may become dependent on model parameters. Indeed, let us assume, without loss of generality, that $\theta_{22}, \theta_{23} < 0$. Then the T-optimal design

$$\xi^* = \left\{ \begin{array}{cc} 1 & \max(-1, -\theta_{22}/2\theta_{23}) \\ \frac{1}{2} & \frac{1}{2} \end{array} \right\}$$

allocates observations at two design points where the discrepancies between the possible values of the second model is largest. The T-optimality of the design is an obvious corollary of Theorem 5.1.

Adaptive discrimination. To address model discrimination problems, adaptive procedures that mimic the numerical construction of T-optimal design may be used. We start with some initial design ξ_{N_0} that allows for finding the unique least squares estimates $\hat{\boldsymbol{\theta}}_{1,N_0}$ and $\hat{\boldsymbol{\theta}}_{2,N_0}$. Starting from these estimates, the following adaptive procedure can be utilized; cf. (5.18) – (5.20):

$$\mathbf{x}_{N+1} = \arg\max_{\mathbf{x}} \ [\eta_1(\mathbf{x}, \hat{\boldsymbol{\theta}}_{1,N}) - \eta_2(\mathbf{x}, \hat{\boldsymbol{\theta}}_{2,N})], \tag{5.61}$$

$$\hat{\boldsymbol{\theta}}_{i,N+1} = \arg\min_{\boldsymbol{\theta}_i \in \Theta_i} \sum_{j=1}^{N+1} [y_j - \eta_i(\mathbf{x}_j, \boldsymbol{\theta}_i)]^2, \quad i = 1, 2. \tag{5.62}$$

The convergence of the adaptive procedure (5.61), (5.62) can be addressed in the same fashion as for the adaptive designs for parameter estimation problems; see Section 5.3. Some examples can be found in Atkinson and Fedorov (1974a,b) [21], [20].

Alternative design problems. In the beginning of this subsection we assumed that the first model is true and that the corresponding regression parameters are known; see (5.55). In what follows we abandon these two assumptions and instead consider the optimization problem

$$\xi^* = \arg\max_{\xi} \min_{\boldsymbol{\theta}_1 \in \boldsymbol{\Theta}_1, \theta_2 \in \boldsymbol{\Theta}_2} \int [\eta_1(\mathbf{x}, \boldsymbol{\theta}_1) - \eta_2(\mathbf{x}, \boldsymbol{\theta}_2)]^2 \xi(dx). \qquad (5.63)$$

Introducing the function $\eta(\mathbf{x}, \boldsymbol{\theta}) = \eta_1(\mathbf{x}, \boldsymbol{\theta}_1) - \eta_2(\mathbf{x}, \boldsymbol{\theta}_2)$ and the vector $\boldsymbol{\theta}^T = (\boldsymbol{\theta}_1^T, \boldsymbol{\theta}_2^T)$, we can rewrite the optimization problem (5.63) as

$$\xi^* = \arg\max_{\xi} \min_{\boldsymbol{\theta} \in \boldsymbol{\Theta}} \int \eta^2(x, \boldsymbol{\theta}) \, \xi(dx), \qquad (5.64)$$

where $\boldsymbol{\Theta} = \boldsymbol{\Theta}_1 \times \boldsymbol{\Theta}_2$. (It may be more natural to use the notation $\Delta\eta(\mathbf{x}, \boldsymbol{\theta})$ instead of $\eta(\mathbf{x}, \boldsymbol{\theta})$ for the difference of the two response functions, but we will use the latter to make notations closer to our standard notations used throughout the book). If

$$\Psi(\xi, \boldsymbol{\theta}) = \int \eta^2(x, \boldsymbol{\theta}) \, \xi(dx), \qquad (5.65)$$

and if $\eta(\mathbf{x}, \boldsymbol{\theta})$ is a continuous function of $\mathbf{x} \in \mathfrak{X}$ for all $\boldsymbol{\theta} \in \boldsymbol{\Theta}$, then we can formulate an analog of Theorem 5.1 and prove that a necessary and sufficient condition for a design ξ^* to be T-optimal is the existence of a measure ζ^* such that for all $\mathbf{x} \in \mathfrak{X}$

$$\varphi'(\mathbf{x}, \xi^*) \leq \min_{\boldsymbol{\theta} \in \boldsymbol{\Theta}} \int \eta^2(\mathbf{x}, \boldsymbol{\theta}) \, \xi^*(dx), \qquad (5.66)$$

where $\varphi'(\mathbf{x}, \xi) = \int_{\boldsymbol{\Theta}(\xi)} \eta^2(\mathbf{x}, \boldsymbol{\theta}) \, \zeta(d\boldsymbol{\theta})$, $\int_{\boldsymbol{\Theta}(\xi)} \zeta(d\boldsymbol{\theta}) = 1$ and

$$\boldsymbol{\Theta}(\xi) = \left\{ \boldsymbol{\theta} \; : \; \boldsymbol{\theta}(\xi) = \arg\min_{\boldsymbol{\theta} \in \boldsymbol{\Theta}} \int \eta^2(\mathbf{x}, \boldsymbol{\theta}) \, \xi(dx) \right\}.$$

To explore links between the optimization problem (5.64) and the optimization problems that were discussed in Chapter 2, consider the linear response $\eta(\mathbf{x}, \boldsymbol{\theta}) = \boldsymbol{\theta}^T \mathbf{f}(\mathbf{x})$. It follows from (5.65) that

$$\Psi(\xi, \boldsymbol{\theta}) = \int \boldsymbol{\theta}^T \mathbf{f}(\mathbf{x}) \mathbf{f}^T(\mathbf{x}) \boldsymbol{\theta} \, \xi(dx) = \boldsymbol{\theta}^T \mathbf{M}(\xi) \boldsymbol{\theta}. \qquad (5.67)$$

where $\mathbf{M}(\xi) = \int \mathbf{f}(\mathbf{x}) \mathbf{f}^T(\mathbf{x}) \, \xi(dx)$. The expression for $\Psi(\xi, \boldsymbol{\theta})$ in (5.67) allows us to state the following results.

Theorem 5.2 *The design problem (5.64) is equivalent to the following minimization problems*

1. $\min_\xi \mathbf{c}^T \mathbf{M}^{-1}(\xi)\mathbf{c}$, *if* $\boldsymbol{\Theta} = \{\boldsymbol{\theta} \; : \; \mathbf{c}^T\boldsymbol{\theta} \geq \delta > 0\}$.

2. $\min_\xi \max_{\mathbf{x} \in \mathfrak{X}} \mathbf{f}^T(\mathbf{x})\mathbf{M}^{-1}(\xi)\mathbf{f}(\mathbf{x})$, *if* $\boldsymbol{\Theta} = \{\boldsymbol{\theta} \; : \; \eta^2(\mathbf{x}, \boldsymbol{\theta}) \geq \delta^2 > 0, \mathbf{x} \in \mathfrak{X}\}$.

3. $\min_\xi \lambda_{\max}\left[\mathbf{M}^{-1}(\xi)\right]$, *if* $\boldsymbol{\Theta} = \{\boldsymbol{\theta} \; : \; \boldsymbol{\theta}^T\boldsymbol{\theta} \geq \delta > 0\}$.

Proof.
1. The first statement can be verified by direct minimization of the Lagrangian $L(\boldsymbol{\theta}, \lambda) = \boldsymbol{\theta}^T\mathbf{M}\boldsymbol{\theta} + \lambda(\mathbf{c}^T\boldsymbol{\theta} - \delta)$ with respect to $\boldsymbol{\theta}$. Indeed,

$$\frac{\partial L}{\partial \boldsymbol{\theta}} = 2\mathbf{M}\boldsymbol{\theta} + \lambda\mathbf{c}, \quad \frac{\partial L}{\partial \lambda} = \mathbf{c}^T\boldsymbol{\theta} - \delta.$$

Equating both partial derivatives to zero leads to

$$\boldsymbol{\theta}^* = -\frac{\lambda^*}{2}\mathbf{M}^{-1}\mathbf{c}, \quad \lambda^* = -\frac{2\delta}{\mathbf{c}^T\mathbf{M}^{-1}\mathbf{c}},$$

and implies that the minimum is attained at $\boldsymbol{\theta}^* = \delta\mathbf{M}^{-1}\mathbf{c}/(\mathbf{c}^T\mathbf{M}^{-1}\mathbf{c})$, and is equal to $L(\boldsymbol{\theta}^*, \lambda^*) = \delta^2(\mathbf{c}^T\mathbf{M}^{-1}\mathbf{c})^{-1}$, which proves the statement. Note that regularity of the information matrix is not required.

2. Since $\eta^2(\mathbf{x}, \boldsymbol{\theta}) = [\boldsymbol{\theta}^T\mathbf{f}(\mathbf{x})]^2$, the proof of the second statement is analogous to that of the first statement, with the substitution of $\mathbf{f}(\mathbf{x})$ for $\mathbf{c}$. Unlike the previous case, the information matrix must be regular to guarantee that $\mathbf{f}^T(\mathbf{x})\mathbf{M}^{-1}\mathbf{f}(\mathbf{x}) < \infty$ for any $\mathbf{x} \in \mathfrak{X}$.

3. The result follows from the identity

$$\lambda_{\min}(\mathbf{M}) = \min_{\boldsymbol{\theta}} \frac{\boldsymbol{\theta}^T\mathbf{M}\boldsymbol{\theta}}{\boldsymbol{\theta}^T\boldsymbol{\theta}}. \; \square$$

In the proof of Theorem 5.2 we have not used any assumptions about the structure of the matrix $\mathbf{M}$. Thus this theorem is valid for both continuous and exact T-optimal designs. If we confine ourselves to continuous designs, then Theorem 5.2 may be extended. It follows from Theorem 2.3 that the following optimization problems are equivalent:

$$(1) \quad \max_\xi \min_{\boldsymbol{\theta}: \; \eta^2(\mathbf{x},\boldsymbol{\theta}) \geq \delta} \int \eta^2(\mathbf{x}, \boldsymbol{\theta}) \, \xi(d\mathbf{x}),$$

$$(2) \quad \min_\xi \max_\mathbf{x} \mathbf{f}^T(\mathbf{x})\mathbf{M}^{-1}(\xi)\mathbf{f}(\mathbf{x}),$$

$$(3) \quad \max_\xi |\mathbf{M}(\xi)|.$$

The above results suggest that D-optimal designs are "good" for model discrimination too. Note that the link between problems of parameter estimation (hypothesis testing) and D-optimality was discussed by Wald (1943) [391].

D-optimal designs may also work well for another class of testing problems. Let us assume that some prior information on the parameters $\boldsymbol{\theta}$ is available in form of the distribution $\pi_0(d\boldsymbol{\theta})$. Then it is reasonable to use the mean of the noncentrality parameter as a criterion of optimality:

$$\Psi_0(\xi) = \int \int \eta^2(\mathbf{x}, \boldsymbol{\theta})\xi(d\mathbf{x})\pi_0(d\boldsymbol{\theta}). \tag{5.68}$$

If $\mathbf{D}_0$ is the variance-covariance matrix of the prior distribution π_0, then for the linear case,

$$\Psi_0(\xi) = \text{tr}[\mathbf{D}_0\mathbf{M}(\xi)].$$

If $\mathbf{D}_0$ is unknown, then one may use the criterion

$$\Psi(\xi) = \min_{|\mathbf{D}_0|\geq d} \text{tr}[\mathbf{D}_0\mathbf{M}(\xi)] = \min_{|\mathbf{D}_0|\geq d} \Psi_0(\xi) \tag{5.69}$$

with some suitable $d > 0$. If the matrix $\mathbf{M}(\xi)$ in nonsingular, then it follows from (10.17) that

$$\Psi(\xi) = m\, d^{1/m}|\mathbf{M}(\xi)|^{1/m}, \tag{5.70}$$

and, therefore, the criterion (5.69) is equivalent to the D-criterion. This result holds for both exact and continuous design problems.

Tchebysheff approximation problem. Let us assume that $\eta^2(\mathbf{x}, \boldsymbol{\theta})$ is a convex function of $\boldsymbol{\theta}$ for any $\mathbf{x} \in \mathfrak{X}$ and that $\boldsymbol{\Theta}$ is compact, i.e., for any unit measure $\zeta(d\boldsymbol{\theta})$,

$$\eta^2(\mathbf{x}, \overline{\boldsymbol{\theta}}) \leq \int \eta^2(\mathbf{x}, \boldsymbol{\theta})\, \zeta(d\boldsymbol{\theta}), \tag{5.71}$$

where $\overline{\boldsymbol{\theta}} = \int \boldsymbol{\theta}\, \zeta(d\boldsymbol{\theta})$. It follows from (5.66) and (5.71) that

$$\min_{\boldsymbol{\theta}\in\boldsymbol{\Theta}} \max_{\mathbf{x}\in\mathfrak{X}} \eta^2(\mathbf{x}, \boldsymbol{\theta}) \leq \max_{\mathbf{x}\in\mathfrak{X}} \eta^2(\mathbf{x}, \overline{\boldsymbol{\theta}}^*)$$

$$\leq \max_{\mathbf{x}\in\mathfrak{X}} \int \eta^2(\mathbf{x}, \boldsymbol{\theta})\, \zeta^*(d\boldsymbol{\theta}) \leq \min_{\boldsymbol{\theta}\in\boldsymbol{\Theta}} \int \eta^2(\mathbf{x}, \boldsymbol{\theta})\, \xi^*(d\mathbf{x})$$

$$\leq \min_{\boldsymbol{\theta}\in\boldsymbol{\Theta}} \max_{\mathbf{x}\in\mathfrak{X}^*} \eta^2(\mathbf{x}, \boldsymbol{\theta}), \tag{5.72}$$

where $\overline{\boldsymbol{\theta}}^* = \int \boldsymbol{\theta}\, \zeta^*(d\boldsymbol{\theta})$, the measure ζ^* is defined in the context of (5.66), and $\mathfrak{X}^* = \text{supp}(\xi^*)$; the second line in (5.72) is the restated inequality (5.66). On the other hand,

$$\min_{\boldsymbol{\theta}\in\boldsymbol{\Theta}} \max_{\mathbf{x}\in\mathfrak{X}} \eta^2(\mathbf{x}, \boldsymbol{\theta}) \geq \min_{\boldsymbol{\theta}\in\boldsymbol{\Theta}} \max_{\mathbf{x}\in\mathfrak{X}^*} \eta^2(\mathbf{x}, \boldsymbol{\theta}) \tag{5.73}$$

because $\mathfrak{X}^* \subset \mathfrak{X}$. Therefore, it follows from (5.72) and (5.73) that

$$\min_{\boldsymbol{\theta} \in \Theta} \max_{\mathbf{x} \in \mathfrak{X}} \eta^2(\mathbf{x}, \boldsymbol{\theta}) = \min_{\boldsymbol{\theta} \in \Theta} \int \eta^2(\mathbf{x}, \boldsymbol{\theta}) \, \xi^*(d\mathbf{x}), \qquad (5.74)$$

and (5.74) implies the following result.

Theorem 5.3 *If $\eta^2(\mathbf{x}, \boldsymbol{\theta})$ is a convex function of $\boldsymbol{\theta}$ for any $\mathbf{x} \in \mathfrak{X}$ and if Θ is compact, then support points of a T-optimal design coincide with the extremal basis $\mathfrak{X}^*$ of the Tchebysheff approximation problem*

$$(\boldsymbol{\theta}^*, \mathfrak{X}^*) = \arg \min_{\boldsymbol{\theta} \in \Theta} \max_{\mathbf{x} \in \mathfrak{X}} |\eta(\mathbf{x}, \boldsymbol{\theta})|. \qquad (5.75)$$

If $\eta(\mathbf{x}, \boldsymbol{\theta}) = \boldsymbol{\theta}^T \mathbf{f}(\mathbf{x})$, the convexity of $\eta^2(\mathbf{x}, \boldsymbol{\theta})$ with respect to $\boldsymbol{\theta}$ is obvious.

Example 5.10 Test for polynomial regression. Let us test a polynomial of degree m versus a polynomial of degree $m - 1$. Let $\mathfrak{X} = [-1, 1]$. To be able to discriminate between the two models, we need to introduce a constraint on the coefficient of the term x^m; cf. constraints in Example 5.9. Assume, without loss of generality that this coefficient is equal to one. Then the optimal design may be defined as

$$\xi^* = \max_{\xi} \min_{\boldsymbol{\theta}} \int \left[x^m - \boldsymbol{\theta}^T \mathbf{f}(\mathbf{x}) \right]^2 \xi(d\mathbf{x}), \qquad (5.76)$$

where $\mathbf{f}(\mathbf{x}) = (1, x, \ldots, x^{m-1})$ and $\boldsymbol{\theta} = (\theta_1, \theta_2, \ldots, \theta_m)^T$. Because of (5.69) and (5.70), the support set of ξ^* can be defined as

$$\mathfrak{X}^* = \arg \min_{\boldsymbol{\theta} \in \Theta} \max_{|x| \leq 1} |x^m - \boldsymbol{\theta}^T \mathbf{f}(\mathbf{x})|. \qquad (5.77)$$

The optimization problem (5.77) is well studied; e.g., see Karlin and Studden (1966) [225]. The support set of the optimal design is

$$\mathfrak{X}^* = \left\{ x_i^* = \cos \frac{m+1-i}{m} \, \pi, \; i = 1, \ldots, m+1 \right\},$$

with the optimal weights $p_i = 1/m$ for $2 \leq i \leq m$, and $p_1 = p_{m+1} = 1/2m$.

Chapter 6

Locally Optimal Designs in Dose Finding

6.1   Comments on Numerical Procedures   151
6.2   Binary Models   154
6.3   Normal Regression Models   156
     6.3.1   Unknown parameters in variance   157
     6.3.2   Optimal designs as a benchmark   160
6.4   Dose Finding for Efficacy-Toxicity Response   161
     6.4.1   Models   163
     6.4.2   Locally optimal designs   165
6.5   Bivariate Probit Model for Correlated Binary Responses   170
     6.5.1   Single drug   172
     6.5.2   Drug combination   180

In this and next three chapters we present examples of optimal experimental designs for nonlinear models arising in various biopharmaceutical applications. We start with examples of optimal designs for dose-response models:

- Binary dose-response models as in Fedorov and Leonov (2001) [141]; see Section 6.2;

- Continuous logistic models, including models with unknown parameters in variance as in Downing et al. (2001) [100]; see Section 6.3;

- Bivariate Gumbel and Cox models that account for both efficacy and toxicity as in Dragalin and Fedorov (2006) [101]; see Section 6.4;

- Bivariate probit models as in Dragalin et al. (2006) [102], Dragalin et al. (2008) [103]; see Section 6.5.

6.1   Comments on Numerical Procedures

We would like to draw the readers' attention to the fact that once the information matrix $\mu(\mathbf{x}, \boldsymbol{\theta})$ is defined for any candidate "observational unit" $\mathbf{x}$ in the design region $\mathfrak{X}$, then the construction of locally optimal designs follows a rather simple routine for

- Either relatively simple models with one measurement per observational unit (or subject in the case of many biopharmaceutical applications), as in the examples of Sections 6.2, 6.3,

- Or more complex models where (a) several responses are measured for the same subject as in the examples of Sections 6.4, 6.5; see also Section 7.5.5; or (b) several measurements are taken for a particular dependent variable (endpoint), as in the examples of serial sampling in pharmacokinetic/pharmacodynamic studies; see Chapter 7.

Indeed, no matter how complex the underlying model is, if the individual information matrix $\mu(\mathbf{x}, \boldsymbol{\theta})$ is defined for all $\mathbf{x} \in \mathfrak{X}$, then the problem of finding the locally optimal design ξ^* is reduced to the optimization problem (2.54) in the space of information matrices $\mathcal{M}(\mathfrak{X})$ for a given optimality criterion Ψ. Moreover, in all examples presented in this book, we solve the optimization problem over the discrete (finite) design region that allows us to calculate individual information matrices prior to running the optimal design algorithm. Specifically, even in the case of continuous design region $\mathfrak{X} = [a, b]$ as in the examples of Sections 6.2, 6.3 and 6.5, we introduce an alternative discrete grid of candidate points,

$$\mathfrak{X} = [a, b] \quad \Longrightarrow \quad \mathfrak{X}_L = \left\{ x_l, \ x_l = a + l\delta, \ \delta = \frac{b - a}{L}, \ l = 0, \ldots, L \right\},$$

and the forward step of the first-order optimization algorithm, as in (3.2) or (3.36), is reduced to optimization over the finite set of information matrices of candidate points $\{x_l\}$. The number L is selected rather large (several hundred) so that the discrete grid $\mathfrak{X}_L$ is rather fine and can serve as a good approximation for the continuous design region $\mathfrak{X}$. Note also that by construction, for all examples of Chapter 7 the design region $\mathfrak{X}$ is the finite set (the set of candidate sequences $\mathbf{x}_l$ of sampling times in pharmacokinetic and pharmacodynamic studies) and, therefore, the forward step of the first-order optimization algorithm also presents a finite optimization problem.

To summarize, the standard routine for the construction of locally optimal designs in all examples of this book is as follows:

1. Select a prior estimate (preliminary guess) $\boldsymbol{\theta} = \widetilde{\boldsymbol{\theta}}$.

2. Select an optimality criterion, $\Psi = \Psi[\mathbf{M}(\xi, \boldsymbol{\theta})]$, e.g., the D-optimality criterion.

3. Choose a penalty (cost) function $\phi(\mathbf{x}, \boldsymbol{\theta})$.

4. Compute information matrices $\mu(\mathbf{x}_l, \boldsymbol{\theta})$ for all candidate points $\mathbf{x}_l$.

5. Start with some nonsingular design ξ_0.

6. Construct a locally optimal design $\xi^*(\boldsymbol{\theta})$ for the selected criterion:

- Utilize the first-order optimization algorithm over the finite set of candidate points $\mathbf{x}_l$ (or, equivalently, over the finite set of candidate information matrices $\boldsymbol{\mu}(\mathbf{x}_l, \widetilde{\boldsymbol{\theta}})$), where the algorithm combines forward and backward steps (see Sections 3.1, 3.1.4, formulae (3.30) – (3.32)) and also uses the merging step (3.33).

- Complete the iterative procedure when the values of the criterion on two consecutive steps differ by less than a preselected threshold; see item (6) in Section 3.1.4.

Other considerations may also be taken into account, such as various utility functions; see Sections 6.4.2 and 9.2. It is recommended that sensitivity analyses are performed, i.e., steps 1 – 6 must be repeated for different $\widetilde{\boldsymbol{\theta}}$ to verify robustness of the design $\xi^*(\widetilde{\boldsymbol{\theta}})$; cf. Atkinson and Fedorov (1988) [22].

In particular, for the D-optimality criterion,

$$\xi^*(\boldsymbol{\theta}) = \arg\max_{\xi} |\mathbf{M}(\xi, \boldsymbol{\theta})|. \tag{6.1}$$

A design ξ^* is locally D-optimal if and only if

$$d(\mathbf{x}, \xi^*, \boldsymbol{\theta}) = \operatorname{tr}\left[\boldsymbol{\mu}(\mathbf{x}, \boldsymbol{\theta})\mathbf{M}^{-1}(\xi^*, \boldsymbol{\theta})\right] \leq m, \tag{6.2}$$

for all $\mathbf{x} \in \mathfrak{X}$, and $d(\mathbf{x}, \xi^*, \boldsymbol{\theta}) = m$ at all support points of the D-optimal design ξ^*; see Section 5.1 and Theorem 2.3 in Section 2.5. At iteration s, first a design point $\mathbf{x}_s^+$ is selected such that

$$\mathbf{x}_s^+ = \arg\max_{\mathbf{x} \in \mathfrak{X}} d(\mathbf{x}, \xi_s, \boldsymbol{\theta}). \tag{6.3}$$

Then either $\mathbf{x}_s^+$ is added to the current design ξ_s, or, if point $\mathbf{x}_s^+$ belongs to the design ξ_s, then its weight is increased according to (3.30), to create an updated design ξ_s^+. Next, the least "informative" point $\mathbf{x}_s^-$ is found, such that

$$\mathbf{x}_s^- = \arg\min_{\mathbf{x} \in X_s} d(\mathbf{x}, \xi_s^+, \boldsymbol{\theta}), \tag{6.4}$$

where X_s is the support set of ξ_s^+, and (3.32) is used to decrease the weight of point $\mathbf{x}_s^-$ and construct design ξ_{s+1}.

When a penalty function $\phi(\mathbf{x}, \boldsymbol{\theta})$ is introduced, one has to consider the optimization problem (6.1) under the constraint Φ^* on the total normalized penalty:

$$\Phi(\xi, \boldsymbol{\theta}) = \int_{\mathcal{X}} \phi(\mathbf{x}, \boldsymbol{\theta})\xi(d\mathbf{x}) \leq \Phi^*; \tag{6.5}$$

cf. (4.8). Recall that the necessary and sufficient condition of D-optimality is now

$$d(\mathbf{x}, \xi^*, \boldsymbol{\theta}) = \operatorname{tr}\left\{\frac{\boldsymbol{\mu}(\mathbf{x}, \boldsymbol{\theta})}{\phi(\mathbf{x}, \boldsymbol{\theta})}\,\mathbf{M}^{-1}(\xi^*, \boldsymbol{\theta})\right\} \leq m/\Phi(\xi^*, \boldsymbol{\theta}); \tag{6.6}$$

cf. (4.16). Consequently, the first-order optimization algorithm must be modified accordingly: the iterative algorithm now uses the sensitivity function

$d(\mathbf{x}, \xi, \boldsymbol{\theta})$ from (6.6) in (6.3) and (6.4); see Remark 4.1 in Section 4.1.1, in particular, formula (4.26). Recall that the optimization problem (6.1), (6.5) is equivalent to the problem of maximizing the information per cost:

$$\xi^*(\boldsymbol{\theta}) = \arg\max_{\xi} |\mathbf{M}(\xi, \boldsymbol{\theta})/\Phi(\xi, \boldsymbol{\theta})|, \qquad (6.7)$$

see (4.9) in Section 4.1.1.

6.2   Binary Models

Binary, or quantal, models arise in various pharmaceutical applications, such as clinical trials with a binary outcome, toxicology studies and quantal bioassays. For a short description and the derivation of the information matrix $\boldsymbol{\mu}(\mathbf{x}, \boldsymbol{\theta})$, see Section 1.5.1, where it is mentioned that the function π in (1.92) is often selected as a probability distribution function. Among the popular choices are the logistic function $\pi_L(z) = e^z/(1 + e^z)$, $z = \boldsymbol{\theta}^T \mathbf{f}(\mathbf{x})$, and the probit function $\pi_P(z) = \mathcal{N}(z)$; see (5.40) and (5.42), respectively. In practice, when properly normalized, the two models lead to virtually identical results; see Agresti (2002) [3], Finney (1971) [155], Hosmer and Lemeshow (2000) [206].

The information matrix for a single observation can be written as $\boldsymbol{\mu}(\mathbf{x}, \boldsymbol{\theta}) = g(\mathbf{x}, \boldsymbol{\theta})g^T(\mathbf{x}, \boldsymbol{\theta})$, where

$$g(\mathbf{x}, \boldsymbol{\theta}) = \frac{\dot{\pi}(z)\mathbf{f}(\mathbf{x})}{\sqrt{\pi(z)[1 - \pi(z)]}}; \qquad (6.8)$$

cf. (1.93), Section 3.1.2, and Example 5.3. Together with the identity (10.10), this leads to the following presentation of the sensitivity functions for the binary model; cf. Table 2.1 and (6.2):

$$\text{D-criterion:}\quad d(\mathbf{x}, \xi, \boldsymbol{\theta}) = g(\mathbf{x}, \boldsymbol{\theta})\mathbf{M}^{-1}(\xi, \boldsymbol{\theta})g^T(\mathbf{x}, \boldsymbol{\theta}), \qquad (6.9)$$

$$\text{A-criterion:}\quad \varphi(\mathbf{x}, \xi, \boldsymbol{\theta}) = g(\mathbf{x}, \boldsymbol{\theta})\mathbf{M}^{-1}(\xi, \boldsymbol{\theta})\mathbf{A}\mathbf{M}^{-1}(\xi, \boldsymbol{\theta})g^T(\mathbf{x}, \boldsymbol{\theta}). \qquad (6.10)$$

As an example, consider a two-parameter binary model (1.92) where $z = \theta_0 + \theta_1 x$, i.e., $\mathbf{f}(x) = (1, x)^T$ and x represents the dose of a drug. For many functions $\pi(z)$, the locally D-optimal designs are two-point designs, with half the measurements at each dose; see Lemma 2.1. For the logistic model (5.40), this result was discussed by Wetherill (1963) [396], White (1975) [398], Kalish and Rosenberger (1978) [223]; see also Silvey (1980) [360], Chapter 6.6; Abdelbasit and Plackett (1983) [1]; Minkin (1987) [285]; Sitter (1992) [363]. We remark that for a sufficiently large range of doses, D-optimal designs are uniquely defined in the z-space. Moreover, for each of the models discussed at

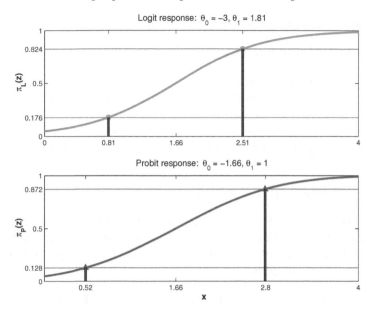

FIGURE 6.1: D-optimal designs for logistic and probit models, $x = (z - \theta_0)/\theta_1$. Upper panel: logistic model, $z = -3 + 1.81x$. Lower panel: probit model, $z = -1.66 + x$.

the beginning of this section, optimal points correspond to certain probabilities of response. For the logistic model (5.40),

$$z_{opt} \approx \pm 1.543, \quad \text{and} \quad \pi_L(-1.543) = 0.176, \quad \pi_L(1.543) = 0.824; \quad (6.11)$$

see Figure 6.1, top. Thus, if x_1 and x_2 are the two optimal doses corresponding to D-optimal design, then

$$\theta_0 + \theta_1 x_1 = -1.543, \quad \theta_0 + \theta_1 x_2 = 1.543.$$

For the probit model (5.42),

$$z_{opt} \approx \pm 1.138, \quad \pi_P(-1.138) = 0.128, \quad \pi_P(1.138) = 0.872; \quad (6.12)$$

see Figure 6.1, bottom. In Figure 6.1, parameters $\boldsymbol{\theta}$ of logit and probit distributions $((-3, 1.81)^T$ and $(-1.66, 1)^T$, respectively) are chosen such that the mean and the variance of the two distributions are the same. For other examples of distribution functions $\pi(z)$, see Ford et al. (1992) [162], Torsney and Musrati (1993) [384].

We postpone a detailed description of adaptive designs to Chapter 8, but mention in passing that formulae (6.11) and (6.12) offer a simple adaptive design algorithm when the information about parameter values $\boldsymbol{\theta}$ is limited:

1. Start with some nonsingular pilot design ξ_0 with n_0 observations.

2. Find the MLE $\hat{\boldsymbol{\theta}}$ based on available observations.

3. Draw the response curve $\eta(x, \hat{\boldsymbol{\theta}})$, draw horizontal lines as in Figure 6.1, and find the x-coordinates x_1^*, x_2^* of the two points at which the curve $\eta(x, \hat{\boldsymbol{\theta}})$ intersects the two horizontal lines. Then split the next cohort equally between x_1^* and x_2^*. (If points x_1^* and/or x_2^* lie outside the design region $\mathfrak{X}$, take a corresponding boundary point of $\mathfrak{X}$ for the support point.)

4. Repeat steps 2 and 3 if needed.

It is worthwhile noting that if x_p is a dose level that causes a particular response in $100p\%$ of subjects, i.e., $\eta(x_p, \boldsymbol{\theta}) = p$, then the normalized variance of the MLE $\widehat{x}_p$ in the two-parameter logistic model is a special case of the c-criterion and can be presented as follows; cf. (2.28):

$$\Psi = \text{Var}(\widehat{x}_p) = \mathbf{c}_p^T \mathbf{D}(\xi, \boldsymbol{\theta}) \mathbf{c}_p = \text{tr}\left[\left(\mathbf{c}_p \mathbf{c}_p^T\right) \mathbf{D}(\xi, \boldsymbol{\theta})\right] \qquad (6.13)$$

with $\mathbf{c}_p = \mathbf{f}(x_p)/\theta_2$; see Wu (1988) [413]. See also an example in Section 8.1.2. For a discussion of c- and A-optimal designs for binary models, see Ford et al. (1992) [162], Sitter and Wu (1993), Zhu and Wong (2000) [426], Mathew and Sinha (2001) [271]. A web-based tool for the analytical construction of locally optimal designs for various nonlinear models is described in Berger and Wong (2009) [44], Chapter 11.6.

6.3 Normal Regression Models

In this section we consider a nonlinear regression model that is utilized in the analysis of dose-, concentration- or exposure-response curves in a large number of clinical and preclinical studies. The model describes the relationship between a continuous response variable, y, and a design variable x (dose, concentration, or exposure level):

$$E(y_{ij}|x_i; \boldsymbol{\theta}) = \eta(x_i, \boldsymbol{\theta}), \quad i = 1, \ldots, n, \quad j = 1, \ldots, r_i; \qquad (6.14)$$

cf. Section 1.4. Observations y_{ij} and $y_{i'j'}$ are often assumed to be independent for $i \neq i'$ and $j \neq j'$, with $\text{Var}(y_{ij}|x_i; \boldsymbol{\theta}) = \sigma^2(x_i)$, i.e., the variance of the response variable may vary across levels of the design variable x. When the response variable y is normally distributed, the variance-covariance matrix of the MLE, $\boldsymbol{\theta}_N$, can be approximated by $\mathbf{D}(\xi, \boldsymbol{\theta}_N)/N$, see (1.89), and the information matrix of a single observation may be derived as the special case of the general formula (1.108):

$$\boldsymbol{\mu}(x_i, \boldsymbol{\theta}) = \mathbf{g}(x_i, \boldsymbol{\theta})\mathbf{g}^T(x_i, \boldsymbol{\theta}), \quad \mathbf{g}(x_i, \boldsymbol{\theta}) = \frac{\mathbf{f}(x_i, \boldsymbol{\theta})}{\sigma(x_i)}, \tag{6.15}$$

where $\mathbf{f}(x, \boldsymbol{\theta})$ is a vector of partial derivatives of the response function $\eta(x, \boldsymbol{\theta})$,

$$\mathbf{f}(x, \boldsymbol{\theta}) = \left[\frac{\partial \eta(x, \boldsymbol{\theta})}{\partial \theta_1}, \frac{\partial \eta(x, \boldsymbol{\theta})}{\partial \theta_2}, \dots, \frac{\partial \eta(x, \boldsymbol{\theta})}{\partial \theta_m}\right]^T; \tag{6.16}$$

cf. Sections 1.5 and 1.7. The construction of optimal designs will be similar to the one for the binary dose-response models of Section 6.2. The difference lies in redefining the $\mathbf{g}(x, \boldsymbol{\theta})$ function that determines the information matrix $\boldsymbol{\mu}(x, \boldsymbol{\theta})$ in (6.15) and the sensitivity function φ in (2.73) for various optimality criteria; cf. (6.8).

6.3.1 Unknown parameters in variance

In various applications it is often assumed that the variance of the error term, σ^2, depends not only on the control variable x, but also on the unknown parameters $\boldsymbol{\theta}$, i.e., $\sigma_i^2 = S(x_i, \boldsymbol{\theta})$. For instance, the variance of the response variable y may depend on its mean, as in the following power model:

$$\mathrm{Var}(y|x, \boldsymbol{\theta}) = S(x, \boldsymbol{\theta}) \sim \eta^\delta(x, \boldsymbol{\theta}), \quad \delta > 0.$$

In cell-based assay studies, the response variable is a cell count and is often assumed to follow a Poisson distribution. Under this assumption and the normal approximation, one can consider the power variance model with $\delta = 1$.

For models with unknown parameters in variance and normally distributed responses, as in (1.107), one can use the general formula (1.108) for the information matrix. In the univariate case, i.e., when $k = 1$, the information matrix $\boldsymbol{\mu}(x, \boldsymbol{\theta})$ permits the following decomposition:

$$\boldsymbol{\mu}(x, \boldsymbol{\theta}) = \mathbf{g}_R(x, \boldsymbol{\theta})\mathbf{g}_R^T(x, \boldsymbol{\theta}) + \mathbf{g}_V(x, \boldsymbol{\theta})\mathbf{g}_V^T(x, \boldsymbol{\theta}), \tag{6.17}$$

where

$$\mathbf{g}_R(x, \boldsymbol{\theta}) = \frac{\mathbf{f}(x, \boldsymbol{\theta})}{\sqrt{S(x, \boldsymbol{\theta})}}, \quad \mathbf{g}_V(x, \boldsymbol{\theta}) = \frac{\mathbf{h}(x, \boldsymbol{\theta})}{\sqrt{2}S(x, \boldsymbol{\theta})},$$

$\mathbf{f}(x, \boldsymbol{\theta})$ is the vector of partial derivatives of $\eta(x, \boldsymbol{\theta})$ as in (6.16), and $\mathbf{h}(x, \boldsymbol{\theta})$ is the vector of partial derivatives of $S(x, \boldsymbol{\theta})$ with respect to $\boldsymbol{\theta}$:

$$\mathbf{h}(x, \boldsymbol{\theta}) = \left[\frac{\partial S(x, \boldsymbol{\theta})}{\partial \theta_1}, \frac{\partial S(x, \boldsymbol{\theta})}{\partial \theta_2}, \dots, \frac{\partial S(x, \boldsymbol{\theta})}{\partial \theta_m}\right]^T. \tag{6.18}$$

In the univariate case, sensitivity functions for the D- and A-optimality criteria can be presented as the sum of two terms too. For example, the sensitivity function for the D-optimality criterion can be written as

$$d(x, \xi, \boldsymbol{\theta}) = \mathbf{g}_R(x, \boldsymbol{\theta})\mathbf{M}^{-1}(\xi, \boldsymbol{\theta})\mathbf{g}_R^T(x, \boldsymbol{\theta}) + \mathbf{g}_V(x, \boldsymbol{\theta})\mathbf{M}^{-1}(\xi, \boldsymbol{\theta})\mathbf{g}_V^T(x, \boldsymbol{\theta}). \tag{6.19}$$

The scalar case, $k = 1$, was extensively discussed by Atkinson and Cook (1995) [17] for various partitioning schemes of parameter vector $\boldsymbol{\theta}$, including separate and overlapping parameters in the variance function.

Example 6.1 *Four-parameter logistic model with power variance*

The four-parameter logistic, or $E_{\max}$ model is used in many pharmaceutical applications, including bioassays of which ELISA, or enzyme-linked immunosorbent assay, and cell-based assays are popular examples:

$$E(y|x; \boldsymbol{\theta}) \ = \ \eta(x, \boldsymbol{\theta}) \ = \ \theta_4 \ + \ \frac{\theta_3 - \theta_4}{1 + (x/\theta_2)^{\theta_1}}, \tag{6.20}$$

where y is the number of cells at concentration x; θ_1 is a slope parameter; parameter θ_2 is often denoted as ED_{50}, i.e., a dose (concentration) at which the response is exactly in between θ_3 and θ_4, so that $\eta(ED_{50}, \boldsymbol{\theta}) = (\theta_3 + \theta_4)/2$; and θ_3 and θ_4 are upper and lower asymptotes, respectively; see Finney (1976) [156], Karpinski (1990) [226], Hedayat et al. (1997) [197], Källén and Larsson (1999) [224]. For other examples of the application of multiparameter logistic models, see Sections 7.5.5, 8.1.2, 8.1.5, 8.1.6.

The model (6.20) provides an example of a *partially* nonlinear model where parameters θ_3 and θ_4 enter the response function in a linear fashion. This, in turn, implies that D-optimal designs do not depend on the values of θ_3 and θ_4; see Hill (1980) [200], Khuri (1984) [227].

To illustrate D-optimal designs for the logistic model (6.20), we use the data from a study on the ability of a compound to inhibit the proliferation of bone marrow erythroleukemia cells in a cell-based assay; see Downing et al. (2001) [100]. In this example, $k = 1$ and the power model of variance is utilized:

$$S(x, \boldsymbol{\theta}) \ = \ \delta_1 \eta^{\delta_2}(x, \boldsymbol{\theta}), \tag{6.21}$$

where $\boldsymbol{\theta} = (\theta_1, \theta_2, \theta_3, \theta_4, \delta_1, \delta_2)^T$. The vector of unknown parameters was estimated by fitting the data collected from a 96-well plate assay, with 6 repeated measurements at each of the 10 concentrations, $\{500, 250, 125, ..., 0.98 \text{ ng/ml}\}$, which represents a twofold serial dilution design with $N = 60$ and weights $w_i = 1/10$, i.e.,

$$\xi_2 \ = \ \{w_i = 1/10, \ x_i = 500/2^i, \ i = 0, 1, ..., 9\}.$$

Thus, the design region was set to $\mathfrak{X} = [-0.02, \ 6.21]$ on the log-scale. Figure 6.2 presents the locally D-optimal design and the variance of prediction for the model defined by (6.20) and (6.21), where $\boldsymbol{\theta} = (1.34, 75.2, 616, 1646, 0.33, 0.90)^T$.

The lower panels of Figure 6.2 present the sensitivity function $d(x, \xi, \boldsymbol{\theta})$ defined in (6.19) for the twofold serial dilution design ξ_2 (left) and D-optimal design ξ^* (right). The solid lines show the function $d(x, \xi, \boldsymbol{\theta})$ while the dashed and dotted lines display the first and second terms on the right-hand side of

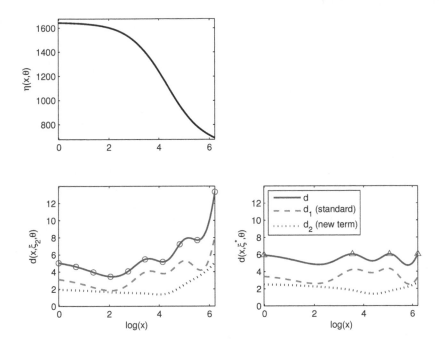

FIGURE 6.2: Plots for Example 6.1. Upper left panel: response function $\eta(x, \boldsymbol{\theta})$. Lower left panel: sensitivity function $d(x, \xi_2, \boldsymbol{\theta})$ for twofold serial dilution design; circles denote serial dilution ξ_2. Lower right: sensitivity function $d(x, \xi^*, \boldsymbol{\theta})$ for optimal design; triangles denote optimal design ξ^*.

(6.19), respectively. Note that the weights of the support points are not equal. In our example $p = \{0.28, 0.22, 0.22, 0.28\}$.

It is worthwhile to note that the optimal design in this example is supported at just four points, which is less than the number of estimated parameters $m = 6$. This happens because the information matrix $\boldsymbol{\mu}(x, \boldsymbol{\theta})$ of a single observation at point x is defined as the sum of the two terms; see (1.108). So even in the case of a single response, $k = 1$, the rank of the information matrix $\boldsymbol{\mu}(x, \boldsymbol{\theta})$ may be greater than one. On the other hand, in the single-response regression models where the variance function does not depend on unknown parameters, the second term on the right-hand side of (1.108) is missing. Therefore, in that case, for the information matrix of any design $\tilde{\xi}$ to be nonsingular, it is necessary to have at least m support points in the design. For other examples, see Fan and Chaloner (2001) [122] and examples in Chapter 7.

6.3.2 Optimal designs as a benchmark

It is worthwhile noting that the direct use of locally optimal designs is not always realistic. As mentioned in Section 6.2, if the logistic model (5.40) is used in the dose-response experiment, then optimal design theory suggests putting half of the patients on each of the two doses, $ED_{17.6}$ and $ED_{82.4}$. Note that dose $ED_{17.6}$ may be too low and not efficacious, while dose $ED_{82.4}$ may be quite toxic and not well tolerated by many patients. Recall also that, although the optimal designs are unique in the z-space, one needs preliminary estimates of parameters $\boldsymbol{\theta}$ to find optimal doses in the original x-space. Hence, appealing to D-optimality of doses in a real-life study may be problematic.

Nevertheless, the importance of locally optimal designs is in that they provide a reference point for the sensitivity analysis and allow one to calculate the relative efficiency of alternative designs.

For instance, in the study described in Section 6.3.1, the scientists were traditionally using the twofold serial dilution design ξ_2, as shown in Figure 6.2. In practice, serial dilution designs can be easily implemented with an arbitrary dilution factor. So the main practical goal was not in constructing optimal designs per se, but to answer the following questions:

- How far is the twofold dilution design from the optimal one?

- Are there "good" serial dilution designs ξ_a with factors a other than 2?

Since there existed a special interest in the estimation of ED_{50}, we compared the relative efficiency of various serial dilution designs with respect to D-optimality and ED_{50}-optimality (i.e., c-optimality for parameter $\theta_2 = ED_{50}$):

$$\text{Eff}_D(\xi_a) = \left[\frac{|\mathbf{M}(\xi_a, \boldsymbol{\theta})|}{|\mathbf{M}(\xi^*, \boldsymbol{\theta})|}\right]^{1/m}, \quad \text{Eff}_{ED_{50}}(\xi_a) = \frac{M_{22}(\xi_a, \boldsymbol{\theta})}{M_{22}(\xi^*, \boldsymbol{\theta})}, \quad (6.22)$$

see (2.24), where by M_{22} we denote the second diagonal element of matrix $\mathbf{M}$. Serial dilution designs are invariant with respect to model parameters, so they serve as a robust alternative to optimal designs. If the efficiency of serial dilutions were close to one, it could provide solid support for the use of such designs in practice.

We fitted the data for over 20 different assays with twofold serial dilution design ξ_2 (concentrations from 500 to 0.98 ng/ml), constructed locally optimal designs, and calculated the relative efficiency of dilution designs. The results could be split into two groups:

1. In most cases design ξ_2 covered the whole range of the logistic curve, and the loss of efficiency was within $10 - 15\%$. This means that $10 - 15\%$ more observations are required to achieve the same efficiency as in the optimal design.

2. In some examples either the left or right end of the curve was not properly covered; e.g., the right end in Figure 6.1, top left panel. Then the

efficiency of designs ξ_2 was less than 0.6, both with respect to D- and c-criteria.

Therefore we suggested trying designs $\xi_{2.5}$ or ξ_3, to start with higher concentrations, and to have 10 different concentrations on the 96-well plate as before, to preserve the logistics of the assays. For example, one of the options with design $\xi_{2.5}$ was to start from 2000 ng/ml, and go down to 800, 320,..., 0.52 ng/ml.

The comparison of designs $\xi_{2.5}$ with the original twofold designs showed that for the cases in Group 1, designs $\xi_{2.5}$ performed similar to designs ξ_2, with essentially the same efficiency. On the other hand, for cases in Group 2 designs $\xi_{2.5}$ were significantly superior, with ratio $\text{Eff}(\xi_{2.5})/\text{Eff}(\xi_2)$ often greater than 1.5 for both optimality criteria. Moreover, designs $\xi_{2.5}$ were relatively close to the optimal ones, with the loss of efficiency not more than 15%. Thus, it was suggested to switch to 2.5-fold serial dilution designs for future studies. For more discussion on robustness issues, see Sitter (1992) [363].

Remark 6.1 In the study discussed above the estimated values of the slope parameter θ_1 were within the interval $[1.2 - 1.5]$, so the logistic curve was not very steep. This was one of the reasons for the good efficiency of 2.5- or 3-fold designs. When parameter θ_1 is significantly greater than 1 (say, 4 and above), then the quality of designs with large dilution factors deteriorates, especially with respect to the estimation of $\theta_2 = ED_{50}$. This happens because when the logistic curve is rather steep, designs ξ_a with larger a will more likely miss points in the middle of the curve, near values $x = ED_{50}$, which in turn may reduce the precision of the parameter estimation.

6.4 Dose Finding for Efficacy-Toxicity Response

In clinical trial analysis, the toxicity and efficacy responses usually occur together and it may be useful to analyze them together. However, in practice the assessment of toxicity and efficacy is sometimes separated. For example, determining the maximum tolerated dose (MTD) is based on toxicity alone and then efficacy is evaluated in Phase II trials over the predetermined dose range. Obviously, the two responses from the same patient are correlated, which will introduce complexity into the analysis. But if one studies these outcomes simultaneously, more information will be gained for future trials, and treatment effects will be understood more thoroughly. In drug-response relationships, the correlation between efficacy and toxicity can be negative or positive, depending on the therapeutic area. To incorporate the two dependent dichotomous outcomes, toxicity and efficacy, several models have been introduced, such as the Gumbel model, see Kotz et al. (2000) [235]; the bivariate binary Cox model, see Cox (1970) [82]; and the probit model, see Finney (1971) [155]; see also Dragalin and Fedorov (2006) [101].

Heise and Myers (1996) [198] were among the first to construct the locally D-optimal design for two correlated binary responses using the Gumbel model. Kpamegan (1998) [238] considered a D-optimal design for the bivariate probit response function in the context of two drugs with two types of distinguishable toxicities. Fan and Chaloner (2001) [122] discussed the locally D-optimal design and Bayesian optimal designs for a continuation-ratio model with ordinal trinomial outcome: efficacy, toxicity, or neutral. Rabie and Flournoy (2004) [331] also studied D-optimal designs for trinomial outcome using the more general contingent response model. These designs, as all D-optimal designs in general, are concerned mainly with *collective ethics*: doing in the dose-finding study what is best for future patients who stand to benefit from the results of the trial.

In contrast, alternative procedures for dose-finding studies have been proposed that are mainly concerned with *individual ethics*: doing what is best for current patients in the trial. In Flournoy (1993) [158], optimal design theory was applied to adaptively allocate treatments addressing individual ethics. Thall and Russell (1998) [373] used a similar method with a proportional odds ratio to model the trinomial outcome case. Also for the trinomial outcome case, Whitehead et al. (2004) [402] considered Bayesian procedures for dose escalation with the objective of determining the therapeutic range of acceptable doses that have a sufficiently large probability of efficacy together with a small enough probability of toxicity. Li et al. (1995) [256] considered sequential maximum likelihood allocations under the general contingent response model, and Kpamegan and Flournoy (2001) [237] used an up-and-down design for the trinomial outcomes model. Similar procedures were considered in Whitehead and Williamson (1998) [401], Whitehead et al. (2001) [400], O'Quigley et al. (2001) [300], Braun (2002) [56], Thall et al. (2003) [372], Thall and Cook (2004) [374], Bekele and Shen (2005) [42], Wang et al. (2005) [394]. Notice, however, that although these designs rely on a noble intention to maximize individual gain by allocating the patient to the "best" known dose, individual ethics may be compromised with such a design by the "poor learning" about the dose-response relationship. Pocock (1983) [312] (see also Palmer and Rosenberger (1999) [304]) points out that each clinical trial involves a balance between individual and collective ethics, and such a balance is rather complex. For further discussion on individual versus collective ethics, or "treatment versus experimentation dilemma," see Section 9.2 and references therein.

In this section we formalize the goal of a dose-finding study as a penalized D-optimal design problem: find the design that maximizes the information (collective, or society ethics) under the control of the total penalty for treating patients in the trial (individual, or all individuals in the trial ethics). Optimal design of experiments can be viewed as a quantitative approach that allows for a compromise between the necessity to accumulate as much information as possible and various constraints (sample size, dose range, cost, ethical concerns, etc.). We present a class of models that can be used in early-phase clinical trials in which patient response is characterized by two dependent binary outcomes: one (Y) for efficacy and one (Z) for toxicity. We view the results of this section as an attempt to quantify the compromise between individual and collective ethics. Whitehead et al. (2006) [403] developed a Bayesian dose-escalation procedure that chooses a dose that minimizes the variance of certain parameter estimates, while satisfying a constraint on the likely risk of overdosing, that is similar to the results presented in this section. For more details, see Dragalin and Fedorov (2006) [101].

6.4.1   Models

In what follows, we consider bivariate responses, but generalizations to higher dimensions are straightforward.

Let Y and Z be the binary 0/1 indicators of efficacy and toxicity response, respectively. Patients have a staggered entry in the trial and are allocated to one of the available doses from some fixed set of doses $\mathfrak{X} = \{x_1, x_2, \ldots, x_n\}$. Throughout this section, doses are expressed on a log scale. Using the location parameter μ ($\mu_E = ED_{50}$, $\mu_T = TD_{50}$) and scale parameter σ, let us standardize doses:

$$x_E = \frac{x - \mu_E}{\sigma_E} \quad \text{for efficacy } Y, \quad x_T = \frac{x - \mu_T}{\sigma_T} \quad \text{for toxicity } Z.$$

Define

$$p_{yz}(x) = p_{yz}(x; \boldsymbol{\theta}) = \Pr(Y = y, Z = z \mid x), \quad y, z = 0, 1;$$

see the table below for an illustration of response probabilities.

		Toxicity		
		1	0	
Efficacy	1	p_{11}	p_{10}	$p_{1.}$
	0	p_{01}	p_{00}	$p_{0.}$
		$p_{.1}$	$p_{.0}$	1

Similar to Section 1.1, assume that r_i independent observations $\{y_{ij}, z_{ij}\}_{j=1}^{r_i}$ are taken at distinct doses x_i and $\sum_i r_i = N$. The log-likelihood function of a single observation (y, z) at dose x is

$$\ell(\boldsymbol{\theta}; y, z, x) = yz \ln p_{11} + y(1 - z) \ln p_{10} + (1 - y)z \ln p_{01} + (1 - y)(1 - z) \ln p_{00},$$

cf. binary response model in Section 1.5.1, and the log-likelihood function of N experiments is given by

$$\mathcal{L}_N(\boldsymbol{\theta}) = \sum_i \sum_{j=1}^{r_i} \ell(\boldsymbol{\theta}; y_{ij}, z_{ij}, x_i). \tag{6.23}$$

The Fisher information matrix of a single observation can be presented as

$$\mu(x, \theta) = \frac{\partial \mathbf{p}}{\partial \theta} \, \nu \, \frac{\partial \mathbf{p}}{\partial \theta^\top}, \qquad (6.24)$$

where

$$\nu = \nu(\mathbf{p}, x, \theta) = \mathbf{P}^{-1} + \frac{1}{1 - p_{11} - p_{10} - p_{01}} \, \mathbf{1} \mathbf{1}^T, \quad \mathbf{1}^T = (1, 1, 1),$$

and

$$\mathbf{p} = (p_{11}, p_{10}, p_{01})^\top, \quad \mathbf{P} = \begin{pmatrix} p_{11} & 0 & 0 \\ 0 & p_{10} & 0 \\ 0 & 0 & p_{01} \end{pmatrix};$$

see Chapter 1.6.2 and Example 5.6 in Section 5.4, specifically formula (5.45).

Gumbel model. In the univariate case, the probability of a response at a given dose is often expressed as an S-shaped curve, or more accurately as a nondecreasing function. Cumulative distribution functions belong to this family, and logistic or normal distributions are popular choices; see Section 6.2. A natural extension in the bivariate case is to express each of the four cell probabilities as the integral of a bivariate cumulative distribution function.

Let us start with the logistic distribution. The individual cell probabilities $p_{yz}(x) = p_{yz}(x, \theta)$ can be derived:

$$p_{11}(x) = G(x_E, x_T),$$
$$p_{10}(x) = G(x_E, \infty) - G(x_E, x_T),$$
$$p_{01}(x) = G(\infty, x_T) - G(x_E, x_T),$$
$$p_{00}(x) = 1 - G(x_E, \infty) - G(\infty, x_T) + G(x_E, x_T),$$

where $G(y, z)$ is the standard Gumbel distribution function given by

$$G(y, z) = F(y)F(z)\{1 + \alpha[1 - F(y)][1 - F(z)]\}, \quad -\infty < y, z < +\infty, \quad (6.25)$$

with $|\alpha| < 1$, and $F(y)$ is a cumulative distribution function, in particular $F(y) = 1/[1 + \exp(-y)]$, i.e., the standard logistic distribution function. Here $\theta^T = (\mu_E, \sigma_E, \mu_T, \sigma_T, \alpha)$. See Kotz et al. (2000) [235], Section 44.13 for more general cases.

Cox model. Another model for efficacy and toxicity can be adapted from Cox's general model of a bivariate binary response as follows:

$$p_{11}(x) = \frac{e^{\alpha_{11} + \beta_{11}x}}{1 + e^{\alpha_{01} + \beta_{01}x} + e^{\alpha_{10} + \beta_{10}x} + e^{\alpha_{11} + \beta_{11}x}},$$

$$p_{10}(x) = \frac{e^{\alpha_{10} + \beta_{10}x}}{1 + e^{\alpha_{01} + \beta_{01}x} + e^{\alpha_{10} + \beta_{10}x} + e^{\alpha_{11} + \beta_{11}x}},$$

$$p_{01}(x) = \frac{e^{\alpha_{01} + \beta_{01}x}}{1 + e^{\alpha_{01} + \beta_{01}x} + e^{\alpha_{10} + \beta_{10}x} + e^{\alpha_{11} + \beta_{11}x}},$$

$$p_{00}(x) = \frac{1}{1 + e^{\alpha_{01} + \beta_{01}x} + e^{\alpha_{10} + \beta_{10}x} + e^{\alpha_{11} + \beta_{11}x}};$$

see Cox (1970) [82], p. 107. Here $\boldsymbol{\theta} = (\alpha_{11}, \beta_{11}, \alpha_{10}, \beta_{10}, \alpha_{01}, \beta_{01})$. The exponential functions in the model can be replaced by any other smooth strictly increasing positive function of x.

Unlike the Gumbel model where the marginal probabilities of Y and Z are logistic in dose, in the Cox model marginal probabilities are, in general, neither logistic nor necessarily monotone with respect to dose. Rather, it is the conditional probabilities of response that are logistic in dose:

$$\Pr(Y = 1 \mid Z = 0; x) = \frac{e^{\alpha_{10} + \beta_{10} x}}{1 + e^{\alpha_{10} + \beta_{10} x}}.$$

As shown in Murtaugh and Fisher (1990) [292], the Cox bivariate binary model has the following properties:

- If $\alpha_{01} + \alpha_{10} = \alpha_{11}$ and $\beta_{01} + \beta_{10} = \beta_{11}$, then the marginal probabilities of Y and Z are logistic in dose;

- If the marginal dependence of Y and Z on x is logistic and $\beta_{10} \neq 0$ or $\beta_{01} \neq 0$, then $\alpha_{01} + \alpha_{10} = \alpha_{11}$ and $\beta_{01} + \beta_{10} = \beta_{11}$;

- Y and Z are independent if and only if $\alpha_{01} + \alpha_{10} = \alpha_{11}$ and $\beta_{01} + \beta_{10} = \beta_{11}$;

- With $u = \alpha_{01} + \beta_{01} x$, $v = \alpha_{10} + \beta_{10} x$ and $w = \alpha_{11} + \beta_{11} x$;

$$\text{Corr}(Y, Z \mid x) = \frac{e^w - e^{u+v}}{\sqrt{(e^w + e^u)(1 + e^u)(e^w + e^v)(1 + e^v)}} \in [-1, 1] .$$

To construct the Fisher information matrix $\boldsymbol{\mu}(x, \boldsymbol{\theta})$ for a single observation at dose x, one has to find partial derivatives $\partial p_{yz}(x, \boldsymbol{\theta}) / \partial \boldsymbol{\theta}$ for the given model (Gumbel or Cox) and apply (6.24); see Dragalin and Fedorov (2006) [101] for details.

6.4.2 Locally optimal designs

Penalized designs. Problems described in this section provide a special case of design problems with constraints that were introduced in Chapter 4. As mentioned at the beginning of Chapter 4, we often interchange the words "penalty" and "costs."

In drug development, there are always ethical concerns and cost constraints associated with different doses. These concerns may be quantified by introducing a penalty function $\phi(x, \boldsymbol{\theta})$, which may depend on unknown parameters, and which reflects ethical and economical burden associated with dose x. A quite flexible penalty function is

$$\phi(x, \boldsymbol{\theta}) = \phi(x, \boldsymbol{\theta}; C_E, C_T) = \{p_{10}(x, \boldsymbol{\theta})\}^{-C_E} \{1 - p_{.1}(x, \boldsymbol{\theta})\}^{-C_T}, \qquad (6.26)$$

which imposes a larger penalty when the probability of success ($Y = 1, Z = 0$) decreases or the probability of toxicity increases. The magnitude of the penalty is controlled by the parameters C_E and C_T. When $C_T = 0$, the penalty affects only those observations that are taken at doses with a low probability of success. When $C_E = 0$, the penalty is imposed only on the observations taken at doses with a high probability of toxicity.

Another popular penalty function is

$$\phi(x, \boldsymbol{\theta}) = K[x - x^*(\boldsymbol{\theta})]^2 + C, \qquad (6.27)$$

where C can be interpreted as the minimal penalty while $x^*(\boldsymbol{\theta})$ is some desirable dose; cf. Lai and Robbins (1978) [244]. For example, $x^*(\boldsymbol{\theta})$ can be defined as the dose at which the probability of success is the largest, i.e.,

$$x^*(\boldsymbol{\theta}) = \arg\max_x \; p_{10}(x, \boldsymbol{\theta}). \qquad (6.28)$$

The solution of (6.28) is often called the *optimal safe dose* (OSD). Other examples of "target dose" x^* include

- *Minimum effective dose* (MED) x_E^*, such that

$$p_{1.}(x, \boldsymbol{\theta}) = \Pr(Y = 1 \mid x) \geq q_E \qquad (6.29)$$

   for all $x \geq x_E^*$, where q_E is the minimum acceptable efficacy response rate. Note that x_E^* depends, in general, on $\boldsymbol{\theta}$.

- *Maximum tolerated dose* (MTD) $x_T^* = x_T^*(\boldsymbol{\theta})$, such that

$$p_{.1}(x, \boldsymbol{\theta}) = \Pr(Z = 1 \mid x) \leq q_T \qquad (6.30)$$

   for all $x \leq x_T^*$, where q_T is the maximum acceptable toxicity rate.

The interval $[x_E^*, x_T^*]$ is usually called the *therapeutic range*.

Haines et al. (2003) [187] considered a penalized optimization problem with

$$\phi(x, \boldsymbol{\theta}) = \begin{cases} 1 & \text{if } p_{1.}(x) \geq q_E \text{ and } p_{.1}(x) \leq q_T \\ \infty & \text{otherwise} \end{cases}. \qquad (6.31)$$

This case can be viewed as a generalization of (6.1) with the design region $\mathfrak{X}(\boldsymbol{\theta})$ that depends on unknown parameters. A similar remark is also valid for the design regions defined by the inequalities in (6.29) and (6.30). Of course, the traditional optimization problem (6.1) is a special case of (6.7), with $\phi(x, \boldsymbol{\theta}) \equiv 1$ for all $x \in \mathfrak{X}$, in the definition of $\Phi(\xi, \boldsymbol{\theta})$ in (6.5).

Example 6.2 *Bivariate Cox model*

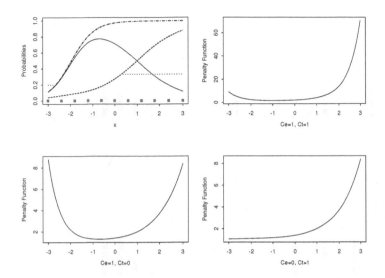

FIGURE 6.3: Cox model with parameter $\boldsymbol{\theta} = (3,3,4,2,0,1)$. Top left: response probabilities. Top right: penalty function (6.26) with $C_E = C_T = 1$. Bottom: penalty function with $C_E = 1$, $C_T = 0$ (left) and $C_E = 0$, $C_T = 1$ (right).

Together with examples of traditional and penalized optimal designs, we present examples of optimal designs with the restricted design region, where doses satisfy constraints (6.29) and (6.30).

As an illustration, we consider the bivariate Cox model with parameters $\boldsymbol{\theta} = (\alpha_{11}, \beta_{11}, \alpha_{10}, \beta_{10}, \alpha_{01}, \beta_{01}) = (3,3,4,2,0,1)$. Figure 6.3, top left panel, shows plots of the probability of success $p_{10}(x, \boldsymbol{\theta})$ (solid line) and two marginal probabilities, of efficacy (dashed line) and toxicity (dotted line), versus dose. The horizontal dotted lines correspond to the minimum acceptable efficacy response rate $q_E = 0.2$ (on the left) and the maximum acceptable toxicity rate $q_T = 1/3$ (on the right), respectively. The set of available doses consists of eleven points equally spaced in the interval $(-3, 3)$ and depicted as filled squares on the horizontal axis, i.e., the design region $\mathfrak{X} = (-3, -2.4, -1.8, ..., 2.4, 3)$. The therapeutic range in this case consists of doses $\{x_2, x_3, x_4, x_5, x_6\}$, and dose x_5 is the optimal safe dose.

Figure 6.3 also presents the penalty function (6.26) for the three sets of parameters (C_E, C_T). One can see that changing the control parameters C_E and C_T leads to different shapes as well as different magnitudes of the penalty. The set $(C_E = C_T = 1)$ penalizes both the lower noneffective and higher toxic doses, but the penalty for toxicity is much higher; see the top right panel. The

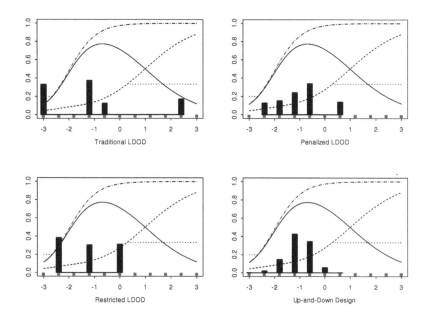

FIGURE 6.4: Locally optimal designs for Cox model with $\theta = (3, 3, 4, 2, 0, 1)$. Top left: traditional. Top right: penalized with penalty function (6.26) with $C_E = 1, C_T = 1$. Bottom left: restricted. Bottom right: up-and-down design.

set $(C_E = 1, C_T = 0)$ penalizes noneffective and toxic doses equally; see the bottom left panel. The set $(C_E = 0, \ C_T = 1)$ penalizes only the toxic doses; see the bottom right panel.

In what follows, we use the following abbreviations: "traditional design" for traditional locally D-optimal design, see (6.1); "penalized design" for penalized locally D-optimal design, see (6.7); "restricted design" for restricted locally D-optimal designs, see (6.29), (6.30) for the constraints on doses. Traditional designs are a special case of penalized designs with $\phi(x, \boldsymbol{\theta}) \equiv const$.

Figure 6.4 shows four designs for the Cox model with parameter $\boldsymbol{\theta} = (3, 3, 4, 2, 0, 1)$. The penalty function is defined by (6.26) with $C_E = C_T = 1$. Each panel plots design points with weights depicted by vertical bars with the respective heights. The traditional design is presented in the top left panel. This is a four-point design at doses $\{x_1, x_4, x_5, x_{10}\}$ with weights $\{0.33, 0.37, 0.13, 0.17\}$. This design requires that a considerable proportion of patients be allocated to a highly toxic dose, which is unlikely to be accepted in practice. The penalized design is a five-point design at doses $\{x_2, x_3, x_4, x_5, x_7\}$ with weights $\{0.13, 0.15, 0.24, 0.34, 0.14\}$; see the top right panel. It allocates

34% of the patients to x_5 (OSD) and 14% to dose x_7 for which the toxicity rate is higher than maximum acceptable, but still much lower than the one for the dose x_{10} recommended by the traditional design. The restricted design allocates 38% and 31% to the two extreme doses $\{x_2, x_6\}$ in the therapeutic range and 30% to dose x_4 in the middle; see the bottom left panel.

For comparison, the bottom right panel shows the stationary distribution for the allocation rule of the up-and-down design considered by Ivanova (2003) [209]. The up-and-down design works as follows. Suppose the ℓ-th patient was treated at dose $x_j = x_{j(\ell)}$ and had a response $\{Y_\ell, Z_\ell\}$. Then the design allocates the next patient to dose

$$
D_{\ell+1} = \begin{cases} x_{j(\ell)-1}, & \text{if } Z_\ell = 1 \\ x_{j(\ell)}, & \text{if } Y_\ell = 1, Z_\ell = 0 \\ x_{j(\ell)+1}, & \text{if } Y_\ell = 0, Z_\ell = 0 \end{cases}
$$

with the appropriate adjustments at the lowest and the highest doses. A slightly different up-and-down design was considered by Hardwick et al. (2003) [192] as a starting rule for their directed walk design.

Given the penalty function $\phi(x, \boldsymbol{\theta})$, one can use the total penalty

$$
\Phi(\xi, \boldsymbol{\theta}) = \sum_{i=1}^{n} w_i \phi(x_i, \boldsymbol{\theta}) \tag{6.32}
$$

as a measure for performance evaluation and comparison of different designs. Another performance measure is the precision of the MLE estimation achieved by a given design, defined as

$$
\mathcal{R}(\xi, \boldsymbol{\theta}) = |\boldsymbol{M}(\xi, \boldsymbol{\theta})|^{-1/m}. \tag{6.33}
$$

Note that $\mathcal{R}(\xi, \boldsymbol{\theta})$ enters the definition of relative D-efficiency in (2.24); see also (6.22). The lower the $\mathcal{R}(\xi, \boldsymbol{\theta})$, the higher the estimation precision. Note that the performance measures (6.32) and (6.33) are normalized in the sense that they do not depend on the number of subjects. The latter is a measure of information obtained by a design, while the former is a measure of the cost (penalty) of getting that information. Obviously, the two performance measures can be combined into one single measure, information per cost:

$$
\Psi_c(\xi, \boldsymbol{\theta}) = \frac{|\boldsymbol{M}(\xi, \boldsymbol{\theta})|^{1/m}}{\Phi(\xi, \boldsymbol{\theta})}; \tag{6.34}
$$

cf. (4.9), where a slightly different motivation was used to introduce the same criterion. A design with higher information per cost is more efficient. This measure can be used to define the relative efficiency of one design with respect to another, similar to relative D-efficiency in (6.22). Thus, if $\Psi_c(\xi')/\Psi_c(\xi'') = k$, then design ξ'' requires k times the number of subjects that design ξ' does to achieve the same information per cost unit. The three performance measures

TABLE 6.1: Performance measures for locally optimal designs

Design	Total Penalty (6.32)	Estimation Precision (6.33)	Info per cost (6.34)
Traditional	8.18	14.99	0.0082
Restricted	2.51	19.23	0.0207
Up-and-Down	1.72	29.42	0.0197
Penalized	2.09	19.86	0.0240

Note: Cox model with parameter $\boldsymbol{\theta} = (3, 3, 4, 2, 0, 1)$. Penalty function (6.26) with $C_E = C_T = 1$.

(6.32) – (6.34) are displayed in Table 6.1. The penalized design is the most efficient among the four considered designs with respect to information per cost (6.34). Obviously, the traditional design is the most accurate with respect to the performance measure (6.33), but it has the highest total penalty. The restricted design reduces the total penalty, but at the price of lower accuracy. The up-and-down design achieves the lowest total penalty, but at the price of the lowest accuracy. The penalized design provides the most efficient trade-off between the two performance measures.

For a discussion of adaptive designs for the bivariate Cox model, see Section 8.2.

6.5 Bivariate Probit Model for Correlated Binary Responses

The Gumbel and Cox models described in Section 6.4 are attractive due to their computational transparency. However, they do not allow for the direct modeling of the correlation between observed responses. In this section we discuss a bivariate probit model that incorporates the correlated responses naturally via the correlation structure of the underlying bivariate normal distribution; see Ashford and Sowden (1970) [13]; Lesaffre and Molenberghs (1991) [255]; Molenberghs and Verbeke (2005) [287]. Adaptive designs for a bivariate probit model are discussed in Section 8.3. For more details, see Dragalin et al. (2006) [102], Dragalin et al. (2008) [103].

Assume that V_1 and V_2 follow the bivariate normal distribution with zero mean and variance-covariance matrix

$$\Sigma = \begin{pmatrix} 1 & \rho \\ \rho & 1 \end{pmatrix},$$

where ρ may be interpreted as the correlation measure between toxicity and efficacy for the same patient; cf. Chib and Greenberg (1998) [75]. This correlation should be specified in advance or treated as an unknown parameter. The correlation can be negative or positive depending on the therapeutic area. For instance, in oncology, the tumor decrease is observed more often for the patients with no side effects than for the patients with side effects, i.e., ρ is negative.

The probit model with correlated responses may be defined via

$$p_{11}(x, \boldsymbol{\theta}) = \mathcal{N}_2[\eta_1(x, \boldsymbol{\theta}_1), \eta_2(x, \boldsymbol{\theta}_2), \rho]$$

$$= \int_{-\infty}^{\eta_1(x,\boldsymbol{\theta}_1)} \int_{-\infty}^{\eta_2(x,\boldsymbol{\theta}_2)} \frac{1}{2\pi|\boldsymbol{\Sigma}|^{1/2}} \exp\left\{ -\frac{1}{2} \mathbf{V}^T \boldsymbol{\Sigma}^{-1} \mathbf{V} \right\} dv_1 dv_2, \qquad (6.35)$$

where $\boldsymbol{\theta}_1$ and $\boldsymbol{\theta}_2$ are unknown parameters, and η_1, η_2 are some functions of dose x and parameters. In the simplest case, η_i are linear functions of parameters:

$$\eta_1(x, \boldsymbol{\theta}_1) = \boldsymbol{\theta}_1^T \mathbf{f}_1(x), \quad \eta_2(x, \boldsymbol{\theta}_1) = \boldsymbol{\theta}_2^T \mathbf{f}_2(x), \qquad (6.36)$$

and $\mathbf{f}_1(x)$ and $\mathbf{f}_2(x)$ contain the covariates of interest. In the simplest case, for modeling a single drug, one may choose $\mathbf{f}_1(x) = \mathbf{f}_2(x) = (1, x)^T$. For modeling a combination of two drugs $\mathbf{x} = (x_1, x_2)$ in the presence of interaction, one may take $\mathbf{f}_1(\mathbf{x}) = \mathbf{f}_2(\mathbf{x}) = (1, x_1, x_2, x_1 x_2)^T$; see Section 6.5.2. Obviously, other choices of η_i are possible when more information is available about drug effects.

The probabilities of efficacy $p_1.$ and toxicity $p_{.1}$ can be expressed as the marginal distributions of the bivariate normal distribution:

$$p_1.(x, \boldsymbol{\theta}) = \mathcal{N}[\boldsymbol{\theta}_1^T \mathbf{f}_1(x)] \qquad (6.37)$$

and

$$p_{.1}(x, \boldsymbol{\theta}) = \mathcal{N}[\boldsymbol{\theta}_2^T \mathbf{f}_2(x)], \qquad (6.38)$$

where $\mathcal{N}(u)$ is the cumulative distribution function of the standard normal distribution; see (5.42).

The other probabilities are defined as

$$p_{10}(x, \boldsymbol{\theta}) = p_1.(x, \boldsymbol{\theta}) - p_{11}(x, \boldsymbol{\theta}), \qquad (6.39)$$

$$p_{01}(x, \boldsymbol{\theta}) = p_{.1}(x, \boldsymbol{\theta}) - p_{11}(x, \boldsymbol{\theta}), \qquad (6.40)$$

$$p_{00}(x, \boldsymbol{\theta}) = 1 - p_1.(x, \boldsymbol{\theta}) - p_{.1}(x, \boldsymbol{\theta}) + p_{11}(x, \boldsymbol{\theta}). \qquad (6.41)$$

We will often suppress arguments x, $\boldsymbol{\theta}$, whenever the interpretation is clear from the context.

Information matrix, known ρ**.** Let $\boldsymbol{\theta}^T = (\boldsymbol{\theta}_1^T, \boldsymbol{\theta}_2^T) \in R^m$, where $m = m_1 + m_2$, $m_s = dim(\boldsymbol{\theta}_s)$, $s = 1, 2$. The information matrix for a single observation at dose x is (cf. Sections 1.6.2 and 5.4)

$$\boldsymbol{\mu}(x, \boldsymbol{\theta}) = \mathbf{C}_1 \mathbf{C}_2 (\mathbf{P} - \mathbf{p}\mathbf{p}^T)^{-1} \mathbf{C}_2^T \mathbf{C}_1^T, \qquad (6.42)$$

where $\mathbf{C}_1$ and $\mathbf{C}_2$ are $m \times 2$ and 2×3 matrices, respectively,

$$\mathbf{C}_1 = \left[\begin{array}{cc} \psi_1(\boldsymbol{\theta}_1^T \mathbf{f}_1)\mathbf{f}_1 & \mathbf{0}_{m_1} \\ \mathbf{0}_{m_2} & \psi_1(\boldsymbol{\theta}_2^T \mathbf{f}_2)\mathbf{f}_2 \end{array} \right], \quad \mathbf{C}_2 = \left[\begin{array}{ccc} \mathcal{N}(u_1) & 1 - \mathcal{N}(u_1) & -\mathcal{N}(u_1) \\ \mathcal{N}(u_2) & -\mathcal{N}(u_2) & 1 - \mathcal{N}(u_2) \end{array} \right],$$

$$u_1 = \frac{\boldsymbol{\theta}_2^T \mathbf{f}_2 - \rho \boldsymbol{\theta}_1^T \mathbf{f}_1}{\sqrt{1 - \rho^2}}, \quad u_2 = \frac{\boldsymbol{\theta}_1^T \mathbf{f}_1 - \rho \boldsymbol{\theta}_2^T \mathbf{f}_2}{\sqrt{1 - \rho^2}},$$

$$\mathbf{P} = \left(\begin{array}{ccc} p_{11} & 0 & 0 \\ 0 & p_{10} & 0 \\ 0 & 0 & p_{01} \end{array} \right), \quad \mathbf{p} = (p_{11} \; p_{10} \; p_{01})^T, \tag{6.43}$$

where $\mathbf{0}_a$ is an $a \times 1$ column vector of zeros and $\psi_1(u)$ denotes the probability density function of the standard normal distribution. For the proof of formula (6.42), see Dragalin et al. (2008) [103]. Note that $m_1 = m_2 = 2$ for the model (6.45) of the single drug; see Section 6.5.1. In the case of two-drug combination, $m_1 = m_2 = 4$ under the model (6.49); see Section 6.5.2.

Unknown ρ. When the correlation between toxicity and efficacy ρ is treated as an unknown parameter, the corresponding information matrix for a single observation at dose x becomes

$$\boldsymbol{\mu}(x, \boldsymbol{\theta}) = \left[\begin{array}{c} \mathbf{C}_1 \mathbf{C}_2 \\ \psi_2 \; -\psi_2 \; -\psi_2 \end{array} \right] (\mathbf{P} - \mathbf{pp}^T)^{-1} \left[\begin{array}{c} \mathbf{C}_1 \mathbf{C}_2 \\ \psi_2 \; -\psi_2 \; -\psi_2 \end{array} \right]^T, \tag{6.44}$$

where matrices $\mathbf{C}_1$, $\mathbf{C}_2$ are introduced in (6.42), matrices $\mathbf{P}$ and $\mathbf{p}$ are defined in (6.43), and $\psi_2 = \psi_2(\boldsymbol{\theta}_1^T \mathbf{f}_1, \boldsymbol{\theta}_2^T \mathbf{f}_2, \rho)$ denotes the probability density function of bivariate normal distribution with means $\boldsymbol{\theta}_1^T \mathbf{f}_1$ and $\boldsymbol{\theta}_2^T \mathbf{f}_2$, variances 1 and correlation coefficient ρ. For derivation, see Dragalin et al. (2008) [103].

6.5.1   Single drug

In clinical trials, investigators often expect that the probability $p_{\cdot 1}$ of toxicity and probability $p_{1 \cdot}$ of efficacy increase as the dose increases. It is also expected that the probability of efficacy without toxicity p_{10} increases as the dose increases at lower doses and then, starting from some dose d', it decreases as the dose gets larger. In this section, several models are considered to illustrate optimal designs. All examples are based on the normalized dose range $[0, 1]$. The general case of a dose range $[d_0, d_{\max}]$ can be reduced to the $[0, 1]$ range by the transformation $x = (d - d_0)/(d_{\max} - d_0)$.

In all examples, the term $\boldsymbol{\theta}_j^T \mathbf{f}_j(x)$ in the probit model (6.35), (6.36) is a linear function of dose x:

$$\boldsymbol{\theta}_1^T \mathbf{f}_1(x) = \theta_{11} + \theta_{12} x, \quad \boldsymbol{\theta}_2^T \mathbf{f}_2(x) = \theta_{21} + \theta_{22} x. \tag{6.45}$$

Known ρ. Here we assume that the correlation coefficient ρ is known

TABLE 6.2: Locally D-optimal designs for the bivariate probit model with $\theta = (-0.9, 10, -1.2, 1.6)$.

		Optimal Design		
Traditional	$\xi_t =$	$\left\{ \begin{array}{ccc} 0 & 0.21 & 1 \\ 0.40 & 0.36 & 0.24 \end{array} \right\}$		
Restricted	$\xi_r =$	$\left\{ \begin{array}{ccc} 0.01 & 0.22 & 0.48 \\ 0.45 & 0.34 & 0.21 \end{array} \right\}$		
Penalized				
$C_E = 0, C_T = 1$	$\xi_{01} =$	$\left\{ \begin{array}{ccc} 0 & 0.21 & 1 \\ 0.49 & 0.40 & 0.11 \end{array} \right\}$		
$C_E = 1, C_T = 0$	$\xi_{10} =$	$\left\{ \begin{array}{ccc} 0.08 & 0.25 & 1 \\ 0.23 & 0.61 & 0.16 \end{array} \right\}$		
$C_E = 1, C_T = 1$	$\xi_{11} =$	$\left\{ \begin{array}{ccc} 0.08 & 0.24 & 0.85 \\ 0.26 & 0.62 & 0.12 \end{array} \right\}$		

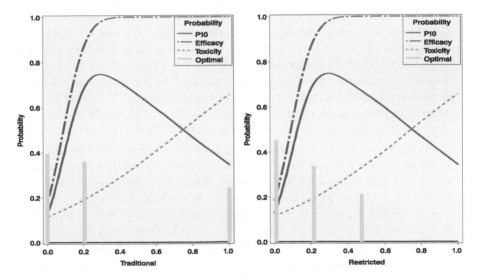

FIGURE 6.5: Response probabilities and locally D-optimal designs for the bivariate probit model with $\theta = (-0.9, 10, -1.2, 1.6)$; traditional locally optimal (left) and restricted locally optimal (right).

(not a parameter to be estimated) and is equal to 0.5. Therefore, the vector of parameters is $\boldsymbol{\theta} = (\theta_{11}, \theta_{12}, \theta_{21}, \theta_{22})^T$.

Figure 6.5 presents locally D-optimal designs together with toxicity, efficacy, and efficacy without toxicity response rates of model (6.45) with parameter values $\boldsymbol{\theta} = (-0.9, 10, -1.2, 1.6)$. Optimal designs are also listed in Table 6.2. If $\mathfrak{X} = [0, 1]$, the optimal design ξ_t is a three-point design with two points at the boundaries of the design region with weights $w_1 = 0.40$ at $x = 0$ and $w_3 = 0.24$ at the highest dose $x = 1$. The remaining support point is located at $x = 0.2$ with $w_2 = 0.36$, close to where the success curve p_{10} reaches its maximum and the efficacy curve has the most pronounced curvature; see Figure 6.5, left panel.

As discussed in Section 6.4.2, it is unethical to assign patients to doses that lead to a high probability of toxicity and a low probability of efficacy. A possible way to address this problem is to use the therapeutic range $[x_E^*, x_T^*]$ as the design region; see (6.29), (6.30). Thus we exclude doses that cause (a) toxicity at a rate higher than $q_T = 0.33$, and (b) efficacy at a rate lower than $q_E = 0.2$. The design region becomes $\mathfrak{X} = [0.01, 0.48]$. The optimal design ξ_r is still a three-point design with two points on the boundaries of the restricted region and one in the middle. The support point inside the design region is almost identical to one of design ξ_t. The weight distribution changes slightly and becomes (0.45, 0.34, 0.21); see Figure 6.5, right panel.

The penalized locally D-optimal designs with the penalty function (6.26) and three sets of pairs (C_E, C_T) are listed in Table 6.2 and plotted in Figure 6.6. The solid convex line denotes the penalty function and the bars denote the optimal design. When $C_E = 0$, $C_T = 1$, the penalty function gets larger as the probability of toxicity increases, so we may expect that a smaller weight will be allocated at the highest dose compared to the nonpenalized optimal design; see Figure 6.6, top panel. The optimal design ξ_{01} is similar to ξ_t with respect to the location of support points. However, the weight of the highest dose $x = 1$ changes to $w_3 = 0.11$ from $w_3 = 0.24$.

When $C_E = 1$, $C_T = 0$, the penalty is imposed on doses where the probability of efficacy without toxicity is low. The penalty reaches its minimum at the dose where p_{10} reaches its maximum. Instead of allocating patients at the boundary $x = 0$ as in ξ_t, the lowest dose in optimal design ξ_{10} is $x = 0.08$, due to the low p_{10} value at $x = 0$, with less weight ($w_1 = 0.23$ vs $w_1 = 0.4$ for ξ_t). The middle point, with high probability of efficacy and no toxicity, has the largest weight $w_2 = 0.61$; see Figure 6.6, bottom left panel.

The penalty function with $C_E = 1$, $C_T = 1$ penalizes observations at doses with high probability of toxicity and low probability of efficacy without toxicity. Thus, it is not surprising that the boundaries are not included in the optimal design; see Figure 6.6, bottom right panel. The lowest and highest dose of the optimal design are now 0.08 and 0.85, respectively. Less weight is assigned to these two support points, while $w_2 = 0.62$ at dose $x = 0.24$ which is close to the point of maximum of p_{10}. Such allocation makes sense from the

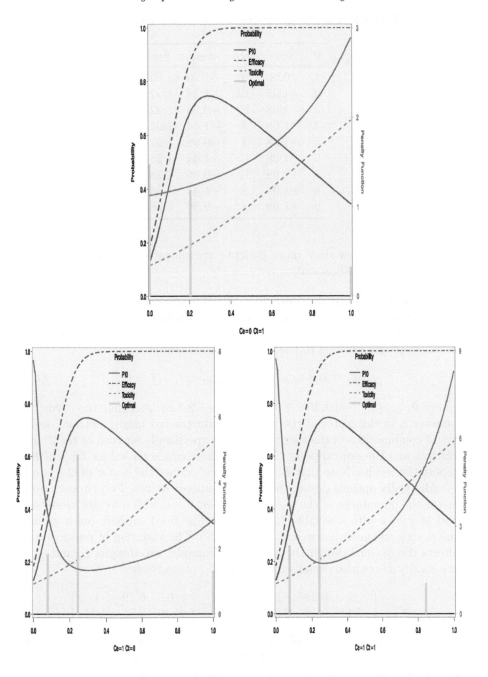

FIGURE 6.6: Response probabilities for the bivariate probit model with $\boldsymbol{\theta} = (-0.9, 10, -1.2, 1.6)$ and penalized locally D-optimal designs; penalty function (6.26) with $C_E = 0, C_T = 1$ (top), $C_E = 1, C_T = 0$ (bottom left), and $C_E = 1, C_T = 1$ (bottom right).

TABLE 6.3: Parameter values used in sensitivity study.

θ	θ_{11}	θ_{12}	θ_{21}	θ_{22}
1	-0.90	10	-1.20	1.60
2	-1.08	12	-1.44	1.92
3	-1.08	12	-0.96	1.92
4	-1.08	8	-1.44	1.92
5	-1.08	8	-0.96	1.92
6	-1.08	12	-1.44	1.28
7	-1.08	12	-0.96	1.28
8	-1.08	8	-1.44	1.28
9	-1.08	8	-0.96	1.28

ethical point of view since more patients are allocated at or near doses that are both safe and efficacious.

Sensitivity analysis, known ρ. In this subsection, we investigate the robustness of the locally optimal designs to variations in, or misspecification of, the unknown parameters. Assume that the investigator can identify that parameter values belong to the four-dimensional cube

$$\theta_{ij} \in [0.8\,\theta_{true,\ ij},\ 1.2\,\theta_{true,\ ij}],\ i,j = 1,2, \tag{6.46}$$

where $\theta_{true,\ 1} = (-0.9, 10)^T$, $\theta_{true,2} = (-1.2, 1.6)^T$, so that the "true" parameter is in the center of the cube. We constructed locally optimal designs for 17 combinations of the four parameters, specifically for each of the $2^4 = 16$ vertices and the central point. Table 6.3 lists parameter values for which we report the results. Note that θ_1 is the "true" value (the center of the cube).

All locally optimal designs have three support points. Two support points are at the boundaries of the design region, at $x = 0$ with a weight close to 0.4 and at $x = 1$ with a weight close to 0.25. The third support point is inside the design region with a weight close to 0.35. The variation of parameter θ_{12} affects the optimal design the most. For example, two designs ξ_5 and ξ_7 are the locally D-optimal designs for θ_5 and θ_7, respectively:

$$\xi_5 = \left\{ \begin{array}{ccc} 0 & 0.28 & 1 \\ 0.42 & 0.36 & 0.23 \end{array} \right\}, \quad \xi_7 = \left\{ \begin{array}{ccc} 0 & 0.19 & 1 \\ 0.40 & 0.36 & 0.24 \end{array} \right\}.$$

The location of the "internal" support point changes from 0.28 to 0.19 when θ_{12} changes from the smaller to the larger value. The variation of the other parameters does not affect the optimal design that much.

To compare designs, a relative deficiency

$$\mathcal{D}(\xi, \theta) = \left\{ \frac{|\mathbf{M}(\xi^*(\theta), \theta)|}{|\mathbf{M}(\xi, \theta)|} \right\}^{1/m} \tag{6.47}$$

TABLE 6.4: Relative deficiency of penalized locally D-optimal designs ξ_{pi} with the penalty function (6.26), $C_E = 1$ and $C_T = 1$; deficiency defined in (6.48).

Design	θ_1	θ_2	θ_3	θ_4	θ_5	θ_6	θ_7	θ_8	θ_9
ξ_{p1}	1.00	1.03	1.19	1.12	1.21	1.11	1.03	1.27	1.16
ξ_{p2}	1.03	1.00	1.08	1.20	1.23	1.13	1.03	1.42	1.28
ξ_{p3}	1.10	1.05	1.00	1.30	1.19	1.28	1.12	1.63	1.41
ξ_{p4}	1.15	1.37	1.57	1.00	1.08	1.46	1.38	1.12	1.03
ξ_{p5}	1.22	1.43	1.40	1.06	1.00	1.68	1.50	1.30	1.13
ξ_{p6}	1.12	1.23	1.98	1.35	1.97	1.00	1.03	1.21	1.19
ξ_{p7}	1.03	1.06	1.40	1.22	1.48	1.04	1.00	1.27	1.20
ξ_{p8}	1.34	1.80	**3.04**	1.20	1.87	1.39	1.49	1.00	1.03
ξ_{p9}	1.20	1.51	2.19	1.07	1.43	1.36	1.37	1.03	1.00

was calculated for each design, where $\xi^*(\boldsymbol{\theta})$ is the locally optimal design for $\boldsymbol{\theta}$. The relative deficiency is the reciprocal of the relative efficiency introduced in (6.22). The value $\mathcal{D}(\xi, \boldsymbol{\theta})$ shows by how much the sample size for the design ξ must be increased to achieve the same accuracy as the locally D-optimal design $\xi^*(\boldsymbol{\theta})$; cf. Section 8.1.4.

We computed relative deficiencies $\mathcal{D}(\xi_i, \boldsymbol{\theta}_j)$ of the locally D-optimal designs ξ_i corresponding to parameters $\boldsymbol{\theta}_j$ in Table 6.3. The largest value is $\mathcal{D}(\xi_5, \boldsymbol{\theta}_7) = 1.21$. This means that if the true parameters $\boldsymbol{\theta}_7$ are misspecified as $\boldsymbol{\theta}_5$, then about 21% more patients are needed for design ξ_5 to achieve the same accuracy of parameter estimation as design ξ_7.

We also conducted a sensitivity analysis for the penalized D-optimal designs with the penalty function (6.26). For a fair comparison, the deficiency is normalized by the total penalty (6.5), and the penalized relative deficiency is defined as

$$\mathcal{D}_p(\xi_{pi}, \boldsymbol{\theta}_j) = \left\{ \left| \frac{\mathbf{M}(\xi_{pj}, \boldsymbol{\theta}_j)}{\Phi(\xi_{pj}, \boldsymbol{\theta}_j)} \right| \Big/ \left| \frac{\mathbf{M}(\xi_{pi}, \boldsymbol{\theta}_j)}{\Phi(\xi_{pi}, \boldsymbol{\theta}_j)} \right| \right\}^{1/4}. \tag{6.48}$$

When $C_E = 1, C_T = 0$, the results are similar to the traditional case discussed above. When $C_E = 0, C_T = 1$, the largest value of $\mathcal{D}_p$ is close to 2.

The results for $C_E = 1$, $C_T = 1$ are listed in Table 6.4. The largest value of $\mathcal{D}_p$ is 3.04: when the true parameters $\boldsymbol{\theta}_3$ are misspecified as $\boldsymbol{\theta}_8$, then about three times more patients are needed when utilizing ξ_{p8} instead of ξ_{p3}, to achieve the same precision.

For design ξ_{p3}, parameters θ_{12} and θ_{22} are at the smallest possible values while for design ξ_{p8}, parameters θ_{12} and θ_{22} are at their largest values. This shows that the penalized D-optimal designs are sensitive to the variation of slope parameters. Figure 6.7 presents the probability of success, marginal probabilities of efficacy and toxicity, the penalty function and penalized locally

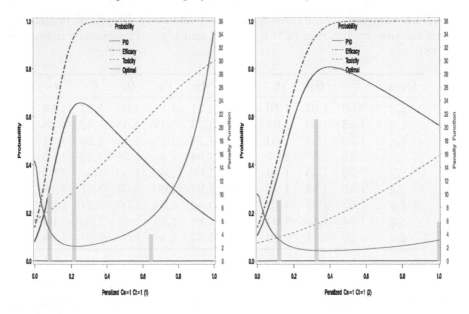

FIGURE 6.7: Probabilities, penalty functions and corresponding penalized locally optimal designs for θ_3 (left) and θ_8 (right).

optimal designs for θ_3 (left panel) and θ_8 (right panel). These two models are quite different. For θ_3, the penalty function has a very large value at $x = 1$; consequently, dose $x = 1$ is not present in the penalized locally D-optimal design; see Figure 6.7, left panel. On the other hand, for θ_8, both toxicity and efficacy increase at a slower rate, and the penalty function increases more slowly, so it is not surprising that $x = 1$ is one of the optimal points; see Figure 6.7, right panel.

Sensitivity analysis, unknown ρ. Now locally optimal designs for the model (6.45) are constructed with the value of ρ varying from -0.8 to 0.8 while the other parameters remain the same as in the example with known ρ. Therefore, the vector of parameters is $\theta = (\theta_{11}, \theta_{12}, \theta_{21}, \theta_{22}; \rho)^T$. We consider the following values of ρ: $(-0.8, -0.5, -0.2, 0, 0.2, 0.5, 0.8)$. For each value of ρ, the traditional locally D-optimal design and the penalized D-optimal design are constructed with penalty function (6.26) with $(C_E, C_T) = (0, 1)$, $(1, 0)$ and $(1, 1)$. The locally D-optimal designs for restricted design regions are not discussed here because the design region depends on ρ and, therefore, it is difficult to compare designs corresponding to different design regions.

When $(C_E, C_T) = (1, 0)$ or $(1, 1)$, the values of the penalty function are relatively stable with respect to varying ρ, so the corresponding penalized D-optimal designs are quite close to the penalized D-optimal designs for known $\rho = 0.5$; see Section 6.5.1 and Figures 6.5, 6.6. Therefore, we focus on tradi-

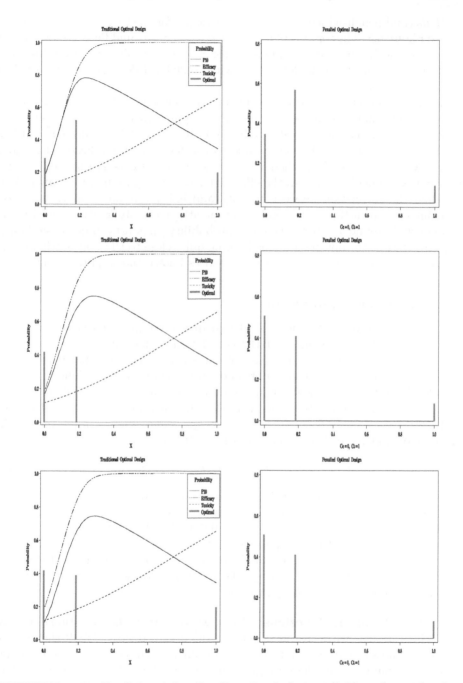

FIGURE 6.8: Traditional locally D-optimal design (left) and penalized locally D-optimal design (right); ρ is an unknown parameter. Top panel: $\rho = -0.8$; middle panel: $\rho = 0$; bottom panel: $\rho = 0.8$.

tional and penalized locally D-optimal designs for the pair $(C_E, C_T) = (0, 1)$; see Figure 6.8. The top two plots are for $\rho = -0.8$, the middle two plots are for $\rho = 0$, and the bottom two plots are for $\rho = 0.8$. Traditional locally optimal designs are shown in the left panel, while penalized designs are presented in the right panel.

The locations of the design points are very close for all three scenarios. On the other hand, the weights change quite significantly. When $\rho = -0.8$, the dose $x = 0.2$ has the largest weight while in Figure 6.5 the dose $x = 0$ has the largest weight. This may be due to the fact that the efficacy curve and p_{10} are almost identical when $x < 0.2$, so more patients are needed around $x = 0.2$ to identify p_{10} from the efficacy curve; see Figure 6.8, top panel. Also when the correlation between toxicity and efficacy is large, more variation is introduced in the model, and, consequently, more observations need to be allocated around $x = 0.2$, where the probability p_{10} starts to decrease. When ρ gets larger, the optimal designs become quite close to those in Section 6.5.1, where the correlation $\rho = 0.5$ was treated as known (not a parameter).

6.5.2 Drug combination

Now we investigate the case of two drugs administered simultaneously. For simplicity, we assume that the correlation coefficient between responses is known: $\rho = 0.5$. As in the case of the single drug, we construct optimal designs with or without constraints and study their robustness. The maximum tolerable rate is increased to 0.5, compared to 0.33 in the single-drug study.

Similar to Section 6.5.1, we consider the bivariate probit model (6.35), (6.36). Now $\mathbf{f}_1(\mathbf{x}) = \mathbf{f}_2(\mathbf{x}) = (1, x_1, x_2, x_1 x_2)^T$. The number of parameters in the model increases from 4 to 8, and $\boldsymbol{\theta}^T = (\boldsymbol{\theta}_1^T, \boldsymbol{\theta}_2^T)$, where

$$\boldsymbol{\theta}_j^T \mathbf{f}_j(\mathbf{x}) = \theta_{j1} + \theta_{j2} x_1 + \theta_{j3} x_2 + \theta_{j4} x_1 x_2, \ j = 1, 2, \tag{6.49}$$

where x_1 denotes a dose of drug 1, x_2 denotes a dose of drug 2, and $x_1 x_2$ denotes the interaction between the two drugs, $x_i \in [0, 1]$, $i = 1, 2$. The unknown parameters are $\boldsymbol{\theta} = (-1.26, 2, 0.9, 14.8; -1.13, 0.94, 0.36, 4)^T$. Figure 6.9 plots surfaces of the probabilities of efficacy/no toxicity (p_{10}), efficacy ($p_{1.}$), and toxicity ($p_{.1}$). The surface p_{10} increases as x_1 and x_2 increase at low dose values; but when both x_1 and x_2 gets larger, p_{10} starts to decrease. Both $p_{1.}$ and $p_{.1}$ increase as x_1 and x_2 increase.

Locally optimal designs. First we construct the traditional locally optimal designs with no constraints on the design region. Recall that in the case of the single drug, the traditional optimal design contains two points on the boundaries of the design region and one point inside; see Table 6.2. The traditional optimal design for a two-drug combination has a similar structure: five of the six support points are located at/near the boundaries of the design region and one point is located inside. Each corner of the design region has optimal points except for the corner $(1,1)$; this happens because the surfaces

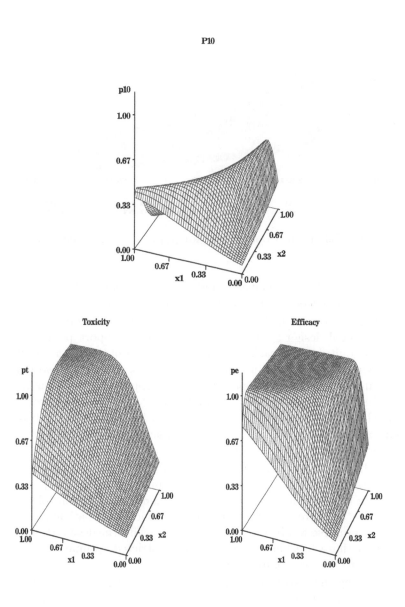

FIGURE 6.9: Response probability surfaces for the drug combination bi-variate probit model.

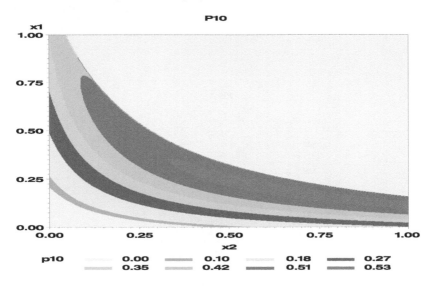

FIGURE 6.10: Contour plot for p_{10} in the restricted region.

of marginal probabilities of efficacy and toxicity are both flat as x_1 and x_2 get very large. The optimal design ξ_t is listed in Table 6.5.

In practice, it may be difficult to assign treatments according to the theoretical optimal design ξ_t. For instance, the two support points (0,1) and (0.08,1) are quite close to each other, and the weight of the latter is only 0.082. That is why we recommend a modified design $\xi_{t,m}$ where the two points are merged and weights of all support points are rounded; cf. the merging procedure described in Section 3.1.4, formula (3.33). The modified design $\xi_{t,m}$ is presented in Table 6.5; its relative deficiency is 1.03 showing that only 3% more patients are needed to obtain the same accuracy of parameter estimation; see (6.47) for the definition of relative deficiency.

Note, however, that both the traditional design ξ_t and its modified version $\xi_{t,m}$ assign 10% of patients to the dose combination (0.44, 0.96), which has a relatively high toxicity rate, much higher than the maximum tolerable rate 0.5. In order to address the individual ethics concern for patients in the trial, a better alternative will be the restricted design with the design region defined by (6.31) with $q_E \geq 0.2$ and $q_T \leq 0.5$. This restricted optimal design is listed as ξ_r in Table 6.5; see Figures 6.10, 6.11.

Comparing the restricted design with the design ξ_t, one may notice that the design point $(0,0)$ of ξ_t is shifted to $(0.16, 0.04)$, a dose combination with higher probability of success. Also, the design point $(0.44, 0.96)$ with high toxicity and low probability of success is moved to $(0.32, 0.48)$, which has a lower probability of toxicity and a higher probability of success.

Penalized locally optimal design. As in Section 6.5.1, we construct

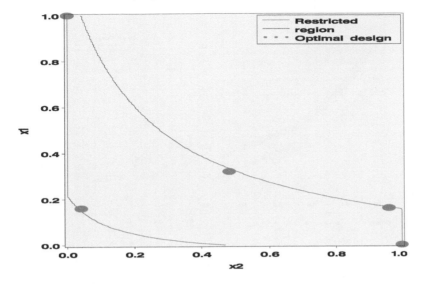

FIGURE 6.11: Locally optimal design and restricted region.

penalized locally D-optimal designs under the penalty function (6.26). When p_{10} or $1 - p_{.1}$ is very small, the penalty function can be very large, which causes computational difficulties. Therefore, we truncated the penalty function at a maximum of 10 units:

$$\phi(x, \boldsymbol{\theta}; C_E, C_T) = min(\{p_{10}(x, \boldsymbol{\theta})\}^{-C_E} \{1 - p_{.1}(x, \boldsymbol{\theta})\}^{-C_T}, 10). \qquad (6.50)$$

Figure 6.12 presents contours of the penalty function (6.50) and penalized optimal designs for pairs $(C_E, C_T) = (0,1)$, $(1,0)$, and $(1,1)$. When $(C_E, C_T) = (0, 1)$, the penalty function increases as both x_1 and x_2 increase. The optimal design ξ_{p01} is a six-point design similar to ξ_t. However, the weights of the support points $(0.12, 1)$ and $(0.32, 0.84)$ are very small; therefore we also list a modified (merged) design $\xi_{p01,m}$ in Table 6.5. The penalized deficiency of the modified design is 1.01; see (6.48).

When $(C_E, C_T) = (1, 0)$, the penalty function has large values when both drugs are either at high or low doses. Design ξ_{p10} does not have $(0,0)$ as a support point. The modified design $\xi_{p10,m}$ has a relative deficiency of 1.16.

When $(C_E, C_T) = (1, 1)$, the behavior of the penalty function is similar to the case when $(C_E, C_T) = (1, 0)$. The locally optimal design ξ_{p11} and its modified version $\xi_{p11,m}$ are listed in Table 6.5. The relative deficiency of the modified design is 1.21. Comparing the three penalty functions, we can see that the penalty functions are rather flat at $x_1 = 1$, $x_2 = 0$, so the point $(1,0)$ is always included in the penalized optimal designs.

Sensitivity analysis. To perform the sensitivity analysis for the model (6.49), we assume that the parameter space is formed by varying the "true"

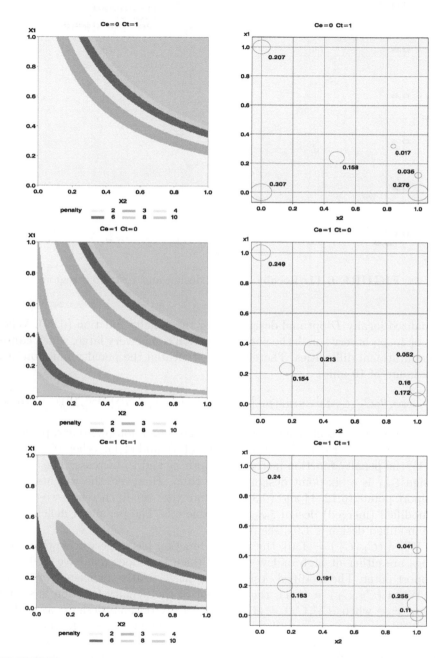

FIGURE 6.12: Penalty functions and penalized locally optimal designs for drug combinations. Top panel: $C_E = 0, C_T = 1$; middle panel: $C_E = 1, C_T = 0$; bottom panel: $C_E = 1, C_T = 1$.

TABLE 6.5: Locally optimal designs for two-drug combination.

	Optimal Design Modified Design					
ξ_t	$(0,0)$ 0.233	$(1,0)$ 0.249	$(0,1)$ 0.211	$(0.08,1)$ 0.082	$(0.28,0.4)$ 0.117	$(0.44,0.96)$ 0.108
$\xi_{t,m}$	$(0,0)$ 0.25	$(1,0)$ 0.25	$(0,1)$ 0.3	$(0.28,0.4)$ 0.10	$(0.44,0.96)$ 0.10	
ξ_r	$(0,1)$ 0.25	$(1,0)$ 0.25	$(0.16,0.96)$ 0.13	$(0.16,0.04)$ 0.23	$(0.32,0.48)$ 0.16	
	Penalized					
ξ_{p01}	$(0,0)$ 0.307	$(1,0)$ 0.207	$(0,1)$ 0.275	$(0.12,1)$ 0.035	$(0.24,0.48)$ 0.158	$(0.32,0.84)$ 0.017
$\xi_{p01,m}$	$(0,0)$ 0.3	$(1,0)$ 0.2	$(0,1)$ 0.3	$(0.24,0.48)$ 0.2		
ξ_{p10}	$(0.23,0.17)$ 0.154	$(1,0)$ 0.249	$(0.03,1)$ 0.172	$(0.1,1)$ 0.16	$(0.3,1)$ 0.052	$(0.37,0.33)$ 0.213
$\xi_{p10,m}$	$(0.23,0.17)$ 0.15	$(1,0)$ 0.25	$(0.1,1)$ 0.35	$(0.37,0.33)$ 0.25		
ξ_{p11}	$(0.2,0.16)$ 0.163	$(1,0)$ 0.24	$(0,1)$ 0.11	$(0.08,1)$ 0.255	$(0.32,0.32)$ 0.191	$(0.44,1)$ 0.041
$\xi_{p11,m}$	$(0.2,0.16)$ 0.2	$(1,0)$ 0.3	$(0.08,1)$ 0.25	$(0.32,0.32)$ 0.25		

parameter values by 20%; cf. (6.46). Instead of using all 2^8 possible combinations of parameters, we consider a fractional factorial design that contains 16 combinations and the central point θ_1; see Table 6.6.

All traditional locally optimal designs contain six to eight support points. Among the support points, the vertices (0,0), (0,1), and (1,0) are always in the optimal designs with weights about 20% each. The other points are located close to (0.1,0) and in the middle of the design region. The weight distribution depends on the parameter values. Only designs ξ_{12}, ξ_{16} and ξ_{17} are eight-point design with two extra support points inside the design region with very small weights ($w_j < 0.1$). By ξ_i we denote the locally optimal design for parameter θ_i in Table 6.6, $i = 1, \cdots, 17$.

The largest value of relative deficiency is 1.58 when the true parameters θ_9 are misspecified as θ_{10}. Designs ξ_9 and ξ_{10} are listed below:

$$\xi_9 = \left\{ \begin{array}{cccccc} (0,0) & (1,0) & (0,1) & (0.07,1) & (0.23,0.33) & (0.57,1) \\ 0.23 & 0.25 & 0.21 & 0.07 & 0.12 & 0.12 \end{array} \right\},$$

$$\xi_{10} = \left\{ \begin{array}{cccccc} (0,0) & (1,0) & (0,1) & (0.16,1) & (0.40,0.44) & (0.36,0.52) \\ 0.24 & 0.25 & 0.23 & 0.12 & 0.10 & 0.06 \end{array} \right\}.$$

It can be seen from Table 6.6 that parameters θ_9 and θ_{10} are quite different.

TABLE 6.6: Parameter values used in the sensitivity analysis

θ	θ_{11}	θ_{12}	θ_{13}	θ_{14}	θ_{21}	θ_{22}	θ_{23}	θ_{24}
1	−1.260	2.0	0.90	14.80	−1.130	0.940	0.360	4.0
2	−1.008	1.6	0.72	11.84	−0.904	0.752	0.288	3.2
3	−1.008	1.6	0.72	17.76	−1.356	1.128	0.432	3.2
4	−1.008	1.6	1.08	11.84	−1.356	1.128	0.288	4.8
5	−1.008	1.6	1.08	17.76	−0.904	0.752	0.432	4.8
6	−1.008	2.4	0.72	11.84	−1.356	0.752	0.432	4.8
7	−1.008	2.4	0.72	17.76	−0.904	1.128	0.288	4.8
8	−1.008	2.4	1.08	11.84	−0.904	1.128	0.432	3.2
9	−1.008	2.4	1.08	17.76	−1.356	0.752	0.288	3.2
10	−1.512	1.6	0.72	11.84	−0.904	1.128	0.432	4.8
11	−1.512	1.6	0.72	17.76	−1.356	0.752	0.288	4.8
12	−1.512	1.6	1.08	11.84	−1.356	0.752	0.432	3.2
13	−1.512	1.6	1.08	17.76	−0.904	1.128	0.288	3.2
14	−1.512	2.4	0.72	11.84	−1.356	1.128	0.288	3.2
15	−1.512	2.4	0.72	17.76	−0.904	0.752	0.432	3.2
16	−1.512	2.4	1.08	11.84	−0.904	0.752	0.288	4.8
17	−1.512	2.4	1.08	17.76	−1.356	1.128	0.432	4.8

For $\boldsymbol{\theta}_9$, all the parameters for the efficacy response take their largest values and all the parameters for the toxicity response take their smallest value, while for $\boldsymbol{\theta}_{10}$ it's just the opposite. So it's not surprising that these two designs differ the most. Also one may notice that the design ξ_1 is quite robust to parameter misspecification.

For the penalty function (6.50) with $(C_E, C_T) = (1,1)$, the locally optimal penalized designs $\xi_{pi}, i = 1, \cdots, 17$, are six- to eight-point designs. Three support points are consistently close to (0,0), (1,0), and (0,1), with weights ranging from 0.1 to 0.25, depending on the value of the penalty function. One or two support points are on the boundary $x_2 = 1$; the other support points are located inside the design region. The largest value of penalized relative deficiency is 1.88. Similar to nonpenalized designs, the maximum is achieved when $\boldsymbol{\theta}_9$ is misspecified as $\boldsymbol{\theta}_{10}$. The corresponding penalized optimal designs are:

$$\xi_{p9} = \left\{ \begin{array}{ccccccc} (0,1) & (1,0) & (0.08,1) & (0.2,0.12) & (0.28,0.28) & (0.6,0.96) \\ 0.15 & 0.29 & 0.22 & 0.15 & 0.16 & 0.03 \end{array} \right\},$$

$$\xi_{p10} = \left\{ \begin{array}{ccccccc} (0,0) & (1,0) & (0,1) & (0.12,1) & (0.2,1) & (0.4,0.44) & (0.36,0.52) \\ 0.25 & 0.25 & 0.21 & 0.08 & 0.04 & 0.13 & 0.04 \end{array} \right\}.$$

In Section 8.3 we will discuss how traditional locally optimal designs are utilized for the construction of adaptive designs for bivariate probit model. For a discussion of optimal designs for correlated binary and continuous responses, see Fedorov et al. (2012) [153].

Chapter 7

Locally Optimal Designs in PK/PD Studies

7.1   Introduction 188
7.2   PK Models with Serial Sampling: Estimation of Model Parameters 191
        7.2.1   Study background 191
        7.2.2   Two-compartment population model 192
        7.2.3   Single dose 195
        7.2.4   Repeated dose administration 197
7.3   Estimation of PK Parameters 199
        7.3.1   Problem setting and model-based designs 200
        7.3.2   PK metrics and their estimation 203
                7.3.2.1   Model-based (parametric) approach 204
                7.3.2.2   Empirical (nonparametric) approach 206
                7.3.2.3   Average PK metrics for one-compartment model 210
        7.3.3   Sampling grid 211
        7.3.4   Splitting sampling grid 215
        7.3.5 MSE of AUC estimator, single and split grids 218
7.4   Pharmacokinetic Models Described by Stochastic Differential Equations 221
        7.4.1   Stochastic one-compartment model I 222
        7.4.2   Stochastic one-compartment model II: systems with positive trajectories 224
        7.4.3   Proof of Lemma 7.1 228
7.5   Software for Constructing Optimal Population PK/PD Designs 230
        7.5.1   Regression models 231
        7.5.2   Supported PK/PD models 232
        7.5.3   Software inputs 232
        7.5.4   Software outputs 234
        7.5.5   Optimal designs as a reference point 236
        7.5.6   Software comparison 241
        7.5.7   User-defined option 245

In this chapter we consider examples of the application of optimal designs in pharmacokinetic studies:

- Pharmacokinetic population models with serial sampling as in Gagnon and Leonov (2005) [167], Fedorov and Leonov (2007) [146]; see Sections 7.2 and 7.3;

- Pharmacokinetic models described by stochastic differential equations as in Anisimov et al. (2007) [12], Fedorov et al. (2010) [147]; see Section 7.4.

In Section 7.5 we describe a MATLAB®-based library for constructing optimal designs for population pharmacokinetic/pharmacodynamic (PK/PD) studies; see Aliev et al. (2009, 2012) [7], [8]; Leonov and Aliev (2012) [253].

As pointed out in Section 6.1, in all examples of this chapter we use the first-order optimization algorithm over the finite (discrete) set of candidate information matrices where individual information matrices are calculated prior to running the optimal design algorithm.

7.1   Introduction

In various PK and PD studies repeated measurements are taken from each patient, and model parameters are estimated from the collected data. The quality of the information in an experiment is reflected in the precision of parameter estimates, which is traditionally expressed by their variance-covariance matrix. Each patient may have several responses measured at several time points, for example, (a) serial measurements of drug concentration, or (b) drug concentration and a PD effect, or (c) concentration of mother drug and its metabolite(s). Such settings lead to nonlinear mixed effects regression models with multiple responses where the sampling scheme for each patient is considered a multidimensional point in the space of admissible sampling sequences. Allocation of predictor variables is vital: how many time points per patient? When?

As noted in Chaloner and Verdinelli (1995) [65], the important work on design of complex PK models was, to very large extent, not in the mainstream statistics literature until the mid-1990s. The absolute majority of publications were in scientific journals on pharmacokinetics and mathematical biology. In particular, a series of papers, utilizing computer simulation, established the importance of optimal allocation of patients to sampling sequences and the impact of this allocation on the precision of parameter estimates. See, for example, Al-Banna et al. (1990) [4]; Ette et al. (1993, 1995, 1998) [117], [118], [119]. Other papers have developed methods based on the Fisher information matrix and optimal design algorithms to generate D-optimal designs, including designs with cost constraints. A number of earlier papers discussed optimal experimental design for individual, or fixed effects, PK studies; see D'Argenio (1981) [86], Atkinson et al. (1993) [16], Pronzato and Pázman (2001) [321]. For papers on population PK studies, see D'Argenio (1990) [87], Mentré et al. (1995, 1997) [278], [277], Retout et al. (2001) [339], Duffull et al. (2002) [107], Retout and Mentré (2003) [340]. In these papers, the authors developed approximations of the Fisher information matrix for nonlinear mixed effects models. See also D'Argenio et al. (2009) [88] for a description of ADAPT 5 software.

It is worthwhile noting that two types of analyses are traditionally used for PK studies:

- Compartmental, when a particular parametric compartmental model is assumed, and model parameters are estimated, such as rate constants, clearances, volume(s) of distribution; see (7.9), (7.23), and (7.81) for examples of compartmental models described by ordinary differential equations (ODEs). Using a compartmental approach, one can also evaluate such PK parameters as area under the curve (AUC), maximal concentration (C_{max}), and time to maximal concentration (T_{max}).

- Noncompartmental, when no specific parametric model is assumed *a priori* and AUC, C_{max} and T_{max} are estimated using the nonparametric approach. Specifically, to estimate AUC, numerical integration algorithms are used based on observed responses. To estimate C_{max} and T_{max}, sample maximum and point of maximum are utilized, respectively. The nonparametric approach is often preferred by regulatory agencies at early stages of drug development.

We focus on the compartmental approach and optimal design for PK compartmental models in Sections 7.2 and 7.5. A comparison of the compartmental and noncompartmental approaches is provided in the example of Section 7.3. Section 7.4 describes optimal designs for compartmental models described by stochastic differential equations (SDEs). In what follows, by model or response parameters we mean rate constants, clearances or volumes of distribution that appear in various compartmental models. By PK parameters or PK metrics we mean AUC, C_{max} and T_{max}, which are discussed in Section 7.3.

A few comments are due about the notations in this chapter where all models have at least two sources of randomness: measurement errors and population variability. The standard model of observations in the context of PK sampling is

$$y_{ij} = \eta(x_{ij}, \gamma_i) + \varepsilon_{ij}, \ i = 1, \dots, N, \quad j = 1, \dots, k_i, \tag{7.1}$$

where N is the number of patients in the study; k_i and x_{ij} are the number of measurements and j-th sampling time, respectively, for patient i; γ_i is the vector of individual parameters of patient i; ε_{ij} are measurement errors with zero mean; cf. (1.130), (2.134).

For an illustration, let random errors $\{\varepsilon_{ij}\}$ be normally distributed with variance σ^2. Let parameters γ_i follow the multivariate normal distribution with mean γ^0 and variance-covariance matrix Ω,

$$\gamma_i \sim \mathcal{N}(\gamma^0, \Omega), \ i = 1, \dots, N, \tag{7.2}$$

and let ε_{ij} and γ_i be mutually independent. Then for a given γ_i, the expectation of y_{ij} with respect to the distribution of ε_{ij} is

$$\mathbf{E}_\varepsilon(y_{ij}|\gamma_i) = \eta(x_{ij}, \gamma_i). \tag{7.3}$$

For examples of response functions $\eta(x, \boldsymbol{\gamma})$, see a two-compartment model in (7.9), (7.10) with the vector of response parameters $\boldsymbol{\gamma} = (K_{12}, K_{21}, K_{10}, V)$, or a one-compartment model (7.23), (7.24) with $\boldsymbol{\gamma} = (K_a, K_e, V)$.

By $\boldsymbol{\theta}$ we denote the combined vector of parameters, which includes population mean response parameters $\boldsymbol{\gamma}^0$, population variance-covariance matrix $\boldsymbol{\Omega}$, and so-called residual variance σ^2, i.e.,

$$\boldsymbol{\theta} = (\boldsymbol{\gamma}^0; \boldsymbol{\Omega}; \sigma^2). \qquad (7.4)$$

The first-order approximation (first-order Taylor expansion in the vicinity of $\boldsymbol{\gamma}^0$) implies the following expression for the mean response:

$$\mathbf{E}(y_{ij}) = \mathbf{E}_{\boldsymbol{\gamma},\varepsilon}(y_{ij}) = \mathbf{E}_{\boldsymbol{\gamma}}[\eta(x_{ij}, \boldsymbol{\gamma}_i)] \approx \eta(x_{ij}, \boldsymbol{\gamma}^0). \qquad (7.5)$$

Note that the expression for $\eta(x_{ij}, \boldsymbol{\gamma}^0)$ does not depend on the values of $\boldsymbol{\Omega}$ and σ^2. Thus, when using the first-order approximation for the mean population response together with (7.4), one can formally write

$$\mathbf{E}(y_{ij}) \approx \eta(x_{ij}, \boldsymbol{\gamma}^0) = \eta(x_{ij}, \boldsymbol{\theta}), \qquad (7.6)$$

where the expression on the right-hand side of (7.6) does not depend on components $\boldsymbol{\Omega}$ and σ^2 of the vector $\boldsymbol{\theta}$. The expression on the right-hand side of (7.5) will be used in our examples to calculate the Fisher information matrix $\boldsymbol{\mu}(\mathbf{x}, \boldsymbol{\theta})$ in (1.108) under the normality assumption. For other examples of approximation of the mean population response, see (7.17) and Section 7.5.6.

In what follows, by $\eta(x, \boldsymbol{\gamma}_i)$ or its multidimensional equivalent $\boldsymbol{\eta}(\mathbf{x}, \boldsymbol{\gamma}_i)$ for the sequence of sampling times $\mathbf{x} = (x_1, \ldots, x_k)$, we mean the analog of (7.3). By $\eta(x, \boldsymbol{\gamma}^0) = \eta(x, \boldsymbol{\theta})$ or its multidimensional equivalent $\boldsymbol{\eta}(\mathbf{x}, \boldsymbol{\gamma}^0) = \boldsymbol{\eta}(\mathbf{x}, \boldsymbol{\theta})$, we mean the analog of (7.5). For an example of the approximation of the variance-covariance matrix $\mathbf{S}(\mathbf{x}, \boldsymbol{\theta})$ in (1.108), see (7.15), (7.16).

Among relevant references on nonlinear mixed models are

- Estimation, including PK/PD applications: Spjotvoll (1977) [367]; Mallet (1986) [263]; Lindstrom and Bates (1990) [259]; Beal and Sheiner (1992) [40]; Wolfinger (1993) [406]; Pinheiro and Bates (1995, 2002) [310], [311]; Delyon et al. (1999) [92]; Demidenko (2004) [93]; Kuhn and Lavielle (2005) [240]; Bauer et al. (2007) [37]; Wang (2007) [395].

- Optimal design and analysis, including Bayesian settings: Chaloner (1984) [64]; Racine-Poon (1985) [332]; Chaloner and Verdinelli (1995) [65] (optimal Bayesian design); Wakefield (1996) [390] (Bayesian analysis for PK studies); Stroud et al. (2001) [369] (design for PK studies); Han et al. (2002) [190] (Bayesian designs in HCV studies); Han and Chaloner (2004) [189]; Atkinson (2008) [15] (design for nonlinear random effects); Dette et al. (2010 [96] (random effects for PK studies with correlated errors).

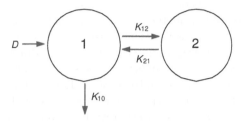

FIGURE 7.1: Diagram of two-compartment model.

7.2 PK Models with Serial Sampling: Estimation of Model Parameters

In this section, we demonstrate how the application of optimal design techniques can lead to a reduction in the per-patient sampling density without significant loss of efficiency, and how cost-based designs can lead to a meaningful comparison of designs with distinct numbers of samples. For further details, see Gagnon and Leonov (2005) [167].

7.2.1 Study background

In Gagnon and Leonov (2005) [167] a clinical trial was considered in which the drug was administered as bolus input D_0 at the beginning of the study, at time $x = 0$, and then bolus inputs D_i were administered at 12- or 24-hour intervals until 72 hours. To describe the concentration of drug at time x, a two-compartment model was used, parameterized via the volume of distribution V, and transfer rate constants K_{12}, K_{21} and K_{10}. Measurements of drug concentration y_{ij} were taken from compartment 1 (central) at times $x_{ij} \equiv x_j$ for each patient, and were assumed to satisfy (7.1), where

$$\eta(x, \gamma_i) = q_1(x, \gamma_i)/V_i, \tag{7.7}$$

$q_1(x, \gamma)$ is the amount of the drug in the central compartment at time x, and $\gamma_i = (V_i, K_{12,i}, K_{21,i}, K_{10,i})$ are individual PK parameters of patient i. See Figure 7.1 for a schematic presentation of the model and Section 7.2.2 for details on the function q_1.

In the trial under consideration $k = 16$ samples were taken from each patient at times from a set $\mathcal{X}_0$,

$$\mathcal{X}_0 = \{5, 15, 30, 45 \text{ min}; 1, 2, 3, 4, 5, 6, 12, 24, 36, 48, 72, 144 \text{ h}\}, \tag{7.8}$$

i.e., the same sampling scheme with 16 sampling times was used for all patients. Obviously, each extra sample provides additional information and increases the precision of parameter estimates. However, the number of samples that may be drawn from each patient is restricted because of blood volume limitations and other logistical and ethical reasons. Moreover, the analysis of each sample is associated with monetary costs. Therefore, it is reasonable to take the cost of drawing samples into account. If $\mathbf{x} = (x_1, ..., x_k)$ is a sequence of sampling times for a particular patient, then $\phi(\mathbf{x})$ will denote the cost of the sampling sequence $\mathbf{x}$. In this section we focus on addressing the following questions:

1. Given restrictions on the number of samples for each patient, what are the optimal sampling times (i.e., how many samples and at which times)?

2. If not all 16 samples are taken, what would be the loss of information/precision?

3. If costs are taken into account, what is the optimal sampling scheme?

In all examples of this section we construct locally D-optimal designs, i.e., by an optimal sampling scheme we mean a sequence, or a combination of sequences, that allow us to obtain the best precision of parameter estimates with respect to the D-criterion. Note also that the design region $\mathfrak{X}$ is a collection of a finite number of sequences that consist of elements of a prespecified discrete set of candidate sampling times; see (7.8) or (7.21). By a single design "point" we mean a sequence of sampling times $\mathbf{x}_i$ for i-th patient.

First, we need to define the regression model with multiple responses, as in (1.107). In what follows, $\mathbf{x}$ will denote a k-dimensional vector of sampling times, and $\mathbf{Y}$ will be a k-dimensional vector of measurements at times $\mathbf{x}$.

7.2.2   Two-compartment population model

The two-compartment model with bolus input is described by the following system of linear differential equations:

$$\begin{cases} \dot{q}_1(x, \boldsymbol{\gamma}) = -(K_{12} + K_{10})q_1(x, \boldsymbol{\gamma}) + K_{21}q_2(x, \boldsymbol{\gamma}), \\ \dot{q}_2(x, \boldsymbol{\gamma}) = K_{12}q_1(x, \boldsymbol{\gamma}) - K_{21}q_2(x, \boldsymbol{\gamma}), \end{cases} \tag{7.9}$$

for $x \in [t_r, t_{r+1})$ with initial conditions

$$q_1(t_r, \boldsymbol{\gamma}) = q_1(t_r - 0, \boldsymbol{\gamma}) + D_r, \quad q_1(0, \boldsymbol{\gamma}) = D_0, \quad q_2(0, \boldsymbol{\gamma}) = 0,$$

where $q_1(x, \boldsymbol{\gamma})$ and $q_2(x, \boldsymbol{\gamma})$ are amounts of the drug at time x in the central (no.1) and peripheral compartments, respectively; t_r is the time of r-th bolus input, and $t_0 = 0$; D_r is the amount of the drug administered at t_r. The solution $\mathbf{q}(x, \boldsymbol{\gamma}) = [q_1(x, \boldsymbol{\gamma}), q_2(x, \boldsymbol{\gamma})]^T$ of the system (7.9) depends on parameters $\boldsymbol{\gamma}^T = (K_{12}, K_{21}, K_{10}, V)$. More precisely, the amounts q_1, q_2

do not depend on volume V while the concentration $\eta(x, \gamma)$ defined in (7.7) depends on V. Note also that amounts q_1, q_2 are not observed directly; instead we observe the concentration $\eta(x, \gamma_i)$. Function $q_1(x, \gamma)$ has jumps at times t_r because of drug administration, while $q_2(x, \gamma)$ is continuous:

$$\mathbf{q}(x, \gamma) = e^{\lambda_1(x-t_r)} \begin{pmatrix} K_{21} + \lambda_1 \\ K_{12} \end{pmatrix} \left[\frac{q_1(t_r, \gamma)}{\lambda_1 - \lambda_2} + \frac{K_{12} + K_{10} + \lambda_1}{K_{12}(\lambda_1 - \lambda_2)} q_2(t_r, \gamma) \right]$$

$$+ e^{\lambda_2(x-t_r)} \begin{pmatrix} K_{21} + \lambda_2 \\ K_{12} \end{pmatrix} \left[\frac{q_1(t_r, \gamma)}{\lambda_2 - \lambda_1} + \frac{K_{12} + K_{10} + \lambda_2}{K_{12}(\lambda_2 - \lambda_1)} q_2(t_r, \gamma) \right], \quad (7.10)$$

where $x \in [t_r, t_{r+1})$ and

$$\lambda_{1,2} = 0.5 \left[K_{12} + K_{21} + K_{10} \pm \sqrt{(K_{12} + K_{21} + K_{10})^2 - 4K_{21}K_{10}} \right];$$

see Seber and Wild (1989) [357], Chapter 8; Gibaldi and Perrier (1982) [176], Appendix B.

In population modeling it is assumed that the individual response parameters γ_i of patient i are independently sampled from a given population, either normal as in (7.2), or log-normal, i.e.,

$$\gamma_{il} = \gamma_l^0 e^{\zeta_{il}}, \; l = 1, \dots, m_\gamma; \; \zeta_i \sim \mathcal{N}(0, \Omega), \quad (7.11)$$

where m_γ is the dimension of the vector γ^0 (so-called "typical" values, in NONMEM nomenclature; see Beal and Sheiner (1992) [40]), and Ω is the variance-covariance matrix of independent, identically distributed random vectors ζ_i. The vector γ^0 and the matrix Ω are often referred to as population parameters.

It was assumed that the error term ε_{ij} in (7.1) satisfies

$$\varepsilon_{ij} = \varepsilon_{1,ij} + \varepsilon_{2,ij} \, \eta(x_j, \gamma_i), \quad (7.12)$$

where $\varepsilon_{1,ij}$ and $\varepsilon_{2,ij}$ are independent, identically distributed normal random variables with zero mean and variance σ_A^2 and σ_P^2, respectively.

Let $\theta = (\gamma^0; \Omega; \sigma_A^2, \sigma_P^2)$ denote a combined vector of model parameters, cf. (7.4), and let k_i be the number of samples taken for patient i. Let $\mathbf{x}_i = (x_{i1}, x_{i2}, \dots, x_{ik_i})^T$ and $\mathbf{Y}_i = (y_{i1}, y_{i2}, \dots, y_{ik_i})^T$ be sampling times and measured concentrations, respectively, for patient i. Further, let $\eta(x, \gamma_i) = q_1(x, \gamma_i)/V_i$, $\eta(x, \theta) = q_1(x, \gamma^0)/V^0$ and

$$\eta(\mathbf{x}_i, \theta) = [\eta(x_{i1}, \theta), \dots, \eta(x_{ik_i}, \theta)]^T; \quad (7.13)$$

cf. (7.5), (7.6). If $\mathbf{F}$ is a $k_i \times m_\gamma$ matrix of partial derivatives of function $\eta(\mathbf{x}_i, \theta)$ with respect to parameters γ_0,

$$\mathbf{F} = \mathbf{F}(\mathbf{x}_i, \gamma^0) = \left[\frac{\partial \eta(\mathbf{x}_i, \theta)}{\partial \gamma_\alpha} \right]\Bigg|_{\gamma = \gamma^0}, \quad (7.14)$$

then the first-order approximation together with (7.2) and (7.12) imply the following approximation of the variance-covariance matrix $\mathbf{S}(\mathbf{x}_i, \boldsymbol{\theta})$ for $\mathbf{Y}_i$:

$$\mathbf{S}(\mathbf{x}_i, \boldsymbol{\theta}) \simeq \mathbf{F}\boldsymbol{\Omega}\mathbf{F}^T + \sigma_P^2 \text{Diag}[\boldsymbol{\eta}(\mathbf{x}_i, \boldsymbol{\theta})\boldsymbol{\eta}^T(\mathbf{x}_i, \boldsymbol{\theta}) + \mathbf{F}\boldsymbol{\Omega}\mathbf{F}^T] + \sigma_A^2 \mathbf{I}_{k_i}, \quad (7.15)$$

where $\mathbf{I}_k$ is a $k \times k$ identity matrix, and $\text{Diag}(\mathbf{A})$ denotes a diagonal matrix with elements a_{ii} on the diagonal. If the $\boldsymbol{\gamma}$ parameters are assumed to be log-normally distributed, then the matrix $\boldsymbol{\Omega}$ on the right-hand side of (7.15) must be replaced with

$$\boldsymbol{\Omega}_1 = \text{Diag}(\boldsymbol{\gamma}^0) \, \boldsymbol{\Omega} \, \text{Diag}(\boldsymbol{\gamma}^0); \quad (7.16)$$

for derivation, see Leonov and Aliev (2012) [253]. Therefore, for any candidate sequence $\mathbf{x}_i$, the response vector $\boldsymbol{\eta}(\mathbf{x}_i, \boldsymbol{\theta})$ and variance-covariance matrix $\mathbf{S}(\mathbf{x}_i, \boldsymbol{\theta})$ are defined, and one can use (1.108) to approximate the Fisher information matrix $\boldsymbol{\mu}(\mathbf{x}_i, \boldsymbol{\theta})$ for each individual sequence and then run the optimal design algorithm.

Remark 7.1 If one uses the Taylor expansion for $\eta(x, \boldsymbol{\gamma})$ up to the second-order terms,

$$\eta(x, \boldsymbol{\gamma}) = \eta(x, \boldsymbol{\gamma}^0) + \left[\frac{\partial \eta(x, \boldsymbol{\gamma}^0)}{\partial \gamma_\alpha}\right]^T [\boldsymbol{\gamma} - \boldsymbol{\gamma}^0] + \frac{1}{2}[\boldsymbol{\gamma} - \boldsymbol{\gamma}^0]^T \mathbf{H}(\boldsymbol{\gamma}^0)[\boldsymbol{\gamma} - \boldsymbol{\gamma}^0] + \dots$$

where

$$\mathbf{H}(\boldsymbol{\gamma}^0) = \left[\frac{\partial^2 \eta(x, \boldsymbol{\gamma})}{\partial \gamma_\alpha \partial \gamma_\beta}\right]\bigg|_{\boldsymbol{\gamma} = \boldsymbol{\gamma}^0},$$

then it follows from (7.2) that the expectation of $\eta(x, \boldsymbol{\gamma}_i)$ with respect to the distribution of parameters $\boldsymbol{\gamma}_i$ can be approximated as

$$\mathbf{E}_{\boldsymbol{\gamma}}[\eta(x, \boldsymbol{\gamma}_i)] \approx \eta(x, \boldsymbol{\gamma}^0) + \frac{1}{2}\text{tr}[\mathbf{H}(\boldsymbol{\gamma}^0)\boldsymbol{\Omega}]. \quad (7.17)$$

If model (7.11) is used for $\boldsymbol{\gamma}_i$, then matrix $\boldsymbol{\Omega}$ in (7.17) must be replaced with matrix $\boldsymbol{\Omega}_1$ defined in (7.16). In our example the second term on the right-hand side of (7.17) is relatively small compared to $\eta(x, \boldsymbol{\gamma}^0)$. Thus, disregarding this term does not significantly affect the results. However, if the second term is not negligible, some adjustments are needed to incorporate the additional term. For further discussion of the approximation options, see Section 7.5.6.

To obtain parameter estimates $\hat{\boldsymbol{\theta}}$ for the construction of locally D-optimal designs, data from 16 samples from the set $\mathcal{X}_0$ and $N = 27$ subjects were used. To fit the data, parameters K_{12} and K_{21} were assumed known, i.e., they were not accounted for in the information matrix $\boldsymbol{\mu}(\mathbf{x}, \boldsymbol{\theta})$ in (1.108). Model (7.11) was used for random effects $\boldsymbol{\gamma}_i$, and the combined vector of unknown parameters $\boldsymbol{\theta}$ was defined as

$$\boldsymbol{\theta} = (\gamma_1^0, \gamma_2^0; \, \Omega_{11}, \Omega_{22}, \Omega_{12}; \, \sigma_A^2, \sigma_P^2),$$

where

$$\gamma_1^0 = CL, \ \gamma_2^0 = V, \ \Omega_{11} = \mathrm{Var}(\zeta_{CL}), \ \Omega_{22} = \mathrm{Var}(\zeta_V), \ \Omega_{12} = \mathrm{Cov}(\zeta_{CL}, \zeta_V),$$

where CL is the plasma clearance and $K_{10} = CL/V$. So, in this example $m_\gamma = 2$ and the total number of unknown parameters is $m = 7$. NON-MEM software (see Beal and Sheiner (1992) [40]) was used to obtain estimates $\hat{\theta} = (0.211, 5.50; 0.0365, 0.0949, 0.0443; 8060, 0.0213)^T$. Drug concentrations were expressed in micrograms/liter (μg/L), elimination rate constant K_{10} in liters/hour (L/h) and volume V in liters (L). The estimates used for other parameters were $K_{12} = 0.400$ and $K_{21} = 0.345$.

Optimal designs were constructed using the first-order optimization algorithm described in Chapter 3, which was implemented independently in MATLAB and SAS® IML. For more details on MATLAB stand-alone tool for constructing optimal population designs for PK models, see Section 7.5.

7.2.3 Single dose

Here we consider the model (7.9) with the single dose $D_0 = 42$ mg. For a design region we take

$$\mathfrak{X}_1 = \{\mathbf{x} = (x_1, ..., x_k); \ x_j \in \mathcal{X}^0, \ j = 1, 2, ..., k; \ 5 \le k \le 8\};$$

i.e., we allow any combination of k sampling times for each patient from the original sequence $\mathcal{X}^0$ defined in (7.8); $5 \le k \le 8$. No costs are introduced, which means that taking 5 samples costs the same as taking 8 samples, etc. Then it is obvious that taking the maximum number of samples is better with respect to the precision of parameter estimates; the D-optimal design is a single sequence of 8 sampling times,

$$\xi_8^* = \{w_1 = 1, \ \mathbf{x}_1 = (5, 15, 30, 45 \ \mathrm{min}, \ 36, 48, 72, 144 \ \mathrm{h}) \}.$$

If by ξ_{16} we denote the design that utilizes all 16 samples from $\mathcal{X}^0$, then the relative D-efficiency of design ξ_8^* is $\mathrm{Eff}_{8,16} = 0.84$; see (6.22). Thus, we lose about 16% of the precision of parameter estimates when taking the 8 best samples instead of all possible 16 samples. On the other hand, we reduce the number of samples by a factor of 2 and lose only 16% of the information. Note also that routine laboratory analysis of each sample requires certain monetary spending; the use of design ξ_8^* would reduce monetary spending by 50%.

We compared nonnormalized variance-covariance matrices $\mathbf{D}(\xi_8^*)$ and $\mathbf{D}(\xi_{16})$, where $\mathbf{D}(\xi) = \mathbf{M}^{-1}(\xi, \boldsymbol{\theta})/N$, $\mathbf{M}(\xi, \boldsymbol{\theta})$ is the normalized information matrix of design ξ, and $N = 27$ is the number of subjects in the study. The increase in the number of samples from 8 to 16 does not essentially change the precision of estimation of parameters $\theta_1, ..., \theta_6$, but affects mainly $\theta_7 = \sigma_P^2$. In particular,

$$\underline{D}_{11}(\xi_{16}) = 7.05e - 5, \ \underline{D}_{11}(\xi_8^*) = 7.17e - 5;$$

TABLE 7.1: Single dose, D-efficiency of k-point designs.

k	5	6	7	8	9	16
No cost	0.69	0.75	0.79	0.84	0.87	1
$\phi_1(\mathbf{x})$	1.19	1.22	1.22	1.21	1.19	1
$\phi_2(\mathbf{x})$	4.00	3.53	3.06	2.66	2.31	1

Note: Row 1 - no costs; row 2 - cost (7.19); row 3 - cost (7.20).

$$\underline{D}_{22}(\xi_{16}) = 1.01e - 1, \ \underline{D}_{22}(\xi_8^*) = 1.05e - 1;$$
while
$$\underline{D}_{77}(\xi_{16}) = 7.86e - 6, \ \underline{D}_{77}(\xi_8^*) = 1.31e - 5;$$
for more details on the comparison, see Gagnon and Leonov (2005) [167]. It is not surprising that the increase in the number of samples leads to a more precise estimate of residual error variance, while it seems rather surprising that this increase contributes very little to better estimation of other parameters. However, the discussion in Section 7.3.5 sheds further light on why this may happen.

Optimal k-sample designs, no costs. We compared optimal k-sample designs ξ_k^* with the 16-sample reference design ξ_{16}, where designs ξ_k^* are D-optimal for design region $\mathfrak{X}_k$,

$$\mathfrak{X}_k = \{\mathbf{x} = (x_1, ..., x_k); \ x_j \in \mathcal{X}^0, \ j = 1, 2, ..., k\}. \tag{7.18}$$

Note that there is no restriction on the number of distinct sequences, or elementary designs, in D-optimal design. It turns out that for $5 \leq k \leq 9$, D-optimal designs consist of a single sequence. Specifically,

$$\xi_5^* = \{5, 15 \, \text{min}; \ 48, 72, 144 \, \text{h}\}, \ldots, \ \xi_9^* = \{5, 15, 30, 45 \, \text{min}; \ 1, 36, 48, 72, 144 \, \text{h}\}.$$

The efficiency results are presented in Table 7.1, first row. Similar to ξ_8^*, variance-covariance matrices of the above designs have a visible change in row/column 7, which corresponds to the residual error variance σ_P^2.

Cost-based designs. Let us assume that the cost increases with the number of samples as in

$$\phi_1(\mathbf{x}_k) = C_v + C_s * k, \tag{7.19}$$

where k is the number of samples taken, C_s is the cost of taking/analyzing a single sample and C_v is associated with the overall cost of the study/patient visit; $C_s = 0.1$, $C_v = 1$ in the examples below. Then one can consider the optimization problem (4.9). We use the cost-normalized information matrix $\mathbf{M}(\xi_c)$ as in (4.19) and the sensitivity function as in (4.24). The results of an efficiency comparison for optimal k-point designs are given in Table 7.1, second row. As expected, once the costs of analyzing samples are taken into account, the designs with smaller numbers of samples become more efficient: first, because they cost less, and second, because they still allow one to collect sufficient information about the model parameters.

A more radical cost function is when the cost of the j-th consecutive sample is proportional to j, for example $C_s * j$, which in turn leads to the quadratic cost function

$$\phi_2(\mathbf{x}_k) = C_v + C_s k(k+1)/2. \tag{7.20}$$

For this cost function, the efficiency of designs with a larger number of samples will obviously deteriorate more rapidly; see row 3 in Table 7.1.

Sensitivity analyses. As discussed in Section 6.3, for nonlinear regression problems, optimal designs depend on prior estimates of unknown parameters. This necessitates various sensitivity analyses to see how robust optimal designs are. We constructed optimal designs for perturbed values of prior estimates and observed the same trend as in the original example, i.e., the changes in the variance-covariance matrix are substantial only for the residual variance parameter $\theta_7 = \sigma_P^2$.

7.2.4 Repeated dose administration

The results in this section are presented for the repeated dose schedule, with the starting dose of 31.5 mg and the maintenance dose of 7 mg repeated every 24 hours. Some sampling times may be "forced" in the design, which mimics forced variables in stepwise regression procedures; see Draper and Smith (1998) [106], Chapter 19; cf. composite designs in Section 2.7. As an example, in this section we consider forced trough time points, i.e., immediately preceding the next dose. This means that samples are always taken at 24, 48 and 72 hours. Therefore, if we select the best three sampling times, then in fact we take six samples: three forced troughs and three "best" time points with respect to the optimization criterion. Compared to the original candidate sampling times from $\mathcal{X}_0$ in (7.8), here we added two extra times at 60 and 84 hours, i.e., 12 hours after drug administration. Thus, candidate sampling times in this section belong to

$$\mathcal{X}^R = \{5, 15, 30, 45 \text{ min}; \ 1, 2, 3, 4, 5, 6, 12, 36, 60, 84, 144 \text{ h}\}. \tag{7.21}$$

Standard normalization, no costs. From the discussion of single dose analysis, it may be expected that taking the 3 or 4 best samples will be enough for a reasonable estimation of model parameters. Indeed, the relative D-efficiency of design ξ_3^R compared to ξ_6^R is $\textit{Eff}_{3,6} = 0.816$, where ξ_k^R is the D-optimal k-sample design for the design region (7.21) with three trough samples,

$$\xi_3^R = \{5, 15 \text{ min}, 144 \text{ h}\}, \quad \xi_6^R = \{5, 15, 30, 45 \text{ min}, 84, 144 \text{ h}\}.$$

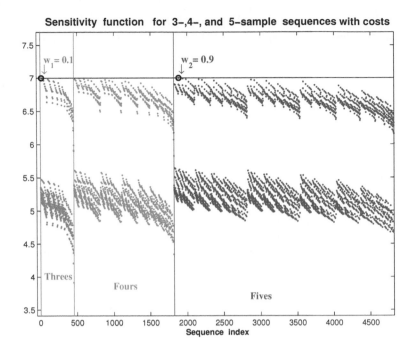

FIGURE 7.2: Sensitivity function for cost-based design.

As before, the substantial differences are in the elements corresponding to residual variances. For all other model parameters, after having taken 6 samples (3 forced and 3 best "flexible"), additional measurements add little to improve the precision of estimating θ_{1-5}. This confirms that essentially all the difference in the estimation of the seven parameters (D-criterion, or generalized variance) is coming from the difference in the estimation of residual variance parameters, as in the case of the single dose.

Cost-based designs. We use the numerical procedure based on (4.24), with the cost function (7.19), where $C_v = 1$, $C_s = 0.1$. The design region is defined as

$$\mathfrak{X} = \{\mathbf{x} = (x_1, ..., x_r); \ x_j \in \mathcal{X}^R, \ j = 1, 2, ..., r; \ 3 \le r \le 5\},$$

with three forced troughs. The cost-based D-optimal design is a combination of two sampling sequences,

$$\xi^* = \{\mathbf{x}_1^* = (5, 15 \text{ min}, \ 144 \text{ h}), \ \mathbf{x}_2^* = (5, 15, 30 \text{ min}, \ 84, 144 \text{ h})\},$$

with weights $w_1 = 0.1$ and $w_2 = 0.9$, respectively. Recall that to calculate frequencies r_i for cost-based designs, the cost function $\phi_1(\mathbf{x})$ must be taken into account; see formula (4.28). This leads to

$$\frac{r_2}{r_1} = \frac{0.9}{0.1} \times \frac{1.3}{1.5} = 7.8;$$

therefore about 11.4% of patients should be randomized to a 3-sample sequence $\mathbf{x}_1^*$ and 88.6% of patients should be randomized to a 5-sample sequence $\mathbf{x}_2^*$.

To demonstrate how the Equivalence Theorem (Theorem 2.3) can be used for this example, we enumerate all candidate sampling sequences and plot the sensitivity function $d(\mathbf{x}_i, \xi^*, \boldsymbol{\theta})$ as a function of index i. Note that $C(15, 3) = 455$ (number of all candidate sequences of 3 sampling times from $\mathcal{X}^M$), $C(15, 4) = 1365$, $C(15, 5) = 3003$, and the total number of candidate sequences is $N = \sum_{k=3}^{5} C(15, k) = 4823$. To order candidate sequences, we start with three-sample sequences and first vary third sampling time, then repeat this procedure for second and first sampling times, and for four- and five-sample sequences; cf. Section 7.5.5. So

$$\mathbf{x}_1 = (5, 15, 30 \text{ min}), \quad \mathbf{x}_2 = (5, 15, 45 \text{ min}), \quad \mathbf{x}_3 = (5, 15 \text{ min}, 1 \text{ h}), \ \dots$$
$$\dots \ \mathbf{x}_{454} = (36, 84, 144 \text{ h}), \quad \mathbf{x}_{455} = (60, 84, 144 \text{ h});$$

$$\mathbf{x}_{456} = (5, 15, 30, 45 \text{ min}), \quad \mathbf{x}_{457} = (5, 15, 30 \text{ min}, 1 \text{ h}), \dots$$
$$\dots \ \mathbf{x}_{1820} = (36, 60, 84, 144 \text{ h});$$

$$\mathbf{x}_{1821} = (5, 15, 30, 45 \text{ min}, 1 \text{ h}), \dots \ \dots, \ \mathbf{x}_{4823} = (12, 36, 60, 84, 144 \text{ h}).$$

Figure 7.2 serves as an illustration of the Equivalence Theorem. The sensitivity function $d(\mathbf{x}_i, \xi^*, \boldsymbol{\theta})$ hits the reference line $m = 7$ at two D-optimal sequences: $\mathbf{x}_{13} = \mathbf{x}_1^*$ and $\mathbf{x}_{1886} = \mathbf{x}_2^*$.

7.3 Estimation of PK Parameters

In many pharmaceutical studies, including clinical PK and bioavailability assessment, multiple blood samples are taken for each enrolled patient, but instead of estimating the model parameters as in Section 7.2, the focus is on the estimation of various average population PK metrics, such as area under the curve (AUC)), maximal concentration (C_{max}) and time to maximal concentration (T_{max}). We will use the terms "PK parameter" and "PK metric" interchangeably for AUC, C_{max} and T_{max}. The goals of this section are as follows:

- Comparison of a model-based approach, when parameters of a compartmental model are estimated and the explicit formulae for PK metrics are used, and an empirical approach, when numerical integration algorithms based on observed responses are used for estimating AUC, and sample values of estimators – for C_{max} and T_{max}. We focus on the empirical approach, namely, the method E2 introduced in Section 7.3.2.2, while using the model-based approach as a benchmark.

- Analysis of alternative sampling grids. Usually in PK studies more samples are taken immediately after administering the drug, and sampling times become less dense after the anticipated T_{max}; see examples in Section 7.2. We show that sampling grids generated by a uniform grid on the vertical (response) axis with respect to values of either the response function or the AUC curve, lead to competitive estimators and allow us to utilize prior information about PK curves.

- Demonstration of how to "split" a single sampling grid into two (or more) subsets, so that the number of patients in the study does not change, while the number of samples per each patient is reduced by half. We demonstrate that such a split often has little effect on the precision of estimation of PK metrics and has a negligible effect on the bias term and terms associated with population variability for AUC estimation.

- Introduction of costs, in particular the costs of patient's enrollment and costs of analyzing samples, and comparison of sampling grids under cost constraints.

In Section 7.3.1 we introduce the model of measurements and briefly discuss population model-based designs, with the design region different from the one discussed in Section 7.2. In Section 7.3.2 the two approaches for the estimation of PK metrics, parametric and nonparametric, are discussed. Sections 7.3.3 and 7.3.4 present the results of simulations for different grids of sampling times. These results demonstrate that (a) when the model is correctly specified, the model-based approach outperforms the traditional empirical one in terms of precision of PK metrics' estimation, but not by much; and that (b) split grids perform competitively. In Section 7.3.5 we present closed-form solutions for the mean squared error (MSE) of the empirical estimator of AUC for a simple case of quadratic regression with random intercept and discuss the behavior of the MSE under cost constraints. For further details, see Fedorov and Leonov (2007) [146].

7.3.1   Problem setting and model-based designs

Our main focus is on an *empirical* (*model-independent, noncompartmental, or nonparametric*) approach, when the only assumptions made about the response function are about its smoothness properties, such as continuity and differentiability of the function itself and its derivatives. In this case no assumptions are made about the shape of the response function, i.e., no parametric model is used for the estimation of average PK parameters. As a benchmark, we consider a *model-based* (*compartmental, or parametric*) approach, when a specific parametric model is correctly assumed for the response function, and average PK metrics are obtained on the second step of the estimation procedure, after model parameters are estimated.

Data in our simulations are generated via the model (7.1), where sampling times $x_{ij} \in [a, b]$, $x_{ij} < x_{i,j+1}$, $j = 0, 1, \ldots, k_i$. Parameters γ_i of patient i are sampled from the multivariate normal distribution (7.2), and measurement errors ε_{ij} are i.i.d. normal variables with mean zero and variance σ^2.

In practice, it is often assumed that response parameters γ_i follow the log-normal distribution; see formula (7.11) in Section 7.2. Other models may be considered for measurements errors: for example, the error variance may depend on the mean response, as in (7.12), or the log-normal distribution of residual errors ε_{ij} may be introduced, as in Gagnon and Peterson (1998) [168]. However, the main goal of examples in this section is to show how the ideas utilized for the construction of optimal model-based designs can be extended to the empirical approach. That is why we provide results under the assumption of normality and mention in passing that these techniques can be used in more general settings.

The example of Section 7.2 demonstrated how to optimize sampling schemes for population PK studies using optimal experimental design techniques for parametric models. Here we show how to bridge the earlier results with the nonparametric approach. In Section 7.2, the design region $\mathfrak{X}$ was formed by the combinations of k sampling times from the sequence $\mathcal{X}_0$ in (7.8). The cost function was introduced in (7.19). It was shown that once the cost C_s of taking/analyzing a single sample becomes positive, then sequences with smaller number of samples may become optimal. Moreover, it may happen that optimal design is a "mix" of several sequences with distinct number of samples, i.e., different sampling schemes will be used for different cohorts; see Section 7.2.4. This fact motivated us to consider "split" grids in Section 7.3.4.

Here we select candidate sequences differently from those in Section 7.2. The particular choice of these sequences will become justified when we discuss splitting sampling grids in Section 7.3.4. Let $\mathcal{X} = \{x_1, x_2, \ldots, x_n\}$ be a set of length n of all candidate sampling times.

- For some patients, say n_1, samples are taken at all times from $\mathcal{X}$, i.e., $\mathbf{x}_1 = \mathcal{X}$.

- Second-order split: for some patients, say $n_2/2$, samples are taken at times $\mathbf{x}_{2,1} = \{x_1, x_3, \ldots, x_{2s-1}, \ldots\}$, and for another $n_2/2$ patients samples are taken at $\mathbf{x}_{2,2} = \{x_2, x_4, \ldots, x_{2s}, \ldots, x_n\}$ (without loss of generality we may assume that n is even). Then a generalized candidate "point" $\mathbf{x}_2$ is the combination of two half-sequences $\mathbf{x}_{2,1}$ and $\mathbf{x}_{2,2}$.

- Third-order split: for $n_3/3$ patients, samples are taken at times $\mathbf{x}_{3,1} = \{x_1, x_4, \ldots, x_{3s+1}, \ldots\}$; a second cohort of $n_3/3$ patients will have sampling times $\mathbf{x}_{3,2} = \{x_2, x_5, \ldots, x_{3s+2}, \ldots\}$; and the last one-third will have samples at $\mathbf{x}_{3,3} = \{x_3, x_6, \ldots, x_{3(s+1)}, \ldots\}$. In this case a candidate "point" $\mathbf{x}_3$ is a combination of three sequences $\mathbf{x}_{3,1}$, $\mathbf{x}_{3,2}$, and $\mathbf{x}_{3,3}$, and so forth with the introduction of higher-order splits. In practice, n is not always even or divisible by 3. In such cases, we can split, say a 17-point grid into 8- and 9-point grids for the second-order split, and 6-,6- and 5-point grids for the third-order split.

The information matrix corresponding to the s-th order split $\mathbf{x}_s$ can be written as $\boldsymbol{\mu}(\mathbf{x}_s, \boldsymbol{\theta}) = \sum_{l=1}^{s} \boldsymbol{\mu}(\mathbf{x}_{s,l}, \boldsymbol{\theta})/s$, where to calculate $\boldsymbol{\mu}(\mathbf{x}_{s,l}, \boldsymbol{\theta})$ we use the techniques described in Section 7.2. If we use the analog of the cost function from (7.19), then the cost of observations at a single generalized "point" $\mathbf{x}_s$ is

$$\phi(\mathbf{x}_s) = C_v + C_s n/s. \qquad (7.22)$$

To illustrate optimal designs and for simulations described later in this section, we selected a one-compartment model with first-order absorption and linear elimination that is described by the following system of ordinary differential equations:

$$\begin{cases} \dot{q}_0(x) = & -K_a q_0(x), & q_0(0) = D, \\ \dot{q}_1(x) = & K_a q_0(x) & - K_e q_1(x), & q_1(0) = 0, \end{cases} \qquad (7.23)$$

where q_0 is the amount of drug at the site of administration, q_1 is the amount of drug in the central compartment, and K_a and K_e are absorption and elimination rate constants, respectively; D is the administered dose. By $\eta(x, \boldsymbol{\gamma}) = q_1(x)/V$ we denote the drug concentration in the central compartment where measurements are taken; see Gibaldi and Perrier (1982) [176], Chapter 1, or Bonate (2010) [49], Chapter 1:

$$\eta(x, \boldsymbol{\gamma}) = \frac{DK_a}{V(K_a - K_e)} \left(e^{-K_e x} - e^{-K_a x}\right), \quad \boldsymbol{\gamma} = (K_a, K_e, V)^T, \qquad (7.24)$$

where V is the volume of distribution, and it is assumed that $K_a > K_e$; see also examples in Sections 7.4 and 7.5. Without loss of generality we take $D = 1$ and $x \in [0, 1]$ (normalized time scale).

To avoid numerical problems with the constraint $K_a > K_e$ when running the nonlinear least squares algorithm for estimating individual parameters $\boldsymbol{\gamma}_i$ in the model-based approach (see Section 7.3.2.1), we reparameterized the model (7.24) with the new set of parameters:

$$\boldsymbol{\gamma} = (\gamma_1, \gamma_2, \gamma_3), \ \gamma_1 = K_e, \ \gamma_2 = K_a - K_e > 0, \ \gamma_3 = 1/V, \qquad (7.25)$$

so that $K_a = \gamma_1 + \gamma_2$, $K_e = \gamma_1$ and $\boldsymbol{\gamma}^0 = (6, 40, 10)$, which mimics the data from a real clinical study. Variance parameters were selected as

$$\sigma = 0.5, \ \boldsymbol{\Omega} = \text{Var}(\boldsymbol{\gamma}) = \text{diag}(\Omega_\alpha) \text{ with } \sqrt{\Omega_\alpha} = 0.15 \, \gamma_\alpha, \ \alpha = 1, 2, 3, \qquad (7.26)$$

and the combined vector of parameters is $\boldsymbol{\theta} = (\gamma_1, \gamma_2, \gamma_3; \Omega_1, \Omega_2, \Omega_3; \sigma^2)$.

To construct locally D-optimal designs, the first-order optimization algorithm was used; see Chapter 3. For the set $\mathcal{X}$ we took a grid with 16 samples generated by the mean AUC curve; see Section 7.3.3:

$$\mathcal{X} = \{0.026,\ 0.041,\ 0.055,\ 0.070,\ 0.085,\ 0.101,\ 0.119,\ 0.138, \qquad (7.27)$$

$$0.160,\ 0.186,\ 0.216,\ 0.253,\ 0.300,\ 0.367,\ 0.478,\ 1\}.$$

The design region is $\mathfrak{X} = \{\mathbf{x}_1, \mathbf{x}_2, \mathbf{x}_3\}$, i.e., all splits up to the third order are included.

When standard normalized designs are considered, it is not surprising that the locally D-optimal design is the single sequence $\mathbf{x}_1$. Indeed, the determinant of the information matrix increases with the number of observations. Once costs of the patient's enrollment and costs of analyzing samples are taken into account, the situation may change and the single sequence may lose its optimality. Let $C_v = 5$ in (7.22):

- If $C_s = 0.45$, then the cost-based D-optimal design is the single sequence $\mathbf{x}_1$;

- If $C_s = 0.7$, then the optimal design is the collection of two "points," $\mathbf{x}_1$ and $\mathbf{x}_2$, with 22% of patients having samples taken at times $\mathbf{x}_1$ and 78% of patients allocated to $\mathbf{x}_2$, i.e., 39% to sequence $\mathbf{x}_{2,1}$ and 39% to sequence $\mathbf{x}_{2,2}$;

- If $C_s = 1$, then the optimal design is the single "point" $\mathbf{x}_2$;

- If $C_s = 2$, then $\xi_{opt} = \{\mathbf{x}_2,\ \mathbf{x}_3\}$, with 15.5% of patients allocated to each of the two sequences $\mathbf{x}_{2,1}$ and $\mathbf{x}_{2,2}$, and 23% of patients allocated to each of the three sequences $\mathbf{x}_{3,1}, \mathbf{x}_{3,2}$ and $\mathbf{x}_{3,3}$.

As mentioned in Section 7.1, regulatory agencies usually require the noncompartmental analysis in the early stages of drug development, such as empirical estimation of average PK parameters, e.g., AUC and C_{max}. This is the reason for us focusing on the empirical approach and using the model-based approach as a benchmark. We exploit the earlier findings from optimal model-based designs to address the question of whether it is cost-expedient to reduce the number of samples for the nonparametric approach. In pursuing this goal we introduce sampling schemes that mimic the above designs. For a discussion of optimal model-based designs for the estimation of individual PK parameters, see Atkinson et al. (1993) [16].

7.3.2 PK metrics and their estimation

To describe estimation procedures used in our simulations, we start with the simplest case when sampling times are the same for all patients:

$$x_{ij} \equiv x_j, \quad k_i \equiv k \ \text{ for all } i = 1, \dots, N, \qquad (7.28)$$

and then comment on how to adjust the estimators when sampling times may differ from patient to patient; see (7.43). The discussed methods involve calculating PK metrics and averaging over the population, yet differ in the order of the two operations. We concentrate on the nonparametric approach and method E2 where one starts with averaging responses at each time point over all patients and then gets estimates of PK parameters for the "averaged" curve; see Section 7.3.2.2 for details. This method is applicable in the case of sparse sampling.

7.3.2.1 Model-based (parametric) approach

In our exposition, all model-based methods start with obtaining individual parameter estimates $\hat{\gamma}_i$ for model (7.1) for each patient (via nonlinear least squares, maximum likelihood, etc.). However, in general, the problem may be tackled using nonlinear mixed effects models; e.g., see Beal and Sheiner (1992) [40], Demidenko (2004) [93], Bonate (2010) [49], Chapter 7. See also Section 2.11.

We consider three types of average PK metrics.

Type I, method M1 (averaging PK parameters). Explicit formulae are used to get

$$\widehat{AUC}_i = \int_a^b \eta(x, \hat{\gamma}_i)dx, \quad \widehat{T}_i = \arg\max_x \eta(x, \hat{\gamma}_i), \quad \widehat{C}_i = \max_x \eta(x, \hat{\gamma}_i); \quad (7.29)$$

for details, see Section 7.3.2.3. Next, when (7.28) is satisfied, the individual estimators are averaged across all patients to obtain population estimators

$$\widehat{AUC}_{M1} = \frac{1}{N}\sum_{i=1}^N \widehat{AUC}_i, \quad \widehat{T}_{M1} = \frac{1}{N}\sum_{i=1}^N \widehat{T}_i, \quad \widehat{C}_{M1} = \frac{1}{N}\sum_{i=1}^N \widehat{C}_i. \quad (7.30)$$

The estimators in (7.30) are strongly consistent estimators, as $N \to \infty$, of

$$AUC_1 = E_\gamma\left[\int_a^b \eta(x, \gamma)dx\right], \quad T_1 = E_\gamma\left[\arg\max_x \eta(x, \gamma)\right],$$

$$C_1 = E_\gamma\left[\max_x \eta(x, \gamma)\right]. \quad (7.31)$$

Instead of arithmetic means as in (7.30), geometric means may be considered; see Lacey et al. (1997) [241], Julious and Debarnot (2000) [222].

Type II, method M2 (direct averaging of responses). One may be interested in the characteristics of the "average" PK curve that would lead to the following estimators:

$$\widehat{AUC}_{M2} = \int_a^b \hat{\eta}_N(x)dx, \quad \widehat{T}_{M2} = \arg\max_x \hat{\eta}_N(x), \quad \widehat{C}_{M2} = \max_x \hat{\eta}_N(x), \quad (7.32)$$

with $\widehat{\eta}_N(x) = \frac{1}{N}\sum_i \eta(x, \widehat{\gamma}_i)$, which consistently estimate population metrics

$$AUC_2 = \int_a^b \bar{\eta}(x)dx, \ T_2 = \arg\max_x \bar{\eta}(x), \ C_2 = \max_x \bar{\eta}(x), \qquad (7.33)$$

where $\bar{\eta}(x) = E_\gamma [\eta(x, \gamma)]$. Note that $AUC_1 = AUC_2$ and $\widehat{AUC}_{M1} = \widehat{AUC}_{M2}$. In practice, to evaluate $\widehat{T}_{M2}$ and $\widehat{C}_{M2}$, the optimization of function $\widehat{\eta}_N(x)$ may be performed numerically; see Section 7.3.2.3.

Type III, method M3 (averaging model parameters). Alternatively, one may first average the individual $\widehat{\gamma}_i$ across patients to get an average model parameter estimate $\widehat{\gamma} = \sum_{i=1}^N \widehat{\gamma}_i/N$, and then calculate estimators

$$\widehat{AUC}_{M3} = \int_a^b \eta(x, \widehat{\gamma})dx, \ \widehat{T}_{M3} = \arg\max_x \eta(x, \widehat{\gamma}), \ \widehat{C}_{M3} = \max_x \eta(x, \widehat{\gamma}),$$
$$(7.34)$$

which consistently estimate

$$AUC_3 = \int_a^b \eta(x, E\gamma)dx, \ T_3 = \arg\max_x \eta(x, E\gamma), \ C_3 = \max_x \eta(x, E\gamma). \ (7.35)$$

The metrics defined in (7.31), (7.33), and (7.35) will be referred to as Type I, Type II and Type III metrics, respectively. We show in Section 7.3.2.2 that methods M1 and M2 have natural analogs in the nonparametric approach with respect to metrics of Type I and II, respectively. We are unaware of an analog of method M3 for the nonparametric approach. As noted above, $AUC_1 = AUC_2$ while all other types of metrics for AUC, T_{max} and C_{max} are, in general, different in the presence of population variability ("larger" Ω lead to a more pronounced difference, while all three types coincide when $\Omega = 0$). To evaluate metrics AUC_1, T_1 and C_1 in (7.31), and T_2 and C_2 in (7.33), we used the Monte Carlo method; see Section 7.3.2.3.

If condition (7.28) is violated, i.e., when sampling times differ for different patients, then individual estimates from (7.29) must be weighted properly. For example,

$$\widehat{AUC}_{M1} = \sum_{i=1}^N w_i \widehat{AUC}_i, \ \text{where} \ \sum_{i=1}^N w_i = 1, \ \text{and} \ w_i^{-1} \sim \text{Var}\left(\int_a^b \eta(x, \widehat{\gamma}_i)dx\right).$$

To describe the quality of any estimator $\widehat{\beta}$, we use its mean squared error (MSE):

$$MSE(\widehat{\beta}) = E\left[\widehat{\beta} - \beta_{true}\right]^2 = \text{Var}(\widehat{\beta}) + \left[E(\widehat{\beta}) - \beta_{true}\right]^2 = Var + Bias^2.$$
$$(7.36)$$

In the parametric approach the second term on the right-hand side of (7.36) is often negligible if the model is specified correctly and the number of observations, i.e., k and N, is large enough. Still, the main focus of this section is the selection of sampling grids that are efficient for the nonparametric approach. Values of model-based estimates and their MSEs are needed as benchmarks.

7.3.2.2 Empirical (nonparametric) approach

As in the parametric case, we start with the estimation procedure under condition (7.28); otherwise, see (7.43).

Type I, method E1. For each patient, find

$$\widehat{T}_i = x_{j^*(i)}, \quad \text{where} \quad j^*(i) = \arg\max_j y_{ij}, \quad \widehat{C}_i = y_{i,j^*(i)}.$$

To get individual estimators $\widehat{AUC}_i$, use one of the numerical integration procedures described later in this subsection. Then average individual estimators to obtain population estimators $\widehat{AUC}_{E1}$, $\widehat{T}_{E1}$ and $\widehat{C}_{E1}$, similar to (7.30); here, the subscript E stands for "empirical." If the sampling grid $\{x_j\}$ is rather fine and N is large, these estimators would be reasonable estimators of the metrics of Type I; see (7.31).

If the number of samples for some individuals is small, then method E1 is not recommended for obvious reasons (cf. sparse sampling often encountered in toxicology; see Nedelman and Gibiansky (1996) [294] or Gagnon and Peterson (1998) [168]). In what follows we concentrate on method E2 which is applicable in the case of sparse sampling.

Type II, method E2. Average responses at each time point across all patients,

$$\hat{\eta}_j = \hat{\eta}_{jN} = \frac{1}{N} \sum_{i=1}^{N} y_{ij}, \quad j = 0, 1, \ldots, k, \tag{7.37}$$

and build estimators for the "population curve" $\{\hat{\eta}_j\}$:

$$\widehat{T}_{E2} = x_{j^*}, \quad \widehat{C}_{E2} = \hat{\eta}_{j^*}, \quad \text{where} \quad j^* = \arg\max_j \hat{\eta}_j.$$

Then use numerical integration algorithms to estimate AUC:

$$\widehat{AUC}_{E2} = \sum_{j=1}^{k} \int_{x_{j-1}}^{x_j} g(x, \mathbf{a}_j) dx, \tag{7.38}$$

where g is an interpolating function (interpolant) whose parameters $\mathbf{a}_j$ are chosen so that g passes exactly through $\hat{\eta}_{j-1}$ and $\hat{\eta}_j$. By construction, estimators $\widehat{AUC}_{E2}$, $\widehat{T}_{E2}$ and $\widehat{C}_{E2}$ may be expected to provide good estimates of the metrics of Type II in (7.33) for a rather fine sampling grid $\{x_j\}$ and large N; see Section 7.3.3 for details and Figure 7.3 for a schematic presentation of AUC estimators for methods M2 and E2.

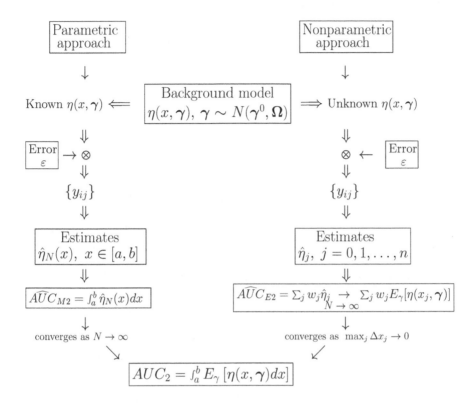

FIGURE 7.3: Schematic presentation of type II AUC estimators; see (7.33). See (7.32) for method M2 (parametric) and (7.38) for method E2 (nonparametric).

Remark 7.2 Instead of arithmetic means at each time point, as in (7.37), sometimes geometric means are interpolated to estimate AUC. Such averaging may be beneficial under the assumption of log-normally distributed data; for details, see Gagnon and Peterson (1998) [168].

Numerical integration procedures.

(1) A trapezoidal rule is the simplest and most widely used procedure in PK studies. The linear trapezoidal rule provides an example of the first-order spline; see Bailer and Piegorsch (1990) [28], Evans and Swartz (2000) [121], and Krommer and Ueberhuber (1998) [239]. The interpolant in (7.38) is a piece-wise linear function,

$$g(x, \mathbf{a}_j) = a_{1j} + a_{2j}(x - x_{j-1}) \text{ for } x \in [x_{j-1}, x_j],$$

where $a_{j1} = \hat{\eta}_{j-1}$, $a_{j2} = (\hat{\eta}_j - \hat{\eta}_{j-1})/(x_j - x_{j-1})$. Consequently,

$$\widehat{AUC}_{E2,\, lin} = \sum_{j=1}^{k} \Delta x_j \widehat{F}_{j,\, lin}, \ \ \text{where} \ \ \widehat{F}_{j,\, lin} = \frac{\hat{\eta}_{j-1} + \hat{\eta}_j}{2}, \ \Delta x_j = x_j - x_{j-1},$$

(7.39)

and the estimator can be written as the weighted sum of averaged observations,

$$\widehat{AUC}_{E2,\, lin} = \sum_{j=0}^{k} w_j \hat{\eta}_j, \ \text{with} \ w_0 = \frac{\Delta x_1}{2}; \ w_k = \frac{\Delta x_n}{2}; \ w_j = \frac{\Delta x_j + \Delta x_{j+1}}{2},$$

(7.40)

where $j = 1, \ldots, k - 1$. Because of that, when observations are uncorrelated, formulae for variance and bias terms may be rather easily obtained. On the other hand, the linear interpolant has zero curvature and in cases where changes in curvature between time points are excessive or when the intervals between sampling times are quite large, this method may lead to substantial errors; see Yeh and Kwan (1978) [420], Chiou (1978) [76].

The use of more advanced methods of numerical integration, like classical Gaussian quadratures, improves the precision of integration but makes it difficult to analyze the statistical properties of computed integrals for noisy observations; see Whittaker and Robinson (1967) [404]. This explains why we prefer to stay with the trapezoidal method and its modifications for the remainder of this section.

Remark 7.3 It can be shown that if function $\bar{\eta}(x)$, introduced in (7.33), has a continuous second derivative, then the bias of the estimator (7.40) is given by

$$Bias = E\left[\widehat{AUC}_{E2,\, lin}\right] - AUC_2 \approx \frac{1}{12} \sum_{j=1}^{k} \bar{\eta}\,''(x_{j-1})(\Delta x_j)^3, \quad (7.41)$$

where the expectation is taken with respect to both between-patient (or population, in γ_i) and within-patient (in ε_{ij}) variability; see Evans and Swartz (2000) [121], Chapter 5. If the population variability vanishes, then the variance component on the right-hand side of (7.36) is equal to

$$Var\left[\widehat{AUC}_{E2,\, lin}\right] = \frac{\sigma^2}{2N}\left[\sum_{j=1}^{k}(\Delta x_j)^2 + \sum_{j=1}^{k-1}\Delta x_j \Delta x_{j+1}\right]; \quad (7.42)$$

see Fedorov and Leonov (2006) [145] for a discussion of optimization problems generated by (7.41) and (7.42). Note, however, that in the nonparametric approach no assumptions are made about the functional form of the response function, and, second, the assumption about population variability is inherent in population PK modeling. The ultimate goal is to minimize the MSE of the estimator and not the bias or variance terms separately. Moreover, when the population variability cannot be ignored, the expression for the variance term would be much more complicated than (7.42). Thus, in general, it is impossible to derive the expression for the MSE in a closed form. We use simulations to compare the performance of various methods for more general settings, see Sections 7.3.3 and 7.3.4, and derive explicit formulae for the MSE for some simple scenarios, see Section 7.3.5.

If the assumption of equal sampling times as in (7.28) does not hold, then the estimation of $\hat{\eta}_j$ in (7.37) must be modified as follows. Order all sampling times from smallest to largest, $a = x_0 < x_1 < \cdots < x_k = b$, and let N_j be the number of patients with sampling time x_j, i.e., $N_j = \{$number of patients such that $x_{ij'} = x_j$ for some $j'\}$. Then

$$\hat{\eta}_j = \frac{1}{N_j} \sum_{i,j':\, x_{ij'}=x_j} y_{ij'}. \qquad (7.43)$$

Among other popular numerical integration methods in pharmacokinetics are

(2) A "hybrid" method in which the linear trapezoidal rule (7.39) is used for the ascending and "plateau" portions of the time-concentration curve and a log-trapezoidal rule is applied for the descending portion (elimination phase):

$$\widehat{AUC}_{E2,H} = \sum_{j=1}^{k} \Delta x_j \widehat{F}_{j,H}, \text{ where } \widehat{F}_{j,H} = \begin{cases} \widehat{F}_{j,\,lin}, & \text{if } x_j \le t^*, \\ \widehat{F}_{j,\,log}, & \text{if } x_j > t^*, \end{cases} \qquad (7.44)$$

where t^* is selected in the right tail of the curve and $\widehat{F}_{j,\,log} = (\hat{\eta}_j - \hat{\eta}_{j-1})/\ln(\hat{\eta}_j/\hat{\eta}_{j-1})$; see Yeh and Kwan (1978) [420], and Purves (1992) [330]. For model (7.24), plasma concentrations increase during the absorption phase and then decline after T_{max}. Thus, as suggested by Chiou (1978) [76], the hybrid method is a reasonable choice for that model.

(3) Cubic spline method: $g(x, \mathbf{a}_j)$ is a piecewise cubic polynomial at each of the intervals $[t_{j-1}, t_j]$, $j = 1, \ldots, k$; see Yeh and Kwan (1978) [420], Wahba (1990) [389], and Wald (1974) [392]. For knots t_j of the spline, one may select sampling times $\{x_j\}$. In addition to continuity conditions, we use the following constraints to define the spline uniquely:

$$g(x_1, \mathbf{a}_1) = g(x_2, \mathbf{a}_2), \quad g(x_{k-1}, \mathbf{a}_{k-1}) = g(x_k, \mathbf{a}_k); \qquad (7.45)$$

see Yeh and Kwan (1978) [420], p. 85. Estimators of T_2 and C_2 are defined as

$$\widehat{T}_{2,S} = \arg\max_x g(x, \mathbf{a}_{j^*}), \quad \widehat{C}_{2,S} = \max_x g(x, \mathbf{a}_{j^*}),$$

where $j^* = \arg\max_j [\max_x g(x, \mathbf{a}_j)]$.

For our simulation studies, we used the hybrid method because of its rather wide applicability and acceptance by regulatory agencies, and the cubic spline method because of its popularity in numerical analysis and function approximation. For notational brevity, in the sequel we use abbreviations MA, EA and SA for the model-based, empirical hybrid (trapezoidal/ log-trapezoidal), and spline methods, respectively.

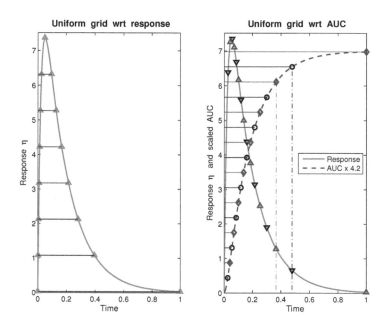

FIGURE 7.4: Uniform grid with respect to values of response (left) and AUC (right). Inverted triangles: odd samples on the mean response curve; circles: odd samples on the scaled AUC curve. Triangles: even samples on the mean response curve; diamonds: even samples on the scaled AUC curve.

7.3.2.3   Average PK metrics for one-compartment model

For the one-compartment model (7.24) over the interval [0,1],

$$
\begin{aligned}
\beta_1(\boldsymbol{\gamma}) &= \int_0^1 \eta(x,\boldsymbol{\gamma})dx = \frac{K_a}{V(K_a - K_e)}\left[\frac{1 - e^{-K_e}}{K_e} - \frac{1 - e^{-K_a}}{K_a}\right], \\
\beta_2(\boldsymbol{\gamma}) &= \arg\max_x \eta(x,\boldsymbol{\gamma}) = \frac{\ln(K_a/K_e)}{K_a - K_e}, \\
\beta_3(\boldsymbol{\gamma}) &= \max_x \eta(x,\boldsymbol{\gamma}) = \frac{1}{V}\left(\frac{K_a}{K_e}\right)^{-K_e/(K_a - K_e)};
\end{aligned}
\tag{7.46}
$$

see Figure 7.4, left panel. The PK parameters in (7.31) were evaluated via 10^6 Monte Carlo simulations. Under (7.25) and (7.26),

$$AUC_1 = 1.836, \quad T_1 = 0.0546, \quad C_1 = 7.342. \tag{7.47}$$

We also evaluated these metrics using the Taylor expansion for functions $\beta_r(\gamma)$, $r = 1, 2, 3$, up to the second-order terms; cf. (7.17):

$$E_\gamma\left[\beta_r(\gamma)\right] \approx \beta_r(\gamma^0) + \frac{1}{2}\,\mathrm{tr}[\mathbf{\Omega}\mathbf{H}_r(\gamma^0)], \quad \mathbf{H}_r(\gamma^0) = \left[\frac{\partial^2\beta(\gamma)}{\partial\gamma\,\partial\gamma^T}\right]\Bigg|_{\gamma=\gamma^0},$$

where $\mathbf{H}_r(\gamma^0)$ is the matrix of second partial derivatives of function β_r with respect to parameters γ. This approximation gave $\widehat{AUC}_1 = 1.803$, $\widetilde{T}_1 = 0.0538$, and $\widetilde{C}_1 = 7.346$. To evaluate T_2 and C_2 in (7.33), we used 10^6 simulations: the maximum of function $\bar{\eta}(x) = E_\gamma\left[\eta(x,\gamma)\right]$ was found by the modified grid method with step 10^{-4} in the vicinity of T_1:

$$T_2 = 0.0521, \quad C_2 = 7.210. \tag{7.48}$$

The average PK parameters in (7.35) can be calculated directly via $\beta_r(\gamma^0)$:

$$AUC_3 = 1.662, \quad T_3 = 0.0509, \quad C_3 = 7.367. \tag{7.49}$$

Although from a practical point of view the discrepancies between (7.47) – (7.49) may be small, we want to reemphasize that the average metrics of Types I - III are, in general, different. To illustrate the difference, in Figure 7.5 we present curves $\eta(x,\gamma^0)$ and $\bar{\eta}(x) = E_\gamma\left[\eta(x,\gamma)\right]$ for different values of the coefficient of variation $CV = \sqrt{\Omega_\alpha}/\gamma_\alpha = \{0.15, 0.3 \text{ or } 0.5\}$; see (7.26). To avoid negative values of model parameters, which may occur for large CV ($CV = 0.5$ in our case), we truncated parameter values by the threshold 0.001.

In practice it is often necessary to estimate the area under the curve from zero to infinity, $AUC_{[0,\infty]}$, given observations in a finite time interval, say $[0, x_k]$. For details on how to handle the estimation of $AUC_{[0,\infty]}$, see Gabrielsson and Weiner (2001) [165], Section 3.2, or Gibaldi (1984) [175]. In particular, the estimate of the area under the curve from x_k to infinity is usually obtained as C_k/K_{el}, where C_k is the measurement (concentration) at time x_k. In our example, the value of the response curve at $x_k = 1$ is very close to zero, $\eta(1, \gamma^0) = 0.0285$, so the difference between $AUC_{[0,\infty]}$ and $AUC_{[0,x_k]}$ is negligible.

7.3.3 Sampling grid

Traditionally in PK studies more samples are taken at the left end of the sampling interval, immediately after administering the drug, and then samples become more sparse after the anticipated T_{max}. We consider two alternative grids that possess this property:

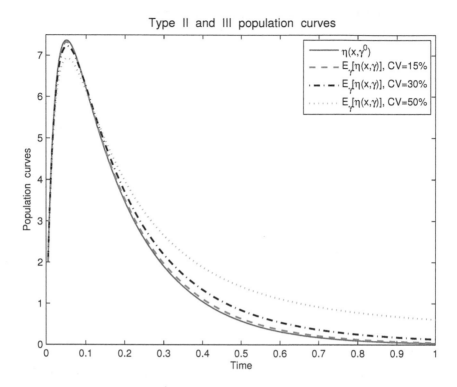

FIGURE 7.5: Type III population curve $\eta(x, \gamma^0)$, solid line. Type II population curves $\bar{\eta}(x) = E_\gamma [\eta(x, \gamma)]$ for different values of coefficient of variation CV: 15% (dashed), 30% (dash-dotted), and 50% (dotted).

- Take a uniform grid on the vertical axis with respect to values of the response function and then project points on the response curve to the x-axis, to obtain sampling times; see Figure 7.4, left panel. Such grids are called "inverse linear" in López-Fidalgo and Wong (2002) [261].

- A uniform grid on the vertical axis may be selected with respect to values of AUC accumulated up to each time; see Figure 7.4, right panel, and (7.27). More precisely, we take a uniform grid on the vertical axis for the AUC curve $A(t) = \int_0^t \eta(x, \gamma^0) dx$ and then project points on the AUC curve to the horizontal axis. The triangles on the response curve correspond to these sampling times; see dash-dotted vertical lines in the right panel. To make ranges of response η and AUC comparable, we plotted values of AUC multiplied by 4.2; see the legend of the right panel.

The construction of such grids requires the knowledge of model parameters that we exploited in our simulations. However, preliminary information is needed for using traditional sampling schemes too. For example, if T_{max} is expected during the first 2 to 3 hours after administering the drug, then it would be natural to have quite a dense sampling frequency over that period of time and then reduce the number/frequency of samples. On the other hand, when it is expected from clinical/pharmacological considerations that the drug concentration may peak over the first 30 to 40 minutes after the dose, then it would be reasonable to reduce the sampling frequency after, say, 1 hour.

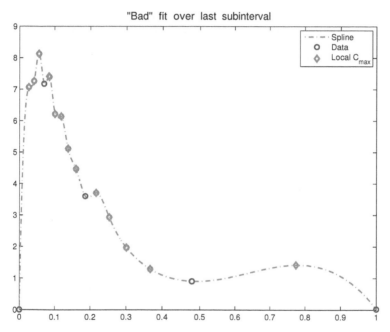

FIGURE 7.6: Example of cubic spline overfitting.

In the selected model, values of the mean response and all its derivatives are very close to zero at the right end of the sampling interval $x_k = 1$, while sampling point x_{k-1} is rather far away from x_k and values of the mean response and its derivatives at x_{k-1} do not vanish. Therefore, fitting data with cubic splines satisfying condition (7.45) may often lead to the situation presented in Figure 7.6, where this condition prevents the smoothing spline from being sufficiently "flat" at $x = x_k$. Thus, instead of using splines over the whole interval we use them over $[0, x_{k-1}]$ and then use the log-trapezoidal rule in the last subinterval $[x_{k-1}, x_k]$; see Yeh and Kwan (1978) [420] for a discussion of similar combination methods. In our simulations the two grids had very similar performance, so we discuss results for the AUC-based grid only.

Expected values of AUC estimator for method E2. The estimator $\widehat{AUC}_{E2,lin}$ in (7.39) is the consistent estimator, as $N \to \infty$, of the integral sum

$$S_{AUC} = \sum_{j=1}^{k} \frac{E_\gamma \eta(x_j, \gamma) + E_\gamma \eta(x_{j-1}, \gamma)}{2} \Delta x_j.$$

For the selected grid, the linear trapezoidal rule overestimates integrals $\int E_\gamma \eta(x, \gamma) dx$ or $\int \eta(x, E\gamma) dx$, over the last interval $[x_{n-1}, x_n]$ because of the curvature. Indeed,

$$I_{1,k} = \int_{x_{k-1}}^{x_k} E_\gamma \eta(x, \gamma) dx = 0.199, \quad I_{3,k} = \int_{x_{k-1}}^{x_k} \eta(x, \gamma^0) dx = 0.104, \quad (7.50)$$

while

$$\widehat{I}_{1,k} = E_\gamma \left[\frac{\eta(x_{k-1}, \gamma) + \eta(x_k, \gamma)}{2} \right] \Delta x_k = 0.275, \qquad (7.51)$$

$$\widehat{I}_{3,k} = \frac{\eta(x_{k-1}, \gamma^0) + \eta(x_k, \gamma^0)}{2} \Delta x_k = 0.177,$$

where to estimate $I_{1,k}$ and $\widehat{I}_{1,k}$ in (7.50) and (7.51), respectively, we used the Monte Carlo method. Because of (7.50) and (7.51), and to match the hybrid method with splines, we selected $t^* = x_{15} = 0.478$ in (7.44), so that

$$\widehat{AUC}_{E2,H} = \sum_{j=1}^{15} \Delta x_j \widehat{F}_{j, \, lin} + \Delta x_n \widehat{F}_{n, \, log}, \qquad (7.52)$$

and via Monte Carlo simulations we obtained $E_\gamma \left(\widehat{AUC}_{E2,H} \right) = 1.833$, which just slightly differs from the value of $AUC_1 = AUC_2 = 1.836$.

Original grid. As mentioned earlier in Section 7.3.2.2, the nonparametric approach is used in population PK studies where the number of samples per subject may be rather small and method E1 for Type I metrics (first estimate individual PK parameters for each subject, then average across population) is not applicable. Therefore we discuss simulation results only for Type II metrics. The results of 10,000 simulation runs with $n = 16$ and $N = 20$ are presented in Figures 7.7 – 7.9, left panel, for the estimators of AUC_2, T_2 and C_2, respectively. For the results of simulations for Type I and III metrics, see Fedorov and Leonov (2006) [145].

AUC_2 estimation, see Figure 7.7: bias terms are rather small for all three approaches, but the standard deviation for MA (0.210) is smaller than for EA (0.222) or SA (0.223);

T_2, see Figure 7.8: bias terms are small, but variability of EA/SA estimators is larger. Moreover, with EA it is essentially impossible to exactly "hit" the true T_2 because of discreteness of the sampling grid. This fact explains the allocation of bars on the middle left panel of Figure 7.8; on average, the empirical estimator of T_2 performs quite well, but variability for EA is much larger than for MA: $std_{T,MA} = 0.0028$, $std_{T,EA} = 0.0079$, $std_{T,SA} = 0.0068$.

C_2, see Figure 7.9: all three approaches are comparable, with MA having an advantage with respect to bias.

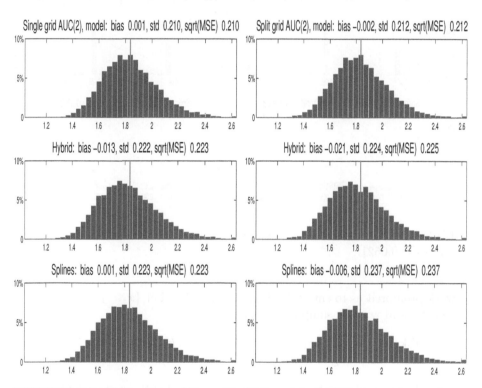

FIGURE 7.7: Estimation of Type II AUC metric: 10,000 runs, 16 sampling times, N=20, AUC_2=1.836 (marked by vertical line). Left panel – single grid, right panel – split grid. Upper plots – model-based, middle plots – empirical (hybrid), lower plots – spline.

7.3.4 Splitting sampling grid

As discussed in Section 7.3.1, when using optimal model-based designs for compartmental models, the number of collected samples may be reduced with minimal loss of precision, and once costs are taken into account, then sampling schemes with smaller number of samples may become optimal. That earlier

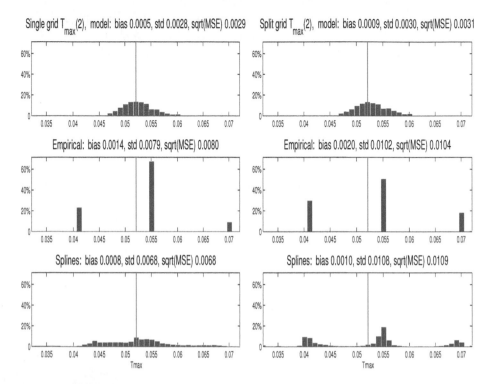

FIGURE 7.8: Estimation of Type II T_{max} metric, same setting as in Figure 7.7, $T_2 = 0.0521$.

work prompted us to entertain the following idea. Let $\{x_j, \ j = 1, \ldots, 2k\}$ be a single grid with $2k$ sampling points.

- Take samples at times $\{x_{2j-1}, \ j = 1, \ldots, k\}$ for the first $N/2$ patients (inverted triangles in Figure 7.4, right panel);

- Take samples at times $\{x_{2j}, \ j = 1, \ldots, k\}$ for the second half of study cohort (triangles in Figure 7.4, right panel);

- When using method E2 for the estimation of AUC_2, average responses in the two series (half-cohorts) separately, then combine the series into a single "population curve" $\{\hat{\eta}_j\}$ and estimate AUC_2 via (7.38).

The results of 10,000 simulations with $2k = 16$ and $N = 20$ are presented in the right panels of Figures 7.7 – 7.9. The combined results (bias, standard deviations and $\sqrt{MSE}$) are given in Table 7.2.

AUC_2 estimation, see Figure 7.7: little change in both bias and standard deviation terms.

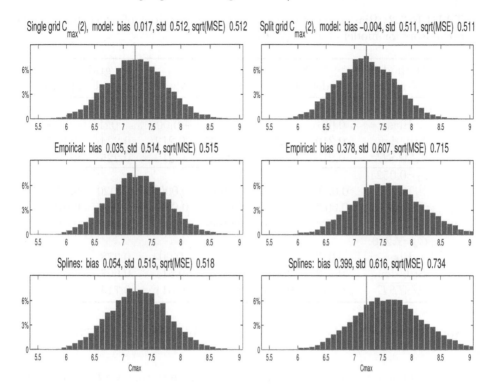

FIGURE 7.9: Method 2: estimation of Type II C_{max} metric, same setting as in Figure 7.7, $C_2 = 7.210$.

T_2, see Figure 7.8: little change with respect to bias, with an increase in standard deviation for EA (29%) and SA (59%).

C_2, see Figure 7.9: visible increase of bias terms for EA and SA, although the relative bias is only on the order of 5%. The explanation for the increase in bias terms for the empirical estimators is as follows. For each time point, average values of responses $\hat{\eta}_j$ from (7.37) would be similar for both single and split grids. However, since the single grid has twice as many patients for each time point compared to the split grid, the variance of $\hat{\eta}_j$ for the single grid, say $\text{Var}(\hat{\eta}_j^{(1)})$, will be twice as small compared to the split grid, say $\text{Var}(\hat{\eta}_j^{(2)})$. Therefore, since there are several points on the grid where the mean response is quite close to C_{max}, then $E\left[\max_j \hat{\eta}_j^{(2)}\right] > E\left[\max_j \hat{\eta}_j^{(1)}\right]$ (under the assumption of independence of $\hat{\eta}_j^{(1)}$ and $\hat{\eta}_j^{(2)}$, this inequality follows from the properties of order statistics; see Lindgren (1993) [257], Chapter 7.6). The above inequality provides a hint as to why the split grid produces a larger positive bias for C_{max} than the single grid.

TABLE 7.2: Bias, standard deviation and square root of MSE for Type II estimators for model (7.24) – (7.26).

Method 2	Single grid			Split grid		
PK metric	Model	Hybrid	Splines	Model	Hybrid	Splines
$AUC_2=1.836$						
Bias	0.001	−0.013	0.001	−0.002	-0.021	−0.006
Std. dev.	0.210	0.222	0.223	0.212	0.224	0.237
$\sqrt{MSE}$	0.210	0.222	0.223	0.212	0.225	0.237
$T_2=0.0521$						
Bias	0.0005	0.0014	0.0008	0.0009	0.0020	0.0010
Std. dev.	0.0028	0.0079	0.0068	0.0030	0.0102	0.0108
$\sqrt{MSE}$	0.0029	0.0080	0.0068	0.0031	0.0104	0.0109
$C_2=7.210$						
Bias	0.017	0.035	0.054	-0.004	0.378	0.399
Std. dev.	0.512	0.514	0.515	0.511	0.607	0.616
$\sqrt{MSE}$	0.512	0.515	0.518	0.511	0.715	0.734

Note: For model-based estimators, see (7.32); for empirical, see (7.37), (7.38).

To summarize these and other simulation results that we have observed, the split grid has a rather small loss of precision compared to the original single grid, and the model-based approach (under the assumption of the correct model) is superior to the empirical approach (EA) with respect to precision of estimation. Still, the EA performs reasonably well, with the exception of variability of T_{max} estimation.

Regulatory agencies usually require the noncompartmental analysis, such as empirical estimation of AUC, in the early stages of drug development. Therefore, it would be beneficial to derive, if possible, explicit formulae for empirical estimators of PK metrics. Since sparse sampling grids are often encountered in practice, we concentrate on Type II metrics and method E2. Even though in the general case it is not feasible to obtain closed-form solutions for bias and variance of the estimators, in Section 7.3.5 we present analytical expressions for a simple quadratic model with random intercept. We hope that this first step may shed some light on the future development for more complex settings.

7.3.5 MSE of AUC estimator, single and split grids

In this section we discuss a simple example to illustrate the statistical expediency of split grids in the presence of population variability and observational errors. We consider the empirical approach introduced in Section 7.3.2.2 and present closed-form expressions for the MSE of the estimator $\widehat{AUC}_{E2,\ lin}$, see

(7.39), when the response is approximated by a polynomial of second order with random intercept

$$\eta(x_j, \boldsymbol{\gamma}_i) = \gamma_{0i} + \gamma_1 x_j + \gamma_2 x_j^2, \qquad (7.53)$$

where $\boldsymbol{\gamma}_i = (\gamma_{0i}, \gamma_1, \gamma_2)$, $\mathrm{E}(\gamma_{0i}) = \gamma_0$ and $\mathrm{Var}(\gamma_{0i}) = u^2$. Let MSE_1 and MSE_2 be the mean squared error of $\widehat{AUC}_{E2,\,lin}$ for the single and split grids, respectively. Let $Bias_k$ and Var_k be the corresponding bias and variance terms in the decomposition of MSE_k,

$$MSE_r = Bias_r^2 + Var_r, \ r = 1, 2,$$

and let the grid be uniform, $\{x_j = jT/(2k), \ j = 0, 1, \ldots, 2k\}$. Without loss of generality assume that $T = 1$. Then for the single grid

$$Bias_1 = \frac{\gamma_2}{6}\frac{1}{4k^2}, \quad Var_1 = \frac{1}{N}\left[\frac{\sigma^2(2k - 0.5)}{4k^2} + u^2\right] \sim \frac{\sigma^2}{2Nk} + \frac{u^2}{N}, \quad (7.54)$$

while for the split grid

$$Bias_2 \equiv Bias_1, \quad Var_2 = \frac{(2k - 1.5)\, 2\sigma^2}{4k^2\ N} + \frac{u^2}{N}\left(1 - \frac{1}{2k^2}\right) \sim \frac{\sigma^2}{Nk} + \frac{u^2}{N}; \tag{7.55}$$

see Fedorov and Leonov (2006) [145] for the proof.

It follows from (7.54) and (7.55) that there is a twofold increase in measurement variability for the split grid, which is not surprising since the total number of samples is reduced by half. However, the bias terms are exactly the same for the two grids, and the population component in the variance term does not change either. Therefore, when the population variance u^2 dominates the measurement error variance σ^2, then $MSE_1 \approx MSE_2$, in spite of the twofold reduction in the number of samples for the split grid. Note also that the bias term in (7.41) will not change if the grid is split into more than two subsets.

Comparison of MSE under cost constraints. It follows from (7.54) and (7.55) that for given k and N the single grid with $2k$ samples per patient will always be better than the split grid in terms of MSE of AUC estimation. How much better depends on the values of η'', σ^2 and u^2. When cost constraints are introduced, the situation may change.

Following examples from Section 7.3.1, we assume that C_v is the cost of the patient's enrollment, C_s is the cost of analyzing a single sample and C_{total} is the upper bound for the study budget. Then the overall costs may be expressed as

$$2kNC_s + NC_v \le C_{total} \quad \text{for the single grid}, \qquad (7.56)$$

$$kNC_s + NC_v \le C_{total} \quad \text{for the split grid}. \qquad (7.57)$$

So under the cost constraint C_{total}, we may either select N and then find the maximal admissible $k = k(N, C_{total})$, or vice versa, first select k and then find the maximal $N = N(k, C_{total})$. In this setting, values of k and N are not independent.

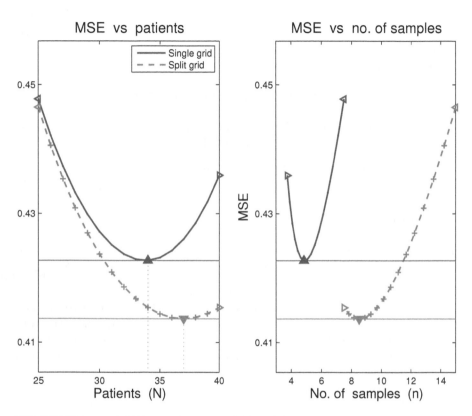

FIGURE 7.10: MSE as a function of N and k, $u = 2.4$, $\sigma = 9$, $25 \leq N \leq 40$.

For our illustrative example, we used $|\eta''| = 100$, $\sigma = 9$, $u = 2.4$, $C_s = 1$, $C_v = 5$, $C_{total} = 500$; for a rationale of the selection of these values, see Fedorov and Leonov (2006) [145]. We selected N between 25 and 40, and for each N found k satisfying (7.56) for the single grid and (7.57) for the split grid. Figure 7.10 presents plots of MSE_1 (solid line) and MSE_2 (dashed line) when $u = 2.4$ and $\sigma = 9$. It demonstrates that once costs are taken into account, the split grid may outperform the original grid in terms of MSE of AUC estimation. For the single grid, the minimum $MSE_{1,min} \approx 0.425$ is attained at $N_1 = 34$ and $k_1 = 5$, which corresponds to $2k_1 = 10$ samples per subject. For the split grid, the minimum $MSE_{2,min} \approx 0.415$ is attained at $N_2 = 37$ and $k_2 = 8$. The total number of samples is $2k_1 N_1 = 340$ and $k_2 N_2 = 296$ for the single and split grids, respectively. So for the same overall cost, the split grid generates smaller MSE than the single grid: once cost constraints are introduced, the increase in k will lead to the decrease in N. Vice versa, when N increases, then k should decrease because of the constraints. This explains the shape of the curves in Figure 7.10.

To conclude the discussion in this section, we mention that our focus here is on the model-independent, or nonparametric approach. We exploit the ideas from the work on the selection of sampling schemes for parametric compartmental models; see Section 7.2. We show that these ideas are also applicable to the nonparametric approach in that

- The number of sampling times may be reduced without significant loss of efficiency (for model-based designs, the quality of different sampling schemes is measured by design optimality criteria, such as D-optimality; for the nonparametric approach, the mean squared error of estimators of PK metrics is used for comparison of designs);

- Once the costs of analyzing samples and costs of patient's enrollment are taken into account, then sampling schemes with smaller number of samples may become optimal.

In the introduction of split grids, as in Section 7.3.4, we use a simple split of sampling times between two (or more) subsets. In principle, such a split may be implemented in a more subtle way. For example, for one group of patients most samples may be taken immediately after administering the drug. For another group, sampling times may be more dense closer to the end of the sampling interval. In that case the costs of running a study may be reduced, especially if patients have to visit the clinic to have samples taken.

The example of a closed-form solution for the mean squared error of AUC estimation discussed in Section 7.3.5 is rather simple. Nevertheless, it allows us to demonstrate explicitly that sampling schemes with smaller numbers of sampling times may outperform more dense grids when costs are incorporated into the designs. This example also helps us better understand the interdependence between population and measurement components of variability.

7.4 Pharmacokinetic Models Described by Stochastic Differential Equations

In Sections 7.2 and 7.3 we discussed examples of PK compartmental models described by ordinary differential equations (ODEs) as in (7.9) and (7.23). Two sources of variability were considered: population, or between-patient, variability as in (7.2), (7.11); and measurement, or observational, error as in (7.12); see also formula (7.1). Now we focus on the third source, namely within-patient variability or an "intrinsic variability of the metabolic system," as stated in Picchini et al. (2006) [308]. This intrinsic variability suggests a move from ODEs to stochastic differential equations (SDEs). Once expressions for the mean and covariance functions of the solution of the SDE system are derived, one can address the optimal design problem: indeed, the general formula (1.108) may be used in the same fashion as in Sections 7.2 and 7.3 to calculate individual information matrices $\boldsymbol{\mu}(\mathbf{x}, \boldsymbol{\theta})$ of sequences $\mathbf{x}$ of sampling times. In this section we focus on the design problem; for a discussion on parameter estimation in stochastic PK models, see Overgaard et al. (2005) [303].

For all examples in this section, we use the one-compartment model (7.23) as the deterministic analog of stochastic systems. In Section 7.4.1 we introduce one of the simplest stochastic analogs of the model (7.23), and then in Section 7.4.2 discuss stochastic systems with positive trajectories. Note that in a number of previous publications on stochastic PK models, no attention was given to the fact that trajectories of the continuous stochastic systems may become negative with positive probability; see Overgaard et al. (2005) [303] or Tornoe et al. (2004a, 2004b) [378], [377].

7.4.1   Stochastic one-compartment model I

To illustrate optimal design techniques for stochastic PK models, Anisimov et al. (2007) [12] introduced a system of SDEs with additional noise terms described by Wiener processes:

$$\begin{cases} dz_0(x) = & -\theta_1 z_0(x)dx & +\sigma_0(x)dw_0(x), & z_0(0) = D, \\ dz_1(x) = & \theta_1 z_0(x)dx & -\theta_2 z_1(x)dx & +\sigma_1(x)dw_1(x), & z_1(0) = 0, \end{cases}$$
$$(7.58)$$

where $\sigma_r(x) \geq 0, r = 0, 1$, are deterministic functions, and $w_r(x)$ are independent Wiener processes, for which $\mathbf{E}[w_r(x)] = 0$, and $\mathrm{Cov}[w_r(x)w_r(s)] = \min(x, s)$. Parameters θ_1 and θ_2 correspond to rate constants K_a and K_e in (7.23). We use Îto's concept, so that for any given deterministic function g, the process $\xi(x) = \int_0^x g(u)dw(u)$ is a Gaussian process satisfying conditions

$$\mathbf{E}[\xi(x)] = 0, \ \mathrm{Cov}[\xi(x), \xi(x + s)] = \int_0^x g^2(u)du, \ s > 0;$$

see, for example, Gardiner (2003) [170]. The solution of system (7.58) is given by

$$\begin{cases} z_0(x) = & q_0(x) + \frac{1}{D}\int_0^x q_0(x - u)\sigma_0(u)dw_0(u), \\ z_1(x) = & q_1(x) + \frac{1}{D}\int_0^x q_1(x - u)\sigma_0(u)dw_0(u) + \int_0^x e^{-\theta_2(x-u)}\sigma_1(u)dw_1(u), \end{cases}$$
$$(7.59)$$

where q_0, q_1 are the solutions of the deterministic ODE system (7.23):

$$\begin{cases} q_0(x) = & De^{-\theta_1 x}, \\ q_1(x) = & \frac{\theta_1 D}{\theta_1 - \theta_2}\left(e^{-\theta_2 x} - e^{-\theta_1 x}\right); \end{cases}$$
$$(7.60)$$

cf. (7.24). Denote $\tilde{S}(x, x+s) = \mathbf{Cov}[q_1(x), q_1(x+s)]$. Using properties of Îto's integral and the independence of $w_0(x)$ and $w_1(x)$, it is straightforward to show that the solution (7.59) is unbiased,

$$\mathbf{E}[z_0(x)] = q_0(x), \ \ \mathbf{E}[z_1(x)] = q_1(x),$$

and

$$\tilde{S}(x, x+s) = \frac{\theta_1^2}{(\theta_2 - \theta_1)^2} \int_0^x \sigma_0^2(u)du \left[e^{-\theta_1 s} e^{2\theta_1(u-x)} + e^{-\theta_2 s} e^{2\theta_2(u-x)} - \right.$$

$$\left. - \left(e^{-\theta_1 s} + e^{-\theta_2 s} \right) e^{(\theta_1+\theta_2)(u-x)} \right] + e^{-\theta_2(2x+s)} \int_0^x \sigma_1^2(s) e^{2\theta_2 u} \, du, \ \ s > 0.$$

$$(7.61)$$

If

$$\sigma_r(x) = \sigma_r e^{-\nu_r x}, \ \ r = 0, 1, \tag{7.62}$$

then the integrals in (7.61) can be taken explicitly. For example, if $\nu_0 \neq \theta_j, j = 1, 2; \ \nu_1 \neq \theta_2$, and $\nu_0 \neq (\theta_1 + \theta_2)/2$, then

$$\tilde{S}(x, x+s) = \frac{\theta_1^2 \sigma_0^2}{(\theta_1 - \nu_0)^2} \left[e^{-\theta_1 s} \frac{e^{-2\nu_0 x} - e^{-2\theta_1 x}}{2(\theta_1 - \nu_0)} + e^{-\theta_2 s} \frac{e^{-2\nu_0 x} - e^{-2\theta_2 x}}{2(\theta_2 - \nu_0)} \right.$$

$$\left. - \left(e^{-\theta_1 s} + e^{-\theta_2 s} \right) \frac{e^{-2\nu_0 x} - e^{-(\theta_1+\theta_2)x}}{\theta_1 + \theta_2 - 2\nu_0} \right] + \sigma_1^2 \, e^{-\theta_2 s} \frac{e^{-2\nu_1 x} - e^{-2\theta_2 x}}{2(\theta_2 - \nu_1)} \ . \tag{7.63}$$

When $\nu_r > 0$, then $\mathrm{Var}[z_1(x)] \to 0$ as $x \to \infty$, and $\tilde{S}(x, x+s) \to 0$ as $s \to \infty$ for any fixed $x > 0$. However, if at least one $\nu_i = 0$, then it follows from (7.63) that $\mathrm{Var}[z_1(x)] \to v^* > 0$, even though $\mathbf{E}[z_1(x)] \to 0$ as $x \to \infty$. That seems counterintuitive from physiological considerations, since in this case the trajectories of the process $z_1(x)$ become negative with positive probability.

Optimal designs. Let $x_1, \ldots, x_k$ be a sequence of k sampling times and $\tilde{\mathbf{S}} = \{\tilde{S}_{j_1 j_2}\} = \left\{ \tilde{S}(x_{j1}, x_{j2}), \ j_1, j_2 = 1, \ldots, k \right\}$. Anisimov et al. (2007) [12] considered an additive error model with independent i.i.d. errors $\varepsilon_{ij} \sim N(0, \sigma_{obs}^2)$, so that measurements y_{ij} satisfy

$$y_{ij} = z_1(x_j)/V_i + \varepsilon_{ij}, \tag{7.64}$$

with normal population distribution $\gamma_i \sim N(\gamma^0, \mathbf{\Omega})$, with $\gamma = (\theta_1, \theta_2, V)^T$. Under the assumption of "small" variance $\sigma_r(x)$, the first-order approximation techniques lead to the following formula for the variance-covariance matrix of the process $\{Y(x), x = x_1, \ldots, x_k\}$, cf. (7.15):

$$\mathbf{S} \approx \tilde{\mathbf{S}}/V^2 + \sigma_{obs}^2 \mathbf{I}_k + \mathbf{F} \, \mathbf{\Omega} \, \mathbf{F}^T, \tag{7.65}$$

where $\mathbf{I}_k$ is a $k \times k$ identity matrix, and $\mathbf{F}$ is a $k \times m_\gamma$ matrix of partial

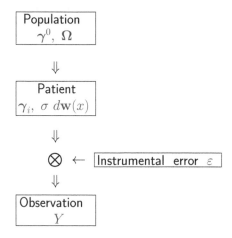

FIGURE 7.11: Three sources of variability in SDE models.

derivatives of function $\eta(x, \boldsymbol{\gamma}) = q_1(x)/V$ with respect to parameters γ_l; cf. (7.14). See Figure 7.11 for a schematic representation of the three sources of variability.

Using formulae (1.108) and (7.65), we constructed examples of optimal sampling schemes for stochastic PK models under the assumption (7.62) with positive ν_r, $r = 0, 1$. Still it was acknowledged that the assumption (7.62) of the diminishing variability of the noise process was rather restrictive and it has not fully accomplished the goal of having positive solutions of the SDE system. Indeed, the process $z_1(x)$ is Gaussian, see (7.59), and therefore the probability $\tilde{P}_x$ that trajectories $z_1(x)$ may become negative is nonzero for any fixed x. Moreover, if at least one $\nu_r = 0$, then $\text{Var}[z_1(x)] \to v^* > 0$, and $\tilde{P}_x \to 0.5$ as $x \to \infty$ because $\mathbf{E}[z_1(x)] \to 0$.

Nevertheless, models similar to (7.58) are popular due to their relative simplicity and Gaussian distribution of its solutions. For instance, Overgaard et al. (2005) [303] considered an exponential decay model analogous to the first equation in (7.58) with $\sigma_0(x) \equiv \sigma_w > 0$, and then took logarithms of the solution in the discrete-time model of observations. Because of the potential negativeness of z_0, such a model seems counterintuitive from physiological considerations, and taking logs is formally incorrect.

7.4.2 Stochastic one-compartment model II: systems with positive trajectories

Given the discussion in the previous section, it would be desirable from a physiological perspective to consider stochastic models with positive solutions z_r. Fedorov et al. (2010) [147] considered the analog of the system (7.58) where the noise terms $\sigma_r(x)dw_r(x)$ on the right-hand side of the equations were replaced with $\sigma_r z_r(x)dw_r(x)$, $\sigma_r > 0$; i.e., the noise terms were proportional to the signal:

$$\begin{cases} dz_0(x) = & -\theta_1 z_0(x)dx & + \sigma_0 z_0(x)dw_0(x), & z_0(0) = D, \\ dz_1(x) = & \theta_1 z_0(x)dx & - \theta_2 z_1(x)dx & + \sigma_1 z_1(x)dw_1(x), & z_1(0) = 0. \end{cases}$$
(7.66)

The noise terms in (7.66) are analogs of a proportional component of variance on the right-hand side of (7.12). The closed-form solution of the system (7.66) and its covariance function $\tilde{S}$ are provided in the following Lemma; for details, see Fedorov et al. (2010) [147].

Lemma 7.1 *(a) The solution of system (7.66) is given by*

$$\begin{cases} z_0(x) = & De^{-(\theta_1 + \frac{\sigma_0^2}{2})x + \sigma_0 w_0(x)}, \\ z_1(x) = & \theta_1 De^{-(\theta_2 + \frac{\sigma_1^2}{2})x + \sigma_1 w_1(x)} \cdot \int_0^x e^{(\theta_2 - \theta_1 + \frac{\sigma_1^2 - \sigma_0^2}{2})s + \sigma_0 w_0(s) - \sigma_1 w_1(s)} ds. \end{cases}$$
(7.67)

(b) The solution is unbiased: $\mathbf{E}z_r(x) = q_r(x)$, $r = 0, 1$, *with* $q_r(x)$ *defined in (7.60).*

(c) The covariance function of the solution is

$$\begin{aligned} \tilde{S}(x, x+s) = & \ \theta_1^2 D^2 \{ a_1 e^{(-2\theta_1 + \sigma_0^2)x - \theta_2 s} + a_2 e^{(-2\theta_1 + \sigma_0^2)x - \theta_1 s} \\ + & \ a_3 e^{(-2\theta_2 + \sigma_1^2)x - \theta_2 s} + a_4 e^{-(\theta_1 + \theta_2)x - \theta_1 s} \\ + & \ a_5 e^{-(\theta_1 + \theta_2)x - \theta_2 s} + a_6 (e^{-2\theta_1 x - \theta_1 s} + e^{-2\theta_2 x - \theta_2 s}) \}, \end{aligned}$$
(7.68)

where

$$a_1 = \frac{\sigma_1^2 - \sigma_0^2}{\Delta\theta(\Delta\theta + \sigma_0^2)[2\Delta\theta - \sigma_1^2 + \sigma_0^2]}, \quad \Delta\theta = \theta_2 - \theta_1,$$

$$a_2 = \frac{1}{\Delta\theta(\Delta\theta + \sigma_0^2)}, \quad a_3 = \frac{2}{(\Delta\theta - \sigma_1^2)[2\Delta\theta - \sigma_1^2 + \sigma_0^2]},$$

$$a_4 = \frac{\sigma_0^2}{(\Delta\theta)^2(\Delta\theta + \sigma_0^2)}, \quad a_5 = \frac{(\sigma_0^2 - 2\sigma_1^2)\Delta\theta - \sigma_0^2\sigma_1^2}{(\Delta\theta)^2(\Delta\theta + \sigma_0^2)(\Delta\theta - \sigma_1^2)}, \quad a_6 = \frac{-1}{(\Delta\theta)^2}.$$

For the proof of Lemma 7.1, see Section 7.4.3. Note that (7.67) immediately implies that z_0, z_1 are positive, and it follows from (7.68) that

$\tilde{S}(x, x+s) \to 0$ as $x \to \infty$ for any fixed $s \geq 0$ if $\theta_1 > \sigma_0^2/2$ and $\theta_2 > \sigma_1^2/2$;
$\tilde{S}(x, x+s) \to 0$ as $s \to \infty$ for any fixed $x \geq 0$.

Optimal designs. We use the measurement model as in (7.64) but assume a fixed effects model $\gamma_i \equiv \gamma^0$ (i.e., no population variability), so that the approximation formula (7.65) for the variance-covariance matrix $\mathbf{S}$ is reduced to

$$\mathbf{S} \approx \tilde{\mathbf{S}}/V^2 + \sigma_{obs}^2 \mathbf{I}_k.$$
(7.69)

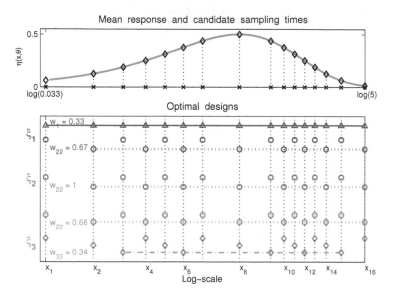

FIGURE 7.12: Sampling times and examples of optimal designs for stochastic PK model.

Similar to the examples in Sections 7.3.1 and 7.3.3, for candidate sampling times we first take a uniform grid on the y-axis (response) and then project points on the response curve to the x-axis to obtain times $\mathcal{X}$; see Figure 7.12, top panel (cf. Figure 7.4). Then we select splits $\mathbf{x}_i$ of different orders as in Section 7.3.1 but allow for different numbers of patients (different weights p_{sl}) on sequences $\mathbf{x}_{s,l}$ of an s-th order split $\mathbf{x_s}$. Therefore, in this case the normalized information matrix is

$$\mathbf{M}(\xi, \boldsymbol{\theta}) = \sum_s \sum_{l=1}^s p_{sl}\boldsymbol{\mu}(\mathbf{x}_{s,l}, \boldsymbol{\theta}). \tag{7.70}$$

For the examples in this section we take $\boldsymbol{\theta} = (\theta_1, \theta_2, V; \sigma_0^2, \sigma_1^2; \sigma_{obs}^2)^T$, where $\theta_1 = 2$, $\theta_2 = 1$, $V = 1$; $\sigma_1 = \sigma_2 = 0.4$; $\sigma_{obs} = 0.05$, and $D = 1$ in (7.66). The set $\mathcal{X}$ of sampling times is the same as in Anisimov et al. (2007) [12]:

$$\mathcal{X} = [x_1, \dots, x_{16}] = [0.033, \ 0.069, \ 0.111, \ 0.158, \ 0.215, \dots \ 2, 703, \ 3.433, \ 5].$$

For the design region, we take all splits up to the 3rd order:

$$\mathfrak{X} = \{\mathbf{x}_1; \ \mathbf{x}_{2,1}, \mathbf{x}_{2,2}; \ \mathbf{x}_{3,1}, \mathbf{x}_{3,2}, \mathbf{x}_{3,3}\}. \tag{7.71}$$

We use the cost function $\phi(\mathbf{x})$ as in (7.22) with $C_v = 1$.

When standard normalized designs are constructed, then as expected the optimal design is the full sequence $\mathbf{x}_1 = \mathcal{X}$. Once costs are incorporated, the full sequence may lose its optimality.

- If $C_s = 0.1$, then the cost-based locally D-optimal design is the full sequence $\mathbf{x}_1$.

- If $C_s = 0.15$, then the optimal design is a combination of two sequences: $\xi_1 = \{(\mathbf{x}_1, \tilde{p}_1 = 0.43), (\mathbf{x}_{2,2}, \tilde{p}_{22} = 0.57)\}$. Recall that to calculate frequencies r_i for cost-based designs, the cost function $\phi(\mathbf{x}_{ij})$ must be taken into account; cf. the example in Section 7.2.4. According to (4.28) and (7.22), this leads to

$$\frac{r_{22}}{r_1} = \frac{\tilde{p}_{22}}{\tilde{p}_1} \times \frac{1 + 0.15 \times 16}{1 + 0.15 \times 8} = 2.05;$$

thus about 33% of subjects should be randomized to the full sequence $\mathbf{x}_1$ and 67% to the sequence $\mathbf{x}_{2,2}$.

- If $C_s = 0.25$, then the optimal design ξ_2 is the sequence $\mathbf{x}_{2,2}$.

- If $C_s = 0.3$, then $\xi_3 = \{(\mathbf{x}_{2,2}, \tilde{p}_{22} = 0.73), (\mathbf{x}_{3,3}, \tilde{p}_{33} = 0.27\}$; thus

$$\frac{r_{22}}{r_{33}} = \frac{\tilde{p}_{22}}{\tilde{p}_{33}} \times \frac{2.5}{3.4} = 2.15,$$

and the relative weights of selected sequences in the cost-based design are $w_{22} \approx 0.66$ and $w_{33} \approx 0.34$; see Figure 7.12, bottom panel.

It is interesting to compare the standard relative D-efficiency (i.e., when $C_s = 0$) of constructed designs to the ratio Φ_ξ of relative costs; cf. (6.32) – (6.34):

$$\text{Eff}_D(\xi_1) = 0.77, \quad \text{Eff}_D(\xi_2) = 0.65, \quad \text{Eff}_D(\xi_3) = 0.59,$$

$$\Phi(\xi_1) = 0.76; \quad \Phi(\xi_2) = 0.6; \quad \Phi(\xi_3) = 0.53,$$

where

$$\text{Eff}_D(\xi_s) = [|\mathbf{M}(\xi, \boldsymbol{\theta})| \,/\, |\boldsymbol{\mu}(\mathbf{x}_1, \boldsymbol{\theta})|]^{1/6}, \quad \Phi(\xi_s) = \sum_{l=1}^{s} w_{sl} \phi(\mathbf{x}_{s,l}) \,/\, \phi(\mathbf{x}_1).$$

For practical reasons, one may force equal weights for subsequences in the same split, i.e., $p_{21} = p_{22}$, $p_{31} = p_{32} = p_{33}$ as in the example of Section 7.3.1. This restriction has essentially no effect in the example of this section since the D-efficiency of such restricted designs drops by less than 0.01.

7.4.3   Proof of Lemma 7.1

(a) The derivation of (7.67) is a simple exercise in the application of general results of stochastic calculus; see Gardiner (2003) [170], Chapter 4.4.7, and Îto's formula: if $Z = Z(z, x)$, where $dz = F dx + G dw$, and $F = F(z, x)$, $G = G(z, x)$ and u are sufficiently smooth functions, then

$$dZ = \left(\frac{\partial u}{\partial x} + \frac{\partial u}{\partial z} F + \frac{1}{2} \frac{\partial^2 u}{\partial z^2} G^2 \right) dx + \frac{\partial u}{\partial z} G \, dw. \qquad (7.72)$$

For z_0, use (7.72) with $u(z_0, x) = \ln z_0$, $F = -\theta_1 z_0$, $G = \sigma_0 z_0$, which leads to

$$d(\ln z_0) = -(\theta_1 + \sigma_0^2/2) dx + \sigma_0 dw_0(x),$$

and z_0 is obtained by integration.

For z_1, first solve a homogeneous equation

$$d\tilde{z}_1(x) = -\theta_2 \tilde{z}_1 dx + \sigma_1 \tilde{z}_1 dw_1(x), \quad \tilde{z}_1(0) = 1,$$

which is structurally identical to the equation for z_0, and thus its solution is $\tilde{z}_1(x) = e^{-(\theta_2 + \sigma_1^2/2)x + \sigma_1 w_1(x)}$. Then search for $z_1(x)$ as the product

$$z_1(x) = z(x)\tilde{z}_1(x), \quad \text{or} \quad z(x) = z_1(x) V(x), \quad \text{where } V(x) = \tilde{z}_1^{-1}(x), \quad (7.73)$$

and use Îto's product rule: if

$$dU_1(x) = F_1(x)dx + G_1 dw, \quad dU_2(x) = F_2(x)dx + G_2 dw,$$

then for sufficiently smooth functions F_r, G_r,

$$d(U_1 U_2) = U_2 dU_1 + U_1 dU_2 + G_1 G_2 dx. \qquad (7.74)$$

It follows from Îto's formula that $dV(x) = \left[(\theta_2 + \sigma_1^2) dx - \sigma_1 dw_1 \right] / \tilde{z}_1(x)$, which together with the second equation in (7.66) and (7.74) imply that

$$dz = \frac{z_1 \left[(\theta_2 + \sigma_1^2) dx - \sigma_1 dw_1 \right] + \left[(\theta_1 z_0 - \theta_2 z_1) dx + \sigma_1 z_1 dw_1 \right] - \sigma_1^2 z_1 \, dx}{\tilde{z}_1(x)},$$

or $dz = \theta_1 z_0(x)/\tilde{z}_1(x) \, dx$, and by direct integration

$$z(x) = z_0 + \int_0^x \theta_1 z_0(s) e^{(\theta_2 + \sigma_1^2/2)s - \sigma_1 w_1(s)} \, ds.$$

The second equation in (7.67) now follows from (7.73) and the first equation in (7.67).

(b) The unbiasedness of solutions z_r follows from the independence of increments $w_r(v) - w_r(u)$ and $w_r(u) - w_r(s)$, $0 \le s < u < v$, and the equality

$$\mathbf{E} e^{a\xi} = e^{a^2/2}, \qquad (7.75)$$

for a standard normal random variable $\xi \sim \mathcal{N}(0,1)$ and any number a.

(c) It follows from (7.67) that $z_1(x+s) = \alpha(x,s)z_1(x) + \beta(x,s)e^{\sigma_0 w_0(x)}$ for any $s > 0$, where

$$
\begin{aligned}
\alpha(x,s) &= e^{-(\theta_2 + \frac{\sigma_1^2}{2})s + \sigma_1[w_1(x+s) - w_1(x)]}, \quad \beta(x,s) = \theta_1 D e^{-(\theta_2 + \frac{\sigma_1^2}{2})(x+s)} \\
&\times \int_x^{x+s} e^{(\theta_2 - \theta_1 + \frac{\sigma_1^2}{2} - \frac{\sigma_0^2}{2})u + \sigma_0[w_0(u) - w_0(x)] + \sigma_1[w_1(x+s) - w_1(u)]} du.
\end{aligned}
$$

Using (7.75), one can calculate the following conditional mathematical expectations:

$$
\mathbf{E}\left[\alpha(x,s)|z_1(x)\right] = \tilde{\alpha}(s), \quad \mathbf{E}\left[\beta(x,s)|w_0(x), z_1(x)\right] = \tilde{\beta}(x,s),
$$

where $\tilde{\alpha}(s) = e^{-\theta_2 s}$, $\tilde{\beta}(x,s) = (\theta_1 D / \Delta\theta) \cdot e^{-(\theta_1 + \frac{\sigma_0^2}{2})x} \cdot \left(e^{-\theta_1 s} - e^{-\theta_2 s}\right)$. Therefore,

$$
\tilde{S}(x, x+s) = \tilde{\alpha}(s) \cdot \mathbf{E}z_1^2(x) + \tilde{\beta}(x,s) \cdot \mathbf{E}e^{\sigma_0 w_0(x)}z_1(x) - \mathbf{E}z_1(x) \cdot \mathbf{E}z_1(x+s). \quad (7.76)
$$

Next it follows from (7.67), (7.75) and the independence of increments of $w_0(x)$ that

$$
\mathbf{E}e^{\sigma_0 w_0(x)}z_1(x) = \theta_1 D e^{-(\theta_2 + \frac{\sigma_1^2}{2})x} \cdot \int_0^x e^{(\theta_2 - \theta_1 + \frac{\sigma_1^2 - \sigma_0^2}{2})s} \cdot \mathbf{E}e^{\sigma_0[w_0(x) - w_0(s)]}
$$

$$
\cdot \mathbf{E}e^{2\sigma_0 w_0(s)} \cdot \mathbf{E}e^{\sigma_1[w_1(x) - w_1(s)]} ds = \frac{\theta_1 D}{\Delta\theta + \sigma_0^2} \left[e^{-(\theta_1 - \frac{3\sigma_0^2}{2})x} - e^{-(\theta_2 - \frac{\sigma_0^2}{2})x}\right].
$$
$$(7.77)$$

Similarly, to calculate $\mathbf{E}z_1^2(x)$, introduce notation $M = \max(s,u)$ and $m = \min(s,u)$:

$$
\mathbf{E}z_1^2(x) = \theta_1^2 D^2 e^{-2(\theta_2 + \frac{\sigma_1^2}{2})x} \cdot \int_0^x \int_0^x e^{(\theta_2 - \theta_1 + \frac{\sigma_1^2 - \sigma_0^2}{2})(s+u)} \cdot \mathbf{E}e^{\sigma_0[w_0(M) - w_0(m)]}
$$

$$
\cdot \mathbf{E}e^{2\sigma_0 w_0(m)} \cdot \mathbf{E}e^{2\sigma_1[w_1(x) - w_1(M)]} \cdot \mathbf{E}e^{\sigma_1[w_1(M) - w_1(m)]} ds \, du
$$

$$
= \frac{\theta_1^2 D^2}{\Delta\theta + \sigma_0^2} \left[\frac{2e^{(-2\theta_1 + \sigma_0^2)x}}{2\Delta\theta + \sigma_0^2 - \sigma_1^2} - \frac{2e^{-(\theta_1 + \theta_2)x}}{\Delta\theta - \sigma_1^2} + \frac{2e^{(-2\theta_2 + \sigma_1^2)x}(\Delta\theta + \sigma_0^2)}{(\Delta\theta - \sigma_1^2)(2\Delta\theta + \sigma_0^2 - \sigma_1^2)}\right].
$$

The expression for the function $\tilde{S}(x, x+s)$ now follows from (7.76), (7.77). $\square$

7.5 Software for Constructing Optimal Population PK/PD Designs

In Sections 7.2 and 7.3 we introduced examples of population pharmacokinetic (PK) studies. Optimal design of experiments for such studies is an important practical problem that has received considerable attention in the literature and software development over the past decade. In 2006, an annual workshop was initiated on the theory of optimal experimental design for nonlinear mixed effects models and its applications in drug development. The worskhop adopted the name PODE (Population Optimum Design of Experiments); see

   http://www.maths.qmul.ac.uk/~bb/PODE/PODE.html.

A special session was organized at the PODE 2007 Meeting to present different software tools for population PK/PD optimal designs, and presentations at this session were summarized at the PAGE 2007 meeting (Population Approach Group Europe); see Mentré et al. (2007) [276]. The discussed software packages included, in alphabetical order,

PFIM (developed in INSERM, Université Paris 7, France); see Retout and Mentré (2003) [340], Bazzoli et al. (2009) [38];

PkStaMp (the development started when the authors of the book were with GlaxoSmithKline, Collegeville, PA); see Aliev et al. (2009, 2012) [7], [8], Leonov and Aliev (2012) [253];

PopDes (CAPKR, School of Pharmacy and Pharmaceutical Sciences, University of Manchester, UK); see Gueorguieva et al. (2007) [183];

PopED (Department of Pharmaceutical Biosciences, Uppsala University, Sweden); see Nyberg et al. (2011) [296];

WinPOPT (School of Pharmacy, University of Otago, New Zealand); see Duffull et al. (2005) [108].

The discussion of software packages continued at PODE 2009 – 2011 meetings.

In this section we describe the PkStaMp library for constructing optimal population PK/PD optimal designs (PharmacoKinetic Sampling Times Allocation/STand-Alone Application, MATLAB Platform). The library is intended for constructing locally D-optimal designs for compartmental PK and PK/PD models. It is compiled as a single executable file that does not require a MATLAB license. In Sections 7.5.1 and 7.5.2 we provide a short description of implemented models. Software inputs and outputs are outlined in Sections 7.5.3 and 7.5.4. Section 7.5.5 describes how the library was used to validate the design of a combined PK/PD study. Sections 7.5.6 and 7.5.7 present examples that were used for the comparison of different software tools. Section 7.5.7 also outlines a user-defined option of the PkStaMp library.

7.5.1 Regression models

We assume that measurements of PK or PD endpoints are taken at times x_{ij} for patient i and satisfy the model (7.1) where residual errors ε_{ij} may have both additive and proportional components of variability as in (7.12):

$$\varepsilon_{ij} = \varepsilon_{1,ij} + \varepsilon_{2,ij}\, \eta(x_{ij}, \gamma_i), \qquad (7.78)$$

where $\varepsilon_{1,ij}$, $\varepsilon_{2,ij}$ are independent identically distributed random variables with zero mean and variance σ_A^2 and σ_P^2, respectively. In compartmental modeling, the amounts of drug at different compartments satisfy the system of ordinary differential equations (ODEs), and for linear systems the solution exists in a closed form. See the example of the one-compartment model with first-order absorption and linear elimination in (7.23) and its solution (7.24), where $\gamma = (K_a, K_e, V)^T$ is the vector of *response* parameters. The individual response parameters γ_i are independently sampled from a given population, either normal as in (7.2) or log-normal as in (7.11). As before, γ^0 is an $m_\gamma \times 1$ vector of population means (typical values, in NONMEM nomenclature, see Beal and Sheiner (1992) [40]), and Ω is an $m_\gamma \times m_\gamma$ variance-covariance matrix of i.i.d. random vectors γ_i in (7.2) or ζ_i in (7.11). By $\theta = (\gamma^0, \Omega; \sigma_A^2, \sigma_P^2)$ we denote the combined vector of model parameters to be estimated, and by m its length.

The formula (1.108) is used for the approximation of individual information matrices $\mu(\mathbf{x}, \theta)$, where $\mathbf{x}$ is a sequence of k sampling times. If the first-order approximation (first-order Taylor expansion) is used, then the mean response η is calculated as in (7.13), and the variance function $\mathbf{S}$ is calculated as in (7.15) and (7.16) for normal and log-normal population distribution, respectively. Note that formula (7.15) may be rewritten as

$$\mathbf{S}(\mathbf{x}_i, \theta) \simeq \mathbf{F}\,\Omega\,\mathbf{F}^T + \Sigma_P \operatorname{Diag}[\eta(\mathbf{x}_i, \theta)\,\eta^T(\mathbf{x}_i, \theta) + \mathbf{F}\,\Omega\,\mathbf{F}^T] + \Sigma_A, \quad (7.79)$$

where $\Sigma_P = \sigma_P^2 \mathbf{I}_{k_i}$, $\Sigma_A = \sigma_A^2 \mathbf{I}_{k_i}$, and $\mathbf{I}_k$ is a $k \times k$ identity matrix. Once the variance function $\mathbf{S}$ is defined/approximated, one can approximate (a) the information matrix $\mu(\mathbf{x}, \theta)$ for any sequence $\mathbf{x}$, and (b) the Fisher information matrix $\mathbf{M}(\xi, \theta) = \sum_u w_u \mu(\mathbf{x}_u, \theta)$ for any continuous design $\xi = \{(\mathbf{x}_u, w_u)\}$, where $\sum_u w_u = 1$.

When using the first-order approximation, the function $\eta(\mathbf{x}, \theta)$ in (7.13) depends only on response parameters γ; see also (7.5). Therefore, all partial derivatives of $\eta(\mathbf{x}, \theta)$ with respect to variance parameters Ω_{ij} and σ^2 are equal to zero.

In our software we construct locally D-optimal designs

$$\xi^* = \underset{\xi \in \mathfrak{X}}{\arg\min} |\mathbf{M}^{-1}(\xi, \theta)|, \qquad (7.80)$$

where the optimization is performed with respect to continuous designs ξ, and sequences $\mathbf{x}_u$ belong to a prespecified design region $\mathfrak{X}$. We implement the first-order optimization algorithm with forward and backward steps as described in Section 3.1; see also Fedorov et al. (2007) [133], Section 7.1.5.

7.5.2   Supported PK/PD models

The list of currently supported models includes

- Linear one- or two-compartment PK models with various routes of administration (oral, bolus, continuous infusion). These models are generated by linear systems of ODEs and thus admit a closed-form solution for $\eta(\mathbf{x}, \boldsymbol{\theta})$; see (7.9), (7.10) in Section 7.2, and (7.23), (7.24) in Section 7.3.

- Models with direct parameterization, for example, a bi-exponential model:

$$\eta(x, \boldsymbol{\gamma}) \;=\; A_1 e^{-\alpha_1 x} \;+\; A_2 e^{-\alpha_2 x}.$$

- Combined models, e.g., one-compartment PK and E_{max} PD models; see Section 7.5.5.

- Nonlinear PK models such as a two-compartment model with first-order absorption and Michaelis-Menten elimination:

$$\begin{cases} \dot{q}_0(x) = -K_a q_0(x) \\ \dot{q}_1(x) = K_a q_0(x) - (K_{10} + K_{12})q_1(x) - \frac{(V_m/V)q_1(x)}{K_m + q_1(x)/V} + K_{21}q_2(x), \\ \dot{q}_2(x) = K_{12}\, q_1(x) \phantom{-(K_{10}+K_{12})q_1(x)-\frac{(V_m/V)q_1(x)}{K_m+q_1}xx} - K_{21}q_2(x), \end{cases}$$
$$\tag{7.81}$$

where $q_0(0) = D$, $q_1(0) = q_2(0) = 0$, and $\eta(x, \boldsymbol{\gamma}) = q_1(x)/V$. For nonlinear systems such as (7.81), closed-form solutions do not exist, and thus we resort to numeric solution of such systems via MATLAB build-in ODE solver `ode45`.

7.5.3   Software inputs

For each of the supported models, the user can modify a number of fields on the screen, in particular,

- *Response* parameters: rate constants, clearances, and volume of distribution. There are three options for response parameter effects:

  1. "Random effect," which allows for population variability: corresponding elements of the population matrix $\boldsymbol{\Omega}$ become enabled and may be edited.

  2. "Fixed effect," i.e., the parameter is assumed the same across all patients, but still must be estimated.

  3. "Constant," i.e., no estimation is required and this effect is not included in the information matrix (partial derivatives in (1.108) are not taken).

Models may be parameterized either via rate constants such as elimination rate K_e (microparameters) or via clearance CL (macroparameters). In the example described in Section 7.2, the "random effect" option would be selected for CL and volume V, and the "constant" option for K_{12} and K_{21}.

- *Population covariance* matrix $\boldsymbol{\Omega}$: elements of this matrix are enabled for "random effect" parameters only, with an option of selecting either the diagonal or the full matrix. Two choices of the distribution of random effects are supported, either normal or log-normal.

- *Residual variances* σ_A^2, σ_P^2: each of the two can be selected as a parameter or a given constant. In the latter case this component is not included in the information matrix, i.e., partial derivatives in (1.108) are not taken.

- Doses: starting dose and dosing schedule if necessary (maintenance dose, frequency, length of infusion for continuous infusion administration).

- Candidate sampling times/design region: there are two options that we consider rather practical.

    1. The user selects the number k of samples ($k_{min} \leq k \leq k_{max}$) and a finite set of candidate sampling times (say, every hour, every half-hour, etc. over the specified time window), and then the program enumerates all possible sequences of length k from this set and uses these sequences as the design region $\mathfrak{X}$; cf. Retout and Mentré (2003) [340] and the example in Section 7.2. In the current version, $k_{min} \geq 1$ and $k_{max} \leq 12$. To avoid samples taken too "close" to each other, a positive time lag may be selected (minimal delta time between consecutive samples).

    Forced samples: the user may want to always use certain times for sampling, e.g., at the end of the dosing interval or at baseline. In this case forced sampling times are included in all candidate sequences; see the example in Section 7.2.4.

    Cost-based design option: when cost $\phi(\mathbf{x})$ is associated with measurements at times $\mathbf{x}$, one can introduce cost-normalized information matrices $\boldsymbol{\mu}_c(\mathbf{x}, \boldsymbol{\theta}) = \boldsymbol{\mu}(\mathbf{x}, \boldsymbol{\theta})/\phi(\mathbf{x})$ and construct cost-based designs, which, in general, lead to a more meaningful comparison of sampling sequences; see (4.19) to (4.24) in Chapter 4. The currently implemented cost function is $\phi(\mathbf{x}_k) = C_v + C_s k$, where k is the length of sequence $\mathbf{x}_k$, and C_V, C_s correspond to costs of the visit (initiation) and analyzing each sample, respectively; cf. Sections 7.2.4, 7.3.1, 7.4.2.

    2. Candidate sequences may be loaded from a specific file; in this case the optimal design will be selected from those sequences. This

option also allows the user to select different costs for different sequences, with an arbitrary cost function, not necessarily depending on the length of the sequence.

Note that by construction, the design region $\mathfrak{X}$ is finite for both options. Such selection allows us to calculate information matrices of candidate sequences prior to running the optimal design algorithm, and reduce the forward step (3.2) of the optimization algorithm to a finite optimization problem; see Section 6.1.

- Tuning parameters of the algorithm: number of iterations, number of sequences in the initial design, stepsize for forward/backward steps, value of δ for numerical differentiation, limit of detection LoD (sampling times for which the response is less than the LoD may be excluded from the analysis). For details, see Section 3.1; see also Fedorov et al. (2007) [133], Section 7.1.5.

Figure 7.13 presents the input screen of the one-compartment PK model (7.23), (7.24) with multiple dosing.

7.5.4   Software outputs

- Plot of response function $\eta(x, \boldsymbol{\gamma}^0)$, regular and log-scale.

- Optimal design which, in general, may have more than one sequence. Since in practice the allocation of patients to different sampling schemes may have logistical issues, we also report five best single-sequence designs if available, i.e., if they produce nonsingular information matrices.

- Sensitivity function of the optimal design, see Section 2.5: a diagnostic plot that illustrates the Equivalence Theorem; see Figure 6.2 in Section 6.3.1, Figure 7.2 in Section 7.2.4, and Figure 7.15 in Section 7.5.5.

- *Sampling windows*: in practice it may be problematic to use exact sampling times derived by the algorithm. We have implemented the following Monte Carlo "sampling windows" design to check how robust the optimal design is with respect to "small" deviations from optimal sampling times, cf. Graham and Aarons (2006) [182], Patan and Bogacka (2007) [305], Ogungbenro and Aarons (2009) [297].

  Assume, without loss of generality, that the optimal design is a single sequence with k samples, $\mathbf{x} = (x_1, x_2, ..., x_k)$. Specify Δ, size of the vicinity around the optimal times, and n, the number of runs.

  - Generate a perturbed sequence $\tilde{\mathbf{x}}_r = (x_1 + \xi_{r1}, x_2 + \xi_{r2}, ..., x_k + \xi_{rk})$ for each run r, where ξ_{rl} are uniform r.v. in $[-\Delta, \Delta]$, $r = 1, \ldots, n$.
  - Calculate information matrices $\boldsymbol{\mu}(\tilde{\mathbf{x}}_r, \boldsymbol{\theta})$ and the information matrix of the average sampling window design, $\boldsymbol{\mu}_\Delta = \frac{1}{n} \sum_{r=1}^n \boldsymbol{\mu}(\tilde{\mathbf{x}}_r, \boldsymbol{\theta})$.

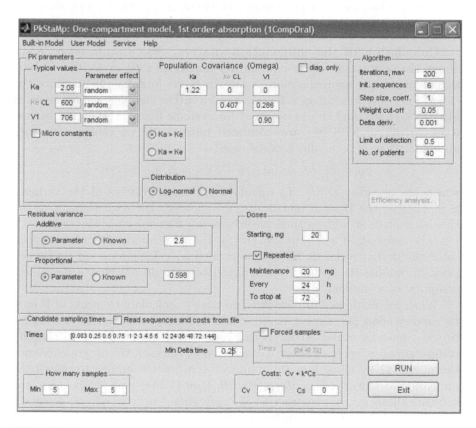

FIGURE 7.13: Typical input screen: one-compartment model with first-order absorption and linear elimination.

     – Get the efficiency of the average design, i.e., compare determinants, average (Monte Carlo) vs. optimal design.

- *User-defined sampling windows*: this option is similar to the previous one except that users can use own sampling windows by loading their low and upper bounds from a file.

- Any user-defined design from a file can be compared with the optimal one, or two user-defined designs can be compared directly to each other.

Calculation of the information matrix. We provide some details about the calculation of the information matrix $\boldsymbol{\mu}(\mathbf{x}, \boldsymbol{\theta})$ in (1.108), in particular about the approximation of matrix $\mathbf{S}$ via formula (7.79). Since the closed-form solutions for $\boldsymbol{\eta}(\mathbf{x}, \boldsymbol{\theta})$ (a) may be rather cumbersome for systems like (7.9), (7.10), and (b) do not exist for systems like (7.81), partial derivatives $\partial\boldsymbol{\eta}/\partial\theta_\alpha$ and $\partial\mathbf{S}/\partial\theta_\alpha$ are calculated numerically via central difference approximation: in a one-dimensional case,

$$d\eta(x_i, \theta)/d\theta \approx [\eta(x_i, \theta + \delta) - \eta(x_i, \theta - \delta)]/2\delta,$$

which has accuracy $O(\delta^2)$. To calculate partial derivatives of the variance $\mathbf{S}$ in (1.108), the Hessian matrix of η's is needed. For each element of the Hessian matrix at a given time x_i, in general, four values of the response η must be determined and thus $2m_\gamma(m_\gamma + 1)$ values for the full matrix. Still, since the design region is finite in our setting, calculations are performed prior to running the optimal design algorithm and do not constitute a large computational burden.

    When calculating (7.79), formally we have to calculate elements of $\mathbf{F}$ only for random effect parameters. On the other hand, in (1.108) partial derivatives $\partial\boldsymbol{\eta}/\partial\theta_\alpha$ must be evaluated for both random and fixed effects. To simplify computations, when fixed effects are selected by the user, the program extends the matrix $\boldsymbol{\Omega}$ by filling it with "dummy" zero rows/columns, to match the dimension of matrices $\mathbf{F} = [\partial\boldsymbol{\eta}(\mathbf{x}, \boldsymbol{\theta})/\partial\boldsymbol{\theta}_\alpha)]$ in (1.108) and (7.79). Also, the software allows for the construction of "individual," or fixed effects, designs if one selects all response parameters as "fixed."

7.5.5   Optimal designs as a reference point

    There are many practical situations when the direct use of locally optimal designs is not the only or the primary goal of the study. Instead, optimal designs are used for sensitivity analyses to compare the relative efficiency of alternative designs; e.g., see Ford et al. (1992) [162] or the example in Section 6.3.2. In this section we provide an example of a combined PK/PD study where optimal design methodology was utilized in this fashion.

    The study evaluated patients with high-risk cardiovascular disease, and one of the goals was to investigate PK and PD properties of the new drug. The dose

of 250 mg of the investigational drug was to be administered daily for the duration of the study to 30 patients on active arm. The one-compartment model
(7.23), (7.24), adjusted for repeated dosing, was used to describe drug concentration $\eta_{pk}(x, \gamma_{pk})$, parameterized via absorption rate K_a, volume of distribution V and clearance CL, so that $K_e = CL/V$ and $\gamma_{pk} = (K_a, V, CL)^T$.
(More precisely, the model was parameterized via apparent volume of distribution V/F and apparent systemic clearance CL/F, where F is oral bioavailability, so that $K_e = (CL/F)/(V/F) = CL/V$ and volume F in the denominator
on the right-hand side of (7.24) must be replaced with V/F).

An E_{max} model was used for a PD endpoint,

$$E_{z_{pd}}[y_{pd}(x)] = \eta_{pd}(x, \gamma) = E_0 \left[1 - \frac{\eta_{pk}(x, \gamma_{pk})}{IC_{50} + \eta_{pk}(x, \gamma_{pk})} \right], \qquad (7.82)$$

where $\gamma = (\gamma_{pk}^T, \gamma_{pd}^T)^T$, $\gamma_{pd} = (E_0, IC_{50})^T$; E_0 is the baseline PD response,
IC_{50} is the drug plasma concentration causing 50% inhibition of PD response,
and residual errors v_{pd} may have both additive and proportional components
of variance as in (7.78).

The following sampling scheme was considered by the clinical team because
of the logistics of the study:

- Take four pairs of PK and PD samples: first pair at week 4, between
  0.5 and 5 hours (absorption phase); second at week 6, between 9 and
  22 h (elimination phase); third at week 8, between 0.5 and 5 h (absorption phase); and fourth at week 10, between 5 and 9 h (around peak
  concentration).

- Take pre-dose (trough) measurements at weeks 4 and 8, both PK and
  PD samples.

- Take a PD sample at baseline, $t = 0$.

Our main goal was to find out how sensitive the proposed study design
was with respect to variation of sampling times within four sampling windows. Given study constraints, we proposed the following design region for
the construction of optimal design:

- Two forced PK and PD samples at 504 h (start of week 4) and 1176 h
  (start of week 8).

- One forced PD sample at baseline, $t = 0$.

- Four "flexible" PK and PD sampling times using the proposed hourly
  windows at day 1 of weeks 4, 6, 8 and 10. For this model, we created a
  special panel for candidate sampling times; see Figure 7.14. This panel
  includes individual sampling windows for each of the four flexible times
  (week/day/hours) and a frequency field: given the value of $Freq$ in this
  field, candidate sampling times for window s are

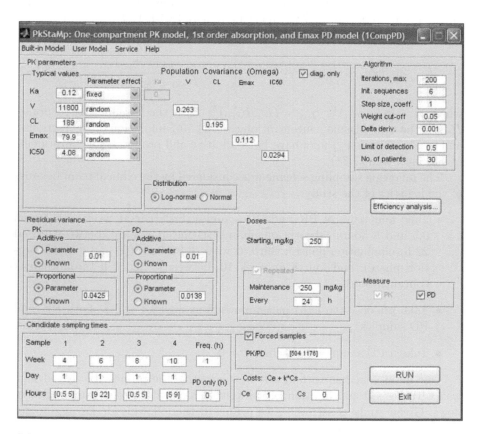

FIGURE 7.14: Input screen for one-compartment PK model and E_{max} PD model.

$$t \in \{t_{s,min}; \ t_{s,min} + jFreq, \ j = 1, 2, \ldots; \ t_{s,max}\},$$

where $[t_{s,min}, \ t_{s,max}]$ are boundaries of the sampling window for the s-th sample, $s = 1, 2, 3, 4$. For example, with hourly boundaries $[0.5,5]$, $[9,22]$, $[0.5,5]$, $[5,9]$, as in the proposed design, and $Freq = 1$ h, the total number of candidate sequences is $6 \times 14 \times 6 \times 5 = 2520$. The "flexible" candidate sequences $\{\mathbf{x}_i\}_{i=1}^{2520}$ are ordered as follows (cf. Section 7.2.4): first, the fourth sampling time point varies as in

$$\mathbf{x}_1 = (0.5, 9, 0.5, \mathbf{5}), \quad \mathbf{x}_2 = (0.5, 9, 0.5, \mathbf{6}), \quad \ldots, \quad \mathbf{x}_5 = (0.5, 9, 0.5, \mathbf{9}).$$

Then this procedure is repeated similarly for the third, second and first sampling time points up to final sequences

$$\mathbf{x}_{2516} = (5, 22, 5, \mathbf{5}), \quad \mathbf{x}_{2517} = (5, 22, 5, \mathbf{6}), \quad \ldots, \quad \mathbf{x}_{2520} = (5, 22, 5, \mathbf{9}).$$

In total, there were six PK samples and seven PD samples collected, and $k = 13$ in the analog of formula (7.79), where

$$\mathbf{x}_i = \left(\begin{array}{c} \mathbf{x}_{6,pk} \\ \mathbf{x}_{7,pd} \end{array} \right), \ \boldsymbol{\eta}(\mathbf{x}_i, \boldsymbol{\theta}) = \left[\begin{array}{c} \boldsymbol{\eta}_{pk}(\mathbf{x}_{6,pk}, \boldsymbol{\theta}) \\ \boldsymbol{\eta}_{pd}(\mathbf{x}_{7,pd}, \boldsymbol{\theta}) \end{array} \right],$$

$$\boldsymbol{\Sigma}_P = \left(\begin{array}{cc} \sigma_{P,pk}^2 \mathbf{I}_6 & \mathbf{0}_{6,7} \\ \mathbf{0}_{7,6} & \sigma_{P,pd}^2 \mathbf{I}_7 \end{array} \right), \ \boldsymbol{\Sigma}_A = \left(\begin{array}{cc} \sigma_{A,pk}^2 \mathbf{I}_6 & \mathbf{0}_{6,7} \\ \mathbf{0}_{7,6} & \sigma_{A,pd}^2 \mathbf{I}_7 \end{array} \right),$$

where $\mathbf{0}_{m,n}$ is an $m \times n$ matrix of zeros.

Preliminary parameter estimates were obtained by fitting data from a previous study of this drug in healthy volunteers using NONMEM software under the assumption of a log-normal distribution of individual response parameters $\boldsymbol{\gamma}_i$ and a diagonal covariance matrix $\boldsymbol{\Omega}$. Specifically, typical values $\boldsymbol{\gamma}^0 = (0.12, 11800, 189, 79.9, 4.08); \quad \boldsymbol{\Omega} = \text{Diag}(0, 0.263, 0.195, 0.112, 0.0294)$, i.e., parameter K_a was taken as a fixed effect; and residual error variances $\sigma_{pk,A}^2 = \sigma_{pd,A}^2 = 0; \ \sigma_{pk,P}^2 = 0.0425, \ \sigma_{pd,P}^2 = 0.0138$.

We selected small values of additive residual variances for regularization purposes, to protect against singularity of the variance-covariance matrix $\mathbf{S}$ in (7.79): $\sigma_{A,pk}^2 = \sigma_{A,pd}^2 = 0.01$, and considered them as given constants. In total, there were $m = 11$ unknown parameters in the model, with $m_\gamma = 5$ (one fixed and four mixed effects), four elements of the diagonal matrix $\boldsymbol{\Omega}$ and two proportional residual variances, $\sigma_{P,pk}^2$ and $\sigma_{P,pd}^2$.

The D-optimal design is a two-sequence design, with hourly times

$$\xi^* = \{\mathbf{x}_1^* = (4.5, 9, 3.5, 8), \ w_1 = 0.58, \ \mathbf{x}_2^* = (5, 22, 3.5, 7), \ w_2 = 0.42\},$$

in addition to forced PK and PD samples. For both optimal sequences, samples are to be taken at the end of the 1st sampling window, middle of the 3rd and end of the 4th. The sequences differ in the location of the second sample (beginning of the window for $\mathbf{x}_1^*$ and the end of the window for $\mathbf{x}_2^*$). In practice, with the given sample size N, weights w_1 and w_2 must be multiplied by N, and then frequencies $n_i = Nw_i$ rounded to the nearest integer keeping $n_1 + n_2 = N$. When $N = 30$, then $n_1 = 17$ and $n_2 = 13$; for more details on rounding and approximate designs, see Section 3.3.

In our example many individual sequences produce a D-efficiency greater than 0.99, in particular, both sequences of the optimal design. Thus, these sequences are essentially as good as the two-sequence optimal design with respect to the precision of parameter estimation, but may be simpler with respect to practical implementation; see the comment in Section 7.5.4 about selection of best single-sequence designs. The worst sampling sequence out of 2520 candidates has a D-efficiency of 0.7; this was sequence $\tilde{\mathbf{x}} = (1.5, 19, 1.5, 5)$, i.e., measurements closer to the start of the 1st window, end of 2nd, start of 3rd, and start of 4th. The mean efficiency of individual sequences is 0.861, with a median value of 0.865, and the D-efficiency of the average design is 0.886. Moreover, if the full 24-hour sampling windows were allowed, i.e., if samples could be taken once daily at any hour of the four days, then the increase in efficiency of the optimal design for such an extended design region, compared to ξ^*, was only about 4%.

It is worthwhile to examine coefficients of variation (CV) of estimated parameters. For $N = 30$, CVs for the optimal design are (2.27, 0.86, 1.10, 0.78)% for random effects; 3.9% for k_a; (22.7, 5.1, 5.6, 9.7)% for diagonal elements of the matrix $\mathbf{\Omega}$ and (2.8, 3.1)% for residual variances. If we consider only the first sequence of the optimal design as the alternative design, then coefficients of variation are essentially the same as for the optimal design: the largest increase is for volume V (from 2.27% to 2.42%) and absorption rate k_a (from 3.9% to 4.1%). If we consider the worst sequence $\tilde{\mathbf{x}} = (1.5, 19, 1.5, 5)$, then the increase in CV is observed for V (from 2.27% to 7.26%), K_a (from 3.9% to 8.5%), and variance of V (from 22.7% to 42.1%); the CV for the other 8 parameters changes by no more than several hundredths of a percent.

These results confirmed that the sampling scheme proposed by the study team was efficient, and also suggested some improvements with respect to specific sampling times within each window.

Sensitivity function. As mentioned in Section 7.5.4, the Equivalence Theorem (Theorem 2.3) provides an excellent diagnostic tool for testing whether or not the numerical algorithm has converged to the optimal design; see Section 2.5 and examples in Sections 6.3.1 and 7.2.4. In Figure 7.15 we plot the sensitivity function $d(\mathbf{x}_i, \boldsymbol{\theta}, \xi^*)$ as a function of index i, $i = 1, \ldots, 2520$. This figure serves as an illustration of Theorem 2.3. The sensitivity function hits the reference line $m = 11$ at two D-optimal sequences:

$$\mathbf{x}_{1699} = \mathbf{x}_1^* = (4.5, 9, 3.5, 8); \quad \mathbf{x}_{2508} = \mathbf{x}_2^* = (5, 22, 3.5, 7).$$

Remark 7.4 For the selected values of response parameters, the steady state for both PK and PD endpoints was reached during week 2 of the study, and then the PK and PD trajectories became essentially periodic functions. Therefore, it is not surprising that when we changed week values to arbitrary num-

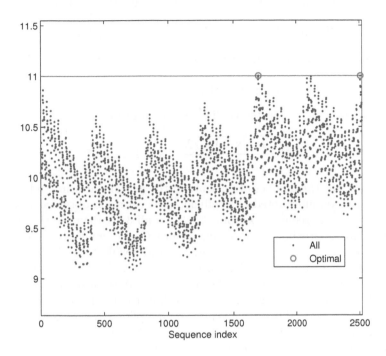

FIGURE 7.15: Sensitivity function for optimal two-sequence design.

bers greater than 2, used arbitrary values for days (not necessarily 1) and constructed optimal designs with the same hourly windows, the results (optimal design and efficiencies) were almost identical, which follows from the general results about optimal designs for periodic functions; in particular, for trigonometric regression, see Fedorov (1972) [127], Chapter 2.4.

7.5.6 Software comparison

In 2009 – 2011 participants of the PODE workshop performed a comparison of different software tools using the one-compartment model (7.24) as an example. The settings were proposed by Nick Holford and France Mentré and were based on data from the earlier warfarin study. The model was parameterized via clearance CL, so that $K_e = CL/V$. It was assumed that the individual response parameters $\boldsymbol{\gamma}_i = (K_{ai}, CL_i, V_i)$ follow the log-normal distribution (7.11) with the mean vector $\boldsymbol{\gamma}^0 = (1, 0.15, 8)$ and the diagonal covariance matrix $\boldsymbol{\Omega} = \mathrm{Diag}(\Omega_r) = \mathrm{Diag}(0.6, 0.07, 0.02)$. It was also assumed that the additive component of residual variance vanishes, $\sigma_A^2 = 0$, and that

$\sigma_P^2 = 0.01$. So the combined vector of parameters for this example was

$$\boldsymbol{\theta} = (k_a^0,\ CL^0,\ V^0;\ \Omega_{k_a},\ \Omega_{CL},\ \Omega_V;\ \sigma_P^2)^T. \qquad (7.83)$$

The goal was to compare the Fisher information matrix for the 8-sample sequence

$$\mathbf{x} = (0.5, 1, 2, 6, 24, 36, 72, 120)\ \text{hours}. \qquad (7.84)$$

All software developers reported coefficients of variation CV_s,

$$CV_s = \frac{\sqrt{[\boldsymbol{\mu}^{-1}(\mathbf{x}, \boldsymbol{\theta})]_{ss}/N}}{\theta_s}, \quad s = 1, 2, \ldots, 7,$$

where $N = 32$ was the number of patients in the actual warfarin study. Thus, values CV_s can be interpreted as coefficients of variation obtained from the design that uses the sequence $\mathbf{x}$ from (7.84) for all 32 patients in the study.

To validate approximate formulae, Monte Carlo simulations were performed in NONMEM (by Joakim Nyberg) and MONOLIX (by Caroline Bazzoli); for references on MONOLIX software, see Lavielle and Méntre (2007) [250], or [288]. Sample estimates of the coefficients of variation were obtained: for a single run, data were generated according to the model (7.1), (7.11), (7.78), with parameters $\boldsymbol{\theta}$ from (7.83) and the sampling sequence $\mathbf{x}$ from (7.84) for 32 patients. Model parameters were estimated using the nonlinear mixed effects models estimation algorithm from either NONMEM or MONOLIX. Then after 1000 runs, sample statistics and coefficients of variations were calculated.

After comparing the outputs, it turned out that all population design tools produced similar coefficients of variation for all model parameters except the absorption rate K_a: $CV(K_a) = 0.052$ for PkStaMp and PopDes, while $CV(K_a) = 0.139$ for other tools. Simulations in both NONMEM and MONOLIX resulted in estimates $CV(K_a) = 0.12 \div 0.13$. The discrepancy between the outputs suggested to look closer at how calculations were implemented by the different software developers.

The matrix $\boldsymbol{\mu}$ in (1.108) can be partitioned as follows, cf. Retout and Mentré (2003) [340]:

$$\boldsymbol{\mu}(\mathbf{x}, \boldsymbol{\theta}) = \left\{ \begin{array}{cc} \mathbf{A} & \mathbf{C} \\ \mathbf{C}^T & \mathbf{B} \end{array} \right\}, \quad \mathbf{A} = \mathbf{A}_1 + \mathbf{A}_2, \ \mathbf{A}_1 = \mathbf{F}^T \mathbf{S}^{-1} \mathbf{F}, \qquad (7.85)$$

where for our specific example

$$\mathbf{A}_{2,\alpha\beta} = \frac{1}{2}\,\text{tr}\left[\mathbf{S}^{-1} \frac{\partial \mathbf{S}}{\partial \theta_\alpha} \mathbf{S}^{-1} \frac{\partial \mathbf{S}}{\partial \theta_\beta} \right], \ \alpha, \beta = 1, 2, 3; \qquad (7.86)$$

$$\mathbf{C}_{\alpha\beta} = \frac{1}{2}\,\text{tr}\left[\mathbf{S}^{-1} \frac{\partial \mathbf{S}}{\partial \theta_\alpha} \mathbf{S}^{-1} \frac{\partial \mathbf{S}}{\partial \theta_\beta} \right], \ \alpha = 1, 2, 3, \ \beta = 4, .., 7; \quad (7.87)$$

$$\mathbf{B}_{\alpha\beta} = \frac{1}{2}\,\text{tr}\left[\mathbf{S}^{-1} \frac{\partial \mathbf{S}}{\partial \theta_\alpha} \mathbf{S}^{-1} \frac{\partial \mathbf{S}}{\partial \theta_\beta} \right], \ \alpha, \beta = 4, .., 7.$$

So $\mathbf{A}$ is the 3×3 matrix that contains partial derivatives with respect to response parameters γ_α; $\mathbf{C}$ is the 3×4 matrix that contains mixed derivatives with respect to response parameters γ_α and variance parameters $(\Omega_\beta, \sigma_M^2)$; and $\mathbf{B}$ is the 4×4-matrix that contains derivatives with respect to all variance parameters $(\Omega_\beta, \sigma_M^2)$.

In PkStaMp we used the first-order approximation (7.15), (7.16) and the full matrix $\boldsymbol{\mu}(\mathbf{x}, \boldsymbol{\theta})$ in (7.85). It turned out that the other software tools (PFIM, PopED, WinPOPT) used the following settings:

- "Exclude" matrix $\mathbf{A}_2$ in the calculation of the matrix $\mathbf{A}$ in (7.85) and use $\mathbf{A}_2 = \mathbf{0}$,

- Exclude matrix $\mathbf{C}$ in the calculation of the matrix $\boldsymbol{\mu}$ in (7.85) and use $\mathbf{C} = \mathbf{0}$ instead,

- Exclude the term $\mathbf{F}\,\boldsymbol{\Omega}\,\mathbf{F}^T$ in the square brackets on the right-hand side of (7.15).

These differences led to quite visible differences in the elements of the information matrix $\boldsymbol{\mu}$ that correspond to the absorption rate K_a. Once we made the initial settings identical, the output results coincided too. Still, several questions remained, in particular (a) what are the consequences of the first-order approximation in (7.15) and (7.16), and (b) which option is preferable, the "full" where the matrices $\mathbf{A}_2$, $\mathbf{C}$ are preserved, or the "reduced" where $\mathbf{A}_2 = \mathbf{C} = \mathbf{0}$?

Linearization for log-normal population distribution. Suppose that ζ is a normal random variable, $\zeta \sim \mathcal{N}(0, \Omega)$, and that $\gamma = e^\zeta$. Then the first-order approximation leads to

$$\gamma \approx 1 + \zeta, \quad \mathrm{E}\gamma \approx 1, \quad \mathrm{Var}(\gamma) \approx \mathrm{E}\zeta^2 = \Omega. \tag{7.88}$$

On the other hand, the exact moments of the log-normally distributed random variable γ are

$$\mathrm{E}\gamma = e^{\Omega/2}, \quad \mathrm{Var}(\gamma) = e^\Omega(e^\Omega - 1), \tag{7.89}$$

and, therefore, when Ω is not too small, the first-order approximation may lead to substantial distortion of the distribution in general, and moments in particular. In our example $\Omega_{K_a} = 0.6$, and the analogs of (7.88) and (7.89) are

$$\mathrm{E}K_{ai} \approx 1, \quad \mathrm{Var}(K_{ai}) \approx 0.6, \tag{7.90}$$

and

$$\mathrm{E}K_{ai} = 1.35, \quad \mathrm{Var}(K_{ai}) = 1.5, \tag{7.91}$$

respectively. For more discussion on linearization options, see Mielke and Schwabe (2010) [283].

Using $\mathbf{A}_2 = \mathbf{0}$ in (7.85). To get an idea of the effect of setting $\mathbf{A}_2 = \mathbf{0}$ in

(7.85), consider a single-response fixed effects model (7.1), i.e., $\boldsymbol{\Omega} = \mathbf{0}$. Let $\{\varepsilon\}$ in (7.78) be normally distributed, with known residual variances $\sigma_A^2 = 0$ and σ_P^2. In this case $\mathrm{Var}(y_{ij}) = \sigma_P^2 \eta^2(x_{ij}, \gamma^0)$, so the term $\mathbf{A}_2$ in (7.86) reduces to $\mathbf{A}_2 = 2 \frac{\mathbf{F}^T \mathbf{F}}{\eta^2}$, and formula (1.108) for the Fisher information matrix becomes

$$\boldsymbol{\mu}_F(x, \boldsymbol{\theta}) = \frac{1}{\sigma_P^2} \frac{\mathbf{F}^T \mathbf{F}}{\eta^2} + 2 \frac{\mathbf{F}^T \mathbf{F}}{\eta^2} = \left(\frac{1}{\sigma_P^2} + 2 \right) \frac{\mathbf{F}^T \mathbf{F}}{\eta^2}. \tag{7.92}$$

When the term $\mathbf{A}_2$ is not used, then the "reduced" information matrix is

$$\boldsymbol{\mu}_R(x, \boldsymbol{\theta}) = \frac{1}{\sigma_P^2} \frac{\mathbf{F}^T \mathbf{F}}{\eta^2}. \tag{7.93}$$

To evaluate the effect of the missing term $\mathbf{A}_2$ on the coefficient of variation, one can check the ratio

$$\sqrt{\frac{\mu_{\alpha\beta,\, F}}{\mu_{\alpha\beta,\, R}}} = \sqrt{\frac{2 + 1/\sigma_P^2}{1/\sigma_P^2}} = \sqrt{1 + 2\sigma_P^2} \sim 1 + \sigma_P^2 \text{ for small } \sigma_P^2. \tag{7.94}$$

So (7.94) suggests that for our example with $\sigma_P^2 = 0.01$, the effect of dropping the term $\mathbf{A}_2$ may be minimal. Once the proportional residual variance σ_P^2 becomes larger, then the effect of the missing term $\mathbf{A}_2$ may be more pronounced.

For an example where accounting for the term $\mathbf{A}_2$ in (7.85) leads to overestimation of the information and underestimation of the variance, see Mielke and Schwabe (2010) [283], Section 4.

Note also that in the considered example the Fisher information matrix $\boldsymbol{\mu}_F(x, \boldsymbol{\theta})$ coincides, up to the coefficient of proportionality, with the information (moment) matrix $\boldsymbol{\mu}_R(x, \boldsymbol{\theta})$ that corresponds to the iteratively reweighted least squares estimator $\hat{\boldsymbol{\theta}}_{IRLS}$; see Section 1.7.1. While the variance-covariance matrix of $\hat{\boldsymbol{\theta}}_{IRLS}$ is larger than the one of the maximum likelihood estimator $\hat{\boldsymbol{\theta}}_{MLE}$, the optimal design for the two methods is the same.

Linearization and using $\mathbf{C} = \mathbf{0}$ in (7.85). We do not have a good explanation of why the reduced version of the information matrix $\boldsymbol{\mu}(\mathbf{x}, \boldsymbol{\theta})$ with $\mathbf{C} = \mathbf{0}$ led to a "better" approximation that was closer to the simulations in NONMEM and MONOLIX. A possible heuristic explanation is that setting $\mathbf{C} = \mathbf{0}$ helped in some way to balance the effect of the distortion due to the first-order approximation; see (7.90), (7.91). From a practical point of view, taking $\mathbf{C} = \mathbf{0}$ and, therefore, using the simpler covariance structure may simplify the estimation algorithm. However, in general, we do not see any solid reason for using $\mathbf{C} = \mathbf{0}$ instead of considering the full matrix with $\mathbf{C}$ defined in (7.87).

Other types of approximation. If one uses the second-order approximation of the response function $\eta(x, \gamma_i)$ in the vicinity of γ^0, then the expectation of $\eta(x, \gamma_i)$ with respect to the distribution of parameters γ_i can be approximated by the formula (7.17); see Remark 7.1. Since the formula

(7.15) for the variance-covariance matrix $\mathbf{S}$ utilizes first derivatives $\mathbf{F}$ of the response $\boldsymbol{\eta}$, calculation of the derivatives of $\mathbf{S}$ in (1.108) in the case of first-order approximation requires second-order derivatives of $\boldsymbol{\eta}$. Thus, with the second-order approximation (7.17), one will require fourth-order derivatives of the response function $\boldsymbol{\eta}$, which numerically will be rather tedious.

One of potential ways of improving the calculation of the information matrix $\boldsymbol{\mu}(\mathbf{x}, \boldsymbol{\theta})$ and avoiding numerical approximation as in (7.15), (7.16) or (7.17) is to calculate the mean and variance via Monte Carlo simulations at each candidate sampling time x_j:

- Generate L independent realizations of response parameters $\boldsymbol{\gamma}_i$ from a given distribution (normal or log-normal), $i = 1, \dots, L$.

- Generate values $\mathbf{Y}_i = \{y_{ij}\}$ according to (7.1) and (7.78), with $x_{ij} \equiv x_j$ for all i.

- Calculate empirical mean and variance:

$$\widehat{\boldsymbol{\eta}} = \widehat{\boldsymbol{\eta}}(\mathbf{x}, \boldsymbol{\theta}) = \widehat{\mathbb{E}}_{\boldsymbol{\theta}}(\mathbf{Y}) = \frac{1}{L} \sum_{i=1}^{L} \mathbf{Y}_i,$$

$$\widehat{\mathbf{S}} = \widehat{\mathbf{S}}(\mathbf{x}, \boldsymbol{\theta}) = \widehat{\mathrm{Var}}_{\boldsymbol{\theta}}(\mathbf{Y}) = \frac{1}{L-1} \sum_{i=1}^{L} (\mathbf{Y}_i - \widehat{\boldsymbol{\eta}})\,(\mathbf{Y}_i - \widehat{\boldsymbol{\eta}})^T. \qquad (7.95)$$

- Use (1.108) to calculate $\boldsymbol{\mu}(\mathbf{x}, \boldsymbol{\theta})$ with values $\{\widehat{\boldsymbol{\eta}},\ \widehat{\mathbf{S}}\}$ from (7.95).

Note that the described Monte Carlo approach will eliminate the need to calculate second- and higher-order derivatives of the response function since the formula (7.15) or its analogs will not be used. The limitation of this approach is that it still relies on the normal approximation (1.108).

Figure 7.16 illustrates three different types of approximation of the response function η; cf. Figure 7.5. The solid line presents $\eta(x, \boldsymbol{\gamma}^0)$, i.e., the first-order approximation; see (7.88). The dashed line shows $\eta(x, \boldsymbol{\gamma}_{log}^0)$, where $\boldsymbol{\gamma}_{log}^0$ is the true mean of the log-normal distribution; see (7.89). The dotted line presents $\hat{\eta}(x)$, which is obtained via the Monte Carlo approach as in (7.95). The differences between the three curves are most pronounced during the absorption phase and at the beginning of the elimination phase (before and after the peak concentration, respectively). These differences can lead to differences in the computation of the information matrix $\boldsymbol{\mu}(\mathbf{x}, \boldsymbol{\theta})$.

7.5.7 User-defined option

A second example for software comparison was discussed at the PODE 2011 meeting; see Mentré et al. (2011) [279]. The example was based on a hepatitis C viral dynamics model (HCV); see Neumann et al. (1998) [295]. The model includes two components. The PK component is a one-compartment

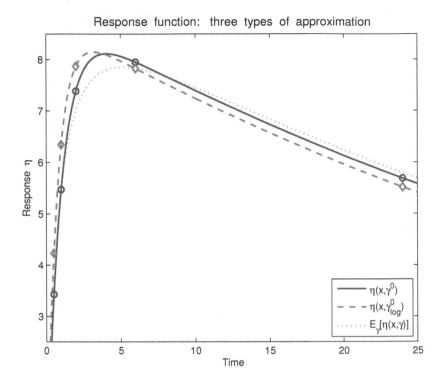

FIGURE 7.16: Mean response curves: first-order approximation (solid line), computed at mean values of log-normal distribution (dashed), and Monte Carlo average (dotted). Locations of circles and diamonds correspond to sampling times from the sequence **x** in (7.84).

model that is similar to (7.24), but with continuous drug infusion of dose $D = 180$ mg for the duration of one day, repeated every week. Thus, the first equation in (7.23) must be replaced with

$$\dot{q}_0(x) = -K_a q_0(x) + r(x), \quad r(x) = \{D, \text{ if } x \in [x_l, x_l + 1], \text{ or } 0 \text{ otherwise}\},$$

where x_l are starting times of infusion, $x_l = 0, 7, 14, \ldots$ (days). The PD model describes the dynamics of the number of "target cells" T, infected cells I and the viral load v:

$$
\begin{cases}
\dot{T}(x) = & -C_1 T(x) - C_2\, T(x)\, v(x) + C_3, \\
\dot{I}(x) = & -\delta I(x) + C_2\, T(x)\, v(x), \\
\dot{v}(x) = & -C_4 \left\{ 1 - \frac{1}{1 + [EC_{50}/\eta_1(x)]^n} \right\}\, I(x) - c\, v(x),
\end{cases}
\tag{7.96}
$$

where $\eta_1(x) = \eta_1(x, \boldsymbol{\gamma}) = q_1(x)/V$ is the drug concentration in the central compartment. The measured PD endpoint is $\eta_2(x) = \eta_2(x, \boldsymbol{\gamma}) = \log_{10} v(x)$.

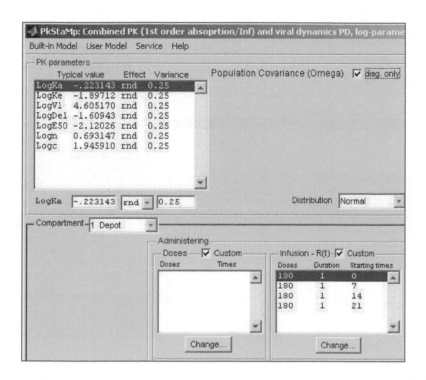

FIGURE 7.17: User-defined option, input screens: parameters and dosing regimen.

For the purposes of software comparison, it was assumed that the measurement error model (7.78) had the additive component only, and $\sigma_P^2 = 0$ for both PK and PD responses. It was also assumed that C_1, C_2, C_3, C_4 were fixed constants. In total, there were seven response parameters: three PK parameters (K_a, K_e, V) and four PD parameters (δ, EC_{50}, n, c). The log-parameterization was used for response parameters, i.e., $\boldsymbol{\gamma} = (\gamma_1, \ldots, \gamma_7) = (\ln K_a, \ldots, \ln c)$, with the normal distribution of parameters γ_i and the diagonal covariance matrix $\boldsymbol{\Omega} = 0.25 \, \mathbf{I}_7$. The goal was to compare the Fisher information matrix for the 12-sample sequence

$$\mathbf{x} = (0, 0.25, 0.5, 1, 2, 3, 4, 7, 10, 14, 21, 28) \text{ days}, \tag{7.97}$$

with the simultaneous measurement of PK and PD responses η_1 and η_2.

To run the HCV example, we implemented a user-defined option in the PkStaMp library. This option allows the user to perform the following actions:

- Similar to built-in models, input model parameters $\boldsymbol{\gamma}^0$ and $\boldsymbol{\Omega}$; cf. Figure

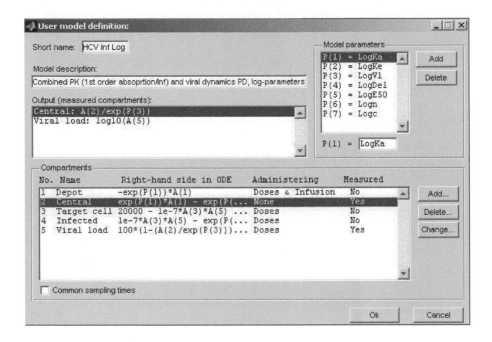

FIGURE 7.18: User-defined option, input screens: specifying differential equations and measured compartments.

7.13 and Figure 7.17. In the HCV example, $K_a = 0.8$; so because of log-parameterization we used $\theta_1 = \log(0.8) = -0.223143$, etc.

- Input different types of dosing. For example, continuous infusion can be specified by starting times and durations; see Figure 7.17, bottom right corner.

- Similar to built-in models, specify residual error model and candidate sampling times for measured compartments.

- Type algebraic expressions on the right-hand side of differential equations into corresponding fields; see Figure 7.18. In the algebraic expressions, by $\{A\}$ we denote amounts in different compartments, i.e., $A(1) = q_0, A(2) = q_1, \ldots, A(5) = v$, and by $\{P\}$ we denote model parameters.

The user-defined option utilizes the numerical solution of the system of ODEs via MATLAB built-in solver *ode*45.

In the PkStaMp run that was reported at the PAGE 2011 meeting, we did not account for the dependence of the initial conditions of the system (7.96) on model parameters that led to minor differences in the reported coefficients of variation compared to other software tools; see Example 2 in Mentré et al. (2011) [279]. This inconsistency was later corrected, and the resulting CVs from PkStaMp became identical to those from the other tools under the same assumptions.

Discussion and future work. Compared to other software tools for optimal population design, the PkStaMp library has some useful extra features, in particular

- Efficient numerical procedure that includes forward and backward steps and computes optimal designs in the space of Fisher information matrices of candidate sequences.

- Flexibility in the selection of candidate sampling sequences, either from all possible subsequences of a predefined sequence of sampling times, or from a prespecified set of candidate sequences with user-defined cost functions; see Section 7.5.3.

- Convergence diagnostics via the sensitivity plot; see Section 7.5.5.

Among potential extensions of the PkStaMp library that we plan to address are the use of Monte Carlo simulations (7.95) to approximate the individual information matrix $\boldsymbol{\mu}(\mathbf{x}, \boldsymbol{\theta})$ in (1.108), and optimal designs for PK models described by stochastic differential equations; see Section 7.4. It is also worthwhile to explore various measures of nonlinearity when using different approximation options; see Bates and Watts (1988) [33], Merlé and Todd (2001) [280], Pázman (1993) [307], Ratkowsky (1983) [336].

Chapter 8

Adaptive Model-Based Designs

8.1   Adaptive Design for E_{max} Model 253
    8.1.1   Study background 254
    8.1.2   Model 254
    8.1.3   Adaptive dose selection with constraints 256
    8.1.4   Simulation studies 257
    8.1.5   Generalized E_{max} model 266
    8.1.6   Extensions 268
    8.1.7   Technical details 272
8.2   Adaptive Designs for Bivariate Cox Model 275
    8.2.1   Progress of the trial: single simulation 277
    8.2.2   Multiple simulations 278
8.3   Adaptive Designs for Bivariate Probit Model 282
    8.3.1   Single drug 282
    8.3.2   Combination of two drugs 287

As discussed in previous chapters, for nonlinear regression models the information matrix depends, in general, on the values of unknown parameters, which leads to the concept of locally optimal designs: first, a preliminary estimate $\tilde{\theta}$ must be specified, and then the optimization problem in (2.8) can be addressed. The misspecification of the preliminary estimates may result in the poor performance of locally optimal designs. Therefore, for nonlinear design problems the use of an adaptive, or sequential, approach can be beneficial; see Section 5.3. In this chapter we provide examples of the application of model-based adaptive designs in biopharmaceutical problems.

The most attractive feature of adaptive sequential experiments is their ability to optimally utilize the dynamics of the learning process associated with experimentation, data analysis and inference. As noted in Chaudhuri and Mykland (1995) [69], at the beginning scientists do not have much information, and hence an initial experiment is bound to be somewhat tentative in nature. As the experiment continues and more and more observations are obtained, scientists are able to form a more precise impression of the underlying theory, and this more definite perception is used to design a more informative experiment in the future that is expected to give rise to more relevant and useful data.

Adaptive designs have become quite popular in biopharmaceutical applications over the past two decades. The vast majority of the literature deals with sequential designs that originate in classic sequential analysis and that have received considerable attention in the pharmaceutical industry due to developments in the area of group sequential designs; see Jennison and Turnbull (2000) [211], Proschan et al. (2006) [326], Chang (2008) [67]. In recent years adaptive designs have drawn further attention due to the development of flexible designs; see Bauer and Brannath (2004) [36], Bauer (2008) [35], Gaydos et al. (2009) [172]. Special issues of several statistical journals were devoted to adaptive designs and their application in drug development; see

Journal of Statistical Planning and Inference, 136(6), 2006;

Journal of Biopharmaceutical Statistics, 16(2), 2006, with several papers on adaptive designs in dose-response studies; and 16(3), 2006, with a paper by Gallo et al. [169], describing the findings of the PhRMA Working Group on adaptive designs in clinical drug development; and 17(6), 2007;

Statistics in Medicine: 27(10), 2008;

Statistics in Biopharmaceutical Research, 2(4), 2010;

Journal of Biopharmaceutical Statistics, 20(6), 2010, where a number of papers were published that discussed a draft guidance issued by the Food and Drug Administration (FDA) entitled "Adaptive Design Clinical Trials for Drugs and Biologics" [124]. The guidance addresses topics such as aspects of adaptive design trials calling for special consideration; tips for when to approach the FDA while planning and conducting adaptive design studies; suggested contents in the submission to the FDA for review; and considerations for the evaluation of a completed adaptive design study.

Most often, adaptive designs are studied within the framework of normally distributed means, or settings that may be reduced to this; control variables, such as dose level, are not introduced. Nonlinear regression models where the experimenter can select different levels of control variables have received less attention, most likely because taking control variables into account leads to increased complexity of the problem. However, in recent years more papers have been published that introduce and study model-based adaptive designs in drug development; for a list of references, see Rosenberger and Haines (2002) [342], Dragalin and Fedorov (2006) [101], Bornkamp et al. (2007) [50], Dragalin et al. (2008) [103], Wang et al. (2012) [393].

In the context of dose-response studies, the adaptive designs are performed in cohorts/stages in order to update dose levels for each cohort and approach doses that are optimal with respect to a given optimality criterion. The adaptive approach relies on the iteration of two steps: estimation and dose selection; see Section 5.3.

(S0) Initial doses are chosen, first experiments are performed and preliminary parameter estimates are obtained.

(S1) Additional doses are selected from the current admissible range of doses $\mathfrak{X}$ to provide the biggest improvement in the design with respect to the selected criterion and current parameter estimates.

(S2) New experiments are performed, data are collected and the estimates of unknown parameters are refined given additional observations.

Steps (S1) and (S2) are repeated given available resources, for instance, the maximal number of subjects to be enrolled in the study, or the maximal number of cohorts n_{coh}. For a fully adaptive design, as described in (5.18) – (5.20), where both estimation and design are performed after each collected observation, if $\xi_N = \{x_1, \ldots, x_N\}$ is the design for the first N patients and if $\hat{\boldsymbol{\theta}}_N$ is the current parameter estimate, then for D-optimality criterion a dose x_{N+1} is defined as

$$x_{N+1} = \arg\max_{x \in \mathfrak{X}} \; d(x, \xi_N, \hat{\boldsymbol{\theta}}_N) = \arg\max_{x \in \mathfrak{X}} \; \mathrm{tr}\,[\boldsymbol{\mu}(x, \hat{\boldsymbol{\theta}}_N)\mathbf{M}^{-1}(\xi_N, \hat{\boldsymbol{\theta}}_N)]. \quad (8.1)$$

In the case of penalized designs, the next dose is defined as

$$x_{N+1} = \arg\max_{x \in \mathfrak{X}} \; \mathrm{tr}\, \left[\frac{\boldsymbol{\mu}(x, \hat{\boldsymbol{\theta}}_N)}{\phi(x, \hat{\boldsymbol{\theta}}_N)} \, \mathbf{M}^{-1}(\xi_N, \hat{\boldsymbol{\theta}}_N) \right]; \quad (8.2)$$

see (4.26).

For a discussion of other approaches, including Bayesian designs, that tackle the problem of unknown parameters in dose-finding studies, see Rosenberger et al. (2001) [344], Berry et al. (2002) [47], Rosenberger and Haines (2002) [342], Haines et al. (2003) [187], Whitehead et al. (2006) [403], Miller et al. (2007) [284], Dragalin et al. (2007) [104], Ivanova et al. (2012) [210]. Fedorov and Leonov (2005) [144], Section 5.6, described adaptive designs for dose-response studies with a restricted dose range. Note that a continual reassessment method (CRM) provides an example of an adaptive Bayesian procedure for finding dose ED_p in one-parameter models; see O'Quigley et al. (1990) [301], O'Quigley (2001) [298], Garrett-Mayer (2006) [171], Cheung (2011) [73]; cf. Section 6.2.

The structure of this chapter is as follows. Section 8.1 describes an adaptive design for the E_{max} model and its application in a clinical study. In Section 8.2 we discuss adaptive designs for the bivariate Cox model, which was introduced in Section 6.4. Section 8.3 describes adaptive designs for the bivariate probit model, which was introduced in Section 6.5.

8.1 Adaptive Design for E_{max} Model

In this section we discuss optimal adaptive designs for a popular nonlinear regression model and its application in a clinical study; for details, see Leonov and Miller (2009) [254].

8.1.1   Study background

The primary objectives of the first-time-in-human study which is discussed here, are focused on confirming the safety of a new drug. The drug is hoped to halt or reverse the progression of Alzheimer's disease, but there is also the opportunity to investigate the effect of the drug on a plasma biomarker. The mechanism of action of the compound should result in decreased levels of this biomarker in the plasma. Characterizing the dose-response relationship in humans will help guide dose selection in future studies.

The reduction of the biomarker is measured as the percent inhibition, i.e., the percentage reduction from baseline (time 0) at a fixed timepoint (t) after dosing, or $100(B_0 - B_t)/B_0$, where B_t is the biomarker assay result at time t. Preclinical experiments suggest that inhibition will be zero for low doses, will increase monotonically with dose, and will plateau at higher doses at a value close to 100%. That is, the endpoint is expected to follow an S-shaped, or E_{max} model similar to that shown in Figure 8.4. Note that because of the way the endpoint is defined the lower asymptote of the curve is zero, and the upper asymptote is constrained to be no greater than 100%. Further, variability in response is predicted to be largest in the middle of the dose range. Details on the E_{max} model are given in Section 8.1.2.

Safety and logistical factors impose constraints on the study design with respect to subject numbers and doses allocated. Subjects must be dosed in cohorts that are large enough to satisfy the Data Safety Monitoring Board that it is safe to proceed to a higher dose, but not so large that unnecessary numbers of subjects are dosed at pharmacologically inactive doses. Three subjects will therefore receive active compound in each of the first two cohorts, with six subjects on active treatment in subsequent cohorts. Two subjects will receive placebo in every cohort.

Initial and maximum permissible doses were selected on the basis of data from preclinical toxicology experiments. Within this range all doses can theoretically be given because the drug is administered intravenously. However, the maximal dose for each cohort is further restricted for safety reasons. A full description of the constraints is given in Leonov and Miller (2009) [254], Section 2.3.

The goal of the study is to maximize the precision of the estimate of the dose that achieves 90% inhibition, since this is expected to be sufficient to drive the mechanism of the compound. The model and optimality criteria are formalized in Section 8.1.2.

8.1.2   Model

The model of observations fits within the nonlinear regression framework (6.14) and provides a special case of the multiparameter logistic model; cf. (6.20):

$$y_i = \eta(x_i, \gamma) + \varepsilon_i, \quad i = 1, \ldots, N, \tag{8.3}$$

where $\{y_i\}$ are measurements, i is a subject's index, x_i is the dose for subject i, N is the total number of subjects in the study, η is the response function:

$$\eta(x,\gamma) = \frac{E_{max}\, x^{\beta}}{ED_{50}^{\beta} + x^{\beta}} = \frac{E_{max}}{1 + (ED_{50}/x)^{\beta}}, \tag{8.4}$$

where $\gamma = (\beta, ED_{50}, E_{max})^T$ is the vector of response parameters; E_{max} is the maximal response (the limit as the dose increases, in percent), ED_{50} is the dose at which the mean response is half of E_{max}, and β is the slope parameter that characterizes how steep the response curve is. For data fitting, it is often recommended to log-transform dose and use $\gamma_2 = \ln(ED_{50})$ in (8.4) instead of ED_{50}, which leads to the following parameterization:

$$\eta(x,\gamma) = \frac{E_{max}}{1 + \exp[\beta(\gamma_2 - \ln x)]}, \tag{8.5}$$

which has better properties with respect to various nonlinearity measures; see Ratkowsky and Reedy (1986) [338].

Remark 8.1 Compared to the E_{max} model of Example 6.1 in Chapter 6, here we selected the lower asymptote as zero, which corresponds to the parameter $\theta_4 = 0$ in (6.20); see the discussion at the beginning of Section 8.1.1. Note also that parameter β in (8.4) corresponds to $-\theta_1$ in (6.20). For other examples of multiparameter logistic models, see Sections 8.1.5 and 8.1.6.

Measurement errors ε_i are independent normal random variables with zero mean and variance that may depend on the response as in

$$\text{Var}(\varepsilon_i) = \sigma_A^2 + \sigma_M^2 \eta(x_i, \gamma), \tag{8.6}$$

or

$$\text{Var}(\varepsilon_i) = \sigma_A^2 + \sigma_M^2 \eta(x_i, \gamma)[E_{max} - \eta(x_i, \gamma)], \tag{8.7}$$

where σ_A^2 and σ_M^2 are the additive and multiplicative components of variance, respectively; cf. (6.21) or (7.12). In model (8.6) the variance increases with the response, while in model (8.7) the variance attains its maximum at dose ED_{50}. By $\theta = (\beta,\ ED_{50},\ E_{max};\ \sigma_A^2,\ \sigma_M^2)^T$ we denote the combined vector of model parameters; cf. (7.4). The variance functions in (8.6) or (8.7) can be written as functions of dose x_i and parameters θ: $\text{Var}(\varepsilon_i) = S(x_i, \theta)$.

In our application the response η was bounded by 100%, and therefore $\max_x \eta(x,\gamma)[E_{max} - \eta(x,\gamma)] = 50^2$. So to make the selection of variance parameter σ_M^2 compatible for models (8.6) and (8.7), we introduced a normalizing coefficient of $1/50$ for the multiplicative component in (8.7), so that for the second variance model

$$\text{Var}(\varepsilon_i) = \sigma_A^2 + \frac{\sigma_M^2}{50} \eta(x_i, \gamma)[E_{max} - \eta(x_i, \gamma)]. \tag{8.8}$$

The goal of the study is to find a dose ED_{90} that attains 90% of the maximal response. If parameterization (8.5) is used, then solving equation $\eta(x, \gamma) = 0.9\, E_{max}$ for x, one gets

$$ED_{90} = \zeta(\boldsymbol{\theta}) = e^{\gamma_2}\, 9^{1/\beta} = ED_{50}\, 9^{1/\beta}, \tag{8.9}$$

which is a nonlinear function of model parameters.

Once the mean response $\eta(x, \boldsymbol{\theta})$ and the variance function $S(x, \boldsymbol{\theta})$ are defined, one can calculate the information matrix $\boldsymbol{\mu}(x, \boldsymbol{\theta})$ via (1.108) and use numerical techniques to find locally optimal designs for a given $\boldsymbol{\theta}$. The peculiarity of the problem discussed in this section is that the design region $\mathfrak{X}$ to which the admissible control variable (dose) belongs, may change from stage to stage (cohort to cohort).

We address two optimality criteria: D-optimality ($\Psi = |\mathbf{D}(\xi, \boldsymbol{\theta})|$) and c-optimality ($\Psi = \mathrm{Var}(ED_{90})$). The variance of the MLE of ED_{90} may be approximated by

$$\mathrm{Var}\left(\widehat{ED}_{90}\right) \approx \frac{\partial \zeta}{\partial \boldsymbol{\theta}^T}\, \mathrm{Var}(\hat{\boldsymbol{\theta}}_N)\, \frac{\partial \zeta}{\partial \boldsymbol{\theta}} = \mathrm{tr}[\mathbf{A}_\zeta \mathrm{Var}(\hat{\boldsymbol{\theta}}_N)], \quad \mathbf{A}_\zeta = \frac{\partial \zeta}{\partial \boldsymbol{\theta}}\, \frac{\partial \zeta}{\partial \boldsymbol{\theta}^T}; \tag{8.10}$$

cf. (2.28) and (6.13). Direct calculations show that

$$\frac{\partial \zeta}{\partial \boldsymbol{\theta}} = \left(\frac{-ED_{90}\ln(9)}{\beta^2},\, ED_{90},\, 0,\, 0,\, 0\right)^T.$$

8.1.3   Adaptive dose selection with constraints

In practice it is often difficult to provide in advance accurate "guesses" of $\boldsymbol{\theta}$ for the construction of locally optimal designs for nonlinear models. Therefore it is expedient to utilize the adaptive approach that is briefly outlined in the beginning of this chapter, while a formal description is given in Section 8.1.7.

It is important to ensure that sufficient data are collected in the initial stage to provide reasonable parameter estimates. In our study the response at the low doses will very likely lie on the lower horizontal portion of the dose-response curve, and at least three different doses are needed to estimate the response parameters γ; see Section 8.1.7. Let $n_{FIX} \geq 3$ be the number of cohorts with "fixed" doses, i.e., when no adaptation is performed. Specifically, in our examples all subjects in cohort 1 get the minimal dose x_{MIN}, while in cohort 2 all subjects get $10 \times x_{MIN}$, with an escalation factor of 5 for the remaining $n_{FIX} - 2$ cohorts.

Often the admissible range of doses $\mathfrak{X}$ is considered fixed for the duration of the study, so $\mathfrak{X} = [\, x_{MIN},\, x_{MAX}\,]$, where x_{MIN} and x_{MAX} are the minimal and maximal allowed doses, respectively. However, in the context of an early dose-escalation study, with limited knowledge about the drug, a more appropriate range may be defined for each cohort j as $\mathfrak{X}_j = [\, x_{MIN},\, x_{MAX,j}\,]$. The dose $x_{MAX,j}$ could be fully prespecified before the start of the study (e.g., increasing by a common factor for each cohort), but our approach has been to define each $x_{MAX,j}$ adaptively, once sufficient data have been observed after the first n_{FIX} cohorts.

The selection of $x_{MAX,j}$ depended on the current estimate of ED_{10}, the dose that achieves 10% of the maximal response. We allowed a tenfold increase of the current maximal allowed dose at doses with no safety signals and little biological response (no inhibition), but reduced the dose escalation factor to fivefold above the dose that exceeds $ED_{10,j}$ which, similar to (8.9), may be expressed as $ED_{10,j} = ED_{50,j} (1/9)^{1/\beta_j}$, where $ED_{50,j}$ and β_j are current estimates of parameters ED_{50} and β, respectively. For further details on dose constraints, see Leonov and Miller (2009) [254], Section 2.3.

Since our drug was administered intravenously, we used the continuous design region $\mathfrak{X}_j$. However, in practice, a fixed number of doses may be specified in advance, and then the design region for cohort j is a discrete set of doses $\{x_{j,\ell}\}$ that belong to $\mathfrak{X}_j$. The latter selection may be driven by practical considerations when only a limited number of dosage levels is available, e.g., for orally administered drugs. See Section 8.1.6 for examples where the design region $\mathfrak{X}$ was restricted to the discrete set of doses.

8.1.4 Simulation studies

The adaptive optimal design algorithm was implemented in MATLAB®, and MATLAB Compiler was utilized to create a stand-alone application that allows the program to run in stand-alone mode; cf. Section 7.5. There are two general options in the software: (1) run simulations to explore the performance of the design for future studies (within the simulation option, one can either run a single simulation with detailed output after each cohort, or run many simulations within a loop, which then produces various tables and histograms for different cohorts as summary statistics); or (2) estimate parameters from the existing data and construct the adaptive optimal design for the next cohort. See Figure 8.1 for a screenshot of the software.

Users can modify such inputs as total number of cohorts in the study and the number of cohorts n_{FIX} with fixed dose selection; cohort size and the number of patients on placebo in each cohort; minimal and maximal admissible doses; choice of optimality criterion, either D- or c-criterion; and choice of dose selection within the given cohort, i.e., whether the same dose is selected for all patients (a common practical constraint), or doses may be different within the cohort; model of variance for the study, either (8.6) or (8.8); values of model parameters $\boldsymbol{\theta} = (\beta, \ ED_{50}, \ E_{max}; \ \sigma_A^2, \ \sigma_M^2)^T$. Note that variance parameters σ_A^2 and σ_M^2 for models (8.6) or (8.8) may be selected either as unknown parameters or as fixed constants. In the latter case $\boldsymbol{\theta} \equiv \boldsymbol{\gamma}$, i.e., the information matrix depends only on response parameters $\boldsymbol{\gamma}$.

For the example used to generate Figures 8.2 – 8.6, we selected the variance model (8.8) (unknown parameters), with the design region $[x_{MIN}, \ x_{MAX}] = [0.001, \ 20]$ and parameter values $\boldsymbol{\theta} = [2, \ 0.4, \ 95; 1, \ 0.5]^T$. Fixed dose alloca-

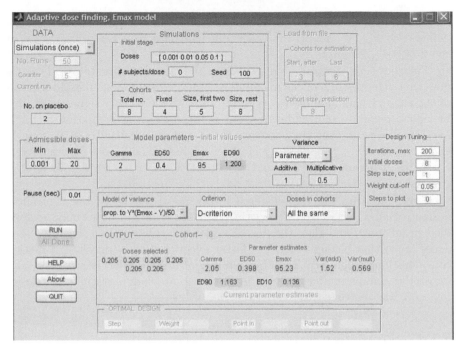

FIGURE 8.1: Screenshot, E_{max} model.

tion was used for cohorts 1 to 4, and all subjects in each subsequent cohort were constrained to receive the same dose.

Single simulation. Both simulation options start with the optimal design algorithm, which constructs the locally D- or c-optimal design. The D-optimal doses are $(0.195, 0.820, 20)$, or $(-1.635, -0.198, 2.996)$ on the log-scale, with weights $(0.3, 0.3, 0.4)$, respectively. Figure 8.2 illustrates the Equivalence Theorem and shows that for the D-optimal design, the sensitivity function reaches its maximum value of $m = 5$ at optimal doses, where m is the number of unknown parameters in the model; cf. Figures 7.2 and 7.15.

Results are presented graphically after dose selection for each cohort:

- Selected doses; see Figure 8.3. Horizontal reference lines correspond to optimal doses and true values of ED_{10} and ED_{90}, to better visualize the selection procedure. Vertical lines separate different cohorts.

- Parameter estimates.

- Actual observations and estimated dose-response curves; see Figure 8.4. Here, vertical reference lines correspond to optimal doses for the selected criterion.

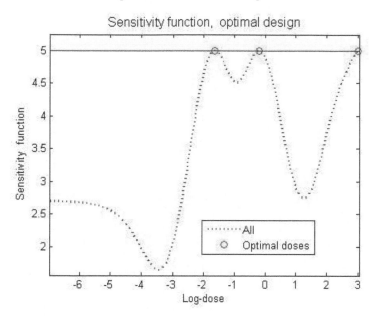

FIGURE 8.2: Sensitivity function, D-optimal design.

After the initial four fixed cohorts, fivefold (i.e., the maximum possible) increases in dose are recommended for cohorts 5 and 6; see Figure 8.3. Doses recommended for cohorts 7 and 8 are then very close to two of the optimal doses. Estimates of ED_{10} and ED_{90} are seen to improve as more data are collected.

As a result of rather slow dose escalation at the beginning of the simulated study, measurements for the first few cohorts lie on the lower horizontal portion of the dose-response curve. Because of this, model parameters are not precisely estimated after cohort 4 prior to cohort 5, and there is a substantial difference between the true and estimated curves; see Figure 8.4, top panel. However, once higher doses are selected by the adaptive algorithm, the estimated curves approach the true curve (see Figure 8.4, bottom panel).

When using actual trial data, the algorithm follows the same estimation and optimization steps as for a single simulation (except that the true parameter values and optimal doses are obviously unknown).

Multiple simulations. One thousand simulations were run with the same settings as for the single simulation described earlier in this section. In these simulations, because of the restrictions on dose escalation (see Section 8.1.3) doses for cohort 5 cannot be selected beyond $\tilde{x}_5 = 1250 \times x_{MIN}$; and in 100% of cases this dose $\tilde{x}_5$ was selected. For cohort 6 the highest available dose was then selected in about 95% of simulations, with lower doses recommended

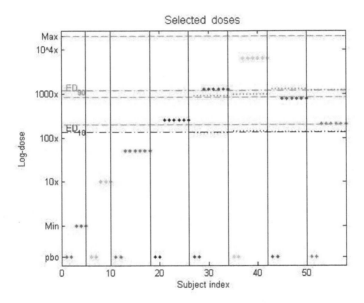

FIGURE 8.3: Simulations, single run: selected doses. Log-dose is shown on the y-axis as a multiple of $x_{MIN} = 0.001$. Dashed horizontal lines correspond to optimal doses, with dash-dotted lines showing true values of ED_{10} and ED_{90}. Short dotted lines give estimated ED_{10} and ED_{90} for each cohort.

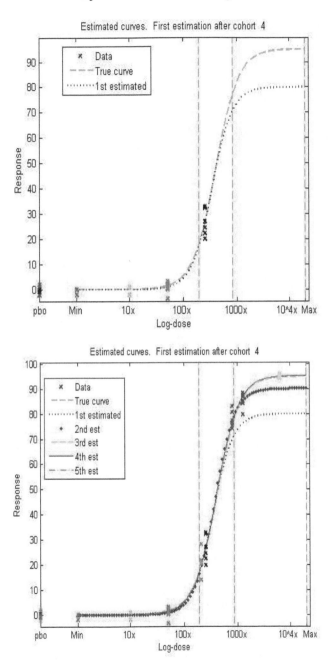

FIGURE 8.4: Simulations, single run: estimated dose-response curves, after four (top) and eight (bottom) cohorts. Vertical dashed lines correspond to the optimal doses. The true dose-response curve is shown with a heavy gray dashed line.

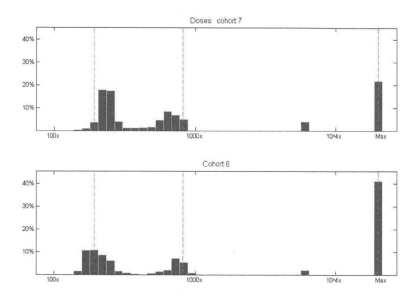

FIGURE 8.5: Selected doses after 1000 simulations, cohort 7 (top) and cohort 8 (bottom). Vertical dashed lines correspond to the optimal doses.

occasionally. Figure 8.5 presents selected doses after cohorts 7 and 8. Here, vertical reference lines correspond to optimal doses. For these cohorts doses close to the three optimal doses are generally chosen; see top and bottom panels of Figure 8.5, respectively. We note that for this particular setting, with 8 cohorts in total and 6 active doses for cohorts 5 – 8, the optimal design algorithm will not necessarily lead to the fastest possible dose escalation, or necessarily allocate any subjects to x_{MAX}, in contrast to a traditional dose-escalation study design. Note that for cohort 8 (bottom panel) the percentages of selected doses in each cluster are close to the optimal weights 0.3, 0.3 and 0.4.

To compare the performance of the adaptive and locally D-optimal designs, in Tables 8.1 and 8.2 we present some sample statistics from these 1000 simulation runs. For the D-optimal design, with the total number of subjects $N = 58$, we rounded $N \times (0.3, 0.3, 0.4)$ to (17, 18, 23), so that 17, 18 and 23 subjects are allocated to optimal doses (0.195, 0.820, 20), respectively. We also compared the results for a simple dose-escalation ("fixed") design, and for a composite design that combines elements of both the fixed and D-optimal designs; cf. Section 2.7 (motivation and detailed description of this design are provided later in this section). The fixed design has the same structure as adaptive designs (5 patients in the first two cohorts and 8 patients in the remaining cohorts, 2 patients on placebo for each cohort), with prescribed doses 0.001, 0.005, 0.02, 0.08, 0.4, 2, 10, and 20 units.

For each of the four designs, for each of the five parameters and ED_{90}, in Table 8.1 we present mean, variance, bias and square root of the mean squared error (MSE); for sample order statistics, see Table 1 in Leonov and Miller (2009) [254]. For the majority of entries the designs are naturally ranked, in terms of bias, variance and spread of the percentiles: the D-optimal design is best, while the adaptive design outperforms the fixed design. Only for parameter σ_A^2 can one observe an opposite ranking when the optimal design is the worst, both with respect to bias and variance of the estimation. This is not surprising: both fixed and adaptive designs are "forced" to place a substantial number of patients on placebo (16 in total, 2 for each cohort), where according to the model the mean response is zero. This leads to a better estimation of the additive variance.

TABLE 8.1: Sample statistics of 1000 simulation runs.

Designs				
	Mean	Var	Bias	$\sqrt{MSE}$
$\gamma = 2$				
Fixed	2.013	0.014	0.013	0.120
Adaptive	2.008	0.009	0.008	0.094
Composite	2.005	0.007	0.005	0.084
Optimal	1.999	0.004	-0.001	0.063
$\ln(ED_{50}) = -0.916$				
Fixed	-0.919	0.002	-0.003	0.041
Adaptive	-0.916	0.001	-0.000	0.031
Composite	-0.920	0.001	-0.003	0.031
Optimal	-0.918	0.000	-0.002	0.022
$E_{max} = 95$				
Fixed	94.992	0.116	-0.008	0.341
Adaptive	95.014	0.161	0.014	0.402
Composite	94.971	0.140	-0.029	0.375
Optimal	94.997	0.043	-0.003	0.208
$\sigma_A^2 = 1$				
Fixed	0.971	0.054	-0.029	0.235
Adaptive	0.960	0.058	-0.040	0.244
Composite	0.952	0.063	-0.048	0.256
Optimal	0.965	0.083	-0.035	0.291
$\sigma_M^2 = 0.5$				
Fixed	0.421	0.045	-0.079	0.227
Adaptive	0.451	0.023	-0.049	0.160
Composite	0.441	0.029	-0.059	0.180
Optimal	0.466	0.015	-0.034	0.126
$ED_{90} = 1.2$				
Fixed	1.196	0.009	-0.004	0.092
Adaptive	1.200	0.007	-0.000	0.081
Composite	1.198	0.005	-0.002	0.073
Optimal	1.201	0.003	0.001	0.051

<u>Note</u>: Estimation performed after 8 cohorts (58 patients).

Figure 8.6 presents the data from the last section of Table 8.1 visually,

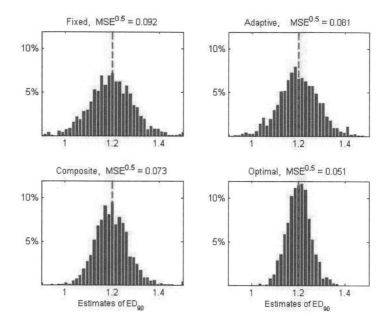

FIGURE 8.6: Histogram of estimates of ED_{90}. Top left – fixed design, top right – adaptive, bottom left – composite, bottom right – D-optimal. The dashed vertical line represents the true value of ED_{90}.

showing histograms of estimates of ED_{90} for each of the four designs. Bias is negligible for all designs, and the natural ordering of the designs in terms of improving precision of estimation can be seen: fixed – adaptive – composite – optimal.

In Table 8.2 we compare variances of parameter estimates calculated from

(1) Empirical sample estimates, and

(2) An analytical closed-form expression using the variance-covariance matrix $\mathbf{D}_N(\xi, \boldsymbol{\theta})$ as in (1.89).

These results demonstrate that, first, the sample and analytical values are reasonably matched, and, second, the designs are again naturally ranked, with D-optimal serving as a "goal post" and the adaptive design outperforming the fixed one. As expected, the only exception is the additive variance σ_A^2.

Another way to compare different designs is via their relative efficiencies with respect to the optimal one, $\mathrm{Eff}_D(\xi, \boldsymbol{\theta}) = [|\mathbf{D}(\xi^*, \boldsymbol{\theta})|/|\mathbf{D}(\xi, \boldsymbol{\theta})|]^{1/m}$; see (2.24), (6.22). The inverse of D-efficiency, or relative deficiency as in (6.47), shows by how much the sample size for the design ξ must be increased to achieve the same accuracy as the D-optimal design. Using (6.22), one can directly compare two arbitrary designs by taking the ratio of their efficiencies.

TABLE 8.2: Empirical vs. analytical variance from 1000 simulations.

					PARAMETERS				
	γ		ED_{50}		E_{max}		σ_A^2		σ_M^2
E	A	E	A	E	A	E	A	E	A
F	0.013	0.012	0.0016	0.0014	0.11	0.10	0.052	0.058	0.043	0.042
A	0.009	0.009	0.0009	0.0010	0.16	0.16	0.058	0.071	0.023	0.027
		(0.001)		(0.0002)		(0.07)		(0.007)		(0.003)
C	0.007	0.006	0.0010	0.0008	0.14	0.12	0.063	0.065	0.029	0.025
O	0.004	0.004	0.0005	0.0005	0.04	0.05	0.083	0.094	0.015	0.017

Note: Empirical (E): sample values for the estimates after eight cohorts (58 patients). Analytical (A): corresponding elements of the variance-covariance matrix $\mathbf{M}^{-1}(\xi_N, \boldsymbol{\theta})$. Standard deviations of analytical variances for adaptive designs are also presented (in parentheses).

The D-efficiency of the fixed design is 0.532, and the mean D-efficiency of adaptive designs is 0.617, with a standard deviation of 0.012. However, it is important to note that both fixed and adaptive designs "force" many patients on placebo and low doses, which makes the direct comparison with locally optimal design rather unfair. Therefore, we find it useful to calculate a composite D-optimal design; see Sections 2.7 and 5.3:

- 16 patients are allocated to placebo (which corresponds to 2 patients in each of the eight cohorts).

- Two groups of 3 patients are allocated to 0.001 and 0.01 units.

- Two groups of 6 patients are allocated to 0.05 and 0.25 units; in total, 34 patients will have preallocated dose levels, as in adaptive designs.

- The remaining 24 patients are assigned according to composite D-optimality criterion: first introduce the initial, or "first-stage" design

$$\xi_0 = \{\text{doses } (0,\ 0.001,\ 0.01,\ 0.05,\ 0.25),\ \text{weights } (16,\ 3,\ 3,\ 6,\ 6)/34 \}$$

and then solve the following optimization problem:

$$\xi_{C,\delta}^* = \arg\min_\xi \left| \left[\delta \mathbf{D}^{-1}(\xi_0, \boldsymbol{\theta}) + (1-\delta)\mathbf{D}^{-1}(\xi, \boldsymbol{\theta}) \right]^{-1} \right|, \qquad (8.11)$$

where $\delta = 34/58$; cf. (2.107) and (2.109).

The composite D-optimal design is

$$\xi_{C,\delta}^* = \{\text{doses } (0.190,\ 0.841,\ 20),\ \text{weights } (0.17,\ 0.43,\ 0.4)\},$$

and after rounding $24 \times (0.17, 0.43, 0.4)$, for simulations we use the allocation $(4,11,9)$ to doses $(0.190, 0.841, 20)$, respectively.

It is not surprising that compared to the locally D-optimal design, the composite design loses some precision with respect to parameter E_{max}, since only 9 patients are allocated to the highest dose (compared with 23 patients for the locally D-optimal design). On the other hand, the composite design is better for the estimation of the additive variance σ_A^2, as expected; cf. Tables 1 and 2 in Leonov and Miller (2009) [254]. Compared to the locally optimal composite design, the relative efficiency of fixed design is 0.770, and the mean relative efficiency of adaptive designs is 0.893 (standard deviation of 0.018). This confirms that adaptive designs quite quickly recover from the lack of information in the initial stages.

In addition to the simulation described above, we investigated altering the adaptive design settings in two ways: first by allowing subjects within each cohort to receive different doses, and second by treating the variance parameters σ_A^2 and σ_M^2 as fixed constants (i.e., they do not enter the information matrix and $m = 3$). Performance of the adaptive design was not altered significantly as a result of either of these changes, in terms of mean, variance, bias or square-root of MSE.

8.1.5 Generalized E_{max} model

An extended logistic model $E_{\max}$, sometimes referred to as the Richards function, can be found in the literature; see Pronzato and Pázman (1994) [320]; Huet et al. (2004) [208], Chapter 1.1.2:

$$\eta_2(x, \tilde{\gamma}) = \frac{E_{max}}{\left[1 + (c_2/x)^{\beta_2}\right]^{\alpha}}, \quad \tilde{\gamma} = (\beta_2, \ c_2, \ E_{max}, \ \alpha)^T, \qquad (8.12)$$

which differs from model (8.4) by the introduction of an additional parameter α in the denominator. For model (8.12), the actual $ED_{50}^{(2)}$, i.e., the dose at which the response is equal to half of E_{max}, is different from c_2,

$$ED_{50}^{(2)} = c_2 \left(2^{1/\alpha} - 1\right)^{-1/\beta_2}, \qquad (8.13)$$

and the function (8.12) loses its symmetry with respect to $ED_{50}^{(2)}$. It seems plausible that the addition of the extra parameter α may increase model flexibility, since there is no biological reason to expect the curve to be symmetric.

To investigate whether this hypothesis holds in practice, we have explored how different the two models are over the whole range of doses. More precisely, we addressed the following question: what is the behavior of $|\eta(x, \gamma) - \eta_2(x, \tilde{\gamma})|$ under the following constraints?

1. $ED_{50} = ED_{50}^{(2)}$

2. The slopes of the two functions at ED_{50} are the same on the log-scale, i.e., the two functions have identical derivatives, $\partial \eta / \partial x = \partial \eta_2 / \partial x \big|_{x=ED_{50}}$

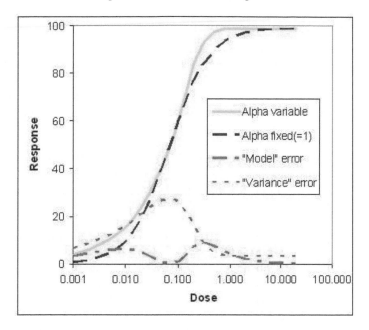

FIGURE 8.7: Screenshot of the tool to compare models (8.4) and (8.12).

The second constraint leads to the following relation:

$$\beta = 2\alpha\beta_2 \left(1 - 2^{-1/\alpha}\right). \tag{8.14}$$

Thus we specify parameters of the function (8.12) first, then get the parameters of function (8.4) from (8.13) and (8.14), and compare the two curves. We created a simple tool to make this comparison; see Figure 8.7. By exploring a variety of plausible parameter values it became evident that the difference between the models was unlikely to ever be large in magnitude, rarely larger than 10% at a maximum across the entire dose range. Further, we compared this "model error" to the potential magnitude of variation due to the combined variance parameters given in (8.8), and found that this was generally larger than the "model error."

Taking this into account together with the additional instability of parameter estimation introduced by the inclusion of this highly nonlinear parameter, we decided that any minor benefits of model flexibility were outweighed by the practical problems it would cause. For more details on this subject, see Ratkowsky (1990) [337], in particular Chapter 2.5.4, which is titled "The Trap of Overgenerality" and discusses, among other issues, the increase of various nonlinearity measures for model (8.12).

8.1.6　Extensions

The stand-alone MATLAB tool for the E_{max} model was developed for a specific clinical scenario with dose-escalation constraints. However, the core adaptive model-based design algorithm can be tailored for other clinical scenarios and other background models where various practical constraints can be implemented. Below we briefly describe two other examples of clinical studies for which we developed MATLAB-based stand-alone adaptive applications.

Adaptive design for constrained binary model. Here we describe a software tool that we created for a study where the primary interest of the study team was in a binary endpoint, which suggested considering a binary logistic model as in (1.92) and (5.40):

$$\eta(x,\boldsymbol{\theta}) = e^z/(1+e^z), \text{ with } z = \boldsymbol{\theta}^T \mathbf{f}(x),\ \boldsymbol{\theta} = (\theta_0,\theta_1)^T,\ \mathbf{f}(x) = (1,x)^T, \quad (8.15)$$

for which the information matrix $\boldsymbol{\mu}(x,\boldsymbol{\theta})$ is defined in (5.41). Note that the probability of response for model (8.15) tends to 1 or 0 when $|x| \to \infty$ (often doses are transformed to log-scale, which justifies the use of negative x). However, in practice it is often reasonable to assume that the maximal probability of response is less than one, and/or the minimal probability of response is greater than zero. Under such circumstances, one can introduce alternative lower and upper bounds for the probability of response, and model the probability as

$$\tilde{\eta}(x,\boldsymbol{\theta}) = \theta_L + (\theta_U - \theta_L)\eta(x,\boldsymbol{\theta}), \quad (8.16)$$

where $\eta(x,\boldsymbol{\theta})$ is defined in (8.15) and $0 \le \theta_L < \theta_U \le 1$. For simulations, bounds θ_L and θ_U may be selected as given constants or unknown parameters. In the latter case, these bounds enter the information matrix and must be estimated in the estimation step of the adaptive algorithm.

Figure 8.8 presents a screenshot of the optimal adaptive design tool that we created for this study. Compared to the stand-alone tool for the E_{max} model, we added several new options, such as

- Calculation of composite adaptive D-optimal design for each stage of the simulated study; see (2.107), (2.109), (8.11). For this project we implemented stage-wise estimation and design, as described in option (b) of Section 5.3. Note that because some doses, including placebo, may be "forced" into the design on stage $j + 1$, the number N_j of observations that correspond to the current "first"-stage design includes not only observations from the first j stages, but also forced doses on stage $j + 1$.

- Choice of either a continuous design region (with minimal and maximal allowable doses specified similar to the E_{max} model), or a discrete set of allowable doses that must be entered in a corresponding field. The latter option is useful in the case of an orally administered drug when the limited number of dosage levels is available.

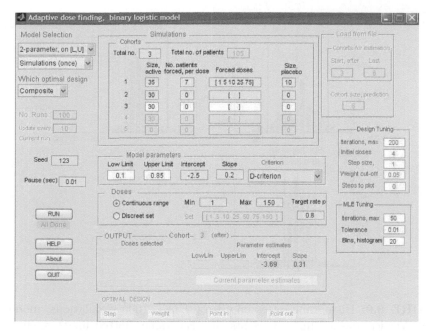

FIGURE 8.8: Screenshot, multiparameter binary logistic model.

- Choice of a target percentile p that defines the target dose ED_p; cf. (6.13), (8.9).

- When running multiple simulations, we present empirical distributions (histograms) of parameter estimates and estimates of the target dose ED_p together with corresponding empirical confidence intervals.

A histogram for the estimates of the target dose ED_p is provided in Figure 8.9. As seen from this figure, the quality of estimation improves with each extra cohort: medians get closer to the true values, and the empirical confidence intervals become tighter as the number of cohorts/patients increases. The information from multiple simulations is stored in the output file (bias, variance, mean squared error, percentiles of empirical distribution of parameter estimates and ED_p, empirical confidence intervals) and can be used to evaluate the operating characteristics of the adaptive algorithm under different simulation scenarios.

Four-parameter E_{max} model. The next example deals with a phase 2a study for a cardiovascular indication. Similar to the example in Section 8.1.2, it was expected that the endpoint would follow the E_{max} model. However, there was no reason to assume that the lower asymptote would be equal to zero. Therefore, for the response function we used a four-parameter E_{max}

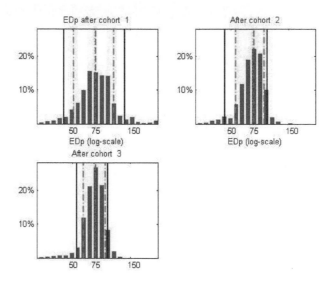

FIGURE 8.9: Histograms of estimates of ED_{80}, 1000 simulations, model (8.15). Vertical dashed line represents the true value; dotted line – median; solid line – boundaries of empirical 90% confidence interval; dash-dotted lines – boundaries of empirical 80% confidence interval.

model instead of (8.4); cf. (6.20):

$$\eta(x, \gamma) = E_0 \; + \; \frac{E_{max} - E_0}{1 + (ED_{50}/x)^\beta}, \tag{8.17}$$

where E_0 is the lower asymptote, and $\gamma = (\beta, ED_{50}, E_{max}, E_0)^T$. Figure 8.10 presents a screenshot of the optimal adaptive design tool for this study. Compared to the MATLAB tool of Section 8.1.4, we provided all the new options listed for the constrained binary model. Following the request of the study team, here we define the target dose not via the percentile of the distribution, but via the difference (called "Delta" in the tool) from the lower asymptote. For example, if $E_0 = -0.5$ and $\Delta = 1$, then this means that the target dose should achieve the response of 0.5 units.

Unlike the example of Section 8.1.2, we did not have to follow strict dose escalation constraints. However, we introduced specific restrictions on doses at the bottom and top of the dose-response curve:

- We do not want to select those doses the response on which is too close to the upper asymptote E_{max} (this may lead to safety issues). Thus, we introduced a field with a top cut-off level ("Delta, top cut-off"): doses for which the response exceeds the current estimate of $E_0 + \Delta_{top}$, cannot be selected for the next cohort.

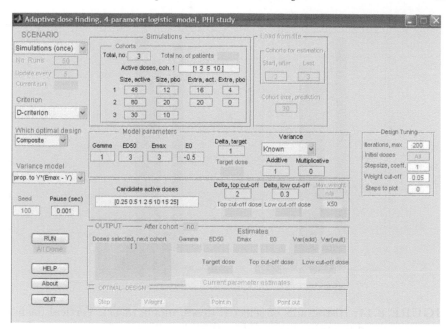

FIGURE 8.10: Screenshot, four-parameter E_{max} model.

- We do not want to put too many patients on doses with little biological response. Thus, we introduced a field with a low cut-off level ("Delta, low cut-off"): doses for which the response is below the current estimate of $E_0 + \Delta_{low}$ will have an upper bound on the number of patients.

Also, we introduced an "enrollment buffer" (fields "Extra, active" and "Extra, placebo") to mimic a potentially slow patient enrollment: parameter estimation and dose selection for the next cohort may be carried out before data from all patients in the current cohort are collected and analyzed.

As more and more patients are enrolled in the study, one may expect that the distribution of optimal doses would become closer to the locally optimal design. This phenomenon is illustrated in Figure 8.11, which shows the selection of optimal doses for the discrete design region (doses are labeled as d_1, d_3 ...). For this example, there were eight candidate doses (0.25, 0.5, 1, 2, 5, 10, 15, 25), and the composite locally D-optimal design was calculated as

$$\xi_C^* = \{\text{doses } (0.5, 2, 5); \quad \text{weights } (0.42, 0.27, 0.31)\}.$$

As seen in Figure 8.11, the "cluster" weights of selected doses for cohorts 2 and 3 are not that far from the optimal weights for doses $d_2 = 0.5$, $d_4 = 2$, $d_5 = 5$. This behavior is in accordance with what we observed in Figure 8.5.

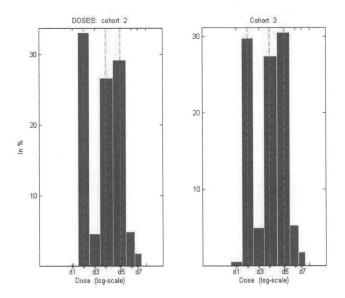

FIGURE 8.11: Histograms of selected doses, model (8.17). Vertical dashed lines correspond to optimal doses: $d_2 = 0.5$, $d_4 = 2$, $d_5 = 5$.

8.1.7 Technical details

D-optimal vs *c*-optimal designs. The variance-covariance matrix of *c*-optimal designs may be singular, in particular when the variance of errors ε_i does not depend on unknown parameters and matrix $\mathbf{A}_\zeta$ in (8.10) is singular; see a discussion on singular cases in Sections 1.1.2 and 2.8. Note that since $\partial \zeta / \partial \boldsymbol{\theta}$ in (8.10) is a vector, the rank of matrix $\mathbf{A}_\zeta$ is one at most. Therefore the calculation of *c*-optimal designs may be computationally unstable; adding or removing a dose with a very small weight may dramatically change the value of the optimality criterion. We have observed such cases in our simulations, when doses with weights of several percent made a substantial impact on the trace of the variance-covariance matrix. Therefore, for our particular example, the search of optimal designs where some doses may have very small weight is not practical because such designs will be essentially impossible to implement in cohorts of six subjects on active treatment. In another setting, with a larger number of subjects, the *c*-optimality criterion could be feasible, and could more directly address the scientific question of the study. For regularized versions of the numerical algorithms, see comments on regularization in Section 3.2.

Computation of information matrix When the variance of measurement errors ε depends on unknown parameters as in (8.6) or (8.8), then in the normal case the information matrix $\boldsymbol{\mu}(x, \boldsymbol{\theta})$ consists of two terms as in

(1.108). In the case of single measurement per subject,

$$\mu(x,\theta) = \frac{1}{S(x,\theta)} \mathbf{f}(x,\theta)\mathbf{f}^T(x,\theta) + \frac{1}{2\,S^2(x,\theta)} \mathbf{h}(x,\theta)\mathbf{h}^T(x,\theta), \quad (8.18)$$

where $\mathbf{f}(x,\theta)$ and $\mathbf{h}(x,\theta)$ are vectors of partial derivatives of $\eta(x,\theta)$ and $S(x,\theta)$, introduced in (6.16) and (6.18); cf. (6.15). As pointed out in Section 6.3.1, the rank of the information matrix $\mu(x,\theta)$ may be greater than 1. This, in turn, may lead to the situation where the number of support points in the optimal design is less than the number m of unknown parameters as in the example presented in Figure 8.2, with $m = 5$ and 3 support points. Note also that for the variance models (8.6) or (8.8), the first three elements of the vectors $\mathbf{f}(x,\theta)$ and $\mathbf{h}(x,\theta)$ are proportional to each other. Thus one needs at least three distinct doses to estimate the response parameters $\gamma = (\beta, ED_{50}, E_{max})^T$.

Adaptive design algorithm. For a formal introduction of adaptive designs, it is convenient to revert to the unnormalized information matrix $\underline{\mathbf{M}}(\xi_N,\theta)$ introduced in (1.87), and unnormalized designs. For the example described in Section 8.1.4 we implemented option (a) of Section 5.3, i.e., model parameters were estimated cohort by cohort (stage by stage) while doses were added after each observation. Because of the relatively small sizes of the proposed cohorts and potential rounding issues, we did not implement option (b) on each stage of the simulated study, which would require the calculation of normalized designs. Still, we allowed for two options for dose selection, either the same dose is chosen for all subjects in the cohort, or doses within the cohort may be different.

Introduce the following notations; cf. Section 5.3. Let n_j be the number of subjects in cohort j, $j = 1,2,\ldots,n_{coh}$, where n_{coh} is the maximal number of cohorts in the study. Let $\Xi_j = \{x_{j,1},\ldots,x_{j,n_j}\}$ be the design for cohort j, let $\xi_{N_j} = \Xi_1 \bigcup \Xi_2 \bigcup \cdots \bigcup \Xi_j$ be the combined design for cohorts $1,\ldots,j$, and let $N_j = n_1 + n_2 + \cdots + n_j$ be the combined number of subjects. The numerical algorithm relies on the equivalence theorem and calculation of the sensitivity function $\varphi(x,\xi,\theta)$ of the selected criterion as in (2.73) and Table 2.1.

Step 1. Initial experiments are performed according to some initial (regular) design ξ_1 with n_1 observations, i.e., $Ey_i^1 = \eta(x_{1,i},\theta)$, $i = 1,2,...,n_1$. Then an initial parameter estimate $\hat{\theta}^1 = \hat{\theta}_{N_1}$ is obtained from model fitting. For details on model fitting, see the end of this section.

Step j, $j > 1$. There are two options for dose selection:

(a) *Same dose is selected for all subjects in cohort j.* Introduce

$$x_j = \arg\max_{x\in\mathfrak{X}_j} \varphi\left(x,\xi_{N_{j-1}},\hat{\theta}^{j-1}\right),$$

where $\mathfrak{X}_j$ is the set of all admissible doses for cohort j; see Section 8.1.3. Then $x_{j,k} \equiv x_j$, $k = 1,2,\ldots,n_j$.

(b) *Doses may be different within a given cohort* and are selected according to the following formulae:

$$x_{j,1} = \arg\max_{x \in \mathfrak{X}_j} \varphi\left(x, \xi_{N_{j-1}}, \hat{\boldsymbol{\theta}}^{j-1}\right),$$

$$x_{j,2} = \arg\max_{x \in \mathfrak{X}_j} \varphi\left(x, \xi_{N_{j-1}+1}, \hat{\boldsymbol{\theta}}^{j-1}\right), \ldots,$$

$$x_{j,n_j} = \arg\max_{x \in \mathfrak{X}_j} \varphi\left(x, \xi_{N_{j-1}+n_j-1}, \hat{\boldsymbol{\theta}}^{j-1}\right),$$

where $\xi_{N_{j-1}+k}$ denotes a design that combines $\xi_{N_{j-1}}$ and doses $x_{j,1}, \ldots, x_{j,k}$.

After all n_j doses are selected, new experiments at dose levels $x_{j,1}, \ldots, x_{j,n_j}$ are carried out, and an updated parameter estimate $\hat{\boldsymbol{\theta}}^j = \hat{\boldsymbol{\theta}}_{N_j}$ is obtained from model fitting. Then go to step $j+1$.

Estimation algorithm. For parameter estimation we used the CIRLS algorithm described in Section 1.7; see (1.118) – (1.121):

$$\hat{\boldsymbol{\theta}}_N = \lim_{s \to \infty} \boldsymbol{\theta}_s, \quad \text{where } \boldsymbol{\theta}_s = \arg\min_{\boldsymbol{\theta}} V_N(\boldsymbol{\theta}, \boldsymbol{\theta}_{s-1}), \tag{8.19}$$

$$V_N(\boldsymbol{\theta}, \boldsymbol{\theta}') = \sum_{i=1}^{N} \frac{[y_i - \eta(x_i, \boldsymbol{\theta})]^2}{S(x_i, \boldsymbol{\theta}')} \tag{8.20}$$

$$+ \sum_{i=1}^{N} \left\{ \frac{[y_i - \eta(x_i, \boldsymbol{\theta}')]^2 - \Delta\eta(x_i; \boldsymbol{\theta}, \boldsymbol{\theta}') - S(x_i, \boldsymbol{\theta})}{\sqrt{2}\, S(x_i, \boldsymbol{\theta}')} \right\}^2,$$

and $\Delta\eta(x_i; \boldsymbol{\theta}, \boldsymbol{\theta}') = [\eta(x_i, \boldsymbol{\theta}) - \eta(x_i, \boldsymbol{\theta}')]^2$.

Because of the structure of the variance function $S(x_i, \boldsymbol{\theta})$, we use a two-step minimization of the function $V_N(\boldsymbol{\theta}, \boldsymbol{\theta}')$. Let

$$z_i = [y_i - \eta(x_i, \boldsymbol{\theta}')]^2 - \Delta\eta(x_i; \boldsymbol{\theta}, \boldsymbol{\theta}'), \quad w_i = S(x_i, \boldsymbol{\theta}'), \quad \sigma^2 = (\sigma_A^2, \sigma_M^2)^T,$$

and let $\mathbf{X}$ be an $N \times 2$ matrix with the first column of ones and

$$X_{i2} = \begin{cases} \eta(x_i, \boldsymbol{\theta}), & \text{for the model (8.6),} \\ \eta(x_i, \boldsymbol{\theta})\,[\theta_3 - \eta(x_i, \boldsymbol{\theta})]/50, & \text{for the model (8.8),} \end{cases} \quad i = 1, \ldots, N.$$

Then first we use weighted least squares to obtain the estimate of variance parameters,

$$\hat{\sigma}^2 = (\mathbf{X}^T \mathbf{W}^{-1} \mathbf{X}^T)^{-1} \mathbf{X}^T \mathbf{W}^{-1} \mathbf{Z}, \quad \text{where } \mathbf{W} = \text{diag}(w_i), \ \mathbf{Z} = (z_1, ..., z_N)^T,$$

and finally take elements of $\hat{\sigma}^2$ for θ_4, θ_5 in $V_N(\boldsymbol{\theta}, \boldsymbol{\theta}')$ and optimize $V_N(\boldsymbol{\theta}, \boldsymbol{\theta}')$ with respect to response parameters $\theta_1, \theta_2, \theta_3$.

8.2   Adaptive Designs for Bivariate Cox Model

In this section we continue the discussion of the bivariate Cox model introduced in Section 6.4. For more details on the examples presented in this section, see Dragalin and Fedorov (2006) [101].

As outlined in the beginning of Chapter 8, the implementation of adaptive design typically begins with some "reasonable" initial design. Then, using observations from the initial portion of patients accrued and treated in the trial, an estimate of θ is formed from the initial design. This value of θ is then used by the corresponding locally D-optimal design to select dose level(s) for the patients to be allocated in the next cohort, leading to a new parameter estimate. This process is repeated until the total number of patients in the study have been allocated, i.e., we consider the noninformative stopping rule.

For the standard D-criterion, at step $N+1$ of the adaptive procedure the dose x_{N+1} is selected according to (8.1). For penalized adaptive D-optimal designs (PAD), the optimal dose at each step is defined in (8.2); cf. (6.6).

In Figure 8.12 we present the behavior of the three performance measures introduced in (6.32) – (6.34). Results for the PAD are presented in the left column. Results for penalized locally D-optimal designs (PLD) are presented in the right column; see (6.6). The same 11 doses were used as in the example of Section 6.4.2. The initial design ξ_{10} that is used to generate data from 10 observations and get initial parameter estimates, uses equal allocation over the first 5 doses, i.e., 2 patients per dose. After the first 10 observations, the maximum likelihood estimate $\hat{\theta}_{10}$ is obtained and the next design point for the PAD is determined according to (8.2). The PLD uses the sensitivity function (6.6), where the parameter value θ is assumed known. In the middle column of Figure 8.12 we present trajectories of the modified PAD where the next dose cannot be selected more than one dose level above the current maximum level. Such modification allows for avoiding substantial fluctuations of the penalty function in the early stages of the simulated trial that may be caused by a rather poor parameter estimation for small sample sizes; compare corresponding middle rows for fully adaptive design (PAD, left column) and modified PAD and PLD (middle and right columns, respectively). Moreover, the modified dose allocation allows us to avoid significant dose increases, which can be unethical in medical practice. The limiting values of the three performance measures for the PAD are close to those of the PLD; see the last row in Table 6.1. Let us emphasize again that the described modification of the adaptive design is in accordance with recommendations on practical implementation of dose escalation; see Faries (1994) [123], Goodman et al. (1995) [178]. See also Section 8.1.3 for an example of similar constraints.

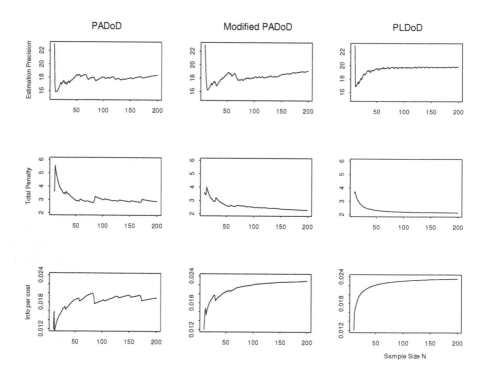

FIGURE 8.12: Convergence of the three performance measures for the three designs: PAD (left column), modified PAD (middle column), and PLD (right column). Cox model with parameter $\theta = (3, 3, 4, 2, 0, 1)$. Penalty function (6.26) with parameters $C_E = C_T = 1$. Top row – criterion (6.33); middle row – (6.32); bottom row – criterion (6.34).

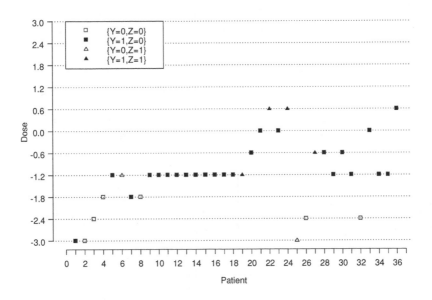

FIGURE 8.13: Graphical summary of the progress of the trial.

8.2.1 Progress of the trial: single simulation

As an illustration of the modified adaptive procedure, we consider simulated data from the Cox model with parameter $\theta = (3, 3, 4, 2, 0, 1)$. We use the up-and-down design of Ivanova (2003) [209] as a start-up procedure; see Section 6.4.2. The up-and-down design will be used for the first 10 patients and will be stopped at the first observed toxicity. At that time, the Cox model will be fitted to obtain the MLE $\hat{\theta}$. The adaptive algorithm will then use all efficacy-toxicity outcomes observed to date to find the next dose according to (8.2). The adaptive design will use 36 patients in total. Figure 8.13 summarizes the progress of the trial. Administered doses are plotted against their order number. The outcome of each patient is represented by the symbol plotted:

$$\square \quad - \quad \{Y = 0, Z = 0\}, \quad \blacksquare - \{Y = 1, Z = 0\},$$
$$\triangle \quad - \quad \{Y = 0, Z = 1\}, \quad \blacktriangle - \{Y = 1, Z = 1\}.$$

The first 19 patients have been allocated according to the up-and-down design (up to the first toxicity response after ten patients). Notice that the up-and-down design would recommend $x_4 = -1.8$ as the next dose. In contrast, the PAD design estimates the unknown parameter θ based on the available responses and utilizes (8.2) to determine the next dose as $x_7 = 0.6$. However,

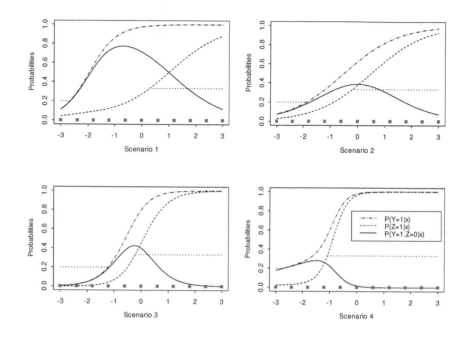

FIGURE 8.14: Four scenarios for multiple simulations.

imposing the restriction of no more than one level higher than the maximum tested dose escalation, the procedure assigns the next subject to $x_5 = -0.6$. Getting two success responses $\{Y = 1, Z = 0\}$ in a row, the design quickly escalates up to dose $x_7 = 0.6$. Notice that the PAD may be quite different from stepwise allocation (one step at a time), and the decision about the next dose is taken based on all previous responses, not just the last one. After all 36 observations are obtained, the Cox model is fitted and the optimal safe dose (OSD) is determined; see (6.28). In this case, the OSD is correctly found to be x_5. The design is also efficient in the following sense: it allocated 27 out of 36 patients to doses that are both safe and efficacious.

8.2.2   Multiple simulations

Here we explore properties of various designs by running 1000 Monte Carlo simulations under four scenarios. The PAD design described in the previous subsection is compared with the up-and-down design. We generated the efficacy-toxicity response from the Cox correlated bivariate binary distribution. For each scenario, the true probability of success $\Pr\{Y = 1, Z = 0\}$, together with two marginal distributions $\Pr(Y = 1)$ and $\Pr(Z = 1)$, as a function of dose are displayed in Figure 8.14. In each plot, eleven points on the horizontal axis represent the set of available doses. The chosen design is used to allocate doses to be administered to the next subject. The efficacy-toxicity response of this subject is then simulated from the Cox model. The allocation procedure is applied to the data collected to date, a new dose for the next subject is determined, and the procedure is repeated. Both designs use 36 subjects. Based on these 36 simulated efficacy-toxicity responses the MLE of the parameter θ in the Cox model is determined and then, using the three fitted curves, the OSD is selected.

Table 8.3 summarizes the simulation results of the four scenarios in terms of the three performance measures (6.32) – (6.34): total penalty, estimation precision and information per cost. The performance measures are determined in each of the simulation runs, together with the selected dose and dose allocation. The relative efficiency of the PAD with respect to the up-and-down design is also reported. Figures 8.15 – 8.18 illustrate the dose allocation and OSD selection for PAD and up-and-down design under Scenarios 1 – 4. PAD design has higher relative efficiency in three scenarios and the same one for Scenario 3. The advantage of the PAD design is clearly illustrated by Scenario 1; see Figure 8.15. While the up-and-down design is very careful in allocating subjects to the safe doses, it may lose considerably in the accuracy of parameter estimation and, consequently, in selecting the optimal safe dose. For example, doses higher than x_6 have not been assigned by the procedure in any of the 1000 simulation runs. However, some of these doses have been selected as OSD in several runs because of bad fit of the three curves in such situations. On the other hand, in similar runs, the PAD design allocated one or two subjects to these doses, improving the accuracy of estimation. As a result, the PAD design has never selected doses higher than x_6 as OSD.

The model for Scenario 1 is the same as the one considered in Section 6.4.2. Notice that the PAD design has similar properties as the PLD, which assumes that the parameter θ is known. For example, the information per cost is 0.0197 for the PAD versus 0.0240 for the PLD; cf. Table 6.1.

In Scenarios 2 and 3 both procedures achieve very high percentage of correct selection of the OSD. Scenario 4 is a difficult case in that both doses x_3 and x_4 have similar probabilities of success. The up-and-down design achieves good accuracy of estimation, but with a great total penalty. It allocates on average about 30% of the subjects to highly toxic doses (x_6 and higher). On the other hand, the PAD design accounts for the penalty and achieves a higher accuracy of estimation with a much lower total penalty. As a result, the relative efficiency of the PAD design is 3.62 times higher, i.e., the up-and-down design requires 3.62 times more subjects in order to achieve the same information per cost as the PAD design.

To summarize, adaptive designs have higher efficacy compared with up-and-down designs. The latter were previously shown to be a good competitor to other available designs; e.g., see Ivanova (2003) [209]. Accounting for both

TABLE 8.3: Performance measures for penalized adaptive D-optimal and up-and-down designs: simulation results for Cox model under Scenarios 1 – 4

Design	Total Penalty (6.32)	Estimation Precision (6.33)	Information per Cost (6.34)	Relative Efficiency
Scenario 1				
PAD	2.75	19.74	0.0197	1.145
Up-and-down	2.13	28.00	0.0172	
Scenario 2				
PAD	6.29	10.34	0.0163	1.025
Up-and-down	5.01	12.82	0.0159	
Scenario 3				
PAD	10.68	27.48	0.0035	1.000
Up-and-down	11.03	26.76	0.0035	
Scenario 4				
PAD	40.48	25.75	0.0043	3.624
Up-and-down	409.59	27.57	0.0012	

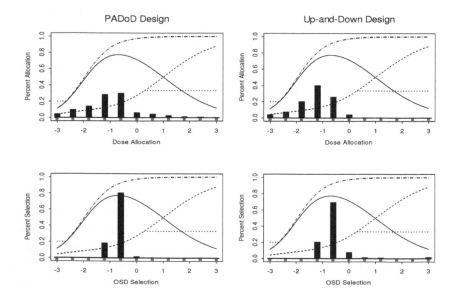

FIGURE 8.15: Scenario 1: Cox model with parameters $\boldsymbol{\theta} = (3, 3, 4, 2, 0, 1)$. Dose allocation (top) and selection of the optimal safe dose (bottom) for the PAD and up-and-down design.

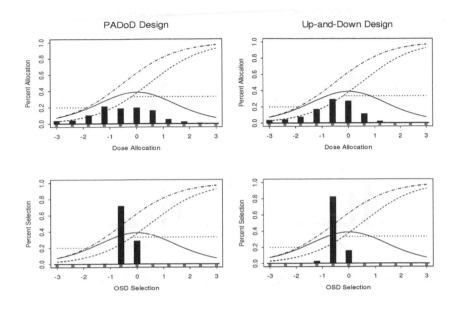

FIGURE 8.16: Scenario 2: Cox model, parameters $\boldsymbol{\theta} = (0, 2, 0.5, 1, -0.5, 1)$.

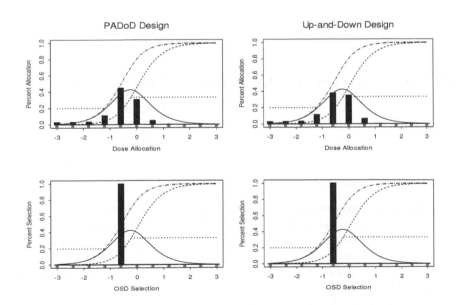

FIGURE 8.17: Scenario 3: Cox model, parameters $\boldsymbol{\theta} = (1, 4, 1, 2, -1, 2)$.

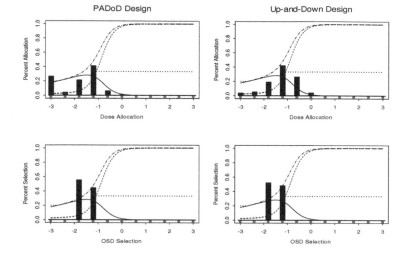

FIGURE 8.18: Scenario 4: Cox model, parameters $\boldsymbol{\theta} = (4, 4, 0, 0.5, -2, 0.5)$.

toxicity and efficacy addresses the ethical concern that as many subjects as possible be allocated at or near doses that are both safe and efficacious.

8.3 Adaptive Designs for Bivariate Probit Model

In this section we continue the discussion of bivariate probit model introduced in Section 6.5. For more details on the examples presented in this section, see Dragalin et al. (2006) [102], Dragalin et al. (2008) [103].

8.3.1 Single drug

Fully adaptive designs. We start with adaptive D-optimal designs and penalized adaptive designs for the model (6.45) with the penalty function (6.26). In each simulation run we use the total of 100 patients. The first 12 patients are allocated equally to the following three doses: $x = 0$, $x = 0.2$, and $x = 0.7$, i.e., 4 patients per dose. After observations from this first cohort are available, the parameters of the probit model (6.45) are estimated and the adaptive design is conducted according to (8.1) or (8.2) until the total number of patients reaches 100. As in Section 6.5.1, we use the value of $\boldsymbol{\theta} = (-0.9, 10, -1.2, 1.6)^T$.

The performance of the adaptive design from one particular simulation

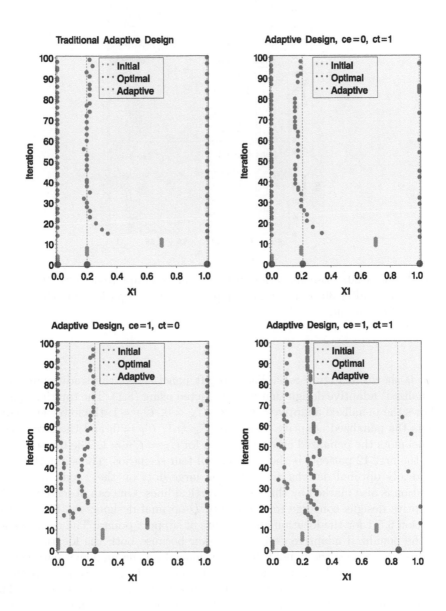

FIGURE 8.19: Progress of adaptive designs under bivariate probit model.

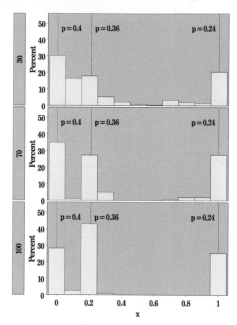

FIGURE 8.20: Dose allocation distribution for adaptive designs; 1000 runs. Top panel – after 30 patients; middle panel – after 70 patients; bottom panel – after 100 patients.

run is shown in Figure 8.19. The top left panel shows the traditional (non-penalized) adaptive design that is constructed using (8.1). The top right panel shows the penalized adaptive design for $C_E = 0$, $C_T = 1$; the lower left panel plots the penalized adaptive design for $C_E = 1$, $C_T = 0$; and the lower right panel plots the penalized adaptive design for $C_E = C_T = 1$. The initial design for the first 12 patients is the same for all four scenarios. The support points of locally optimal designs are shown as large dots on the x-axis, and their location is also marked by thin dotted vertical lines. One can observe that the adaptive designs converge to the locally D-optimal designs; see Table 6.2 in Section 6.5.1 for the location and weights of support points. The convergence of the penalized adaptive designs is slower because both the location of the optimal doses and the penalty function depend on the unknown parameters. When $C_E = C_T = 1$, the penalty function changes the most, so more patients are needed for the adaptive design to converge to the optimal design. The locally optimal design ξ_{11} allocates 12% of patients to the highest optimal dose 0.85 while the adaptive procedure has 5 patients assigned to doses higher than 0.85.

Traditional designs, 1000 Monte Carlo runs. Figure 8.20 reports the dose allocation distribution when 30, 70 and all 100 patients complete the simulated trial. The vertical reference lines mark support points of the locally D-optimal design, and the corresponding optimal weights are labeled next to these lines. As expected, the selected doses are widely spread out in the early stage of the adaptive procedure, after 30 patients. After 70 patients, the dose allocation becomes much closer to the optimal design. At the end of the procedure, almost all selected doses are concentrated around the optimal design points.

The histograms and the asymptotic normal distribution curve of the final parameter estimators are plotted in Figure 8.21. We calculated the asymptotic variances of MLEs based on the locally D-optimal design. The vertical reference lines on each histogram represent the true value of the parameter plus/minus one theoretical standard deviation. One may notice that all estimates are biased; some are really far away from the "true" values. We attributed this to numerical artifacts due to the specific settings of the numerical algorithm. Additionally, for binary models the optimization problem associated with the MLE may not have a unique solution, even when the information matrix of the design is regular. For instance, even in the case of a single-response logit or probit model and fixed sample size N, there exist samples such that the likelihood function does not have a unique maximum with positive probability; see Albert and Anderson (1984) [6].

Composite design. In situations where there is an additional cost for performing interim analyses, multistage designs have practical advantages over fully adaptive designs. The composite designs discussed in this section are examples of two-stage designs; see Sections 5.3, 8.1.4, 8.1.6. As in the case of fully adaptive designs, 100 patients are used in the composite design. The first 48 patients are equally allocated to the initial design points 0, 0.2, and 0.7. For comparison purposes, the same initial design and responses for the first stage are used to construct the composite optimal designs: traditional and penalized.

Locally optimal composite designs are listed in Table 8.4. The traditional composite design is very close to the locally D-optimal design ξ_t, while the penalized designs are slightly different from the corresponding penalized locally optimal design mainly due to poor estimation of the penalty function; see Table 6.2 for locally optimal (noncomposite) designs and Figure 6.6 for the plots of response rate curves and penalty functions. When $C_E = 0$, the final design ξ_{c01} is close to the locally optimal design ξ_{01} with similar dose levels and weights. When $C_E = 1$, the locations of optimal doses do not change much but more weight is assigned to the middle dose. After a closer look at the behavior of the penalty function near $x = 0$, we found that the penalty values for $\hat{\theta}$ are larger than those for the true parameter θ_t. This may be the reason for shifting some weight from the lowest dose $x = 0$ to the optimal dose in the middle of the dose range.

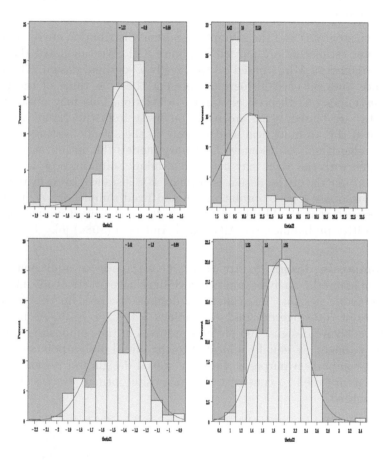

FIGURE 8.21: Histograms of parameter estimates, fully adaptive designs.

TABLE 8.4: Composite traditional and penalized designs with the penalty function (6.26).

	Optimal Design		
Traditional	$\xi_c = \left\{ \begin{array}{ccc} 0 & 0.25 & 1 \\ 0.4 & 0.31 & 0.29 \end{array} \right\}$		
Penalized			
$C_E = 0, C_T = 1$	$\xi_{c01} = \left\{ \begin{array}{ccc} 0 & 0.24 & 1 \\ 0.56 & 0.33 & 0.10 \end{array} \right\}$		
$C_E = 1, C_T = 0$	$\xi_{c10} = \left\{ \begin{array}{ccc} 0.12 & 0.27 & 1 \\ 0.08 & 0.85 & 0.07 \end{array} \right\}$		
$C_E = 1, C_T = 1$	$\xi_{c11} = \left\{ \begin{array}{ccc} 0.12 & 0.27 & 0.92 \\ 0.10 & 0.86 & 0.04 \end{array} \right\}$		

1000 runs, traditional composite design. The parameters were estimated after responses from the first 48 patients were generated. For some simulations, the maximization algorithm did not converge; thus Figure 8.22 plots the histograms of parameter estimates only from 878 simulation runs that did converge. We use the same format as in Figure 8.21, with vertical lines representing true values plus/minus one standard deviation. Now one can see that the parameter estimates are not biased and the mean estimates are very close to the true values. Almost all resulting composite designs are three-point designs, with support points located close to doses 0, 0.2, and 1.

Overall, composite designs perform well with respect to selecting the locally optimal design. However, when the estimation algorithm does not converge, the resulting optimal design will be very doubtful. Comparing these simulation results with those for the fully adaptive procedure, we see that composite designs provide better parameter estimates.

8.3.2 Combination of two drugs

Similar to the example in Section 6.5.2, we use the model (6.49) with eight parameters. The correlation coefficient $\rho = 0.5$ is assumed known (not a parameter to be estimated). We consider the restricted design region that is defined by (6.31) with $q_E \geq 0.2$ and $q_T \leq 0.5$. For all examples in this section, the initial design uses 50 patients. Then the adaptive or composite design algorithm allocates the remaining 67 patients to the best doses. Obviously, the restricted region depends on the unknown parameters. In Figures 8.23 – 8.25 we use the following notation/lines:

- The support points of the initial design are marked as rectangles;

- The support points of the locally optimal design are plotted as big dots;

- Solid lines bound the true restricted design region;

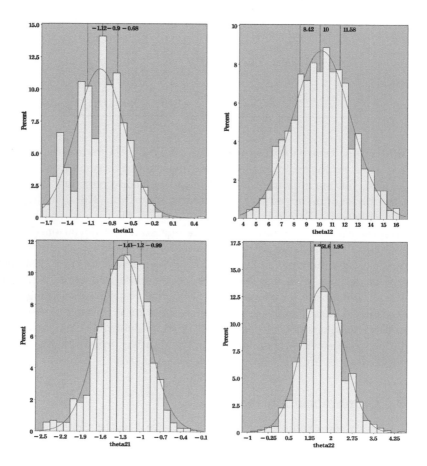

FIGURE 8.22: Histograms of parameter estimates, composite designs.

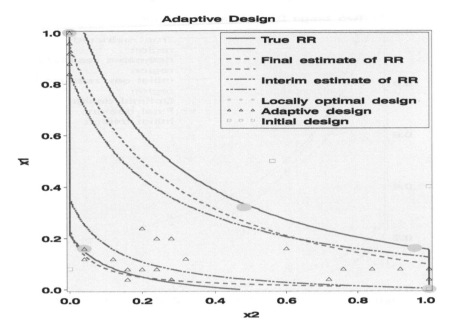

FIGURE 8.23: Adaptive design, restricted design region.

- Dash-dotted lines bound the estimated design region after the data from the first stage are collected and analyzed;

- Dashed lines bound the estimated design region at the end of the study, after all 117 patients are enrolled and analyzed.

Fully adaptive designs. The adaptive design from a particular single run is shown in Figure 8.23. The initial design uses an equal allocation of 50 patients to five doses. The triangles denote design points selected by the adaptive procedure. Most of them are inside the true restricted region. One may notice that the estimated design region after the end of the study (bounded by dashed lines) is quite close to the true region and the design points converge to the locally optimal design. This demonstrates that the adaptive procedure performs reasonably well even when little information about the unknown parameters is available.

Composite designs. We consider two different initial designs: when individual drug information is known and when such information is not available. For composite designs, we assign 67 patients as a single cohort in the second stage.

Before starting drug combination studies, investigators usually complete studies of the individual drugs. In our first example patients in the first stage are allocated to six doses: three doses of drug 1 only and three doses of drug 2

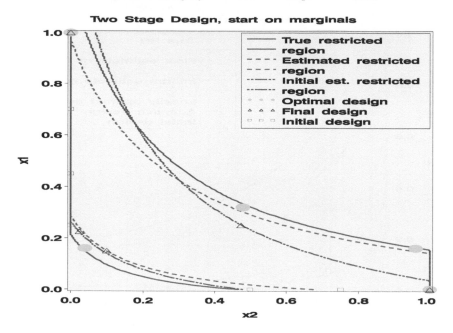

FIGURE 8.24: Composite design for drug combination study; initial design utilizes single drugs only.

only. No observations are collected in the first stage on any drug combination, thus the interaction terms θ_{14}, θ_{24} in the model (6.49) cannot be estimated. Because of this, the reduced model without the interaction terms is fitted after the first stage, and the preliminary parameter values (guesstimates) for the interaction terms are used: $\theta_{14} = 14$ and $\theta_{24} = 4$. Figure 8.24 plots the results of the composite design. The rectangles that denote the initial design are on the marginals. The triangles denote the design points selected by the composite design algorithm. These points are quite close to the locally optimal design marked by big dots. Also, one may notice that the estimated restricted region at the end of the study (bounded by dashed lines) is quite close to the true design region (solid lines). Thus, the composite design procedure performs well if the initial values for the interaction parameters are close to the true values.

If no individual drug information is available, we assign the first 50 patients to the same initial design as in the fully adaptive design example earlier in this section. The results are presented in Figure 8.25. As expected, the design points (triangles) selected at the second stage are inside the true region and are close to the locally optimal design. The estimated restricted regions after the first stage and the second stage are quite close to each other.

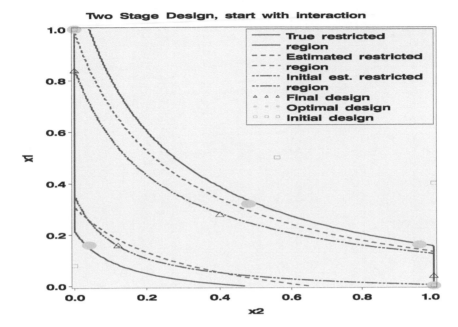

FIGURE 8.25: Composite design for drug combination study; initial design includes drug combinations.

The relative deficiencies of the constructed adaptive and composite designs are 1.02 and 1.01, respectively; see (6.47) for the definition. Thus, both the adaptive and the composite procedures perform quite well in our example.

Chapter 9

Other Applications of Optimal Designs

9.1 Methods of Selecting Informative Variables 293
    9.1.1 Motivating example 295
    9.1.2 Principal component analysis 297
    9.1.3 Direct selection of variables 298
    9.1.4 Model with measurement errors 301
    9.1.5 Clinical data analysis 304
9.2 Best Intention Designs in Dose-Finding Studies 312
    9.2.1 Utility and penalty functions 313
    9.2.2 Best intention and adaptive D-optimal designs 315
    9.2.3 Discrete design region $\mathfrak{X}$ 328

In this chapter we discuss some nontraditional applications of optimal experimental design techniques. In Section 9.1 methods of selecting informative variables are considered as in Fedorov et al. (2006) [138]. In Section 9.2 we discuss and compare several types of adaptive designs, including those that allocate each new patient (or a cohort of patients) to the dose currently viewed as the best one, for example, the seemingly most efficacious. We call this type of allocation "best intention" designs. As it turns out, similar to other areas of life, the best intentions may lead to rather disastrous situations. Theoretical results originating in research on optimal/automatic control strategies suggest that the best intention approach needs modifications to insure convergence to the "best" dose. Monte Carlo simulations presented in Section 9.2 provide corroborating evidence that caution is needed: even for very simple models, best intention designs may converge to a wrong dose with non-zero probability.

9.1 Methods of Selecting Informative Variables

In this section we describe methods for selection of the most informative variables. The information is measured by metrics similar to those discussed in Section 2.2. We discuss methods related to optimal design methodology and compare them with the traditional methods of dimension reduction, such as principal component analysis and methods of direct selection of the most informative variables, which include principal variables and battery reduction.

Suppose we observe a random m-dimensional vector $\mathbf{U} = (u_1, \ldots, u_m)$ with mean $\mathbf{U}_0$ and variance-covariance matrix $\mathbf{K}$, i.e.,

$$E(\mathbf{U}) = \mathbf{U}_0, \quad Var(\mathbf{U}) = \mathbf{K}. \tag{9.1}$$

The goal is to predict the vector $\mathbf{U}$ measuring only a few, n, of its components, $n < m$. Such a problem arises, for example, when an investigator is faced with a collection of variables of equal *a priori* interest. These variables may be related to the health of a patient, where the costs of measuring and monitoring a set of variables depend on the number of variables in the set and may also depend on specific variables. Thus, if a "good," or "most informative," in the sense that will be defined later, subset can be found, it could be considered as characterizing the behavior of the entire system, with obvious cost savings.

For all considered approaches, it is crucial to introduce the concept of an optimality criterion of prediction. The criteria presented are functions of the variance-covariance (dispersion) matrix of prediction for variables that are of interest to a practitioner. All methods provide sets of the "most informative" variables, but each in its own sense:

- Principal components – with respect to the optimization problem in (9.4); see Section 9.1.2.

- Principal variables – with respect to the same optimization problem (9.4), under the additional restriction (9.5); see Section 9.1.3.

- Methods based on optimal design techniques – with respect to the optimization problem (9.15); see Section 9.1.4.

It is assumed that the variance-covariance matrix $\mathbf{K}$ is known. In practice it means that there exist enough data for a reasonable estimation of its elements.

The structure of this section is as follows. A motivating example which presents data from a typical clinical trial is introduced in Section 9.1.1. In Section 9.1.2, the principal component method is discussed and a number of optimality criteria considered. The principal component analysis has a solid mathematical foundation and possesses many optimal properties; see, for example, Jolliffe (2002) [221], McCabe (1984) [272], Section 5. It may lead to the selection of a few linear combinations that perfectly predict the variables of interest. However, the principal components are linear combinations of the measured variables and, therefore, are often difficult to interpret. Moreover, the first principal components may include all the original variables and, consequently, all of them are required to be measured. That is, reduction in the number of variables is not guaranteed.

To overcome this, one can apply the direct search of the most informative variables, which are called "principal variables" in McCabe (1984) [272] and discussed in Section 9.1.3. This method is closely related to battery reduction as discussed in Cureton and D'Agostino (1983) [85], and to the subject of entropy criteria in optimal experimental design; see Shewry and Wynn (1987)

[358], Sebastiani and Wynn (2000) [354]. Numerically the optimization problem is very close to what is called "construction of exact discrete optimal experimental designs"; see, for example, Section 3.3. There exist a number of discrete exchange-type algorithms that usually lead to a significant improvement in an initial design, but do not generally converge to a globally optimal design.

As soon as the selection of the most informative variables is bridged with experimental design theory, the introduction of observational errors and the transition to normalized continuous designs is a natural step; see Section 9.1.4. The numerical algorithms considered were introduced by Batsell et al. (1998) [34] in a different setting (measuring computer network loads) and refined by Fedorov et al. (2003) [137]. These algorithms appear to be a generalized version of the "water-filling" algorithms of the information theory for maximizing information transmitted through noisy channels; see Cover and Thomas (1991) [81], Chapter 13. The model with observational errors allows us to take into account costs of measuring original variables which makes the approach more realistic from a practical point of view. In Section 9.1.5 we apply different approaches to the analysis of clinical laboratory data introduced in Section 9.1.1.

9.1.1   Motivating example

The results of laboratory tests presented in Table 9.1 are from a typical clinical trial. For a detailed description of all tests, see Fedorov et al. (2006) [138].

Multiple samples of these routine tests generally are collected on each patient at baseline and then at regularly scheduled intervals. The trial included a placebo arm and several active treatment arms. The sample variance-covariance matrices differed among the treatment arms; therefore for the purposes of our investigation, only the patients from the placebo arm were considered. The variance-covariance matrix presented is derived from the data of blood and urine samples collected from 93 patients with complete data to ensure that the estimated covariance matrix would be positive definite. Clinicians would view variables in their relevant units of measurement. These units have specific meanings and, as such, we keep them rather than trying to make the variables uniform on some arbitrary scale.

The 35 laboratory tests presented here can be divided into specific categories. These are hematology (quality and quantity of various blood cells); liver function; renal function; urine (constituents including that not normally found in urine such as elements of blood); electrolytes; blood lipids; and blood glucose. The hematology category can be further separated into primary and secondary categories; see Table 9.1. Ranks R_i in column 5 correspond to the ordering of variables with respect to variances K_{ii} in column 4.

TABLE 9.1: Ranking of 35 laboratory tests using mean/variance structure.

No.	Test	Mean $U_{0,i}$	Var K_{ii}	Rank R_i	$K_{ii}/U_{0,i}$	$K_{ii}/U_{0,i}^2$
		HEMATOLOGY (PRIMARY)				
1	HCT	43.14	10.22	14	0.237	0.005
2	HGB	14.66	1.28	26	0.088	0.006
3	PLATE	239.2	4504.4	2	18.83	0.079
4	RBC	4.79	0.163	30	0.034	0.007
5	WBC	6.16	3.47	20	0.564	0.092
		HEMATOLOGY (SECONDARY)				
6	NEUT	56.08	102.4	10	1.82	0.033
7	NEUTS	56.04	103.1	9	1.84	0.033
8	LYMPH	31.24	68.22	11	2.18	0.070
9	EOSIN	4.25	7.25	17	1.70	0.402
10	MONO	7.31	5.58	18	0.763	0.104
11	BASO	0.74	0.272	28	0.365	0.490
		LIVER FUNCTION				
12	ALAT	21.49	149.1	8	6.93	0.323
13	ASAT	19.84	50.68	12	2.55	0.129
14	ALKPH	74.92	417.4	6	5.57	0.074
15	BILTOT	0.76	0.056	33	0.074	0.098
16	ALBT	4.25	0.038	35	0.009	0.002
17	PROT	7.36	0.170	29	0.023	0.003
		LIVER FUNCTION				
18	CREAT	1.09	0.051	34	0.047	0.043
19	BUN	15.33	26.65	13	1.73	0.113
20	URIC	5.31	2.03	25	0.384	0.072
		URINALYSIS				
21	UPROT	0.47	2.29	24	4.88	10.38
22	UBLD	0.71	2.75	22	3.93	5.61
23	URBC	0.58	2.40	23	4.13	7.12
24	UWBC	1.48	2.88	21	1.94	1.31
25	UGLUC	0.19	1.14	27	5.88	30.49
		ELECTROLYTES				
26	K	4.26	0.136	31	0.032	0.008
27	NA	140.6	5.31	19	0.038	0.000
28	CL	102.4	8.99	16	0.088	0.001
29	CO2C	23.92	9.20	15	0.385	0.016
30	CA	9.24	0.136	32	0.015	0.002
		LIPIDS				
31	CHOLF	213.2	1424.3	4	6.67	0.031
32	HDLF	53.76	217.5	7	4.04	0.075
33	LDLF	126.7	1135.7	5	8.95	0.071
34	TRIGF	163.3	6804.8	1	41.66	0.255
		Glucose				
35	GLUCF	111.6	1530.5	3	13.71	0.123

Clinicians generally will want to review all laboratory values for each individual patient in order to monitor most closely each patient's safety. However, a large number of variables can make it difficult to assess trends in the sample as a whole. A technique that discards some of the variables from consideration, but still preserves most of the information contained in the original space would be welcome. Ideally, such a technique would remove a number of the variables, leaving one or two per category, and possibly remove a whole category. From our perspective, the methods that we discuss here may be recommended in the early stages of drug development, i.e., phases I or II.

9.1.2 Principal component analysis

Let us first discuss a problem of selecting the n most informative linear combinations of the original variables $\mathbf{U}$, $n < m$; for the exact meaning of the term "most informative" in this section, see Proposition 9.1. In Sections 9.1.2 and 9.1.3, it is assumed that all variables have zero mean, $\mathbf{U}_0 = 0$, and can be measured without errors. Shifting of the origin, i.e., taking $\tilde{\mathbf{U}} = \mathbf{U} - \mathbf{U}_0$, reduces the problem to the case of zero means.

Principal components are orthogonal linear combinations of the original variables with decreasing variance; see Jolliffe (2002) [221], Rao (1973) [334]. They may be defined via the solution of the eigenvalue-eigenvector problem,

$$\mathbf{V}_\alpha = \mathbf{P}_\alpha^T \mathbf{U},$$

where $\mathbf{P}_\alpha$ is the normalized eigenvector of the covariance matrix $\mathbf{K}$ corresponding to the eigenvalue λ_α,

$$\lambda_\alpha \mathbf{P}_\alpha = \mathbf{K}\mathbf{P}_\alpha, \quad \mathbf{P}_\alpha^T \mathbf{P}_\alpha = 1, \quad \text{and} \quad \lambda_1 \geq \lambda_2 \geq \ldots \geq \lambda_m.$$

For the sake of simplicity, throughout the section it is assumed that the variance-covariance matrix $\mathbf{K}$ is regular.

The role of principal components in statistics may be interpreted as follows. Let the goal be to select $n \leq m$ linear combinations of elements of the vector $\mathbf{U}$ that contain most of the information about the whole vector $\mathbf{U}$. These linear combinations may be presented as $\mathbf{J} = \mathbf{B}^T \mathbf{U}$, where $\mathbf{B}$ is an $m \times n$ matrix of rank n. The best linear unbiased predictor of $\mathbf{U}$ based on $\mathbf{J}$ is

$$\hat{\mathbf{U}}_B = \mathbf{KB}\left(\mathbf{B}^T\mathbf{KB}\right)^{-1}\mathbf{J} \tag{9.2}$$

and its variance-covariance matrix is

$$\mathbf{D}_B = \text{Var}\left(\hat{\mathbf{U}}_B - \mathbf{U}\right) = \mathbf{K} - \mathbf{KB}\left(\mathbf{B}^T\mathbf{KB}\right)^{-1}\mathbf{B}^T\mathbf{K}; \tag{9.3}$$

see, for example, Rao (1973) [334], Chapter 8g. For any linear unbiased predictor $\tilde{\mathbf{U}}_B$,

$$\text{Var}\left(\tilde{\mathbf{U}}_B - \mathbf{U}\right) \geq \text{Var}(\hat{\mathbf{U}}_B - \mathbf{U}),$$

where the inequality is understood in the sense of nonnegative definite matrix ordering; cf. (1.18). In (9.3) and in what follows, whenever the inversion of matrices is involved, we assume the regularity of corresponding matrices. In the case of (9.3), it means that the matrix $\mathbf{B}$ has rank n.

The next natural step is the selection of a matrix $\mathbf{B}^*$ that minimizes $\mathbf{D}_B$ in (9.3). Unfortunately, the best matrix $\mathbf{B}^*$ cannot be selected such that it minimizes the variance-covariance matrix in the sense of nonnegative definite matrix ordering. However, the following statement holds; see Rao (1973) [334], Chapter 8, or Seber (1984) [355], Chapter 5.2.

Proposition 9.1 *Let an $m \times m$ matrix $\mathbf{D}$ be nonnegative definite and let a function $\Psi(\mathbf{D})$ be strictly increasing, i.e., $\Psi(\mathbf{D}_1) > \Psi(\mathbf{D}_2)$ if $\mathbf{D}_1 \geq \mathbf{D}_2$ and $\mathbf{D}_1 \neq \mathbf{D}_2$. Then*

$$(\mathbf{P}_1, \ldots, \mathbf{P}_n) = \mathbf{B}_n^* = \arg\min_B \Psi(\mathbf{D}_B), \qquad (9.4)$$

where $\mathbf{P}_1, \ldots, \mathbf{P}_n$ are eigenvectors of the matrix $\mathbf{K}$ corresponding to its n largest eigenvalues $\lambda_1 \geq \ldots \geq \lambda_n$, and $\mathbf{D}_B$ is given by (9.3).

Functions satisfying the conditions of Proposition 9.1 include $\Psi_1(\mathbf{D}) = \text{tr}(\mathbf{D})$, and $\Psi_2(\mathbf{D}) = |\gamma \mathbf{I}_m + \mathbf{D}|, \gamma > 0$, where $\mathbf{I}_m$ is an $(m \times m)$ identity matrix. So, the first n principal components generate a solution of the optimization problem $\min_B \Psi(\mathbf{D}_B)$ for a number of popular optimality criteria; see McCabe (1984) [272], Section 5, for more examples.

In general, principal components depend upon all components of $\mathbf{U}$. If some of the components of the first n eigenvectors of $\mathbf{K}$ are simultaneously small enough, then the corresponding variables may be discarded and principal component analysis may lead to a reduction in the number of original variables to be measured. Otherwise, the introduction of principal components does not lead to substantial dimensional reduction. Note also that one should be careful in judging the importance of a variable in a principal component by the size of its coefficient, or loading; see Cadima and Jolliffe (2001) [58] for examples when this is not true.

Another fact restricting the practicality of the principal component method is that the selection of principal components is not invariant to linear transformations of the coordinate system. For instance, inflating a scale of any variable (say, moving from centimeters to microns) will very likely place this variable as the main contributor to the first principal component; this fact may be easily verified by considering a diagonal matrix $\mathbf{K}$. One of the ways to tackle this problem is to consider the correlation matrix $\mathbf{C}$ instead of $\mathbf{K}$ and to proceed with eigenvectors of $\mathbf{C}$. However, in this case the above optimal properties of principal components are valid not for the original vector $\mathbf{U}$, but for the vector $\mathbf{Q} = (u_1/\sqrt{K_{11}}, u_2/\sqrt{K_{22}}, \ldots, u_n/\sqrt{K_{nn}})^T$.

9.1.3   Direct selection of variables

The two peculiarities discussed at the end of Section 9.1.2 triggered the development of methods that allow one to minimize any given function of the matrix $\mathbf{D}_B$ through direct selection of subsets of variables, rather than through linear combinations of those variables. The n most "informative" variables $\mathbf{U}_n$ out of m variables $\mathbf{U} = (u_1, \ldots, u_m)^T$ are called "principal variables" in McCabe (1984) [272]. Note that any subvector $\mathbf{U}_n = (u_{i_1}, \ldots, u_{i_n})^T$ admits representation $\mathbf{U}_n = \mathbf{B}_n^T \mathbf{U}$, where $\mathbf{B}_n$ is an $m \times n$ matrix such that its (i, j)-th element

$$[B_n]_{ij} = \begin{cases} 1, & \text{if } i = i_j, \ j = 1, \ldots, n, \\ 0, & \text{otherwise.} \end{cases} \qquad (9.5)$$

So by the "most informative" variables we mean those that provide the solution of the optimization problem on the right-hand side of (9.4) under the additional constraint (9.5). For any $\mathbf{B}_n$ satisfying (9.5) and any Ψ satisfying the conditions of Proposition 9.1,

$$\Psi(\mathbf{D}_{B_n}) \geq \Psi(\mathbf{D}_{B_n^*}).$$

In this sense, the first n principal components provide a lower bound for

$$\min_{B_n \in \mathcal{B}_n} \Psi(\mathbf{D}_{B_n}),$$

where $\mathcal{B}_n$ is a set of all matrices $\mathbf{B}_n$ satisfying (9.5). Of course, the first n principal components allow for a better prediction of the whole vector $\mathbf{U}$ than the first n principal variables, but as mentioned earlier, the former may depend on all components of the vector $\mathbf{U}$.

If $\mathbf{B}_n$ is of the form (9.5), then the rows and columns of $\mathbf{D}_{B_n}$, which correspond to measured variables, equal identically zero. This fact follows from the proof of formula (9.8), which is given at the end of this section. Therefore matrix $\mathbf{D}_{B_n}$ is singular and some caution is needed in introducing the optimality criteria. For example, in this case $|\mathbf{D}_{B_n}| = 0$ no matter how well the measured variables predict the others. That is why it is expedient to consider the following problem:

$$\mathbf{U}_n^* = \arg\min_{U_n} \Psi(\mathbf{D}_{22}), \tag{9.6}$$

where $\mathbf{D}_{22}$ is the submatrix of $\mathbf{D}_{B_n}$ obtained by striking out the rows and columns of $\mathbf{D}_{B_n}$ that correspond to the measured variables. Let us assume, without loss of generality, that the first n variables are measured and the last $(m - n)$ variables are not. Then the variance-covariance matrix $\mathbf{K}$ and the matrix $\mathbf{B}_n$ in (9.5) can be partitioned as

$$\mathbf{K} = \begin{pmatrix} \mathbf{K}_{11} & \mathbf{K}_{12} \\ \mathbf{K}_{21} & \mathbf{K}_{22} \end{pmatrix}, \quad \mathbf{B}_n = \begin{pmatrix} \mathbf{I}_n \\ \mathbf{0}_{m-n,n} \end{pmatrix}, \tag{9.7}$$

and

$$\mathbf{D}_{22} = \mathbf{K}_{22} - \mathbf{K}_{21}\mathbf{K}_{11}^{-1}\mathbf{K}_{12}, \tag{9.8}$$

where $\mathbf{K}_{11}$ is an $n \times n$ submatrix of $\mathbf{K}$ corresponding to the observed variables $\mathbf{U}_{(n)}$; $\mathbf{K}_{22}$ is an $(m - n) \times (m - n)$ submatrix corresponding to unobserved $m - n$ variables to be predicted; submatrix $\mathbf{K}_{21} = \mathbf{K}_{12}^T$ defines covariances between two subvectors $\mathbf{U}_{(n)}$ and $\mathbf{U}_{(m-n)}$; and $\mathbf{0}_{a,b}$ is an $a \times b$ matrix of zeros. For the proof of (9.8), see the end of this section.

Optimization problem (9.6) is a discrete one and can be solved by the exhaustive search, which means that one has to compute $\Psi(\mathbf{D}_{22})$ for all $m!/[n!\,(m - n)!]$ possible choices of matrix $\mathbf{B}_n$. For large m and n, the direct search can be computationally laborious, which suggests the use of various exchange-type procedures; see Shewry and Wynn (1987) [358] or Fedorov et al. (2003 [137]). In general, unlike principal component analysis, the optimization problem (9.6) has a different solution for different criteria. See McCabe (1984) [272], Section 6, for examples of optimality criteria; cf. Section 2.2.

The selection of principal variables is closely related to the method of battery reduction; see Cureton and D'Agostino (1983) [85]. Battery reduction addresses essentially the same problem: how to find n variables from the original m variables that reproduce most of the variability of the original variables. One of the algorithms used for the latter problem relies on the Gram-Schmidt orthogonalization procedure and will lead to the following solution. The first new variable b_1 coincides with one of the original variables u_{i_1}. The second variable b_2 is a linear combination of the previously selected variable u_{i_1} and a new one, u_{i_2}, etc; for details, see Cureton and D'Agostino (1983) [85], Chapter 12. Therefore, the battery reduction algorithm leads to linear combinations of no more than n original variables.

If, similar to the case of principal variables, we assume that new variables b_i are generated by the first n original variables, then

$$\mathbf{b} = \mathbf{B}_{BR}\mathbf{U} , \quad \text{where} \quad \mathbf{B}_{BR} = \begin{pmatrix} \mathbf{T}_n \\ \mathbf{0}_{m-n,n} \end{pmatrix}, \tag{9.9}$$

and $\mathbf{T}_n$ is an $n \times n$ regular upper triangular matrix. It is interesting to note that principal variables and battery reduction methods are equivalent in the sense of (9.6), i.e.,

$$\mathbf{D}_{B_n} \equiv \mathbf{D}_{B_{BR}}. \tag{9.10}$$

For the proof of (9.10), see the end of this section.

It follows from the identity (10.7) that

$$|\mathbf{D}_{22}| = |\mathbf{K}_{22} - \mathbf{K}_{21}\mathbf{K}_{11}^{-1}\mathbf{K}_{12}| = \frac{|\mathbf{K}|}{|\mathbf{K}_{11}|} .$$

Thus to minimize $|\mathbf{D}_{22}|$, one has to maximize $|\mathbf{K}_{11}|$, which is equivalent to choosing a set of the most scattered variables $\mathbf{U}_{(n)}$. In other words, maximizing the retained variation, represented by $|\mathbf{K}_{11}|$, is equivalent to minimizing the lost variation, represented by $|\mathbf{D}_{22}|$; see McCabe (1984) [272] and Shewry and Wynn [358] (1987).

As in the case of the principal component analysis, principal variables or battery reduction methods lead to solutions that are not invariant to scale transformations for some popular optimality criteria such as $\text{tr}(\mathbf{D}_{22})$ or $|\mathbf{D}_{22}|$. However, certain criteria exist that are invariant in this sense. For instance, if one considers a random vector with non-zero mean $\mathbf{U}_0$, then a criterion

$$\Psi(\mathbf{D}_{22}) = \sum_i [\mathbf{D}_{22}]_{ii} U_{0i}^{-2}$$

furnishes such an example. Unfortunately, this criterion does not satisfy the conditions of Proposition 9.1, and therefore the principal component method does not provide a lower bound in this case.

9.1.4   Model with measurement errors

In this section we introduce a model and optimality criteria that may be considered a generalization of (9.1). Let us assume that a random vector $\mathbf{U}$ is measured with a random error ε; then the model of observations is as follows:

$$\mathbf{Y} = \mathbf{U} + \varepsilon, \qquad (9.11)$$

where $\mathbf{Y}$ is a vector of measurements, and $\mathbf{Y}, \mathbf{U}$ and ε have m components. As before, we assume that

$$E(\mathbf{U}) = \mathbf{U}_0, \quad Var(\mathbf{U}) = \mathbf{K}.$$

Additionally, the following assumptions hold:

$$E(\varepsilon) = 0, \quad Var(\varepsilon) = \boldsymbol{\Sigma} = \text{Diag}(\Sigma_{ii}), \quad E(\varepsilon \mathbf{U}^T) = 0,$$

where $\text{Diag}(c_i)$ is a diagonal matrix with values c_i on the diagonal.

The vector $\mathbf{U}$ may represent a collection of variables measuring aspects of the health of a patient (blood cell counts, liver function, cholesterol, etc.). Then by u_{il} we denote an observed value of variable i for patient l. The error in the measurement is given by ε_{ilk}, where the subscript k reflects the case of repeated measurement, for example, measurements of blood pressure.

It must be emphasized that we allow for repeated measurements of components of $\mathbf{U}$. If there are r_i measurements of the i-th component, i.e., $k = 1, \ldots, r_i$, then $\Sigma_{ii} = \sigma_i^2 / r_i$, where σ_i^2 is a variance of a single measurement of the i-th component.

Let $N = \sum_{i=1}^m r_i$ be the total number of observations, and let $p_i = r_i/N$ be the weight, or a fraction of the observations taken to measure the i-th component. Then

$$\Sigma_{ii} = \frac{\sigma_i^2}{N p_i}, \qquad (9.12)$$

and the collection of weights $\xi = \{p_i\}_1^m$ is a direct analog of the normalized design; cf. (2.48). Let $\bar{\mathbf{Y}}(\xi) = (\bar{y}_1(\xi), \ldots, \bar{y}_m(\xi))^T$ be a vector of averaged observations of a given $\mathbf{U}$, where

$$\bar{y}_i(\xi) = \frac{1}{r_i} \sum_{k=1}^{r_i} y_{ik}.$$

Then the estimator

$$\hat{\mathbf{U}}(\xi) = \mathbf{K} \left[\mathbf{K} + \boldsymbol{\Sigma}(\xi) \right]^{-1} \bar{\mathbf{Y}}(\xi) \qquad (9.13)$$

minimizes the mean squared error $E_{u,\varepsilon}\left\{ [\tilde{\mathbf{U}}(\xi) - \mathbf{U}] [\tilde{\mathbf{U}}(\xi) - \mathbf{U}]^T \right\}$ among all estimators $\tilde{\mathbf{U}}(\xi)$ that are linear with respect to y_{ik}. The variance-covariance matrix of $\hat{\mathbf{U}}(\xi)$, under the assumption that $\mathbf{K}$ and $\boldsymbol{\Sigma}$ are positive definite, is given by

$$\mathbf{D}(\xi) = \mathbf{K} - \mathbf{K}[\mathbf{K} + \boldsymbol{\Sigma}(\xi)]^{-1}\mathbf{K} = [\mathbf{K}^{-1} + \boldsymbol{\Sigma}^{-1}(\xi)]^{-1}; \qquad (9.14)$$

see Harville (1997) [195], Chapter 18.2. The numerical procedure discussed later in this section uses the formula on the right-hand side of (9.14) to compute $\mathbf{D}(\xi)$. Thus if $p_i = 0$, which means that the i-th component is not measured, then according to (9.12), we put $\Sigma_{ii}^{-1}(\xi) = 0$, in order that $\mathbf{D}(\xi)$ is correctly defined.

Obviously, a question arises as to how to define $\hat{\mathbf{U}}(\xi)$ in (9.13) when some of the variables are not measured. Following the notation from Section 9.1.3, we assume, without loss of generality, that the first n variables are measured and the last $(m-n)$ variables are not, i.e., $p_i = 0, \quad i = n+1, n+2, \ldots, m$. It is shown in Fedorov et al. (2003) [137] that the estimator $\hat{\mathbf{U}}(\xi)$ can be defined as $\hat{\mathbf{U}}(\xi) = (\hat{\mathbf{U}}_1(\xi), \hat{\mathbf{U}}_2(\xi))^T$, with

$$\hat{\mathbf{U}}_1(\xi) = \mathbf{K}_{11}(\mathbf{K}_{11}+\Sigma_{11}(\xi))^{-1}\bar{\mathbf{Y}}_1(\xi), \quad \hat{\mathbf{U}}_2(\xi) = \mathbf{K}_{21}(\mathbf{K}_{11}+\Sigma_{11}(\xi))^{-1}\bar{\mathbf{Y}}_1(\xi),$$

where $\bar{\mathbf{Y}}_1(\xi) = (\bar{y}_1(\xi), \ldots, \bar{y}_n(\xi))^T$; $\mathbf{K}_{11}$ and $\Sigma_{11}(\xi)$ are $n \times n$ submatrices of $\mathbf{K}$ and $\Sigma(\xi)$, respectively, corresponding to the first n variables; $\mathbf{K}_{21}$ is an $(m-n) \times n$ submatrix of $\mathbf{K}$ that defines covariances between unmeasured and measured components; cf. (9.7).

We can introduce various criteria of optimality $\Psi[\mathbf{D}(\xi)]$ that depend on the collection of weights $\{p_i\}$, or designs ξ, and search for the best combination of N measurements of the components of $\mathbf{U}$,

$$\xi^* = \arg \min_{\xi} \Psi[\mathbf{D}(\xi)]. \tag{9.15}$$

So here by the "most informative" variables we mean those that have large weights in the optimal design ξ^* defined in (9.15). Since $\mathbf{K}$ is positive definite, (9.14) implies that $\mathbf{D}(\xi)$ is also positive definite and, therefore, unlike the methods discussed in Section 9.1.3, we do not need a careful partitioning of the variance-covariance matrix. Moreover, the introduction of observational errors makes (9.15) invariant with respect to scale transforms for many popular criteria including the D-optimality criterion, i.e., minimization of $|\mathbf{D}(\xi)|$. When one deals with the direct search, inflating a scale of any measured variable will lead to the increase of the determinant $|\mathbf{K}_{11}|$ and the subsequent inclusion of this variable in the "optimal" subset. On the other hand, in the situation with observational errors, scale transforms change both elements of $\mathbf{K}$ and related σ_i^2, which makes the solution of (9.15) invariant to such transforms. Formulae (9.16) and (9.17) will further clarify this point.

Numerical algorithms. The convergence results for the first-order algorithms for the construction of continuous optimal designs for various optimality criteria are studied in Fedorov et al. (2003) [137], Theorems 2 – 4; cf. Section 2.5. For illustration purposes, we discuss the algorithm for D-criterion.

First, we noe that in this setting a D-optimal design ξ_D is also a minimax one, i.e.,

$$\xi_D = \arg \min_{\xi} |\mathbf{D}(\xi)| = \arg \min_{\xi} \max_{i} D_{ii}(\xi)/\sigma_i^2.$$

This result is similar to the equivalence theorems of Section 2.5. Next, let ξ_s be the design on step s, and let α_s be a sequence of decreasing positive numbers satisfying (3.7). One of many possible choices is $\alpha_s = 1/(m+s)$. For each s, the algorithm has two intermediate steps, forward and backward; cf. the algorithms described in Section 3.1.4.

1. *Forward step.* Given ξ_s and $\mathbf{D}(\xi_s)$, find

$$\arg \max_i D_{ii}(\xi_s)/\sigma_i^2 \ = \ i_F. \tag{9.16}$$

   Add α_s to the weight of variable u_{i_F}, denote the new design by ξ_s^+ and compute the matrix $\mathbf{D}(\xi_s^+)$. Note that for the design ξ_s^+, the sum of the weights is greater than 1.

2. *Backward step.* Find

$$\arg \min_{i \in I_s} D_{ii}(\xi_s^+)/\sigma_i^2 \ = \ i_B, \tag{9.17}$$

   where I_s is a set of variables with non-zero weights at step s. Delete α_s from the weight of variable u_{i_B}, which brings the sum of weights back to 1; denote new design by ξ_{s+1} and compute $\mathbf{D}(\xi_{s+1})$. To avoid negative weights when the weight of variable u_{i_B} is less than α_s, certain adjustments should be made as discussed in Section 3.1.4.

It is shown in Fedorov et al. (2003) [137] that this iterative procedure converges, i.e., $\xi_s \to \xi_D$ as $s \to \infty$.

The two-step iterative procedure of (9.16) and (9.17) admits various generalizations. One can use a given number $n_F > 1$ of forward steps and the same number of backward steps; cf. Section 3.1.4. To mimic the methods of discrete design construction, one can keep the step length constant for relatively many iterations, $\alpha_s = 1/J$ for $s \leq t_0$ and some integer $J \leq m$, decreasing α_s only after step t_0. Then ξ_{s_0} is a discrete design built for J variables while the D-optimal design ξ_D allows one to evaluate the relative efficiency of ξ_{s_0}. The algorithms with a fixed step length usually lead to a significant improvement of an initial design, but in general do not converge to a globally optimal design. Among other possible modifications are imposing upper and lower bounds on weights p_i, and restricting optimization in (9.16) and (9.17), which forces some variables in or off the optimal design, similar to the stepwise regression procedure; cf. forced sampling times in Section 7.2.4.

Measurement costs and cost constraints. The introduction of continuous designs makes it possible to take costs of measuring different variables into account. When measurements for certain variables are more expensive than for others (say, liver function *versus* cholesterol), then taking costs of measurements into consideration seems reasonable from a practical perspective. In this case the definition of a design may be changed as in Chapter 4.1.

Let ϕ_i be a cost of a single measurement of the i-th component, and let r_i be a number of its measurements, with the restriction

$$\sum_{i=1}^{m} r_i \phi_i \leq \Phi^* \tag{9.18}$$

on the total cost; cf. (4.6). Then weights p_i are defined as $p_i = r_i \phi_i / \Phi^*$. When the optimal design ξ^* is constructed, then to obtain frequencies r_i, values $r_i' = p_i \Phi^* / \phi_i$ must be rounded to the nearest integer r_i subject to (9.18); cf. (4.28).

For the example discussed in Section 9.1.5, we do not have any information on costs of measuring individual variables and therefore do not include examples with cost constraints in our numerical study. However, once such information becomes available, it can be readily used for the selection of the most informative variables.

9.1.5   Clinical data analysis

We compare the performance of various methods as applied to the clinical data introduced in Section 9.1.1.

Principal component analysis. First of all, we note that the ranges of variables in this example differ greatly. Among other statistics, Table 9.1 presents the ranks R_i of the diagonal elements K_{ii}. For example, the variance of variable 34 (triglycerides, fasting) is the largest and equals $K_{34,34} = 6804.8$; thus, $R_{34} = 1$. Next, $K_{3,3} = 4504.4$ (platelets) and $R_3 = 2$, $K_{35,35} = 1530.5$ (glucose, fasting), $K_{31,31} = 1424.3$ (cholesterol, fasting), etc. On the other hand, several variables have low variances, for example, $K_{15,15} = 0.056$ (total bilirubin, $R_{15} = 33$) and $K_{16,16} = 0.038$ (albumin, $R_{16} = 35$). That huge discrepancy can be partially explained by the selection of measurement units.

Not surprisingly, the first eigenvalues and corresponding eigenvectors are tightly related to the variables with the largest diagonal elements of $\mathbf{K}$. Figure 9.1 presents a plot of the logarithms of eigenvalues *versus* the sorted diagonal elements of matrix $\mathbf{K}$. The largest eigenvalues directly correspond to the largest diagonal elements of $\mathbf{K}$. For example, $\lambda_1 = 7102.0$, with the dominating weight of variable 34, $P_{1,34} = 0.97$; $\lambda_2 = 4560.7$ with $P_{2,3} = -0.97$; $\lambda_3 = 2268.4$ with $P_{3,31} = 0.70$, $P_{3,33} = 0.65$; $\lambda_4 = 1514.6$ with $P_{4,35} = -0.96$. (Recall that the eigenvectors are normalized in order that $\mathbf{P}_i^T \mathbf{P}_i = 1$, $i = 1, \ldots, n$.)

In Figures 9.2 and 9.3, variables $\{j\}$ on the x-axis are sorted in descending order with respect to values of K_{ii}, i.e., with respect to ranks R_i; see the data in Table 9.1. For example, $j = 1$ corresponds to variable 34; $j = 2$ corresponds to variable 3, etc. The diamonds in Figure 9.2 show the diagonal elements of the variance-covariance matrix $\mathbf{D}_{B^*(n)}$, where $\mathbf{B}^*(n)$ is defined in

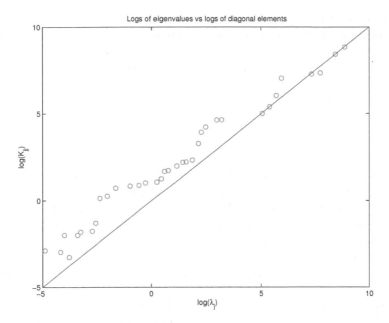

FIGURE 9.1: Logs of eigenvalues versus logs of sorted diagonal elements.

(9.4) and formed by the first n eigenvectors of $\mathbf{K}$, $n = 1, 2, 3, 4$. In Figures 9.2 and 9.3, presented are variables corresponding to the first 15 largest diagonal elements of $\mathbf{K}$. (All other diagonal elements are less than 10.) For $n = 1$, the first eigenvector $\mathbf{P}_1$ is essentially defined by variable 34, which has rank $R_{34} = 1$. Thus, inclusion of the first principal component eliminates most of the variability of this variable, $j = 1$; i.e., $[\mathbf{D}_{B^*(1)}]_{34,34}$ is small enough while the variance of the other variables corresponding to big K_{ii} is comparatively large. Next, the inclusion of $\mathbf{P}_2$ does the same for variable 3 (rank $R_3 = 2$), and so $[\mathbf{D}_{B^*(2)}]_{3,3}$ is small as well as $[\mathbf{D}_{B^*(2)}]_{34,34}$. Since in eigenvector $\mathbf{P}_3$ we have significant coefficients of variables 31 and 33 (ranks 4 and 5, respectively), the inclusion of $\mathbf{P}_3$ drastically reduces the variability of those two variables and so on.

Principal variables. Direct selection of the most informative variables leads to similar results. Obviously, variable 34 is the first principal variable ($K_{34,34}$ being the largest diagonal element of $\mathbf{K}$), the best pair is {34,3}, then a triplet {34,3,35}, etc.

The stars in Figure 9.2 present the diagonal elements of matrices $\mathbf{D}_{B_n}$, $n = 1, 2, 3, 4$, where $\mathbf{B}_n$ are selected according to (9.5), $i_1 = 34, i_2 = 3, i_3 = 35, i_4 = 31$. The only major difference between principal components and principal variables is for $n = 3$: while $\mathbf{P}_3$ includes variables 31 and 33 with significant coefficients, the direct selection method chooses variable 35 (rank $R_{35} = 3$) as the third most significant with respect to (9.6). This makes $[D_{B_3}]_{35,35} = 0$, but does not affect the variance of variables 31 and 33, with $j = 4$ and 5, respectively.

Another way to verify the importance of the selected variables is as follows. Take the first n eigenvectors $\mathbf{P}_j$ and keep only those elements of $\mathbf{P}_j$ that correspond to the first n ranks, i.e.,

$$\tilde{P}_{ji} = \begin{cases} P_{ji}, & \text{if } R_i \leq n, \\ 0, & \text{otherwise} \end{cases} \quad (i = 1, \ldots, m; \quad j = 1, \ldots, n).$$

Next, define an $m \times n$ matrix $\tilde{\mathbf{B}}(n) = (\tilde{\mathbf{P}}_1, \tilde{\mathbf{P}}_2, \ldots, \tilde{\mathbf{P}}_n)$ and compute $\mathbf{D}_{\tilde{B}(n)}$. Our analysis for $n = 1, \ldots, 6$, shows that the difference between $\mathbf{D}_{B_n}$ and $\mathbf{D}_{\tilde{B}(n)}$ is negligible (elements of $\mathbf{D}_{B_n} - \mathbf{D}_{\tilde{B}(n)}$ being less than 10^{-6} in absolute value). Thus, variables with the largest K_{ii} actually define the first principal components in our example. In a sense, the procedure is a version of battery reduction discussed in Section 9.1.3.

We remind the reader that neither the principal component method nor the direct search is invariant with respect to linear variable transformations. For instance, if for variable 4 (red blood cell count; see Table 9.1) one changes units from $10^{12}/L$ to $10^9/L$, then K_{44} would jump to $163 \cdot 10^3$, which would immediately change the rank of variable 4 from $R_4 = 30$ to $R_4 = 1$ and would include this variable in the first principle component with the dominating weight.

Search in the presence of observational errors. To describe optimal design algorithms for the model with measurements errors (9.11), we use the following variance model in (9.12):

$$\sigma_i^2 = \sigma_0^2 \, \delta_i. \tag{9.19}$$

As seen from the expression (9.14) for the variance-covariance matrix $\mathbf{D}(\xi)$, the optimal designs depend on the ratio σ_0^2/N. In the simulation studies we take various values of this ratio. Two scenarios for δ_i are considered: (a) $\delta_i \equiv 1$, and (b) not all δ_i's are equal. In our example, assumption (a) of the homogeneous variance is hardly realistic. However, we run the algorithm for this case for illustration purposes.

For the algorithm with decreasing step length and a comparatively small ratio $\sigma_0^2/N = 0.01$, the weights of the included variables do not exceed 0.045 and are distributed over more than 25 variables. When the ratio σ_0^2/N increases, more weight shifts toward the variables with the large K_{ii}. For example, when $\sigma_0^2/N = 1$, then weights of variables with ranks 1, 2, 3, and 6 (variables 34, 3, 35, 14) are greater than 0.1; see the top panel of Figure 9.3. This is because when σ_0^2/N increases, elements of matrix $\mathbf{\Sigma}^{-1}(\xi)$ in (9.14) become smaller, so that for large σ_0^2/N matrix $\mathbf{D}(\xi)$ becomes closer to the original covariance matrix $\mathbf{K}$. Therefore, according to the selection of variables in forward and backward steps (9.16) and (9.17), more measurements

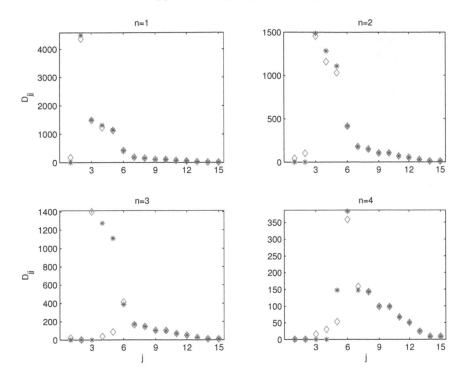

FIGURE 9.2: Variance of prediction based on principal components (diamonds) and principal variables (stars), first 15 sorted variables.

should be placed with the variables that correspond to the largest diagonal elements K_{ii}. We also note that the middle panel of Figure 9.3 serves as an illustration of Theorem 2 from Fedorov et al. [137] (2003), which is an analog of Theorem 2.4 in Section 2.5: variance of prediction attains its maximum at variables with non-zero weights, which in our case corresponds to variables that should be measured. It also reflects the connection of the proposed algorithm with the "water filling" algorithm from information theory; see Cover and Thomas (1991) [81], Chapter 13.

Now if we choose the algorithm with fixed step length $1/J$, where J is a number of variables to be measured, $J < 10$, then variables corresponding to the largest diagonal elements K_{ii} are included in the design. This result holds for all considered values of σ_0^2/N from 0.01 to 1; see Figure 9.3, bottom, where the variance of prediction for the design with eight measured variables is presented. The variables included in the optimal discrete design, all with weight $1/8$, are marked with asterisks: those are variables with rank $1 - 6$, 8, and 10.

Let us now discuss the performance of the algorithms with non-

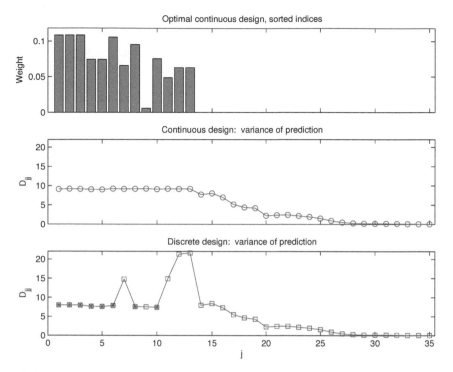

FIGURE 9.3: Sorted variables, homogeneous error variance, $\sigma_0^2/N = 1$. Optimal continuous design (top); variance of prediction for continuous design (middle); variance of prediction for discrete design (bottom), optimal variables marked by asterisks.

homogeneous δ_i, with two power models of variance:

$$\delta_i \ = \ K_{ii}^\gamma \ \ (0 < \gamma \le 1), \tag{9.20}$$

$$\delta_i \ = \ U_{0,i}^\beta \ \ (0 < \beta \le 2); \tag{9.21}$$

see Box and Hill (1974) [52], Finney (1976) [156], Karpinski (1990) [226].

Variance model (9.19), (9.20). If $\gamma < 1$, then the performance of the exchange-type algorithms is similar to that for the model with homogeneous variance, both with decreasing and with fixed step length. (We have studied values of γ up to 0.9). Indeed, if $\Sigma^{-1}(\xi)$ is small enough, then it follows from (9.14) that the ratio $D_{ii}(\xi)/\sigma_i^2$ is approximately proportional to $K_{ii}^{1-\gamma}$, and, thus, variables with large K_{ii} are included in the design.

If $\gamma = 1$, then the performance of the method is exactly the same as for the method applied to the correlation matrix

$$C_{ij} \ = \ K_{ij}/\sqrt{K_{ii}K_{jj}}$$

with homogeneous variance $\sigma_i^2 \equiv \sigma_0^2$. Indeed, let

$$\mathbf{D}_1(\xi) = \left[\mathbf{C}^{-1} + \frac{N}{\sigma_0^2} \operatorname{Diag}(p_i) \right]^{-1}, \text{ and } \mathbf{D}(\xi) = \left[\mathbf{K}^{-1} + \frac{N}{\sigma_0^2} \operatorname{Diag}\left(\frac{p_i}{K_{ii}} \right) \right]^{-1},$$

i.e., $\mathbf{D}(\xi)$ be defined by (9.19) and (9.20) with $\gamma = 1$. Then

$$\arg\min_{\xi} |\mathbf{D}(\xi)| = \arg\min_{\xi} |\mathbf{D}_1(\xi)|. \tag{9.22}$$

The proof of (9.22) is given at the end of this section.

For algorithms with decreasing step length and various choices of σ_0^2/N, the weights are distributed over almost all the variables. The use of continuous design in this case does not lead to actual dimension reduction since almost all variables are present in the optimal design. Still, the continuous design may be used as a reference point for discrete designs, to verify how close optimal discrete designs are to the theoretical optimal ones.

The variance of prediction for the optimal discrete design with 8 selected variables is presented in the top panel of Figure 9.4; here we do not sort the variables according to their ranks R_i and preserve the original ordering. The reference line $D_{ii} = 0.71$ corresponds to the maximal value of the variance of prediction for the optimal continuous design. It shows that the optimal discrete design is not significantly inferior to the continuous one. Note that the choice of variables differs greatly from the model with homogeneous variance. Only variables 34 and 35 relate to the large diagonal elements of $\mathbf{K}$. Also included are variables with very small K_{ii}, for example variable 16 (albumin) with $K_{16,16} = 0.038$. There are three variables included from the secondary hematology category (8, 10, 11), and a single one from five other categories: liver function (16), urine (22), urinary electrolytes (26), blood lipids (34), and blood sugar (35). Only two categories, primary hematology and renal function, are not represented in this design.

Variance model (9.19), (9.21). For continuous designs with $\beta = \{0.5, 1\}$ and $\sigma_0^2/N = 0.01$, the weights are distributed over more than 20 variables. As σ_0^2/N increases, more measurements should be placed with the variables with large values of ratio $K_{ii}/U_{0,i}^\beta$. This happens because as σ_0^2/N becomes larger, $\mathbf{D}(\xi)$ becomes closer to $\mathbf{K}$; thus, according to (9.16), (9.17), and (9.21), variables with large $K_{ii}/U_{0,i}^\beta$ are selected.

The influence of $K_{ii}/U_{0,i}^\beta$ is even more visible for $\beta = 2$. In this scenario, variables 21 to 25 (urinalysis group) have the largest $K_{ii}/U_{0,i}^2$; that is why they all are included in the optimal design; see the last column of Table 9.1 and middle and bottom panels of Figure 9.4.

For discrete designs, values of $K_{ii}/U_{0,i}^\beta$ drive variable selection. Consider an example where $J = 8$. When $\beta = 0.5$ or 1, then among the included are variables 3, 12, 14, 21, 23, 33 – 35, independently of the given σ_0^2/N (0.01, 0.1, or 1).

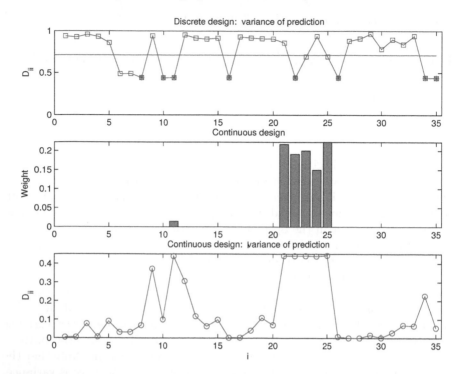

FIGURE 9.4: Top: error variance (9.20), $\gamma = 1$, $\sigma_0^2/N = 0.1$; variance of prediction for discrete design, optimal variables marked by asterisks. Middle and bottom: error variance (9.21), $\beta = 2$, $\sigma_0^2/N = 0.1$. Optimal continuous design (middle), variance of prediction (bottom); original ordering of variables.

When $\beta = 2$, the algorithm chooses all variables from the urinalysis group (21 – 25), and also variables 9, 11, and 12, i.e., all variables with the largest values of $K_{ii}/U_{0,i}^2$.

To conclude the numerical example, we remark that the model should be tailored to the context and needs of the clinician. For instance, for the model implied by (9.21), the choice of $\beta = 2$ has an obvious explanation as to how the algorithm works: it chooses the variables according to the (squared) values of their coefficients of variation. Many times biological variables behave such that their variances are proportional to their mean values. The algorithm with $\beta = 1$ in this case is the more appropriate choice. In other contexts, clinicians may be concerned as to how invariant the results are. Here the model implied by (9.20) with $\gamma = 1$ may be more appropriate, as the results of the algorithm correspond to using the correlation matrix. Use of the correlation matrix is frequently viewed as a natural way of standardizing the variables involved, especially in contexts like the social sciences where variables may be measured in arbitrary units; see Flury (1988) [160]. Both the correlation matrix and the coefficient of variation have the advantage that they are standardized measures. These special cases have intuitive appeal to non-statisticians and they could be imposed on the data according to the context.

Proof of some technical results

Proof of formula (9.8). Using (9.7) and standard formulae for products of partitioned matrices, cf. Harville (1997) [195], Chapter 2.2, one gets:

$$\mathbf{KB}_n = \begin{pmatrix} \mathbf{K}_{11} \\ \mathbf{K}_{21} \end{pmatrix}, \quad \mathbf{B}_n^T \mathbf{KB}_n = \mathbf{K}_{11}, \quad \mathbf{B}_n^T \mathbf{K} = (\mathbf{K}_{11} \ \mathbf{K}_{12}),$$

$$\mathbf{KB}_n \left(\mathbf{B}_n^T \mathbf{KB}_n \right)^{-1} \mathbf{B}_n^T \mathbf{K} = \begin{pmatrix} \mathbf{K}_{11} & \mathbf{K}_{12} \\ \mathbf{K}_{21} & \mathbf{K}_{21} \mathbf{K}_{11}^{-1} \mathbf{K}_{12} \end{pmatrix}, \tag{9.23}$$

which implies that the variance-covariance matrix $\mathbf{D}_{B_n}$ in (9.3) is equal to

$$\mathbf{D}_{B_n} = \begin{pmatrix} \mathbf{0}_{n,n} & \mathbf{0}_{n,m-n} \\ \mathbf{0}_{m-n,n} & \mathbf{K}_{22} - \mathbf{K}_{21} \mathbf{K}_{11}^{-1} \mathbf{K}_{12} \end{pmatrix}. \ \square$$

Proof of formula (9.10). Using (9.9) and the above-mentioned formulae for products of partitioned matrices gives

$$\mathbf{KB}_{BR} = \begin{pmatrix} \mathbf{K}_{11} \mathbf{T}_n \\ \mathbf{K}_{21} \mathbf{T}_n \end{pmatrix}, \quad \left(\mathbf{B}_{BR}^T \mathbf{K} \ \mathbf{B}_{BR} \right)^{-1} = \mathbf{T}_n^{-1} \mathbf{K}_{11}^{-1} \left(\mathbf{T}_n^T \right)^{-1},$$

$$\mathbf{B}_{BR}^T \mathbf{K} = \left(\mathbf{T}_n^T \mathbf{K}_{11} \ \mathbf{T}_n^T \mathbf{K}_{12} \right).$$

Therefore, after routine matrix algebra one gets that the product $\mathbf{KB}_{BR} \left(\mathbf{B}_{BR}^T \mathbf{KB}_{BR} \right)^{-1} \mathbf{B}_{BR}^T \mathbf{K}$ is exactly the same as on the right-hand side of (9.23), which proves (9.10). $\square$

Proof of formula (9.22). Note that the matrix $\mathbf{C}$ can be presented as

$$\mathbf{C} = \text{Diag} \left(K_{ii}^{-1/2} \right) \mathbf{K} \, \text{Diag} \left(K_{ii}^{-1/2} \right).$$

Thus,

$$\mathbf{D}_1^{-1}(\xi) = \text{Diag} \left(K_{ii}^{1/2} \right) \mathbf{K}^{-1} \text{Diag} \left(K_{ii}^{1/2} \right) + \frac{N}{\sigma_0^2} \text{Diag} \left(p_i \right)$$

$$= \text{Diag} \left(K_{ii}^{1/2} \right) \left[\mathbf{K}^{-1} + \frac{N}{\sigma_0^2} \text{Diag} \left(\frac{p_i}{K_{ii}} \right) \right] \text{Diag}(K_{ii}^{1/2})$$

$$= \text{Diag}(K_{ii}^{1/2}) \, \mathbf{D}^{-1}(\xi) \, \text{Diag} \left(K_{ii}^{1/2} \right),$$

which implies that

$$|\mathbf{D}(\xi)| = |\mathbf{D}_1(\xi)| \prod_{i=1}^{m} K_{ii}. \tag{9.24}$$

Since $\mathbf{K}$ does not depend on ξ, (9.22) follows from (9.24). $\square$

9.2   Best Intention Designs in Dose-Finding Studies

In early dose-finding clinical trials, balancing between gathering information and treating patients enrolled in these studies is an everlasting conflict, and it generates a massive literature that gravitates to two contradictory approaches. The first approach targets the most effective gathering of information and is based on the ideas of optimal design theory. The second approach follows a natural intention to allocate patients to doses that are the best according to the current knowledge; cf. a discussion about individual and collective ethics at the beginning of Section 6.4. The genesis of most proposed designs of this type can be found in optimal automatic control theory. Unfortunately, some warnings well known in optimal design and in optimal control theory are not taken seriously in drug development practice. We name designs of the second type "best intention" (BI) designs. In what follows, we discuss potential pitfalls for both approaches and propose some remedies based on the idea of quantifying potential harm.

The allocation of subjects to the dose currently believed to be best, or to doses close to the best one, has become very popular in clinical dose-finding studies, for example, when the intention is to identify the maximum tolerated dose (MTD) or the minimum effective dose (MED); cf. Section 6.4.2. Examples can be found in Wetherill (1963) [396], Lai and Robbins (1978) [244], O'Quigley et al. (1990) [301], Li et al. (1995) [256], and Thall and Cook (2004) [374]. BI designs are promoted as being ethnically attractive and caring about the sampled subjects. However, doubts about the convergence and informativeness of BI designs were raised long ago, and cases were found in which such designs led to allocations converging to the wrong point; see, for example, Lai and Robbins (1982) [246]; Bozin and Zarrop (1991) [55]; Ghosh et al. (1997) [174], Chapter 15; Pronzato (2000) [316]; Shu and O'Quigley (2008) [359]; Chang and Ying (2009) [66]; Azriel et al. (2011) [27].

In Section 9.2.1, we define two types of "best" doses in terms of utility functions. We describe best intention (BI) and penalized adaptive D-optimal (PAD) designs in Section 9.2.2. Although there are a number of alternative approaches to dose-finding in the literature, e.g., see Chevret (2006) [74], in this section we restrict comparisons of BI designs to PAD. We focus on two types of dose-finding problems and consider continuous linear and quadratic response functions. For these models, one can easily understand the drawbacks of naive BI designs and propose remedies that are based on the results from optimal design theory. While in Section 9.2.2 doses are selected from a continuous sample space, in Section 9.2.3 the search is restricted to a finite number of doses. For further details, see Fedorov et al. (2011) [132].

9.2.1 Utility and penalty functions

Consider responses $\mathbf{Y}$ (continuous, dichotomous, or ordinal) that satisfy the regression model

$$E[\mathbf{Y}|x] = \boldsymbol{\eta}(x, \boldsymbol{\theta}),$$

where $\boldsymbol{\eta}$ are known functions of x and $\boldsymbol{\theta}$; x may be a dose or a combination of doses selected from the set $\mathfrak{X}$ (design region), and $\boldsymbol{\theta}$ is an m-dimensional vector of unknown parameters. In general, both $\mathbf{Y}$ and $\boldsymbol{\eta}$ may be vectors as in studies with both efficacy and toxicity endpoints. For instance, binary measures of efficacy and toxicity yield four possible outcomes, and a vector of expected responses can be defined as

$$\boldsymbol{\eta}^{\mathrm{T}}(x, \boldsymbol{\theta}) = [p_{10}(x, \boldsymbol{\theta}), p_{11}(x, \boldsymbol{\theta}), p_{01}(x, \boldsymbol{\theta}), p_{00}(x, \boldsymbol{\theta})],$$

where $p_{10}(x, \boldsymbol{\theta})$ is the probability of efficacy and no toxicity; $p_{11}(x, \boldsymbol{\theta})$ is the probability of efficacy with toxicity, etc.; see Sections 6.4 and 6.5.

A practitioner typically is concerned not with $\boldsymbol{\eta}(x, \boldsymbol{\theta})$ itself, but with a utility function $\zeta(x, \boldsymbol{\theta})$ that describes the potential benefits associated with treatment at a particular dose. Examples of reasonable utility functions in the study of efficacy and toxicity are

$\zeta(x, \boldsymbol{\theta}) = p_{10}(x, \boldsymbol{\theta})$, the probability of efficacy and no toxicity;

$\zeta(x, \boldsymbol{\theta}) = p_{1\cdot}(x, \boldsymbol{\theta}) = p_{10}(x, \boldsymbol{\theta}) + p_{11}(x, \boldsymbol{\theta})$, i.e., the marginal probability of efficacy;

Let $p_{\cdot 1}(x, \boldsymbol{\theta})$ denote the marginal probability of toxicity, and let $p_{1\cdot}^*$ and $p_{\cdot 1}^*$ denote "desirable" values of marginal probabilities. Then a utility function can be defined as $\zeta(x, \boldsymbol{\theta}) = \boldsymbol{\pi}(x, \boldsymbol{\theta})^{\mathrm{T}}\mathbf{W}\boldsymbol{\pi}(x, \boldsymbol{\theta})$, where $\boldsymbol{\pi}^{\mathrm{T}}(x, \boldsymbol{\theta}) = [p_{1\cdot}(x, \boldsymbol{\theta}) - p_{1\cdot}^*, p_{\cdot 1}(x, \boldsymbol{\theta}) - p_{\cdot 1}^*]$ measures the discrepancy between corresponding probabilities at x and the "best" dose. If $\mathbf{W}$ is the identity matrix, toxicity and efficacy are given equal weight, and the utility function is $\zeta(x, \boldsymbol{\theta}) = [p_{1\cdot}(x, \boldsymbol{\theta}) - p_{1\cdot}^*]^2 + [p_{\cdot 1}(x, \boldsymbol{\theta}) - p_{\cdot 1}^*]^2$. Such a utility function is similar to what in engineering and economics is called the desirability function; see Fuller and Scherer (1998) [164].

The two most common problems in dose finding studies are

(1) **Type I**: search for the dose at which the utility function equals a pre-specified value ζ^*,

$$x^*(\boldsymbol{\theta}) = \arg \min_{x \in \mathfrak{X}} |\zeta(x, \boldsymbol{\theta}) - \zeta^*|; \tag{9.25}$$

(2) **Type II**: search for the dose that maximizes the utility function

$$x^*(\boldsymbol{\theta}) = \arg \max_{x \in \mathfrak{X}} \zeta(x, \boldsymbol{\theta}). \tag{9.26}$$

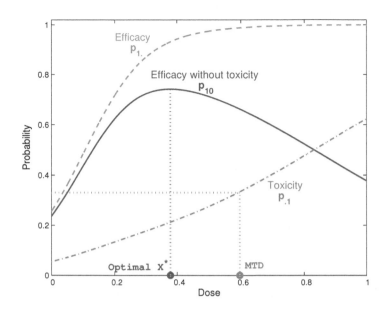

FIGURE 9.5: Illustration of various response probabilities: efficacy without toxicity (solid line), efficacy (dashed), and toxicity (dash-dotted).

Note that a Type I problem can be viewed as a special case of Type II with the utility function $\zeta' = -|\zeta - \zeta^*|$, but we prefer to consider them separately to emphasize the very different properties of BI designs for each of them. In general, $\mathfrak{X}$ can be either continuous or discrete. For the sake of simplicity, we consider the design region $\mathfrak{X} \in R^1$. Multivariate $\mathfrak{X}$ may lead to additional difficulties for Type I problems, where (9.25) may have infinitely many solutions: $x^*(\boldsymbol{\theta})$ is often an isoline in a two-dimensional space or a surface in higher-dimensional spaces. Everywhere, except in Section 9.2.3, $\mathfrak{X}$ is assumed to be continuous and $\mathfrak{X} = [-1, +1]$ if it is not stated differently.

Designs that address (9.25) will be said to be of Type I. The corresponding solution is often called the maximum tolerated dose (MTD); see (6.30) in Section 6.4.2. Identifying the minimum effective dose (MED) is "technically" similar to identifying the MTD. However, search procedures may differ. For example, in searching for the MTD, trials typically start with low doses and escalate avoiding overdosing, whereas, in searching for the MED, trials may start with a high dose. Early examples of Type I dose-finding designs are given, among others, by von Békésy (1947) [387], Dixon and Mood (1948) [99],Robbins and Monro (1951) [341], Derman (1957) [94], Wu (1985) [412], Wetherill and Glazebrook (1986) [397], Durham and Flournoy (1994) [110].

In Figure 9.5, the probability of efficacy with no toxicity P_{10} (solid line) increases as doses become more efficacious and then decreases when doses become more toxic. In this context, a typical goal is to identify the dose which maximizes the probability of efficacy without toxicity, and this is a Type II problem. Examples of Type II designs are found in Kiefer and Wolfowitz (1952) [230], Fedorov and Müller (1989) [149], Gooley et al. (1994) [179], Li et al. (1995) [256], Durham et al. (1998) [112], Hardwick and Stout (2001) [193], Kpamegan and Flournoy (2001) [237], Thall and Cook (2004) [374]. See also examples in Sections 6.4, 6.5, 8.2, 8.3.

Estimating $x^*(\boldsymbol{\theta})$ with the least possible uncertainty (e.g., variance or mean squared error) or with the least harm to patients are popular objectives of early phase studies. Unfortunately, these objectives often "pull" designs in different directions. The phrases "treatment versus experimentation," "treatment versus learning," etc. can be found in numerous publications on dose-finding studies; see Bartroff and Lai (2010) [31], Bartroff et al. (2013) [32]. To quantify the problem, we have to introduce a measure of losses, or harm, or cost, or potential penalty for the wrong prediction of x^*. The situation is similar to what is traditionally used in decision theory and associated with risk, loss or regret functions; cf. Le Cam (1986) [251] and Pratt et al. (1995) [315]. In dose-finding setting, Lai and Robbins (1978, 1979) [244], [245] were probably the first to use a penalty function to measure the quality of the proposed design; see also Dragalin et al. (2008) [103] and Pronzato (2010) [318].

In drug development, there are a few players that loosely can be described as the targeted population, sampled patients, a specific patient, a sponsor (e.g., pharmaceutical company) and various regulatory agencies. For instance, for the n-th in-trial patient, Lai and Robbins (1978) [244] use the quadratic penalty $\phi(x_n) = (x_n - x^*)^2$, where x_n is the dose that the patient is allocated. For the targeted population, the potential loss (harm, or penalty) is determined by the uncertainty of the recommended (predicted) best dose x^*, i.e., $\mathrm{E}[(\hat{x}_N^* - x^*)^2]$. For the sampled patients, the total average penalty $N^{-1}\sum_{n=1}^{N}\phi(x_n)$, or its expected value, might be a sound measure of harm. Fedorov and Wu (2007) [152] added the cost of an observation and used the penalty function $\phi(x_n) = (x_n - x^*)^2 + c$ for a patient and its obvious extensions for the sampled and targeted populations. In this section, we use the same penalty function; cf. examples in Sections 6.4.2, 6.5, 8.2, 8.3, and examples of cost-based PK/PD designs in Sections 7.2.3, 7.2.4, 7.3.5.

9.2.2 Best intention and adaptive *D*-optimal designs

Here we discuss the use of BI and penalized PAD designs for Type I problems with the linear response model and Type II problems with the quadratic model.

Type I problem. To examine the simplest Type I dose-finding problem, consider

$$y = \eta(x, \boldsymbol{\theta}) + \varepsilon, \quad \zeta(x, \boldsymbol{\theta}) = \eta(x, \boldsymbol{\theta}) = \theta_1 + \theta_2 x, \quad x \in \mathfrak{X} = [-1, 1], \quad (9.27)$$

where $E[\varepsilon] = 0$, $Var[y|x] = \sigma^2$. Let $\tilde{x}(\boldsymbol{\theta}) = (\zeta^* - \theta_1)/\theta_2$. The best dose is defined as

$$x^*(\boldsymbol{\theta}) = \arg\min_{x \in \mathfrak{X}} |\zeta(x, \boldsymbol{\theta}) - \zeta^*| = \begin{cases} \tilde{x}(\boldsymbol{\theta}), & |\tilde{x}(\boldsymbol{\theta})| \leq 1, \\ \pm 1, & \pm\tilde{x}(\boldsymbol{\theta}) > 1. \end{cases} \quad (9.28)$$

The model (9.27) may look too simple to be useful in dose-finding studies, where logistic, probit and other nonlinear models dominate; see Section 6.2. However, it provides a local approximation for any dose-finding problem with a "smooth" utility function. Therefore, the asymptotic properties of other BI and PAD designs that are valid for this model will be very much the same as for any other differentiable response model.

In 1951 Robbins and Monro [341] in their seminal paper on stochastic approximation proposed to allocate the n-th subject at

$$x_{n+1} = x_n - \alpha_n(y_n - \zeta^*), \quad (9.29)$$

where $\{\alpha_n\}_{n=1}^{\infty}$ is any deterministic sequence such that $\sum_{n=1}^{\infty} \alpha_n = \infty$ and $\sum_{n=1}^{\infty} \alpha_n^2 \leq \infty$. Under the assumption of bounded variance of measurement errors $\{\varepsilon\}$, this procedure has the optimal convergence rate if $\alpha_n \sim 1/n$, and the best constant governing the convergence rate if $\alpha_n = \theta_2/n$; see Sacks (1958) [346]. One can also verify that if θ_1 is known and $\hat{\theta}_{2n}$ is the least squares estimator for model (9.27), then (9.29) with $\alpha_n = \hat{\theta}_{2n}/n$ is equivalent to

$$x_{n+1} = \bar{x}_n - \hat{\theta}_{2n}^{-1}(\bar{y}_n - \zeta^*) = \frac{\zeta^* - \theta_1}{\hat{\theta}_{2n}}, \quad \text{where } \bar{x}_n = \sum_{i=1}^{n} x_i, \ \bar{y}_n = \sum_{i=1}^{n} y_i; \ (9.30)$$

cf. Wetherill (1963) [396], Anbar (1978) [9]). Thus, while (9.29) looks like a short memory procedure, the opposite is true. On an intuitive level, one can say that x_n carries the cumulative prior information on the experiment. Note that the knowledge of the true value of the slope θ_2 is essential for equating (9.29) with (9.30). However, it was shown by Polyak (1990) [313] and Ruppert (1988) [345] that a simple averaging of the design points $\{x_n\}$ allows one to obtain the best constant governing the optimal convergence rate; see also Polyak and Juditsky (1992) [314].

The idea behind the Robbins-Monro procedure is rather simple; see Figure 9.6 for the illustration. Let $\theta_2 > 0$. If $x_n > x^*$, then because the random errors in (9.27) have zero mean, the observation y_n will be, on average, larger than ζ^*, and according to (9.29) the next point x_{n+1} will be smaller than x_n. By the same token, if $x_{n+1} < x^*$, then the observation y_{n+1} will be smaller than ζ^*, and the next point x_{n+2} will be larger than x_{n+1}. In both cases the procedure "pushes" design points toward the target dose x^* while the decreasing step length α_n prevents the large oscillations.

When both θ_1 and θ_2 are unknown, it seems natural to replace them by the least squares estimators $\hat{\theta}_{1n}$ and $\hat{\theta}_{2n}$:

$$x_{n+1} = \frac{\zeta^* - \hat{\theta}_{1n}}{\hat{\theta}_{2n}}. \quad (9.31)$$

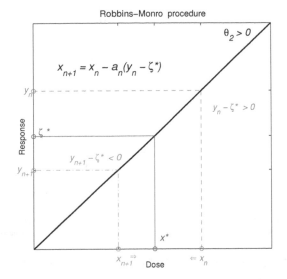

FIGURE 9.6: Illustration of Robbins-Monro procedure (9.29).

Although motivated by the Newton–Raphson method (see Ypma (1995) [422] and Lai (2001) [242]), Robbins and Monro (1951) proposed using a sequence of constants in place of $\hat{\theta}_{2n}/n$. Lai and Robbins (1982) [246] noted that, with a non-zero probability, the sequence $\{x_n\}$ from (9.31) sticks to a boundary point from which it does not move away even if $n \to \infty$. A few simple corrective measures were proposed to make $\{x_n\}$ converge to x^*, and to be asymptotically normally distributed: one has to bound the absolute value of the estimated slope or select a correct sign of the estimated $\hat{\theta}_2$ (the latter is not difficult when searching for the MTD since toxicity usually increases with dose); see also Anbar (1978) [9].

Sequences of predicted best doses may converge to the wrong doses not only for the simple linear response model, but also for more general models. See, for instance, Chang and Ying (2009) [66]); Ghosh et al. (1997) [174], Chapter 15; and Wu (1985) [412], where

$$x_{n+1} = \arg\min_{x \in \mathfrak{X}} \left| \zeta\left(x, \hat{\boldsymbol{\theta}}_n\right) - \zeta^* \right|, \tag{9.32}$$

where $\hat{\boldsymbol{\theta}}_n$ is the maximum likelihood estimator, which coincides with the LSE in the normal case. In Wu (1985) [412], procedures as in (9.31) or (9.32) were called the adaptive Robbins-Monro procedure (ARM). We use the term "naive" ARM when either (9.31) or (9.32) is used directly, i.e., without any adjustments. Otherwise we use the term "tuned" ARM.

To illustrate the potential lack of consistency in the allocation sequence

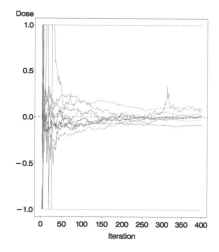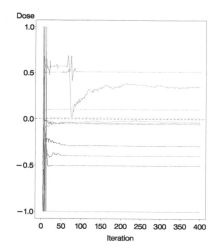

FIGURE 9.7: Sample trajectories of naive ARM, type I dose-finding, linear model (left) and quadratic model (right).

$\{x_n\}$ from (9.31), we resort to Monte Carlo simulations of the model (9.27) with independently normally distributed observations, where $\theta_1 = 0$, $\theta_2 = 1$, $\sigma^2 = 1$, $\zeta^* = 0$; i.e., $x^* = 0$. In addition, doses are restricted to lie in $[-1,1]$. Figure 9.7, left panel, shows exemplary sequences of $\{x_1, \ldots, x_{400}\}$ from (9.31) with an initial cohort of two subjects, one each at ± 1. Most BI designers use the last x_n to estimate x^*, and we do so here, so $\{x_1, \ldots, x_{400}\}$ is also the sequence of predicted best doses. In this and all other examples, 10,000 Monte Carlo simulations were performed. Note that some sequences show early wide variation that simmers down after about 25 trials; convergence then occurs approximately at rate $n^{-1/2}$. Note the lines at ± 1 indicate that some sequences "stick" to boundaries of the design space, and there is no evidence that these sequences will ever converge to the best dose $x^* = 0$. Table 9.2 shows that 1.9% and 1.8% of predicted best dose sequences stuck to the boundaries for $n = 100$ and 400, respectively. That is, increasing the sample size fourfold did not reduce the likelihood of this problem.

In contrast, adaptive optimal design allocates the next subject to the dose

$$x_{n+1} = \arg\max_{x \in \mathfrak{X}} \text{Var}[\eta(x, \hat{\boldsymbol{\theta}}_n)] = \arg\max_{x \in \mathfrak{X}} \mathbf{f}^T(x)\mathbf{M}^{-1}(\xi_n)\mathbf{f}(x), \qquad (9.33)$$

where the variance of the predicted response is the largest, i.e., our knowledge about response function is the worst; cf. (3.2), (5.29), and (8.1). For the linear regression model, the sequence $\{x_n\}$ consists of alternating $+1$ and -1. The selection of x_n for PAD involves both $\text{Var}\left[\eta(x, \hat{\boldsymbol{\theta}}_n)\right]$ and the penalty function

TABLE 9.2: Percent of predicted best dose sequences stuck to the boundaries

		Sample Size $n = 100$		Sample Size $n = 400$	
MODEL	Start-up Sample Size	ARM/BI	PAD with $c = 0.1$	ARM/BI	PAD with $c = 0.1$
Linear	2	1.9	0.0	1.8	0.0
	8	0.0	0.0	0.0	0.0
Quadratic	3	11.3	0.0	10.9	0.0
	12	1.8	0.0	1.5	0.0

$\phi(x, \hat{\boldsymbol{\theta}}_n)$, so

$$x_{n+1} = \arg \max_{x \in \mathfrak{X}} \left\{ \text{Var} \left[\eta(x, \hat{\boldsymbol{\theta}}_n) \right] - \frac{m\phi(x, \hat{\boldsymbol{\theta}}_n)}{\sum_{i=1}^{n} \phi(x_i, \hat{\boldsymbol{\theta}}_n)} \right\}, \qquad (9.34)$$

where m is the number of unknown parameters in the model; cf. (4.17). For PAD designs, typically least squares or maximum likelihood methods are used to estimate the best dose. From Table 9.2, one can see that no PAD-predicted dose sequences stuck to the boundaries in 10,000 simulations for either $n = 100$ or 400. In this and other examples of this section, simulations are performed with $\phi(x, \boldsymbol{\theta}) = [x - x^*(\boldsymbol{\theta})]^2 + c$, $c = 0.1$.

Figure 9.8 shows histograms of predicted best doses for ARM (left panel) and PAD (right panel), respectively. Histograms from each procedure were simulated with start-up sample sizes of 2 (top row) and 8 (bottom row). As expected, histograms for each procedure are much more dispersed for $n = 100$ (left columns) than for $n = 400$ (right columns).

However, the frequency of observations on the boundaries decreases from 1.9% for ARM with a start-up sample size of 2 to 0% with a start-up sample size of 8 (Table 9.2). Comparing top and bottom rows in Figure 9.8, significant improvement can be seen in having a larger fixed start-up cohort. With start-up cohorts of size 2, the standard deviation of ARM predicted doses reduces from 0.17 for $n = 100$ to 0.14 for $n = 400$, but it halves from 0.10 to 0.05 with start-up cohorts of size 8. This observation leads to the obvious recommendation that the size and allocation of the start-up cohorts for ARM should be selected carefully and should be large enough to avoid estimators that stick to boundaries.

In contrast with ARM, PAD predicted dose sequences did not stick to the boundaries (Table 9.2), and their standard deviation halves as expected from 0.10 ($n = 100$) to 0.05 ($n = 400$), regardless of start-up cohort sizes. Note that with the larger initial cohort size, histograms of ARM predicted doses are visually similar to those from PAD designs, and both of them are asymptotically identical to the distribution of x_n from the tuned ARM (the slope θ_2 is bounded and estimates $\hat{\theta}_{2n}$ are correspondingly restricted). More

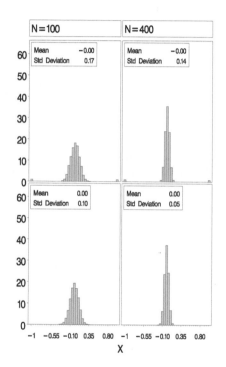

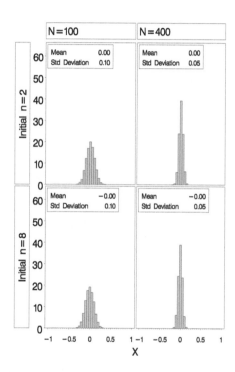

FIGURE 9.8: Histograms of predicted best doses for the linear model (9.27): ARM (left panel) and PAD (right panel); initial cohort sizes of 2 (top rows) and 8 (bottom rows). Left columns: after 100 observations; right columns: after 400 observations.

TABLE 9.3: Risks for different customers

Customers	Risk	Tuned ARM	Locally D-optimal
Targeted population	$E\left(x_N^* - x^*\right)^2$	$\sim (\sigma/\theta_2)^2\, N^{-1}$	$(\sigma/\theta_2)^2\, N^{-1}$
Patient sample	$E\left[\sum_{i=1}^{N}\left(x_i^* - x^*\right)^2\right]$	$\sim (\sigma/\theta_2)^2\, lnN$	N
n-th patient	$E\left(x_n^* - x^*\right)^2$	$\sim (\sigma/\theta_2)^2\, n^{-1}$	1
Sponsor	N	$Q + qN$	$Q + qN$

Note: $\sim$ denotes "asymptotically" (for large N); Q is the cost of a trial initiation; q is the cost of a patient enrollment.

about tuning of ARM may be found in Lai (2001) [242] and Bartroff and Lai (2010) [31]. Again, we emphasize that the initial design and its sample size are critical to ARM performance, but have no noticeable effect on PAD designs.

Table 9.3 compares risks (mean penalties) based on $\phi(x, \boldsymbol{\theta}) = (x - x^*)^2$ from the tuned ARM and the locally D-optimal design for the targeted population, sampled patients, a specific patient and a sponsor. We used $\phi(x, \boldsymbol{\theta}) = (x - x^*)^2$ to make results compatible with the theoretical findings of Lai and Robbins (1978) [244]. Note that the tuned ARM is equally as good as the D-optimal design with respect to gaining information about x^*, but is superior to the D-optimal design with respect to the risk. The tuned ARM has reduced risk for two types of customers, the sample in-study patients and an individual patient, mainly due to the selection of a very specific loss function. As soon as one adds a per-patient cost c to obtain $\phi(x, \boldsymbol{\theta}) = (x - x^*)^2 + c$, the slow logarithmic growth of the ARM risk to a patient sample is replaced with linear growth, putting its convergence rate on par with locally D-optimal designs.

Total penalties, $\sum_{i=1}^{n}\phi(x_i, \boldsymbol{\theta}) = \sum_{i=1}^{n}(x_i - x^*)^2 + nc$, with per-subject cost $c = 0.1$, are shown in Table 9.4 for ARM and PAD designs with $n = 400$. With the continuous linear model, total penalties using ARM have skewed distributions and depend heavily on the start-up cohort size (when increasing start-up size from 2 to 8, the mean drops from 13.1 to 4.2, which is the mean total penalty using the PAD design for both cohort sizes). In comparison, the PAD penalties have relatively little skewness and are independent of start-up cohort size. ARM and PAD procedures have similar penalties with the larger start-up sample.

While the knowledge of x^* and penalties/risks are important components of clinical trial design, the purpose of most trials is also to learn about the local behavior of the dose-response curve in the vicinity of x^*. Figure 9.9 presents scatterplots of estimates $\hat{\theta}_{1n}$ vs. $\hat{\theta}_{2n}$ from the naive ARM (left panel) and PAD designs (right panel) after 100 and 400 observations (left and right columns,

TABLE 9.4: Total penalty $\sum_{i=1}^{n}(x_i - x^*)^2 + nc$ for $c = 0.1$ and $n = 400$

Model	Start-up Size	ARM/BI Mean	ARM/BI Median	PAD Mean	PAD Median
Linear	2	13.1	4.8	4.2	3.0
	8	4.2	3.1	4.2	3.0
Quadratic	3	71.1	18.3	7.2	4.7
	12	29.1	7.2	4.9	2.9

respectively). Estimates from PAD designs are tightly packed, showing small variation, relative to estimates from ARM deigns. With the naive ARM, variation is significantly greater, not ellipsoidal in shape, and distinct clusters of estimates corresponding to sequences stuck to the boundaries are especially evident for designs with small start-up cohorts. We have also observed that a tuned ARM usually eliminates predicted dose sequences from the boundaries, but does not change the general shape of the central "cloud" of parameter estimates.

Figure 9.9 also shows that even though x_n from an ARM with a sufficient initial cohort size will estimate x^* well, the corresponding estimators for $\hat{\theta}_{1n}$ and $\hat{\theta}_{2n}$ behave rather poorly relative to PAD designs. The explanation of this fact is as follows. For polynomial regression of order m, the behavior of $\hat{\theta}_n$ is determined by the elements of the information matrix

$$M_{\alpha\beta}(n) = \sum_{i=1}^{n} x_i^{\alpha+\beta-2}, \quad \alpha, \beta = 0, \ldots, m;$$

see Lai and Wei (1982) [247], Lai (2003) [243]. For the tuned ARM, the allocations x_n converge to $x^* = 0$ at rate $n^{-1/2}$ in terms of standard error, and the element $M_{22}(n)$ determines the asymptotic variance of the slope $\hat{\theta}_{2n}$, which still grows to infinity but very slowly:

$$M_{22}(n) = \sum_{i=1}^{n} x_i^2 \sim \sum_{i=1}^{n} \frac{1}{i} \sim \ln n, \qquad (9.35)$$

while $M_{11} \sim n$. For PAD designs, $M_{22}(n) \sim n$ provides much faster growth than ARM designs with $M_{22}(n) \sim \ln n$; see Anderson and Taylor (1976) [10].

To conclude the discussion of the linear model, we again emphasize that

- For a Type I problem the naive ARM, which can be viewed as the BI design, may fail.

- Simple tuning, like bounding slope estimates, or adding extra variability to x_n, makes the ARM a good method for estimating x^* and allocating subjects near x^*. Details on various improvements/tunings of ARM are given by Lai (2001) [242] and Lai (2003) [243].

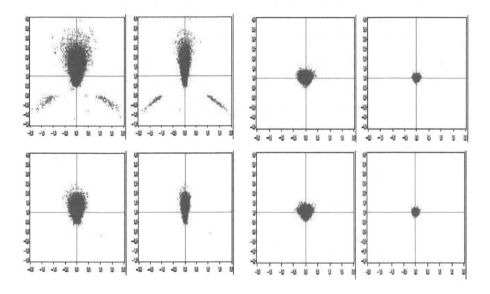

FIGURE 9.9: Scatterplots of estimates $\hat{\theta}_1$ vs $\hat{\theta}_2$ for the linear model (9.27), same setting as in Figure 9.8.

- ARM leads to lower (comparatively to locally D-optimal designs) quadratic risks. However, the penalized adaptive D-optimal designs is a strong alternative.

- ARM provides very poor estimation of the local behavior of the dose-response curve. When the underlying model has more than one parameter and the selected doses are clustered at a given level, this leads to identifiability problems. It is worthwhile noting that in the original CRM paper, O'Quigley et al. (1990) [301] focused on one-parameter models. Careless application of CRM-type methods to multiparameter models often produces erratic results due to the insufficient information for the estimation of all model parameters; see Shu and O'Quigley (2008) [359], O'Quigley and Conoway (2010) [299].

- One can verify that the adaptive penalized c-optimal designs, i.e., designs that minimize $\phi(x, \boldsymbol{\theta}) = \text{Var}[\hat{x}^*]$, where $\hat{x}^* = -\hat{\theta}_1/\hat{\theta}_2$ and $\phi(x, \boldsymbol{\theta}) = (x - x^*)^2 + c$, coincide with naive ARM, and therefore, what is true for ARM is relevant for c-optimal designs as well.

Type II problem. We examine the simplest model for Type II dose-finding experiments:

$$y = \eta(x, \boldsymbol{\theta}) + \varepsilon, \quad \zeta(x, \boldsymbol{\theta}) = \eta(x, \boldsymbol{\theta}) = \theta_1 + \theta_2 x + \theta_3 x^2, \quad x \in \mathfrak{X} = [-1, 1], \quad (9.36)$$

where $\text{E}[\varepsilon] = 0$ and $Var[y|x] = \sigma^2$. The "best" dose is the one that maximizes the quadratic function, i.e., $x^*(\boldsymbol{\theta}) = -\theta_{2n}/2\theta_{3n}$. While (9.36) is simple, it provides a good approximation to any "smooth" function in the vicinity of x^*.

For (9.36), the naive BI procedure is

$$x_{n+1}(\boldsymbol{\theta}) = \arg\max_{x \in \mathfrak{X}} [\zeta(x, \boldsymbol{\theta})] = \begin{cases} \tilde{x}_n & \text{if } |\tilde{x}_n| \leq 1, \\ \pm 1 & \text{if } \tilde{x}_n > 1 \text{ or } < -1, \end{cases} \quad (9.37)$$

where $\tilde{x}_n = -\hat{\theta}_{2n}/2\hat{\theta}_{3n}$. Independent observations were simulated from the normal distribution $\varepsilon \sim \mathcal{N}(\boldsymbol{\theta}, \sigma^2)$ with $\theta_1 = 1$, $\theta_2 = 0$, $\theta_3 = -1$ and $\sigma^2 = 1$, so again the best dose is $x^*(\boldsymbol{\theta}) = 0$. Each simulated sequence begins with a fixed initial cohort of either 3 or 12 patients equally allocated to -1, 0 and 1. As before, simulations of PAD designs include the quadratic penalty with cost $c = 0.1$.

Table 9.2 shows that 11.3% of BI predicted dose sequences stuck to the boundaries when $n = 100$, and this percentage reduced only to 10.9% for $n = 400$. Thus, the boundary problem for BI sequences is significantly worse for quadratic models. In contrast, none of the PAD predicted dose sequences stuck to the boundaries.

Most alarming for BI designs, however, is that predicted best dose sequences may converge to values that are different from x^*. This phenomenon was noted long ago, and a short survey with a number of major references can be found in Pronzato (2008) [317]. More subtle theoretical results, such as the existence of the attractors different from x^*, can be found, for instance, in Bozin and Zarrop (1991) [55]. These results were established for the Kalman-Bucy type of estimators, which are simpler to analyze than the least squares estimators. Our Monte Carlo simulations provide empirical evidence that, in general, BI sequences based on the least squares method do not converge to the best dose. The existence of such attractors may exacerbate problems with applications if an unaware practitioner, observing a convergence to the (wrong) "best" dose, makes a prediction with unfounded confidence.

Histograms of best doses (x_{100} and x_{400}) selected by the naive BI and PAD designs are presented in Figure 9.10, left and right panels, respectively. The top and bottom rows correspond to start-up cohorts of size $n = 3$ and $n = 12$, respectively. BI histograms for x_{100} and x_{400} are almost identical: there is no substantial improvement after 300 observations are added. The standard deviation for the ARM best dose predictions changes from 0.42 to 0.41 for a start-up size of 3, and from 0.27 to 0.26 for a start-up size of 12.

The lack of improvement in parameter estimation with increased sample sizes for BI designs is also seen in the plots of parameter estimates in Figure 9.11. Similar to ARM for the linear model, parameter estimates for the BI design have some clusters; see the left panel. For corresponding PAD designs (right panel), marked improvement is seen with increased sample size.

To provide a heuristic explanation of the poor performance of BI designs, consider the least squares estimates $\hat{\boldsymbol{\theta}}_n$. Let us assume that this estimate is at least as good as a (nonadaptive) estimate generated by some fixed regular design. For the latter, the rate of convergence is $O(n^{-1/2})$. Similar to the ARM for the linear model,

$$M_{22}(n) = \sum_{i=1}^{n} x_i^2 \sim \ln\ n; \tag{9.38}$$

cf. (9.35). This gives us hope for the consistency of $\hat{\theta}_{2n}$. However,

$$M_{33}(n) \ \sim\ \sum_{i=1}^{n} x_i^4 \sim \sum_{i=1}^{n} 1/i^2 \longrightarrow \pi^2/6; \tag{9.39}$$

see Andrews et al. [11], Chapter 1.2. Thus, the convergence of the least squares estimator of $\hat{\theta}_{3n}$ and, subsequently, of $\hat{x}_n^*(\boldsymbol{\theta}) = -\hat{\theta}_{2n}/2\hat{\theta}_{3n}$ to the true value $x^*(\boldsymbol{\theta})$ cannot be guaranteed; cf. Lai and Wei (1982) [247].

The introduction of forced perturbations in dose allocation is a popular remedy for BI procedures; cf. Bozin and Zarrop (1991) [55] and Pronzato (2008) [317]. For instance, $M_{33}(n) \sim \ln n$ if

$$x_{n+1} = \hat{x}_n^* + z_n n^{-1/4},$$

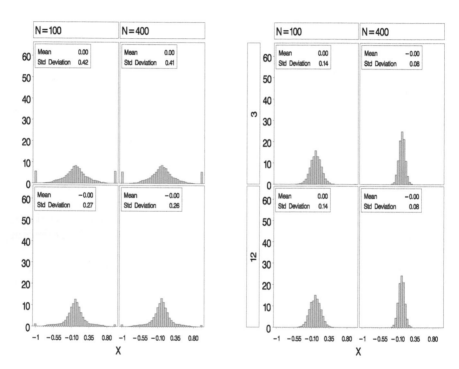

FIGURE 9.10: Histograms of predicted best doses for the quadratic model (9.36): BI (left panel) and PAD (right panel); initial cohort sizes of 3 (top rows) and 12 (bottom rows). Left columns: after 100 observations; right columns: after 400 observations.

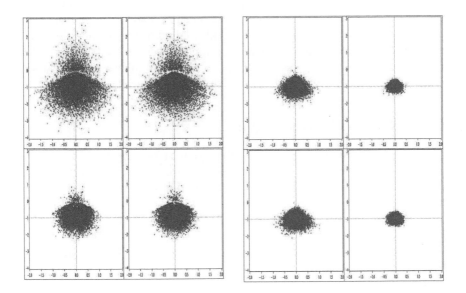

FIGURE 9.11: Scatterplots of estimates $\hat{\theta}_1$ vs $\hat{\theta}_2$ for the quadratic model (9.36), same setting as in Figure 9.10.

where z_n can be any random variable with bounded variance, symmetrically distributed around zero. Therefore, the consistency of $\hat{\theta}_{3n}$, and, consequently, the convergence of $\{\hat{x}_n^*(\boldsymbol{\theta})\}$, is secured; see Lai (2001) [242]. At the same time the sequence $\{x_n\}$ stays close to x^*, keeping risk at a relatively low level. However, we recommend the use of penalized adaptive designs to permit the experimenter to quantify needs and ethical/cost constraints.

To summarize, we would like to emphasize that for a Type II problem the naive BI designs do not work. Their convergence to wrong doses may lead to the false optimism of a practitioner that can result in false prediction of the best dose. The empirical tuning of BI designs leads to estimators that are inferior to what can be found for the penalized adaptive optimal designs. The penalized adaptive design machinery provides routine tools for quantifying trial objectives (through criteria of optimality) and allows for ethical and/or cost constraints through selection of risk/penalty functions.

9.2.3 Discrete design region $\mathfrak{X}$

In clinical dose-finding studies, allocation rules that were adapted from numerical optimization, optimal control, or optimal design usually need some modifications in order to operate on a lattice of doses. For instance, in the one-dimensional case, $\mathfrak{X} = \{x_1, \ldots, x_k\}$ where k is the number of distinct doses. With a discrete design region $\mathfrak{X}$, it is important to distinguish the design region from the prediction space $\tilde{\mathfrak{X}}$. For example, test doses may be sampled from the given doses of currently manufactured pills. Alternatively, one may only be able to study a few doses of some drug, yet be interested in the best dose over a continuous range that includes these doses. Usually, $\tilde{\mathfrak{X}}$ will include $\mathfrak{X}$.

Type I problem. Almost immediately after the publication of the pioneering papers on the Robbins-Monro procedure, it was noted that some modifications are needed to make it work for discrete $\mathfrak{X}$. The introduction of additional randomization, interpolation/extrapolation from $\mathfrak{X}$ to $\tilde{\mathfrak{X}}$, and changing doses not farther than one step away from the current allocation were found useful in transporting major Robbins-Monro ideas to discrete sample spaces. Various amendments and improvements were extensively discussed in the dose-finding community, and many references can be found in Chevret (2006) [74]; see also Cheung (2010) [72].

With regard to naive Type I BI designs, Azriel et al. (2011) [27], Theorem 1, proved that there exists no such design that converges to x^* for all increasing response functions. Our simulations confirm the need for at least some corrective measures with BI procedures. We make a few recommendations to improve the discrete version of ARM:

- With a sparse grid, instead of following the common practice of using the final treatment allocation x_N as a recommended dose (see, for example,

Zacks (2009) [425], Chapter 6), use

$$\tilde{x}_N = \arg\min_{x \in \tilde{\mathfrak{X}}} |\zeta(x, \hat{\boldsymbol{\theta}}_N) - \zeta^*|. \tag{9.40}$$

In practice, when the validity of $\zeta(x, \boldsymbol{\theta})$ is in doubt for the whole set $\tilde{\mathfrak{X}}$, local approximations with any simple function (e.g., linear, sigmoid-shaped or functions used in CRM papers) will work; cf. Dupa and Herkenrath (2007) [109]. For studies with small samples sizes, Stylianou and Flournoy (2002) [370] recommend modeling $\zeta(x, \hat{\boldsymbol{\theta}}_N)$ in (9.40) with isotonic regression and using linear interpolation from $\mathfrak{X}$ to $\tilde{\mathfrak{X}}$ to obtain the recommended dose.

- Introduce extra randomization, for instance, as in Derman (1957) [94], Durham and Flournoy (1994), (1995) [110], [111], or Dupa and Herkenrath (2007) [109]. It is crucial to avoid long "runs" at the same dose that can falsely be viewed as convergence. This can be achieved by treating subjects in cohorts (Gezmu and Flournoy (2006) [173]) or by sampling at a dose until some k successive toxicities are observed (Oron and Hoff (2009) [302]). These procedures can also be used to start-up parametric procedures.

- New allocations should be to one of the neighboring points of the current x_n. This stabilizes the sequence in that only the sign of $\hat{\theta}_n$ (direction, not the actual slope) is important. This restriction also is usually desired by clinical researchers, but our recommendation follows directly from analysis of the procedures.

- We recommend using PAD to get information about the local behavior of dose-response curves near x^*. While using PAD, one may restrict allocations to doses neighboring the current one. We do not recommend c-optimal adaptive design, even though it coincides with ARM for the linear model and also with typically recommended local models like the CRM, because c-optimal designs do not provide sufficient information about the local behavior of dose-response curves near x^*.

Type II problem. Similar to Type I dose-finding, all patterns observed for continuous $\mathfrak{X}$ hold for Type II objectives. Defining dose-finding problems in terms of the two sets $\mathfrak{X}$ and $\tilde{\mathfrak{X}}$ is even more beneficial here than for Type I objectives. It allows for a better understanding of the structure of $\zeta(x, \boldsymbol{\theta})$ near the optimal dose. All recommendations for type I dose-finding hold, but more pronounced emphasis on extra randomization is required.

To conclude this section, let us emphasize once again that we made an attempt to attract the attention of statisticians who are involved in design and analysis of dose-finding trials, to potential flaws in some gaining popularity adaptive designs, which we dubbed here as "best intention" designs. Our extensive Monte Carlo simulations, together with some partially neglected theoretical results developed in the framework of optimal adaptive control theory, show that the reckless application of ethically very sound and attractive ideas may lead to dismal results, especially for Type II problems. Various remedies are readily available for Type I dose-finding, and they lead to procedures that are very close to statistically optimal. Unfortunately, the situation with Type II dose-finding is much worse.

The systematic use of the machinery of optimal design theory and, in particular, penalized adaptive (multistage) designs, leads to designs that for Type I problems are either equivalent to the popular BI designs (like ARM or "naive" CRM) or superior to them. For Type II problems, our simulations confirm the superiority of penalized adaptive optimal designs.

Remark 9.1 In all examples of this section we used the penalty function $\phi(x, \boldsymbol{\theta}) = (x - x^*)^2 + c$. In spite of its simplicity, it approximates a wide and popular class of penalty functions $\phi(x, \boldsymbol{\theta}) = \zeta(x^*, \boldsymbol{\theta}) - \zeta(x, \boldsymbol{\theta}) + c$. Indeed, assuming that $\zeta(x, \boldsymbol{\theta})$ is twice differentiable with respect to x and using the Taylor expansion in the vicinity of x^*, one readily concludes that

$$\phi(x, \boldsymbol{\theta}) \simeq -\frac{1}{2} \frac{\partial^2 \zeta(x, \boldsymbol{\theta})}{\partial x^2} \bigg|_{x=x^*} (x - x^*)^2 + c = A(\boldsymbol{\theta})(x - x^*)^2 + c. \quad (9.41)$$

In (9.37) we search for the maximum of $\zeta(x, \boldsymbol{\theta})$, so it is natural to assume that the second derivative of $\zeta(x, \boldsymbol{\theta})$ is negative, i.e., $A(\boldsymbol{\theta})$ is positive.

Remark 9.2 One of possible alternatives to PAD is an adaptive design based on compound criteria; see Läuter (1974) [249]; cf. Section 2.2.4. A simple compound criterion for (9.36) was proposed by Pronzato (2000) [316]:

$$\Psi[\mathbf{M}(\xi)] = (1 - w) \int_{\mathcal{X}} \zeta(x, \boldsymbol{\theta}) \xi(dx) + w \ln |\mathbf{M}(\xi)|. \quad (9.42)$$

Let us assume that $\eta(x, \boldsymbol{\theta}) = \boldsymbol{\theta}^T \mathbf{f}(x)$, as in all examples of this section. Note that $\max_{x \in \mathcal{X}} \zeta(x, \boldsymbol{\theta}) = \max_\xi \int_{\mathcal{X}} \zeta(x, \boldsymbol{\theta}) \xi(dx)$. The sensitivity function of the criterion (9.42) is

$$\varphi(x, \boldsymbol{\theta}) = (1 - w) \zeta(x, \boldsymbol{\theta}) + w \mathbf{f}^T(x) \mathbf{M}^{-1}(\xi) \mathbf{f}(x). \quad (9.43)$$

Applying results of Chapter 5 leads to the following adaptive design:

$$x_{n+1} = \arg \max_{x \in \mathcal{X}} \left[(1 - w) \zeta(x, \hat{\boldsymbol{\theta}}_n) + w \mathbf{f}^T(x) \mathbf{M}^{-1}(\xi_n) \mathbf{f}(x) \right]. \quad (9.44)$$

The balance between treatment and information gain in (9.44) is controlled by w.

Chapter 10

Useful Matrix Formulae

10.1 Matrix Derivatives 332
10.2 Partitioned Matrices 333
10.3 Equalities 333
10.4 Inequalities 334

In this chapter we provide some matrix formulae that are utilized in various optimal design applications. For useful references on matrix algebra, see Harville (1997) [195], Magnus and Neudecker (1988) [262], Marcus and Minc (1992) [267], Seber (2008) [356].

Symbols and Notation

$\mathbf{A}, \mathbf{B}, \mathbf{C}, \cdots$	capital letters denote matrices
$\mathbf{a}, \mathbf{f}, \mathbf{x}$	lowercase letters denote vectors
$\mathbf{A}^T$	transpose of matrix $\mathbf{A}$
A_{ij}	(i, j)-th element of matrix $\mathbf{A}$
$\mathbf{a}^T$	transpose of vector $\mathbf{a}$
a_i	i-th element of vector $\mathbf{a}$
$\mathbf{I}_m$	identity matrix of order $m \times m$
$\mathrm{tr}(\mathbf{A})$	trace of matrix $\mathbf{A}$ (sum of diagonal elements)
$\mathrm{diag}(\mathbf{A})$	square matrix with elements $a_{11}, a_{22}, \cdots$ on the diagonal and zero elsewhere
$\|\mathbf{A}\|$	determinant of $\mathbf{A}$
$\|\|\mathbf{A}\|\|$	norm of $\mathbf{A}$
$\lambda_i(\mathbf{A})$	i-th eigenvalue of $\mathbf{A}$

Vector and Matrix Norms

	Vector Norm $\|\|\mathbf{x}\|\|$	Matrix Norm $\|\|\mathbf{X}\|\|$
Euclidean or l_2	$\sqrt{\mathbf{x}^T \mathbf{x}}$	$\max_i \lambda_i(\mathbf{X}'\mathbf{X})$
l_1 norm	$\sum_i \|x_i\|$	$\max_j (\sum_{i=1}^{n} \|X_{ij}\|)$
l_∞ norm	$\max_i \|x_i\|$	$\max_i (\sum_{j=1}^{n} \|X_{ij}\|)$

10.1   Matrix Derivatives

Let $\mathbf{M} = \mathbf{M}(\alpha)$ be an $m \times k$ matrix that depends on parameter α. Let $u = u(\mathbf{M})$ be a scalar function of $\mathbf{M}$. Denote

$$\frac{d\mathbf{M}}{d\alpha} = \left\{ \frac{d\mathbf{M}_{ij}}{d\alpha} \right\}, \quad \frac{\partial u}{\partial \mathbf{M}} = \left\{ \frac{\partial u}{\partial M_{ij}} \right\}, \quad i = 1, \ldots, m; \quad j = 1, \ldots, k;$$

i.e., $d\mathbf{M}/d\alpha$ and $\partial u/\partial \mathbf{M}$ are $m \times k$ matrices.

Let $\mathbf{a}$ and $\mathbf{x}$ be $k \times 1$ and $m \times 1$ vectors, respectively. Denote

$$\frac{\partial \mathbf{a}^T}{\partial \mathbf{x}} = \left\{ \frac{\partial a_j}{\partial x_i} \right\}, \quad i = 1, \ldots, m; \quad j = 1, \ldots, k;$$

i.e., $\partial \mathbf{a}^T/\partial \mathbf{x}$ is an $m \times k$ matrix.

Formulae (10.1) and (10.2) are used in the proof of Theorem 1.1.

If $\mathbf{M}$ is a symmetric nonsingular matrix which depends on parameter α, and if u is a scalar function of $\mathbf{M}$, then

$$\frac{du}{d\alpha} = \mathrm{tr}\left[\frac{\partial u}{\partial \mathbf{M}} \frac{d\mathbf{M}}{d\alpha} \right]. \tag{10.1}$$

If $\mathbf{A}$, $\mathbf{M}$, and $\mathbf{B}$ are symmetric matrices of proper dimension, then

$$\frac{\partial}{\partial \mathbf{M}} \mathrm{tr}\left[(\mathbf{A} - \mathbf{M})\mathbf{B} \right]^2 = 2\mathbf{B}(\mathbf{M} - \mathbf{A})\mathbf{B}. \tag{10.2}$$

For proofs, see Harville (1997) [195], Chapter 15.

Formulae (10.3) – (10.5) are used in the derivation of sensitivity functions for D- and A-criteria; see Section 2.5.

$$\frac{d \ln |\mathbf{M}|}{d\alpha} = \mathrm{tr}\left[\mathbf{M}^{-1} \frac{d\mathbf{M}}{d\alpha} \right], \quad \frac{\partial \ln |\mathbf{M}|}{\partial \mathbf{M}} = \mathbf{M}^{-1}, \tag{10.3}$$

$$\frac{d\,\mathrm{tr}[\mathbf{A}\mathbf{M}^{-1}]}{d\alpha} = \mathrm{tr}\left[\mathbf{A}\frac{d\mathbf{M}^{-1}}{d\alpha} \right], \tag{10.4}$$

$$\frac{d\mathbf{M}^{-1}}{d\alpha} = -\mathbf{M}^{-1}\frac{d\mathbf{M}}{d\alpha}\mathbf{M}^{-1}. \tag{10.5}$$

For proofs, see Magnus and Neudecker (1988) [262], Chapters 8.3, 8.4 and 9.9.

The next formula is used in Sections 1.1.1 and 1.5.1: if $\mathbf{x}$ is an $m \times 1$ vector and $\mathbf{A}$ is an $m \times k$ matrix, then

$$\frac{\partial(\mathbf{x}^T\mathbf{A})}{\partial \mathbf{x}} = \mathbf{A}. \tag{10.6}$$

10.2   Partitioned Matrices

If $\mathbf{M} = \begin{pmatrix} \mathbf{A} & \mathbf{B} \\ \mathbf{C} & \mathbf{D} \end{pmatrix}$, where $\mathbf{A}$ and $\mathbf{D}$ are square matrices and $|\mathbf{A}| \neq 0$, then

$$\mathbf{M}^{-1} = \begin{pmatrix} \mathbf{A}^{-1} + \mathbf{A}^{-1}\mathbf{B}\mathbf{H}^{-1}\mathbf{C}\mathbf{A}^{-1} & -\mathbf{A}^{-1}\mathbf{B}\mathbf{H}^{-1} \\ -\mathbf{H}^{-1}\mathbf{C}\mathbf{A}^{-1} & \mathbf{H}^{-1} \end{pmatrix},$$

where $\mathbf{H} = \mathbf{D} - \mathbf{C}\mathbf{A}^{-1}\mathbf{B}$ and $|\mathbf{A}| \neq 0$.

If $|\mathbf{D}| \neq 0$, then

$$\mathbf{M}^{-1} = \begin{pmatrix} \mathbf{K}^{-1} & -\mathbf{K}^{-1}\mathbf{B}\mathbf{D}^{-1} \\ -\mathbf{D}^{-1}\mathbf{C}\mathbf{K}^{-1} & \mathbf{D}^{-1} + \mathbf{D}^{-1}\mathbf{C}\mathbf{K}^{-1}\mathbf{B}\mathbf{D}^{-1} \end{pmatrix},$$

where $\mathbf{K} = \mathbf{A} - \mathbf{B}\mathbf{D}^{-1}\mathbf{C}$, if $|\mathbf{D}| \neq 0$.

$$|\mathbf{M}| = |\mathbf{A}||\mathbf{D} - \mathbf{C}\mathbf{A}^{-1}\mathbf{B}| = |\mathbf{D}||\mathbf{A} - \mathbf{B}\mathbf{D}^{-1}\mathbf{C}|; \qquad (10.7)$$

see Harville (1997) [195], Chapter 13.3.

10.3   Equalities

Formulae (10.8) – (10.10) are used in Section 2.2.1.

For any symmetric $m \times m$ matrix $\mathbf{D}$ there exist an orthogonal matrix $\mathbf{P}$ and diagonal matrix $\mathbf{\Lambda}$, both of order m, such that

$$\mathbf{D} = \mathbf{P}^T \mathbf{\Lambda} \mathbf{P}, \quad \mathbf{P}\mathbf{P}^T = \mathbf{P}^T\mathbf{P} = \mathbf{I}_m \quad \text{and} \quad \mathbf{\Lambda} = diag[\lambda_\alpha], \qquad (10.8)$$

where $\lambda_\alpha = \lambda_\alpha(\mathbf{D})$ are eigenvalues of $\mathbf{D}$; see Harville (1997) [195], Chapter 21.5.

For any square matrices $\mathbf{A}$ and $\mathbf{B}$

$$|\mathbf{A}\mathbf{B}| = |\mathbf{A}|\,|\mathbf{B}|; \qquad (10.9)$$

see Harville (1997) [195], Chapter 13.3.

For any matrices $\mathbf{A}$ and $\mathbf{B}$ of order $m \times s$ and $s \times m$, respectively,

$$\mathrm{tr}[\mathbf{A}\mathbf{B}] = \mathrm{tr}[\mathbf{B}\mathbf{A}]; \qquad (10.10)$$

see Harville (1997) [195], Chapter 5.2.

Formulae (10.11) and (10.12) are used in Section 3.1.2.

If matrices $\mathbf{A}$ and $\mathbf{B}$ are of dimensions $m \times m$ and $m \times k$, respectively, then

$$|\mathbf{A} + \mathbf{B}\mathbf{B}^T| = |\mathbf{A}| \, |\mathbf{I}_k + \mathbf{B}^T\mathbf{A}^{-1}\mathbf{B}|; \qquad (10.11)$$

see Harville (1997) [195], Theorem 18.1.1.

If $\mathbf{A}$ and $\mathbf{D}$ are nonsingular, then

$$(\mathbf{A} + \mathbf{B}\mathbf{D}\mathbf{B}^T)^{-1} = \mathbf{A}^{-1} - \mathbf{A}^{-1}\mathbf{B}(\mathbf{B}^T\mathbf{A}^{-1}\mathbf{B} + \mathbf{D}^{-1})^{-1}\mathbf{B}^T\mathbf{A}^{-1}; \qquad (10.12)$$

see Harville (1997) [195], Theorem 18.2.8.

$$(\mathbf{A} - \mathbf{U}\mathbf{V}^T)^{-1} = \mathbf{A}^{-1} + \frac{\mathbf{A}^{-1}\mathbf{U}\mathbf{V}^T\mathbf{A}^{-1}}{1 - \mathbf{V}^T\mathbf{A}^{-1}\mathbf{U}};$$

$$(\mathbf{A} + \alpha \mathbf{f}\,\mathbf{f}^T)^{-1} = \mathbf{A}^{-1} - \frac{\mathbf{A}^{-1}\mathbf{f}\,\mathbf{f}^T\mathbf{A}^{-1}}{\alpha^{-1} + \mathbf{f}^T\mathbf{A}^{-1}\mathbf{f}} = \mathbf{A}^{-1} - \frac{\alpha\mathbf{A}^{-1}\mathbf{f}\,\mathbf{f}^T\mathbf{A}^{-1}}{1 + \alpha\mathbf{f}^T\mathbf{A}^{-1}\mathbf{f}}. \qquad (10.13)$$

10.4   Inequalities

Inequalities (10.14) – (10.16) are used in Section 2.3. Let $\mathbf{M}$ satisfy (2.45), i.e. $\mathbf{M} = (1 - \alpha)\mathbf{M}_1 + \alpha\mathbf{M}_2$, where $0 \le \alpha \le 1$.

If $\mathbf{M}_1$ and $\mathbf{M}_2$ are nonsingular matrices, then

$$\ln|\mathbf{M}| \ge (1 - \alpha)\ln|\mathbf{M}_1| + \alpha\ln|\mathbf{M}_2|; \qquad (10.14)$$

see Magnus and Neudecker (1988) [262], Chapter 11.22.

If $\mathbf{M}_1$ and $\mathbf{M}_2$ are nonnegative definite $m \times m$ matrices, then

$$|\mathbf{M}|^{1/m} \ge (1 - \alpha)|\mathbf{M}_1|^{1/m} + \alpha|\mathbf{M}_2|^{1/m}; \qquad (10.15)$$

see Marcus and Minc (1992) [267], Chapter 4.1.8, or Magnus and Neudecker (1988) [262], Chapter 11.25.

If $\mathbf{M}_1$ and $\mathbf{M}_2$ are symmetric positive definite matrices, then

$$\mathbf{M}^{-1} \le (1 - \alpha)\mathbf{M}_1^{-1} + \alpha\mathbf{M}_2^{-1}; \qquad (10.16)$$

see Seber (2008) [356], Chapter 10.4.2.

Hadamard's inequality: if $\mathbf{M}$ is an $m \times m$ matrix, then

$$|\mathbf{M}|^2 \le \prod_{i=1}^{m}\sum_{j=1}^{m} M_{ij}^2.$$

Moreover, if $\mathbf{M}$ is positive definite, then

$$|\mathbf{M}| \leq \prod_{i=1}^{m} M_{ii}.$$

If $\mathbf{M}_1$ and $\mathbf{M}_2$ are $m \times m$ positive definite matrices, then

$$\text{tr}(\mathbf{M}_1\mathbf{M}_2) \geq m|\mathbf{M}_1|^{1/m}|\mathbf{M}_2|^{1/m}. \tag{10.17}$$

Thus,

$$|\mathbf{M}_1|^{1/m} = \min_{|\mathbf{M}_2|=1} \text{tr}(\mathbf{M}_1\mathbf{M}_2)/m.$$

Bibliography

[1] K.M. Abdelbasit and R.L. Plackett. Experimental design for binary data. *J. Am. Statist. Assoc.*, 78:90–98, 1983.

[2] M. Abramowitz and I.A. Stegun. *Handbook of Mathematical Functions with Formulas, Graphs and Mathematical Tables*. Dover, New York, 9th edition, 1972.

[3] A. Agresti. *Categorical Data Analysis*. Wiley, New York, 2nd edition, 2002.

[4] M.K. Al-Banna, A.W. Kelman, and B. Whiting. Experimental design and efficient parameter estimation in population pharmacokinetics. *J. Pharmacokin. Biopharmaceut.*, 18(4):347–360, 1990.

[5] A. Albert. *Regression and the Moore-Penrose Pseudoinverse*. Academic Press, New York, 1972.

[6] A. Albert and J.A. Anderson. On the existence of maximum likelihood estimates in logistic regression models. *Biometrika*, 71(1):1–10, 1984.

[7] A. Aliev, V. Fedorov, S. Leonov, and B. McHugh. PkStaMp library for optimization of sampling schemes for PK/PD models. In S.M. Ermakov, V.B. Melas, and A.N. Pepelyshev, editors, *Proceedings of the 6th St. Petersburg Workshop on Simulation*, volume 1, pages 368–374. VVM com Ltd., St. Petersburg, Russia, 2009.

[8] A. Aliev, V. Fedorov, S. Leonov, B. McHugh, and M. Magee. PkStaMp library for constructing optimal population designs for PK/PD studies. *Comm. Stat. Simul. Comp.*, 41(6):717–729, 2012.

[9] D. Anbar. A stochastic Newton-Raphson method. *J. Statist. Plann. Inf.*, 2:153–163, 1978.

[10] T.W. Anderson and J.B. Taylor. Some experimental results on the statistical properties of least squares estimates in control problems. *Econometrica*, 44(6):1289–1302, 1976.

[11] G.E. Andrews, R. Askey, and R. Roy. *Special Functions*. Cambridge University Press, Cambridge, 1999.

[12] V.V. Anisimov, V.V. Fedorov, and S.L. Leonov. Optimal design of pharmacokinetic studies described by stochastic differential equations. In J. López-Fidalgo, J.M. Rodriguez-Diaz, and B. Torsney, editors, *mODa 8 – Advances in Model-Oriented Design and Analysis*, pages 9–16. Physica-Verlag, Heidelberg, 2007.

[13] J.R. Ashford and R. R. Sowden. Multi-variate probit analysis. *Biometrics*, 26:535–546, 1970.

[14] A.C. Atkinson. A segmented algorithm for simulated annealing. *Statist. Computing*, 2(4):221–230, 1992.

[15] A.C. Atkinson. Examples of the use of an equivalence theorem in constructing optimum experimental designs for random-effects nonlinear regression models. *J. Statist. Plann. Inf.*, 36:2595–2606, 2008.

[16] A.C. Atkinson, K. Chaloner, A.M. Herzberg, and J. Juritz. Optimal experimental designs for properties of a compartmental model. *Biometrics*, 49:325–337, 1993.

[17] A.C. Atkinson and R.D. Cook. D-optimum designs for heteroscedastic linear models. *J. Am. Statist. Assoc.*, 90(429):204–212, 1995.

[18] A.C. Atkinson and D.R. Cox. Planning experiments for discriminating between models (with discussion). *J. Royal Statist. Soc. B*, 36:321–348, 1974.

[19] A.C. Atkinson and A. Donev. *Optimum Experimental Design*. Clarendon Press, Oxford, 1992.

[20] A.C. Atkinson and V.V. Fedorov. Optimal design: Experiments for discriminating between several models. *Biometrika*, 62:289–303, 1974.

[21] A.C. Atkinson and V.V. Fedorov. Optimal design: Experiments for discriminating between two rival models. *Biometrika*, 62:57–70, 1974.

[22] A.C. Atkinson and V.V. Fedorov. The optimum design of experiments in the presence of uncontrolled variability and prior information. In Y. Dodge, V.V. Fedorov, and H. Wynn, editors, *Optimal Design and Analysis of Experiments*, pages 327–344. North-Holland, Amsterdam, 1988.

[23] A.C. Atkinson, V.V. Fedorov, A.M. Herzberg, and R. Zhang. Elemental information matrices and optimal experimental design for generalized regression models. *J. Statist. Plann. Inf.*, Early view, http://dx.doi.org/10.1016/j.jspi.2012.09.012, 2012.

[24] A.C. Atkinson, R. Tobias, and A. Donev. *Optimum Experimental Designs, with SAS*. Oxford University Press, 2007.

[25] C.L. Atwood. Sequences converging to *D*-optimal designs of experiments. *Ann. Stat.*, 1:342–352, 1973.

[26] M. Avriel. *Nonlinear Programming: Analysis and Methods*. Dover Publications, Mineola, NY, 2003.

[27] D. Azriel, M. Mandel, and Y. Rinott. The treatment versus experimentation dilemma in dose finding studies. *J. Statist. Plann. Inf.*, 141(8):2759–2768, 2011.

[28] A.J. Bailer and W.W. Piegorsch. Estimating integrals using quadrature methods with an application in pharmacokinetics. *Biometrics*, 46(4):1201–1211, 1990.

[29] R. A. Bailey. *Design of Comparative Experiments*. Cambridge University Press, Cambridge, UK, 2008.

[30] H. Bandemer, A. Bellmann, W. Jung, Le Anh Son, S. Nagel, W. Näther, J. Pilz, and K. Richter. *Theorie and Anwendung der Optimalen Versuchsplanung. I. Handbuch zur Theorie*. Akademie-Verlag, Berlin, 1977.

[31] J. Bartroff and T.L. Lai. Approximate dynamic programming and its application to the design of phase I cancer trials. *Statistical Science*, 25(2):245–257, 2010.

[32] J. Bartroff, T.L. Lai, and M.C. Shih. *Sequential Experimentation in Clinical Trials: Design and Analysis*, volume 298 of *Springer Series in Statistics*. Springer, New York, 2013.

[33] D.M. Bates and D.G. Watts. *Nonlinear Regression Analysis and Its Applications*. Wiley, New York, 1988.

[34] S. Batsell, V.V. Fedorov, and D. Flanagan. Multivariate prediction: Selection of the most informative components to measure. In A.C. Atkinson, L. Pronzato, and H. Wynn, editors, *Proceedings of MODA-5 International Workshop*, pages 215–222. Springer-Verlag, New York, 1988.

[35] P. Bauer. Adaptive designs: Looking for a needle in the haystack – A new challenge in medical research. *Statist. Med.*, 27(10):1565–1580, 2008.

[36] P. Bauer and W. Brannath. The advantages and disadvantages of adaptive designs in clinical trials. *Drug Discov. Today*, 9:351–357, 2004.

[37] R.J. Bauer, S. Guzy, and C. Ng. A survey of population analysis methods and software for complex pharmacokinetic and pharmacodynamic models with examples. *AAPS J.*, 9(1):E60–E83, 2007.

[38] C. Bazzoli, S. Retout, and F. Mentré. Fisher information matrix for nonlinear mixed effects multiple response models: Evaluation of the appropriateness of the first order linearization using a pharmacokinetic/pharmacodynamic model. *Statist. Med.*, 28(14):1940–1956, 2009.

[39] S.L. Beal and L.B. Sheiner. Heteroscedastic nonlinear regression. *Technometrics*, 30(3):327–338, 1988.

[40] S.L. Beal and L.B. Sheiner. *NONMEM User's Guide.* NONMEM Project Group, University of California, San Francisco, 1992.

[41] E.F. Beckenbach and Bellman R.E. *Inequalities.* Springer, Berlin, 1961.

[42] B. N. Bekele and Y. Shen. A Bayesian approach to jointly modeling toxicity and biomarker expression in a phase I/II dose-finding trial. *Biometrics*, 61:343–354, 2005.

[43] R. Bellman. *Introduction to Matrix Analysis.* SIAM, Philadelphia, 1995.

[44] M.P.F. Berger and W.K. Wong. *An Introduction to Optimal Designs for Social and Biomedical Research (Statistics in Practice).* Wiley, Chichester, 2009.

[45] J.M. Bernardo. Expected information as expected utility. *Ann. Statist.*, 7:686–690, 1979.

[46] J.M. Bernardo and A.F.M. Smith. *Bayesian Theory.* Wiley, New York, 1994.

[47] D.A. Berry, P. Müller, A. P. Grieve, M.K. Smith, T. Parke, R. Blazek, N. Mitchard, and M. Krams. Adaptive Bayesian designs for dose-ranging drug trials. In C. Gatsonis, R.E. Kass, B. Carlin, A. Carriquiry, A. Gelman, I. Verdinelli, and M. West, editors, *Case Studies in Bayesian Statistics V*, volume 162 of *Lecture Notes in Statistics*, pages 99–181. Springer, New York, 2002.

[48] I.O. Bohachevsky, M.E. Johnson, and M.L. Stein. Generalized simulated annealing for function optimization. *Technometrics*, 28(3):209–217, 1986.

[49] P. Bonate. *Pharmacokinetic-Pharmacodynamic Modeling and Simulation.* Springer, New York, 2010.

[50] B. Bornkamp, F. Bretz, A. Dmitrienko, G. Enas, B. Gaydos, C.-H. Hsu, F. König, M. Krams, Q. Liu, B. Neuenschwander, T. Park, J. Pinheiro, A. Roy, R. Sax, and F. Shen. Innovative approaches for designing and analyzing adaptive dose-ranging trials. *J. Biopharm. Statist.*, 17:965–995, 2007.

[51] G.E.P. Box and W.J. Hill. Discrimination among mechanistic models. *Technometrics*, 9:327–338, 1967.

[52] G.E.P. Box and W.J. Hill. Correcting inhomogeneity of variance with power transformation weighting. *Technometrics*, 16:385–389, 1974.

[53] G.E.P. Box and W.G. Hunter. Sequential design of experiments for nonlinear models. In J.J Korth, editor, *Proceedings of IBM Scientific Computing Symposium*. IBM, White Plains, NY, 1965.

[54] G.E.P. Box and H.L. Lucas. Design of experiments in nonlinear situations. *Biometrika*, 46:77–90, 1959.

[55] A. Bozin and M. Zarrop. Self-tuning extremum optimizer – Convergence and robustness properties. In *Proceedings of ECC 91, First European Control Conference*, pages 672–677, 1991.

[56] T. Braun. The bivariate continual reassessment method: Extending the CRM to phase I trials of two competing outcomes. *Controlled Clinical Trials*, 23:240–256, 2002.

[57] L.D. Brown, I. Olkin, J. Sacks, and Wynn H.P., editors. *Jack Kiefer. Collected Papers III. Design of Experiments*. Springer, New York, 1985.

[58] J.F.C.L. Cadima and I.T. Jolliffe. Variable selection and the interpretation of principal subspaces. *J. Agricultural, Biological, and Environmental Statistics*, 6:62–79, 2001.

[59] S. Cambanis. Sampling designs for time series. In E.J. Hannan, P.R. Krishnaiah, and M.M. Rao, editors, *Time Series in the Time Domain. Handbook of Statistics*, volume 5, pages 337–362. North-Holland, Amsterdam, 1985.

[60] R.J. Carroll and D. Ruppert. Robust estimation in heteroscedastic linear models. *Ann. Statist.*, 10:429–441, 1982.

[61] R.J. Carroll and D. Ruppert. *Transformation and Weighting in Regression*. Chapman & Hall, New York, 1988.

[62] W.F. Caselton, L. Kan, and J.V. Zidek. Quality data networks that minimize entropy. In A.T. Walden and P. Guttorp, editors, *Statistics in the Environmental and Earth Sciences*, pages 10–38. Arnold, London, 1992.

[63] W.F. Caselton and J.V. Zidek. Optimal monitoring network designs. *Statist. Prob. Lett.*, 2:223–227, 1984.

[64] K. Chaloner. Optimal Bayesian experimental design for linear models. *Ann. Statist.*, 12:283–300, 1984.

[65] K. Chaloner and I. Verdinelli. Bayesian experimental design: A review. *Statistical Science*, 10:273–304, 1995.

[66] H.H. Chang and Z. Ying. Nonlinear sequential designs for logistic item response theory models with applications to computerized adaptive tests. *Ann. Statist.*, 37(3):1466–1488, 2009.

[67] M. Chang. *Adaptive Design Theory and Implementation Using SAS and R.* Chapman & Hall/CRC, Boca Raton, FL, 2008.

[68] P. Chaudhuri and P.A. Mykland. Nonlinear experiments: Optimal design and inference based on likelihood. *J. Am. Stat. Assoc.*, 88:538–546, 1993.

[69] P. Chaudhuri and P.A. Mykland. On efficient designing of nonlinear experiments. *Statistica Sinica*, 5:421–440, 1995.

[70] H. Chernoff. Locally optimal designs for estimating parameters. *Ann. Math. Statist.*, 24:586–602, 1953.

[71] H. Chernoff. *Sequential Analysis and Optimal Design*. SIAM, Philadelphia, 1972.

[72] Y.K. Cheung. Stochastic approximation and modern model-based designs for dose-finding clinical trials. *Statistical Science*, 25(2):191–201, 2010.

[73] Y.K. Cheung. *Dose Finding by the Continual Reassessment Method.* Chapman & Hall/CRC, Boca Raton, FL, 2011.

[74] S. Chevret, editor. *Statistical Methods for Dose-Finding Experiments*. Wiley, New York, 2006.

[75] S. Chib and Greenberg E. Analysis of multivariate probit models. *Biometrika*, 85:347–361, 1998.

[76] W.L. Chiou. Critical evaluation of the potential error in pharmacokinetic studies of using the linear trapezoidal rule method for the calculation of the area under the plasma level-time curve. *J. Pharmacokinet. Biopharm.*, 6(6):539–546, 1978.

[77] W.G. Cochran. Experiments for nonlinear functions (R.A. Fisher Memorial Lecture). *J. Am. Stat. Assoc.*, 68:771–781, 1973.

[78] R.D. Cook. Influential observations in linear regression. *J. Am. Stat. Assoc.*, 74(365):169–174, 1979.

[79] R.D. Cook and V.V. Fedorov. Constrained optimization of experimental design. *Statistics*, 26:129–178, 1995.

[80] R.D. Cook and W.K. Wong. On the equivalence of constrained and compound optimal designs. *J. Am. Stat. Assoc.*, 89(426):687–692, 1994.

[81] T.M. Cover and J.A. Thomas. *Elements of Information Theory.* Wiley, New York, 1991.

[82] D.R. Cox. *The Analysis of Binary Data.* Chapman & Hall, London, 1970.

[83] H. Cramèr. *Mathematical Methods of Statistics.* Princeton University Press, Princeton, NJ, 1946.

[84] J.S. Cramer. *Logit Models from Economics and Other Fields.* Cambridge University Press, Cambridge, 2003.

[85] O. Cureton and D. D'Agostino. *Factor Analysis: An Applied Approach.* Lawrence Erlbaum, Hillsdale, NY, 1983.

[86] D.Z. D'Argenio. Optimal sampling times for pharmacokinetic experiments. *J. Pharmacokin. Biopharmaceut.*, 9(6):739–756, 1981.

[87] D.Z. D'Argenio. Incorporating prior parameter uncertainty in the design of sampling schedules for pharmacokinetic parameter estimation experiments. *Math. Biosci.*, 99:105–118, 1990.

[88] D.Z. D'Argenio, A. Schumitzky, and X. Wang. *ADAPT 5 User's Guide: Pharmacokinetic/Pharmacodynamic Systems Analysis Software.* Biomedical Simulations Resource, University of Southern California, Los Angeles, 2009.

[89] M. Davidian and R.J. Carroll. Variance function estimation. *J. Am. Stat. Assoc.*, 82:1079–1091, 1987.

[90] M. Davidian and D.M. Giltinan. *Nonlinear Models for Repeated Measurement Data.* Chapman & Hall, London, 1995.

[91] A. de la Garza. Spacing of information in polynomial regression. *Ann. Math. Statist.*, 25:123–130, 1954.

[92] B. Delyon, M. Lavielle, and E. Moulines. Convergence of a stochastic approximation version of the EM algorithm. *Ann. Statist.*, 27(1):94–128, 1999.

[93] E. Demidenko. *Mixed Models. Theory and Application.* Wiley, Hoboken, NJ, 2004.

[94] C. Derman. Non-parametric up-and-down experimentation. *Ann. Math. Statist.*, 28:795–798, 1957.

[95] H. Dette and V.B. Melas. A note on the de la Garza phenomenon for locally optimal designs. *Ann. Statist.*, 39(2):1266–1281, 2011.

[96] H. Dette, A. Pepelyshev, and T. Holland-Letz. Optimal designs for random effect models with correlated errors with applications in population pharmacokinetics. *Ann. Appl. Statist.*, 4(3):1430–1450, 2010.

[97] H. Dette, A. Pepelyshev, and A. Zhigljavsky. Improving updating rules in multiplicative algorithms for computing D-optimal designs. *Comput. Statist. Data Anal.*, 53:312–320, 2008.

[98] H. Dette and W.K. Wong. Optimal designs when the variance is a function of the mean. *Biometrics*, 55:925–929, 1999.

[99] W.J. Dixon and A.M. Mood. A method for obtaining and analyzing sensitivity data. *J. Am. Statist. Assoc.*, 13(1):109–126, 1948.

[100] D.J. Downing, V.V. Fedorov, and S.L. Leonov. Extracting information from the variance function: Optimal design. In A.C. Atkinson, P. Hackl, and W.G. Müller, editors, *mODa6 – Advances in Model-Oriented Design and Analysis*, pages 45–52. Physica-Verlag, Heidelberg, 2001.

[101] V. Dragalin and V.V. Fedorov. Adaptive designs for dose-finding based on efficacy-toxicity response. *J. Stat. Plann. Inf.*, 136:1800–1823, 2006.

[102] V. Dragalin, V.V. Fedorov, and Y. Wu. Optimal designs for bivariate probit model. BDS Technical Report 2006-01. GlaxoSmithKline Pharmaceuticals, 2006.

[103] V. Dragalin, V.V. Fedorov, and Y. Wu. Adaptive designs for selecting drug combinations based on efficacy-toxicity response. *J. Stat. Plann. Inf.*, 138(2):352–373, 2008.

[104] V. Dragalin, F. Hsuan, and S.K. Padmanabhan. Adaptive designs for dose-finding studies based on sigmoid E_{max} model. *J. Biopharm. Statist.*, 18:1051–1070, 2007.

[105] N.R. Draper and W.G. Hunter. The use of prior distributions in the design of experiments for parameter estimation in non-linear situations. *Biometrika*, 54:147–153, 1967.

[106] N.R. Draper and H. Smith. *Applied Regression Analysis*. Wiley, New York, 3rd edition, 1998.

[107] S.B. Duffull, S. Retout, and F. Mentré. The use of simulated annealing for finding optimal population designs. *Comput. Methods Programs Biomed.*, 69:25–35, 2002.

[108] S.B. Duffull, T.H. Waterhouse, and J.A. Eccleston. Some considerations on the design of population pharmacokinetic studies. *J. Pharmacokin. Pharmacodyn.*, 32:441–457, 2005.

[109] V. Dupa and U. Herkenrath. Stochastic approximation on a discrete set and the multi-armed bandit problem. *Comm. Statist. Sequential Analysis*, 1(1):1–25, 2007.

[110] S.D. Durham and N. Flournoy. Random walks for quantile estimation. In S.S. Gupta and J.O. Berger, editors, *Statistical Decision Theory and Related Topics, V*, pages 467–476. Springer, New York, 1994.

[111] S.D. Durham and N. Flournoy. Up-and-down designs I: Stationary treatment distributions. In N. Flournoy and W.F. Rosenberger, editors, *Adaptive Designs*, volume 25 of *IMS Lecture Notes - Monograph Series*, pages 139–157. Institute of Mathematical Statistics, Hayward, CA, 1995.

[112] S.D. Durham, N. Flournoy, and W. Li. A sequential design for maximizing the probability of a favourable response. *Canad. J. Statist.*, 26(3):479–495, 1998.

[113] O. Dykstra. The augmentation of experimental data to maximize $|X'X|$. *Technometrics*, 13:682–688, 1971.

[114] G. Elfving. Optimum allocation in linear regression theory. *Ann. Math. Statist.*, 23:255–262, 1952.

[115] S.M. Ermakov, editor. *Mathematical Theory of Experimental Design*. Nauka, Moscow, 1983.

[116] S.M. Ermakov and A.A. Zhigljavsky. *Mathematical Theory of Optimal Experiment*. Nauka, Moscow, 1987.

[117] E.I. Ette, A.W. Kelman, C.A. Howie, and B. Whiting. Interpretation of simulation studies for efficient estimation of population pharmacokinetic parameters. *Ann. Pharmacotherapy*, 27:1034–1039, 1993.

[118] E.I. Ette, A.W. Kelman, C.A. Howie, and B. Whiting. Analysis of animal pharmacokinetic data: Performance of the one point per animal design. *J. Pharmacokin. Biopharmaceut.*, 23(6):551–566, 1995.

[119] E.I. Ette, H. Sun, and T.M. Ludden. Balanced designs in longitudinal population pharmacokinetic studies. *J. Clin. Pharmacol.*, 38:417–423, 1998.

[120] J.W. Evans. Computer augmentation of experimental data to maximize $|X'X|$. *Technometrics*, 21:321–330, 1979.

[121] M. Evans and T. Swartz. *Approximating Integrals via Monte Carlo and Deterministic Methods*. Oxford University Press, Oxford, 2000.

[122] S.K. Fan and K. Chaloner. Optimal design for a continuation-ratio model. In A.C. Atkinson, P. Hackl, and W.G. Müller, editors, *mODa6 – Advances in Model-Oriented Design and Analysis*, pages 77–85. Physica-Verlag, Heidelberg, 2001.

[123] D. Faries. Practical modification of the continual reassessment method for phase I cancer clinical trials. *J. Biopharm. Statist.*, 4:147–164, 1994.

[124] FDA. *Adaptive Design Clinical Trials for Drugs and Biologics, Draft Guidance.* FDA, http://www.fda.gov/downloads/Drugs/GuidanceComplianceRegulatoryInformation/Guidances/UCM201790.pdf, 2010.

[125] V.V. Fedorov. *Theory of Optimal Experiment.* Moscow University Press, Moscow (in Russian), 1969.

[126] V.V. Fedorov. The design of experiments in the multiresponse case. *Theory Probab. Appl.*, 16:323–332, 1971.

[127] V.V. Fedorov. *Theory of Optimal Experiment.* Academic Press, New York, 1972.

[128] V.V. Fedorov. Regression problems with controllable variables subject to error. *Biometrika*, 61:49–56, 1974.

[129] V.V. Fedorov. Parameter estimation for multivariate regression. In V. Nalimov, editor, *Regression Experiments (Design and Analysis)*, pages 112–122. Moscow Universtiy Press, Moscow, 1977.

[130] V.V. Fedorov. Design of model testing experiments. In *Symposia Matematica*, volume XXV, pages 171–180. Instituto Nazionale Di Alta Matematica, 1981.

[131] V.V. Fedorov. Design of spatial experiments: model fitting and prediction. In S. Ghosh and C.R. Rao, editors, *Design and Analysis of Experiments*, volume 13 of *Handbook of Statistics*, pages 515–553. Elsevier, North Holland, 1996.

[132] V.V. Fedorov, N. Flournoy, Y. Wu, and R. Zhang. Best intention designs in dose-finding studies. Preprint NI11065-DAE, http://www.newton.ac.uk/preprints/NI11065.pdf. Isaac Newton Institute for Mathematical Sciences, Cambridge, UK, 2011.

[133] V.V. Fedorov, R. Gagnon, S. Leonov, and Y. Wu. Optimal design of experiments in pharmaceutical applications. In A. Dmitrienko, C. Chuang-Stein, and R. D'Agostino, editors, *Pharmaceutical Statistics Using SAS. A Practical Guide*, pages 151–195. SAS Press, Cary, NC, 2007.

[134] V.V. Fedorov, R. Gagnon, and S.L. Leonov. Design of experiments with unknown parameters in variance. *Appl. Stoch. Models Bus. Ind.*, 18:207–218, 2002.

[135] V.V. Fedorov and P. Hackl. *Model-Oriented Design of Experiments*. Springer, New York, 1997.

[136] V.V. Fedorov, P. Hackl, and W. Müller. Estimation and experimental design for second kind regression models. *Inform. Biom. Epidem. Med. Biol.*, 24(3):134–151, 1993.

[137] V.V. Fedorov, A.M. Herzberg, and S.L. Leonov. Component-wise dimension reduction. *J. Stat. Plann. Inf.*, 114:81–93, 2003.

[138] V.V. Fedorov, A.M. Herzberg, and S.L. Leonov. Methods of selecting informative variables. *Biometrical J.*, 48(1):157–173, 2006.

[139] V.V. Fedorov and B. Jones. The design of multicentre trials. *Statist. Meth. Med. Res.*, 14(3):205–48, 2005.

[140] V.V. Fedorov and V. Khabarov. Duality of optimal designs for model discrimination and parameter estimation. *Biometrika*, 73:183–190, 1986.

[141] V.V. Fedorov and S.L. Leonov. Optimal design of dose-response experiments: A model-oriented approach. *Drug Inf. J.*, 35(4):1373–1383, 2001.

[142] V.V. Fedorov and S.L. Leonov. Optimal designs for regression models with forced measurements at baseline. In A. Di Bucchianico, H. Läuter, and H. Wynn, editors, *mODa 7 – Advances in Model-Oriented Design and Analysis*, pages 61–69. Physica-Verlag, Heidelberg, 2004.

[143] V.V. Fedorov and S.L. Leonov. Parameter estimation for models with unknown parameters in variance. *Comm. Statist. Theory Meth.*, 33(11):2627–2657, 2004.

[144] V.V. Fedorov and S.L. Leonov. Response driven designs in drug development. In W.K. Wong and M.P.F. Berger, editors, *Applied Optimal Designs*, pages 103–136. Wiley, Chichester, 2005.

[145] V.V. Fedorov and S.L. Leonov. Estimation of population PK measures: Selection of sampling grids. BDS Technical Report 2006-02. GlaxoSmithKline Pharmaceuticals, 2006.

[146] V.V. Fedorov and S.L. Leonov. Population pharmacokinetic measures, their estimation and selection of sampling times. *J. Biopharm. Statist.*, 17(5):919–941, 2007.

[147] V.V. Fedorov, S.L. Leonov, and V.A. Vasiliev. Pharmacokinetic studies described by stochastic differential equations: Optimal design for systems with positive trajectories. In A. Giovagnoli, A.C. Atkinson, and B. Torsney, editors, *mODa 9 – Advances in Model-Oriented Design and Analysis*, pages 73–80. Physica-Verlag/Springer, Berlin, 2010.

[148] V.V. Fedorov and M.B. Malyutov. Optimal designs in regression problems. *Math. Operat. Statist.*, 3:281–308, 1972.

[149] V.V. Fedorov and W. Müller. Comparison of two approaches in the optimal design of an observation network. *Statistics*, 20(3):339–351, 1989.

[150] V.V. Fedorov and A. Pázman. Design of physical experiments (statistical methods). *Fortschritte der Physik*, 24:325–345, 1968.

[151] V.V. Fedorov and A.B. Uspensky. *Numerical Aspects of Design and Analysis of Regression Experiments*. Moscow State University Press, Moscow, 1975.

[152] V.V. Fedorov and Y. Wu. Dose finding designs for continuous responses and binary utility. *J. Biopharm. Statist.*, 17(6):1085–1096, 2007.

[153] V.V. Fedorov, Y. Wu, and R. Zhang. Optimal dose-finding designs with correlated continuous and discrete responses. *Statist. Med.*, 31(3):217–234, 2012.

[154] J. Fellman. On the allocation of linear observations. *Soc. Sci. Fenn. Comment. Phys.-Math.*, 44:27–78, 1974.

[155] D.J. Finney. *Probit Analysis*. Cambridge University Press, Cambridge, 1971.

[156] D.J. Finney. Radioligand assay. *Biometrics*, 32:721–740, 1976.

[157] R.A. Fisher. *The Design of Experiments*. Hafner, Ney York, 8th edition, 1971.

[158] N. Flournoy. A clinical experiment in bone marrow transplantation: Estimating a percentage point of a quantal response curve. In C. C. Gatsonis, J.S. Hodges, R.E. Kass, and N.D. Singpurwala, editors, *Case Studies in Bayesian Statistics*, pages 324–336. Springer-Verlag, New York., 1993.

[159] N. Flournoy, W.F. Rosenberger, and W.K. Wong, editors. *New Developments and Applications in Experimental Design*, volume 34 of *IMS Lecture Notes - Monograph Series*. Institute of Mathematical Statistics, Hayward, CA, 1998.

[160] B. Flury. *Common Principal Components and Related Multivariate Models*. Wiley, New York, 1988.

[161] I. Ford and S.D. Silvey. A sequentially constructed design for estimating a nonlinear parametric function. *Biometrika*, 67(2):381–388, 1980.

[162] I. Ford, B. Torsney, and C.F.J. Wu. The use of a canonical form in the construction of locally-optimal designs for nonlinear problems. *J. Roy. Statist. Soc. B*, 54:569–583, 1992.

[163] G.E. Forsythe, M.A. Malcolm, and C.B. Moler. *Computer Methods for Mathematical Computations*. Prentice Hall, Englewood Cliffs, NJ, 1976.

[164] D. Fuller and W. Scherer. The desirability function: Underlying assumptions and application implications. In *Proceedings of 1998 IEEE International Conference on Systems, Man, and Cybernetics*, volume 4, pages 4016–4021. IEEE, 1998.

[165] J. Gabrielsson and D. Weiner. *Pharmacokinetic and Pharmacodynamic Data Analysis, Concepts and Applications*. Swedish Pharmaceutical Press, Stockholm, 3rd edition, 2001.

[166] N. Gaffke and R. Mathar. On a class of algorithms from experimental design. *Optimization*, 24:91–126, 1992.

[167] R. Gagnon and S. Leonov. Optimal population designs for PK models with serial sampling. *J. Biopharm. Statist.*, 15(1):143–163, 2005.

[168] R. Gagnon and J.J. Peterson. Estimation of confidence intervals for area under the curve from destructively obtained pharmacokinetic data. *J. Pharmacokinet. Biopharm.*, 26(1):87–102, 1998.

[169] P. Gallo, C. Chuang-Stein, V. Dragalin, B. Gaydos, M. Krams, and J. Pinheiro. Adaptive designs in clinical drug development – An executive summary of the PhRMA Working Group. *J. Biopharm. Statist.*, 16(3):143–163, 2006.

[170] C.W. Gardiner. *Handbook of Stochastic Methods for Physics, Chemistry and the Natural Sciences*. Springer, Berlin, 3rd edition, 2003.

[171] E. Garrett-Mayer. The continual reassessment method for dose-finding studies: A tutorial. *Clin. Trials*, 3:57–71, 2006.

[172] B. Gaydos, K.M. Anderson, D. Berry, N. Burnham, C. Chuang-Stein, J. Dudinak, P. Fardipour, P. Gallo, S. Givens, R. Lewis, J. Maca, J. Pinheiro, Y. Pritchett, and M. Krams. Good practices for adaptive clinical trials in pharmaceutical product development. *Drug Inf. J.*, 43:539–556, 2009.

[173] M. Gezmu and N. Flournoy. Group up-and-down designs for dose-finding. *J. Statist. Plann. Inf.*, 136(6):1749–1764, 2006.

[174] M. Ghosh, N. Mukhopadhyay, and P.K. Sen. *Sequential Estimation.* Wiley, New York, 1997.

[175] M. Gibaldi. *Biopharmaceutics and Clinical Pharmacokinetics.* Lea & Febiger, Philadelphia, PA, 1984.

[176] M. Gibaldi and D. Perrier. *Pharmacokinetics.* Marcel Dekker, New York, 2nd edition, 1971.

[177] J. Gladitz and J. Pilz. Construction of optimal designs in random coefficient regression models. *Statistics*, 13:371–385, 1982.

[178] S.N. Goodman, M.L. Zahurak, and S. Piantadosi. Some practical improvements in the continual reassessment method for phase I studies. *Statist. Med.*, 14:1149–1161, 1995.

[179] T.A. Gooley, P.J. Martin, D.F. Lloyd, and M. Pettinger. Simulation as a design tool for phase I/II clinical trials: An example from bone marrow transplantation. *Controlled Clinical Trials*, 15:450–460, 1994.

[180] P. Goos and B. Jones. *Optimal Design of Experiments: A Case Study Approach.* Wiley, New York, 2011.

[181] I.S. Gradshteyn and I.M. Ryzhik. *Table of Integrals, Series, and Products.* Academic Press, San Diego, 5th edition, 1994.

[182] G. Graham and L. Aarons. Optimum blood sampling windows for parameter estimation in population pharmacokinetic experiments. *Statist. Med.*, 25:4004–4019, 2006.

[183] I. Gueorguieva, K. Ogungbenro, G. Graham, S. Glatt, and L. Aarons. A program for individual and population optimal design for univariate and multivariate response pharmacokinetic-pharmacodynamic models. *Comput. Methods Programs Biomed.*, 86:51–61, 2007.

[184] P.G. Guest. The spacing of observations in polynomial regression. *Ann. Math. Statist.*, 29:294–299, 1958.

[185] P. Guttorp, N.D. Le, P.D. Sampson, and J.V. Zidek. Using entropy in the redesign of an environmental monitoring network. In G. P. Patil and C.R. Rao, editors, *Multivariate Environmental Statistics*, pages 173–202. North Holland, Amsterdam, 1993.

[186] L.M. Haines. The application of the annealing algorithm to the construction of exact optimal designs for linear-regression models. *Technometrics*, 29(4):439–447, 1987.

[187] L.M. Haines, I. Perevozskaya, and W.F. Rosenberger. Bayesian optimal designs for phase I clinical trials. *Biometrics*, 59:561–570, 2003.

[188] M. Hamada, H.F. Martz, C.S. Reese, and A.G. Wilson. Finding near-optimal Bayesian experimental designs via genetic algorithms. *Am. Statistician*, 55(3):175–181, 2001.

[189] C. Han and K. Chaloner. Bayesian experimental design for nonlinear mixed-effects models with application to HIV dynamics. *Biometrics*, 60:25–33, 2004.

[190] C. Han, K. Chaloner, and A.S. Perelson. Bayesian analysis of a population HIV dynamic model. In C. Gatsonis, A. Carriquiry, A. Gelman, D. Higdon, R. Kass, D. Pauler, and I. Verdinelli, editors, *Case Studies in Bayesian Statistics*, volume VI, pages 223–237. New York, Springer, 2002.

[191] J.W. Hardin and J.M. Hilbe. *Generalized Estimating Equations*. Chapman & Hall, Boca Raton, FL, 2003.

[192] J. Hardwick, M.C. Meyer, and Q.F. Stout. Directed walk designs for dose-response problems with competing failure modes. *Biometrics*, 59:229–236, 2003.

[193] J. Hardwick and Q.F. Stout. Optimizing a unimodal response function for binary variables. In A.C. Atkinson, B. Bogacka, and A. Zhigljavsky, editors, *Optimum Design 2000*, pages 195–208. Kluwer, Dordrecht, 2001.

[194] R. Harman and L. Pronzato. Improvements on removing nonoptimal support points in D-optimum design algorithms. *Statist. Probab. Lett.*, 77:90–94, 2007.

[195] D.A. Harville. *Matrix Algebra From a Statistician's Perspective*. Springer, New York, 1997.

[196] R. Haycroft, L. Pronzato, H.P. Wynn, and A.A. Zhigljavsky. Studying convergence of gradient algorithm via optimal experimental design theory. In L. Pronzato and A.A. Zhigljavsky, editors, *Optimal Design and Related Areas in Optimization and Statistics*, volume 28 of *Springer Optimization and Its Applications*, pages 13–37. Springer, New York, 2009.

[197] A.S. Hedayat, B. Yan, and J.M. Pezutto. Modeling and identifying optimum designs for fitting dose response curves based on raw optical data. *J. Am. Statist. Assoc.*, 92:1132–1140, 1997.

[198] M.A. Heise and R.H. Myers. Modeling and identifying optimum designs for fitting dose response curves based on raw optical data. *Biometrics*, 52:613–624, 1996.

[199] C.C. Heyde. *Quasi-Likelihood and Its Applications*. Springer, New York, 1997.

[200] P.D.H. Hill. *D*-optimal designs for partially nonlinear regression models. *Technometrics*, 22:275–276, 1980.

[201] P.G. Hoel. Efficiency problems in polynomial estimation. *Ann. Math. Statist.*, 29:1134–1145, 1958.

[202] P.G. Hoel. Asymptotic efficiency in polynomial estimation. *Ann. Math. Statist.*, 32:1042–1047, 1961.

[203] P.G. Hoel. Minimax designs in two dimensional regression. *Ann. Math. Statist.*, 36:1097–1106, 1965.

[204] P.G. Hoel. Optimum designs for polynomial extrapolation. *Ann. Math. Statist.*, 36:1483–1493, 1965.

[205] T. Holland-Letz, H. Dette, and D. Renard. Efficient algorithms for optimal designs with correlated observations in pharmacokinetics and dose-finding studies. *Biometrics*, 68(1):138–145, 2012.

[206] D.W. Hosmer and S. Lemeshow. *Applied Logistic Regression*. Wiley, New York, 2000.

[207] I. Hu. On sequential designs in nonlinear problems. *Biometrika*, 85:496–503, 1998.

[208] S. Huet, A. Bouvier, M.-A. Poursat, and E. Jolivet. *Statistical Tools for Nonlinear Regression. A Practical Guide with S-PLUS and R examples.* Springer, New York, 2000.

[209] A. Ivanova. A new dose-finding design for bivariate outcomes. *Biometrics*, 59:1001–1007, 2003.

[210] A. Ivanova, C. Xiao, and Y. Tymofyeyev. Two-stage designs for phase 2 dose-finding trials. *Statist. Med.*, 31(24):1001–1007, 2012.

[211] C. Jennison and B.W. Turnbull. *Group Sequential Methods with Applications to Clinical Trials.* Chapman & Hall, Boca Raton, FL, 2000.

[212] R.I. Jennrich. Asymptotic properties of nonlinear least squares estimators. *Ann. Math. Statist.*, 40:633–643, 1969.

[213] R.I. Jennrich and M.D. Schluchter. Unbalanced repeated-measures models with structured covariance matrices. *Biometrics*, 42:805–820, 1986.

[214] R. Jin, W. Chen, and A. Sudjianto. An efficient algorithm for constructing optimal design of computer experiments. *J. Stat. Plann. Inf.*, 134:268–287, 2005.

[215] J.D. Jobson and W.A. Fuller. Least squares estimation when the covariance matrix and parameter vector are functionally related. *J. Am. Stat. Assoc.*, 75:176–181, 1980.

[216] M.E. Johnson and C.J. Nachtsheim. Some guidelines for constructing exact *D*-optimal designs on convex design spaces. *Technometrics*, 25:271–277, 1983.

[217] N.L. Johnson, A.W. Kemp, and N. Balakrishnan. *Univariate Discrete Distributions*. Wiley, New York, 3rd edition, 2005.

[218] N.L. Johnson, S. Kotz, and N. Balakrishnan. *Continuous Univariate Distributions – 1*. Wiley, New York, 2nd edition, 1994.

[219] N.L. Johnson, S. Kotz, and N. Balakrishnan. *Continuous Univariate Distributions – 2*. Wiley, New York, 2nd edition, 1995.

[220] N.L. Johnson, S. Kotz, and N. Balakrishnan. *Discrete Multivariate Distributions*. Wiley, New York, 1997.

[221] I.T. Jolliffe. *Principal Component Analysis*. Springer-Verlag, New York, 2nd edition, 2002.

[222] S.A. Julious and C.A.M. Debarnot. Why are pharmacokinetic data summarized by arithmetic means? *J. Biopharm. Statist.*, 10(1):55–71, 2000.

[223] L.A. Kalish and J.L. Rosenberger. Optimal designs for the estimation of the logistic function. Technical Report 33, Penn State University, University Park, PA, 1978.

[224] A. Källén and P. Larsson. Dose response studies: How do we make them conclusive? *Statist. Med.*, 18:629–641, 1999.

[225] S. Karlin and W. Studden. *Tchebysheff Systems: With Applications in Analysis and Statisticss*. Wiley, New York, 1966.

[226] K.F. Karpinski. Optimality assessment in the enzyme-linked immunosorbent assay (ELISA). *Biometrics*, 46:381–390, 1990.

[227] A.I. Khuri. A note on *D*-optimal designs for partially nonlinear regression models. *Technometrics*, 26(1):59–61, 1984.

[228] J. Kiefer. Optimum experimental designs V, with applications to systematic and rotable designs. In *Proc. Fourth Berkeley Symp.*, volume 1, pages 381–405. University of California Press, Berkeley, CA, 1961.

[229] J. Kiefer. General equivalence theory for optimum designs (approximate theory). *Ann. Statist.*, 22:849–879, 1974.

[230] J. Kiefer and J. Wolfowitz. Stochastic estimation of the maximum of a regression function. *Ann. Math. Statist.*, 23:462–466, 1952.

[231] J. Kiefer and J. Wolfowitz. Consistency of the maximum likelihood estimator in the presence of infinitely many incidental parameters. *Ann. Math. Statist.*, 27(4):887–906, 1956.

[232] J. Kiefer and J. Wolfowitz. The equivalence of two extremum problems. *Canad. J. Math.*, 12:363–366, 1960.

[233] C.P. Kitsos, D.M. Titterington, and B. Torsney. An optimal design problem in rhythmometry. *Biometrics*, 44:657–671, 1988.

[234] N.P. Klepikov and S.N. Sokolov. *Analysis and Planning of Experiments by the Method of Maximum Likelihood.* Akademie-Verlag, Berlin, 1961.

[235] S. Kotz, N. Balakrishnan, and N.L. Johnson. *Continuous Multivariate Distributions*, volume 1. Wiley, New York, 2nd edition, 2000.

[236] S. Kotz, T. Kozubowski, and K. Podgorski. *The Laplace Distribution and Generalizations: A Revisit with Applications to Communications, Economics, Engineering, and Finance.* Birkhäuser, 2001.

[237] E. Kpamegan and N. Flournoy. An optimizing up-and-down design. In A.C. Atkinson, B. Bogacka, and A. Zhigljavsky, editors, *Optimum Design 2000*, pages 211–224. Kluwer, Dordrecht, 2001.

[238] E.P. Kpamegan. D-optimal design given a bivariate probit response function. In N. Flournoy, W.F. Rosenberger, and W.K. Wong, editors, *New Developments and Applications in Experimental Design*, volume 34 of *IMS Lecture Notes – Monograph Series*, pages 62–72. Institute of Mathematical Statistics, Hayward, CA, 1998.

[239] A.R. Krommer and C.W. Ueberhuber. *Computational Integration.* SIAM, Philadelphia, 1998.

[240] E. Kuhn and M. Lavielle. Maximum likelihood estimation in nonlinear mixed effects models. *Comput. Stat. Data An.*, 49:1020–1038, 2005.

[241] L.F. Lacey, O.N. Keene, J.F. Pritchard, and A. Bye. Common non-compartmental pharmacokinetic variables: Are they normally or log-normally distributed? *J. Biopharm. Statist.*, 7(1):171–178, 1997.

[242] T.L. Lai. Sequential analysis: some classical problems and new challenges. *Statistica Sinica*, 11(2):303–351, 2001.

[243] T.L. Lai. Stochastic approximation. *Ann. Statist.*, 31(2):391–406, 2003.

[244] T.L. Lai and H. Robbins. Adaptive design in regression and control. *Proc. Natl. Acad. Sci. USA*, 75(2):586–587, 1978.

[245] T.L. Lai and H. Robbins. Adaptive design and stochastic approximation. *Ann. Statist.*, 7:1196–1221, 1979.

[246] T.L. Lai and H. Robbins. Iterated least squares in multiperiod control. *Adv. Appl. Math.*, 3(1):50–73, 1982.

[247] T.L. Lai and C.Z. Wei. Least squares estimation in stochastic regression models, with application to identification and control of dynamic systems. *Ann. Statist.*, 10:154–166, 1982.

[248] P.J. Laurent. *Approximation et Optimization.* Hermann, Paris, 1972.

[249] E. Läuter. Experimental design in a class of models. *Math. Oper. Statist., Ser. Statist.*, 5:379–398, 1974.

[250] M. Lavielle and F. Mentré. Estimation of population pharmacokinetic parameters of saquinavir in HIV patients with the MONOLIX software. *J. Pharmacokin. Pharmacodyn.*, 34(2):229–249, 2007.

[251] L. Le Cam. *Asymptotic Methods in Statistical Decision Theory.* Springer, New York, 1986.

[252] E.L. Lehmann and G. Casella. *Theory of Point Estimation.* Springer, New York, 2nd edition, 1998.

[253] S. Leonov and A. Aliev. Optimal design for population PK/PD models. *Tatra Mountains Mathematical Publications*, 51:115–130, 2012.

[254] S. Leonov and S. Miller. An adaptive optimal design for the E_{max} model and its application in clinical trials. *J. Biopharm. Statist.*, 19(2):361–385, 2009.

[255] E. Lesaffre and G. Molenberghs. Multivariate probit analysis: A neglected procedure in medical statistics. *Statist. Med.*, 10:1391–1403, 1991.

[256] Z. Li, S.D. Durham, and N. Flournoy. An adaptive design for maximization of a contingent binary response. In N. Flournoy and W.F. Rosenberger, editors, *Adaptive Designs*, volume 25 of *IMS Lecture Notes – Monograph Series*, pages 139–157. Institute of Mathematical Statistics, Hayward, CA, 1995.

[257] B.W. Lindgren. *Statistical Theory.* Chapman & Hall, London, 4th edition, 1993.

[258] D.V. Lindley. On a measure of the information provided by an experiment. *Ann. Math. Statist.*, 27:986–1005, 1956.

[259] M.J. Lindstrom and D.M. Bates. Nonlinear mixed effects models for repeated measures data. *Biometrics*, 46:673–687, 1990.

[260] R.C. Littell, G.A. Milliken, W.W. Stroup, R.D. Wolfinger, and O. Schabenberger. *SAS for Mixed Models.* SAS Institute, Cary, NC, 2006.

[261] J. López-Fidalgo and W.K. Wong. Design issues for Michaelis-Menten model. *J. Theor. Biol.*, 215:1–11, 2002.

[262] J.R. Magnus and H. Neudecker. *Matrix Differential Calculus with Applications in Statistics and Econometrics*. Wiley, New York, 1988.

[263] A. Mallet. A maximum likelihood estimation method for random coefficient regression models. *Biometrika*, 41:1015–1023, 1986.

[264] M.B. Malyutov. Lower bounds for an average number of sequentially designed experiments. In K. Ito and Yu.V. Prokhorov, editors, *Probability Theory and Mathematical Statistics*, pages 419–434. Springer, Berlin, 1982.

[265] M.B. Malyutov. On asymptotic properties and application of IRGNA-estimates for parameters of generalized regression models. In *Stochastic Processes and Applications*, pages 144–165. Moscow (in Russian), 1982.

[266] M.B. Malyutov. Design and analysis in generalized regression model. In V.V. Fedorov and H. Läuter, editors, *Model-Oriented Data Analysis*, pages 72–76. Springer, Berlin, 1988.

[267] M. Marcus and H. Minc. *A Survey of Matrix Theory and Matrix Inequalities*. Dover, New York, 1992.

[268] R.J. Martin. Spatial experimental design. In S. Ghosh and C.R. Rao, editors, *Design and Analysis of Experiments*, volume 13 of *Handbook of Statistics*, pages 477–514. Elsevier, North Holland, 1996.

[269] R. Martín-Martín, L. Rodríguez-Aragón, and B. Torsney. Multiplicative algorithm for computing D-optimum designs for pVT measurements. *Chemometrics Intell. Lab. Syst.*, 111(1):20–27, 2012.

[270] B. Matérn. *Spatial Variation*. Springer, Berlin, 1986.

[271] T. Mathew and B.K. Sinha. Optimal designs for binary data under logistic regression. *J. Statist. Plann. Inf.*, 93:295–307, 2001.

[272] G.P. McCabe. Optimal designs for binary data under logistic regression. *Technometrics*, 26(2):137–144, 1984.

[273] D.L. McLeish and D. Tosh. Sequential designs in bioassay. *Biometrics*, 46:103–116, 1990.

[274] G. Megreditchan. L'optimization des reseaux d'observation des champs meteorologiques. *La Meterologie*, 6:51–66, 1979.

[275] V.B. Melas. *Functional Approach to Optimal Experimental Design*, volume 184 of *Lecture Notes in Statistics*. Springer, New York, 2006.

[276] F. Mentré, S. Duffull, I. Gueorguieva, A. Hooker, S. Leonov, K. Ogung-benro, and S. Retout. Software for optimal design in population pharmacokinetics and pharmacodynamics: A comparison. In *Abstracts of the Annual Meeting of the Population Approach Group in Europe. ISSN 1871-6032.* PAGE http://www.page-meeting.org/?abstract=1179, 2007.

[277] F. Mentré, A. Mallet, and D. Baccar. Optimal design in random-effects regression models. *Biometrika*, 84(2):429–442, 1997.

[278] F. Mentré, Y. Merlé, J. Van Bree, A. Mallet, and J.-L. Steimer. Sparse-sampling optimal designs in pharmacokinetics and toxicokinetics. *Drug Inf. J.*, 29:997–1019, 1995.

[279] F. Mentré, J. Nyberg, K. Ogungbenro, S. Leonov, A. Aliev, S. Duffull, C. Bazzoli, and A. Hooker. Comparison of results of the different software for design evaluation in population pharmacokinetics and pharmacodynamics. In *Abstracts of the Annual Meeting of the Population Approach Group in Europe (PAGE). ISSN 1871-6032.* PAGE http://www.page-meeting.org/default.asp?abstract=2066, 2011.

[280] Y. Merlé and M. Todd. Impact of pharmacokineticpharmacodynamic model linearization on the accuracy of population information matrix and optimal design. *J. Pharmacokin. Pharmacodyn.*, 28(4):363–388, 2001.

[281] R.K. Meyer and C.J. Nachtsheim. Constructing exact d-optimal experimental designs by simulated annealing. *Amer. J. Math. Manage. Sci.*, 8:329–359, 1988.

[282] C.A. Micchelli and G. Wahba. Design problem for optimal surface interpolation. In Z. Ziegler, editor, *Approximation Theory and Applications*, pages 329–348. Academic Press, New York, 1996.

[283] T. Mielke and R. Schwabe. Some considerations on the Fisher information in nonlinear mixed effects models. In A. Giovagnoli, A.C. Atkinson, and B. Torsney, editors, *mODa 9 – Advances in Model-Oriented Design and Analysis*, pages 129–136. Physica-Verlag/Springer, Berlin, 2010.

[284] F. Miller, O. Guilbaud, and Dette H. Optimal designs for estimating the interesting part of a dose-effect curve. *J. Biopharm. Statist.*, 17:1097–1115, 2007.

[285] S. Minkin. Optimal designs for binary data. *J. Am. Statist. Assoc.*, 82:1098–1103, 1987.

[286] T.J. Mitchell. An algorithm for construction of D-optimal experimental designs. *Technometrics*, 16:203–211, 1974.

[287] G. Molenberghs and G. Verbeke. *Models for Discrete Longitudinal Data.* Springer, New York, 2005.

[288] MONOLIX. *http://www.lixoft.net/monolix/overview/.* Lixoft, 2011.

[289] M. Morris. *Design of Experiments. An Introduction Based on Linear Models.* Chapman & Hall/CRC, Boca Raton, FL, 2010.

[290] R. Muirhead. *Aspects of Multivariate Statistical Theory.* Wiley, New York, 1982.

[291] W.G. Müller. *Collecting Spatial Data (Optimum Design of Experiments for Random Fields).* Springer, Berlin, 2007.

[292] P.A. Murtaugh and L.D. Fisher. Bivariate binary models of efficacy and toxicity in dose-ranging trials. *Commun. Statist. Theory Meth.*, 19:2003–2020, 1990.

[293] C.J. Nachtsheim. Tools for computer-aided design of experiments. *J. Qual. Technol.*, 19:132–160, 1987.

[294] J.R. Nedelman and E. Gibiansky. The variance of a better AUC estimator for sparse, destructive sampling in toxicokinetics. *J. Pharm. Sciences*, 85(8):884–886, 1996.

[295] A.U. Neumann, N.P. Lam, H. Dahari, D.R. Gretch, T.E. Wiley, T.J. Layden, and A.S. Perelson. Hepatitis C viral dynamics in vivo and the antiviral efficacy of interferon-α therapy. *Science*, 282:103–107, 1998.

[296] J. Nyberg, S. Ueckert, E. Strömberg, M.O. Karlsson, and A.C. Hooker. PopED, version 2.12. In *http://poped.sourceforge.net*, 2011.

[297] K. Ogungbenro and L. Aarons. An effective approach for obtaining optimal sampling windows for population pharmacokinetic experiments. *J. Biopharm. Statist.*, 19(1):174–189, 2009.

[298] J. O'Quigley. Dose-finding designs using continual reassessment method. In J. Crowley, editor, *Handbook of Statistics in Clinical Oncology*, pages 35–72. Marcel Dekker, New York, 2001.

[299] J. O'Quigley and M. Conaway. Continual reassessment and related dose-finding designs. *Statist. Sci.*, 25(2):245–257, 2010.

[300] J. O'Quigley, M. Hughes, and T. Fenton. Dose finding designs for HIV studies. *Biometrics*, 57:1018–1029, 2001.

[301] J. O'Quigley, M. Pepe, and L. Fisher. Continual reassessment method: A practical design for phase I clinical trials in cancer. *Biometrics*, 46:33–48, 1990.

[302] A.P. Oron and P.D. Hoff. The k-in-a-row up-and-down design, revisited. *Statist. Med.*, 28(13):1805–1820, 2009.

[303] R.V. Overgaard, N. Jonsson, C.W. Tornoe, and H. Madsen. Non-linear mixed-effects models with stochastic differential equations: implementation of an estimation algorithm. *J. Pharmacokinet. Pharmacodyn.*, 32(1):85–107, 2005.

[304] C.R. Palmer and W.F. Rosenberger. Ethics and practice: Alternative designs for phase III randomized clinical trials. *Controlled Clinical Trials*, 20:172–186, 1999.

[305] M. Patan and B. Bogacka. Efficient sampling windows for parameter estimation in mixed effects models. In J. López-Fidalgo, J.M. Rodriguez-Diaz, and B. Torsney, editors, *mODa 8 – Advances in Model-Oriented Design and Analysis*, pages 147–155. Physica-Verlag, Heidelberg, 2007.

[306] A. Pázman. *Foundations of Optimum Experimental Design*. Reidel, Dordrecht, 1986.

[307] A. Pázman. *Nonlinear Statistical Models*. Kluwer, Dordrecht, 1993.

[308] U. Picchini, S. Ditlevsen, and A. De Gaetano. Modeling the euglycemic hyperinsulinemic clamp by stochastic differential equations. *J. Math. Biol.*, 53:771–796, 2006.

[309] J. Pilz. *Bayesian Estimation and Experimental Design in Linear Regression Models*. Wiley, New York, 1991.

[310] J.C. Pinheiro and D.M. Bates. Approximations to the log-likelihood function in the nonlinear mixed-effects model. *J. Comp. Graph. Stat.*, 4:1235, 1995.

[311] J.C. Pinheiro and D.M. Bates. *Mixed Effects Models in S and S-Plus*. Springer, New York, 2002.

[312] S.J. Pocock. *Clinical Trials*. Wiley, Chichester, 1983.

[313] B.T. Polyak. New method of stochastic approximation type. *Automat. Remote Control*, 51:937–946, 1990.

[314] B.T. Polyak and A.B. Juditsky. Acceleration of stochastic approximation by averaging. *SIAM J. Control Optim.*, 30:838–855, 1992.

[315] J.W. Pratt, H. Raiffa, and R. Schlaifer. *Introduction to Statistical Decision Theory*. MIT Press, Cambridge, MA, 1995.

[316] L. Pronzato. Adaptive optimization and D-optimum experimental design. *Ann. Statist.*, 28(6):1743–1761, 2000.

[317] L. Pronzato. Optimal experimental design and some related control problems. *Automatica*, 44:303–325, 2008.

[318] L. Pronzato. Penalized optimal designs for dose-finding. *J. Statist. Plann. Inf.*, 140(1):283–296, 2010.

[319] L. Pronzato and A. Pázman. Nonlinear experimental design based on the distribution of estimators. *J. Statist. Plann. Inf.*, 33:385–402, 1992.

[320] L. Pronzato and A. Pázman. Second-order approximation of the entropy in nonlinear least-squares estimation. *Kybernetika*, 30(2):187–198, 1994.

[321] L. Pronzato and A. Pázman. Using densities of estimators to compare pharmacokinetic experiments. *Comput. Biol. Med.*, 31(3):179–195, 2001.

[322] L. Pronzato and A. Pázman. *Design of Experiments in Nonlinear Models: Asymptotic Normality, Optimality Criteria and Small-Sample Properties*, volume 212 of *Lecture Notes in Statistics*. Springer, New York, 2013.

[323] L. Pronzato and E. Walter. Robust experiment design via stochastic approximation. *Math. Biosci.*, 75:103–120, 1985.

[324] L. Pronzato and E. Walter. Robust experiment design via maximin optimization. *Math. Biosci.*, 89:161–176, 1988.

[325] L. Pronzato, H. Wynn, and A. Zhigljavsky. *Dynamical Search: Applications of Dynamical Systems in Search and Optimization*. Chapman & Hall/CRC, Boca Raton, FL, 2000.

[326] M.A. Proschan, K.K.G. Lan, and J.T. Wittes. *Statistical Monitoring of Clinical Trials. A Unified Approach*. Springer, New York, 2006.

[327] B.N. Pshenichnyi. *Necessary Conditions for an Extremum*. Marcel Dekker, New York, 1971.

[328] F. Pukelsheim. *Optimal Design of Experiments*. Wiley, New York, 1993.

[329] F. Pukelsheim and B. Torsney. Optimal weights for experimental designs on linearly independent support points. *Ann. Statist.*, 19:1614–1625, 1991.

[330] R.D. Purves. Optmimum numerical integration methods for estimation of area-under-the-curve (AUC) and area-under-the-moment-curve (AUMC). *J. Pharmacokinet. Biopharm.*, 20(3):211–226, 1992.

[331] H.S. Rabie and N. Flournoy. Optimal designs for contingent responses models. In A. Di Bucchianico, H. Läuter, and H. Wynn, editors, *mODa 7 – Advances in Model-Oriented Design and Analysis*, pages 133–142. Physica-Verlag, Heidelberg, 2004.

[332] A. Racine-Poon. A Bayesian approach to non-linear random effects models. *Biometrics*, 41:1015–1024, 1985.

[333] C.R. Rao. The theory of least squares when the parameters are stochastic and its application to the analysis of growth curves. *Biometrika*, 52 (3/4):447–458, 1965.

[334] C.R. Rao. *Linear Statistical Inference and Its Applications*. Wiley, New York, 2nd edition, 1973.

[335] D. Rasch, J. Pilz, L.R. Verdooren, and A. Gebhardt. *Optimal Experimental Design with R*. Chapman & Hall/CRC, Boca Raton, FL, 2011.

[336] D.A. Ratkowsky. *Nonlinear Regression Modeling*. Marcel Dekker, New York, 1983.

[337] D.A. Ratkowsky. *Handbook of Nonlinear Regression Models*. Marcel Dekker, New York, 1990.

[338] D.A. Ratkowsky and T.J. Reedy. Choosing non-linear parameters in the four-parameter logistic model for radioligand and related assays. *Biometrics*, 42:575–582, 1986.

[339] S. Retout, S.B. Duffull, and F. Mentré. Development and implementation of the population Fisher information matrix for the evaluation of population pharmacokinetic designs. *Comp. Meth. Progr. Biomed.*, 65:141–151, 2001.

[340] S. Retout and F. Mentré. Further developments of the Fisher information matrix in nonlinear mixed effects models with evaluation in population pharmacokinetics. *J. Biopharm. Statist.*, 13(2):209–227, 2003.

[341] H. Robbins and S. Monro. A stochastic approximation method. *Ann. Math. Statist.*, 22:400–407, 1951.

[342] W.F. Rosenberger and L.M. Haines. Competing designs for phase I clinical trials: A review. *Statist. Med.*, 21:2757–2770, 2002.

[343] W.F. Rosenberger and J.M. Hughes-Oliver. Inference from a sequential design: Proof of conjecture by Ford and Silvey. *Statist. Prob. Lett.*, 44:177–180, 1999.

[344] W.F. Rosenberger, N. Stallard, A. Ivanova, C. Harper, and M. Ricks. Optimal adaptive designs for binary response trials. *Biometrics*, 57:909–913, 2001.

[345] D. Ruppert. Efficient estimators from a slowly convergent Robbins-Monro procedure. Technical Report 781, School of Operations Research and Industrial Engineering. Cornell University, Ithaca, NY, 1988.

[346] J. Sacks. Asymptotic distribution of stochastic approximation procedures. *Ann. Math. Statist.*, 29:373–405, 1958.

[347] J. Sacks and D. Ylvisacker. Designs for regression problems with correlated errors. *Ann. Math. Statist.*, 37:66–89, 1966.

[348] J. Sacks and D. Ylvisacker. Designs for regression problems with correlated errors, many parameters. *Ann. Math. Statist.*, 39:49–69, 1968.

[349] J. Sacks and D. Ylvisacker. Designs for regression problems with correlated errors, III. *Ann. Math. Statist.*, 39:2057–2074, 1968.

[350] T. Schmelter. Considerations on group-wise identical designs for linear mixed models. *J. Statist. Plann. Inf.*, 137:4003–4010, 2007.

[351] T. Schmelter. The optimality of single-group designs for certain mixed models. *Metrika*, 65:183–193, 2007.

[352] T. Schmelter, N. Benda, and R. Schwabe. Some curiosities in optimal designs for random slopes. In J. López-Fidalgo, J.M. Rodriguez-Diaz, and B. Torsney, editors, *mODa 8 – Advances in Model-Oriented Design and Analysis*, pages 189–195. Physica-Verlag, Heidelberg, 2007.

[353] R. Schwabe. *Optimum Designs for Multi-Factor Models*, volume 113 of *Lecture Notes in Statistics*. Springer, New York, 1996.

[354] P. Sebastiani and Wynn H. Maximum entropy sampling and optimal Bayesian experimental design. *J. Royal Statist. Soc. B*, 62:145–157, 2000.

[355] G.A.F. Seber. *Multivariate Observations*. Wiley, New York., 1984.

[356] G.A.F. Seber. *A Matrix Handbook for Statisticians*. Wiley, Hoboken, NJ, 2008.

[357] G.A.F. Seber and C.I. Wild. *Nonlinear Regression*. Wiley, New York., 1989.

[358] M. Shewry and H. Wynn. Maximum entropy sampling. *J. Appl. Stat.*, 14:165–169, 1987.

[359] J. Shu and J. O'Quigley. Dose-escalation designs in oncology: ADEPT and the CRM. *Statist. Med.*, 27:5345–5353, 2008.

[360] S.D. Silvey. *Optimal Design*. Chapman & Hall, London, 1980.

[361] S.D. Silvey and D.M. Titterington. A geometric approach to optimal design theory. *Biometrika*, 60(1):21–32, 1973.

[362] S.D. Silvey, D.M. Titterington, and B. Torsney. An algorithm for optimal designs on a finite design space. *Comm. Statist. Theory Methods*, 14:1379–1389, 1978.

[363] R.R. Sitter. Robust designs for binary data. *Biometrics*, 48:1145–1155, 1992.

[364] K. Smith. On the standard deviations of adjusted and interpolated values of an observed polynomial function and its constants and the guidance they give towards a proper choice of the distribution of observations. *Biometrika*, 12:1–85, 1918.

[365] S.N. Sokolov. Continuous planning of regression experiments. *Theory Probab. Appl.*, 8:89–96, 1963.

[366] S.N. Sokolov. Continuous planning of regression experiments. II. *Theory Probab. Appl.*, 8:298–304, 1963.

[367] E. Spjotvoll. Random coefficients regression models. A Review. *Statistics*, 8:69–93, 1977.

[368] S.M. Stigler. Gergonne's 1815 paper on the design and analysis of polynomial regression experiments. *Historia Mathematica*, 1(4):431–439, 1974.

[369] J.R. Stroud, P. Müller, and G.L. Rosner. Optimal sampling times in population pharmacokinetic studies. *Appl. Statist.*, 50:345–359, 2001.

[370] M. Stylianou and N. Flournoy. Dose finding using the biased coin up-and-down design and isotonic regression. *Biometrics*, 58(1):171–177, 2002.

[371] M.A. Tanner. *Tools for Statistical Inference. Methods for the Exploration of Posterior Distributions and Likelihood Functions*. Springer, New York, 1996.

[372] P. Thall, R.E. Millikan, P. Mueller, and S.-J. Lee. Dose-finding with two agents in phase I oncology trials. *Biometrics*, 59:487–496, 2003.

[373] P. Thall and K. Russell. A strategy for dose-finding and safety monitoring based on efficacy and adverse outcomes in phase I/II clinical trials. *Biometrics*, 54:251–264, 1998.

[374] P.F. Thall and J.D. Cook. Dose-finding based on efficacy-toxicity trade-offs. *Biometrics*, 60:684–693, 2004.

[375] D.M. Titterington. Algorithms for computing D-optimal design on finite design spaces. In *Proceedings of the 1976 Conference on Information Science and Systems*, pages 213–216. John Hopkins University, Baltimore, MD, 1976.

[376] D.M. Titterington. Estimation of correlation coefficients by ellipsoidal trimming. *J. Appl. Stat.*, 27:227–234, 1978.

[377] C.W. Tornoe, J.L. Jacobsen, and H. Madsen. Grey-box pharmacokinetic/pharmacodynamic modelling of a euglycaemic clamp study. *J. Math. Biol.*, 48:591–604, 2004.

[378] C.W. Tornoe, J.L. Jacobsen, O. Pedersen, T. Hansen, and H. Madsen. Grey-box modelling of pharmacokinetic/pharmacodynamic systems. *J. Pharmacokinet. Pharmacodyn.*, 31(5):401–417, 2004.

[379] B. Torsney. Contribution to discussion of a paper by Dempster, Laird and Rubin. *J. Roy. Statist. Soc. Ser. B*, 39:22–27, 1977.

[380] B. Torsney. A moment inequality and monotonicity of an algorithm. In K.O. Kortanek and A.V. Fiacco, editors, *Proceedings of the International Symposium on Semi-Infinite Programming and Applications*, Lecture Notes in Economics and Mathematical Systems, pages 249–260. Springer, Berlin, 1983.

[381] B. Torsney. W-iterations and ripples therefrom. In L. Pronzato and A.A. Zhigljavsky, editors, *Optimal Design and Related Areas in Optimization and Statistics*, volume 28 of *Springer Optimization and Its Applications*, pages 1–12. Springer, New York, 2009.

[382] B. Torsney and S. Mandal. Two classes of multiplicative algorithms for constructing optimizing distributions. *Comp. Statist. Data Analysis*, 51(3):1591–1601, 2006.

[383] B. Torsney and R. Martín-Martín. Multiplicative algorithms for computing optimum designs. *J. Statist. Plann. Inf.*, 139:3947–3961, 2006.

[384] B. Torsney and A.K. Musrati. On the construction of optimal designs with applications to binary response and to weighted regression models. In W.G. Müller, H.P. Wynn, and A.A. Zhigljavsky, editors, *Model-Oriented Data Analysis*, pages 37–52. Physica-Verlag, Heidelberg, 1993.

[385] J.Y. Tsay. On the sequential construction of D-optimal designs. *J. Am. Stat. Assoc.*, 71(355):671–674, 1976.

[386] G. Verbeke and G. Molenberghs. *Linear Mixed Models for Longitudinal Data*. Springer, New York, 2000.

[387] G. von Békésy. A new audiometer. *Archives of Otolaryngology*, 35:411–422, 1947.

[388] E.F. Vonesh and V.M. Chinchilli. *Linear and Nonlinear Models for the Analysis of Repeated Measurements*. Marcel Dekker, New York, 1997.

[389] G. Wahba. *Spline Models for Observational Data*. SIAM, Philadelphia, 1990.

[390] J.C. Wakefield. The Bayesian approach to population pharmacokinetic models. *J. Am. Statist. Assoc.*, 91:134–140, 1996.

[391] A. Wald. On the efficient design of statistical investigations. *Ann. Math. Statist.*, 14:134–140, 1943.

[392] S. Wald. Spline functions in data analysis. *Technometrics*, 16(1):1–11, 1974.

[393] S.J. Wang, H.M. Hung, and R.T. O'Neill. Paradigms for adaptive statistical information designs: Practical experiences and strategies. *Statist. Med.*, 31:3011–3023, 2012.

[394] W. Wang, R.F. Woolson, and W.R. Clarke. Estimating and testing treatment effects on two binary endpoints and association between endpoints in clinical trial. *Comm. Statist. Simul. Comp.*, 34:751–769, 2005.

[395] Y. Wang. Derivation of various NONMEM estimation methods. *J. Pharmacokin. Pharmacodyn.*, 34(5):575–593, 2007.

[396] G.B. Wetherill. Sequential estimation of quantal response curves (with discussion). *J. Royal Stat. Soc. Ser.B*, 25(1):1–48, 1963.

[397] G.B. Wetherill and K.D. Glazebrook. *Sequential Methods in Statistics*. Chapman & Hall, London, 1986.

[398] L.V. White. *The optimal design of experiments for estimation in nonlinear model*. PhD thesis, University of London, 1975.

[399] L.V. White. An extension of the general equivalence theorem to nonlinear models. *Biometrika*, 60(2):345–348, 1993.

[400] J. Whitehead, S. Patterson, D. Webber, S. Francis, and Y. Zhou. Easy-to-implement Bayesian methods for dose-escalation studies in healthy volunteers. *Biostatistics*, 2:47–61, 2001.

[401] J. Whitehead and D. Williamson. An evaluation of Bayesian decision procedures for dose-finding studies. *J. Biopharm. Statist.*, 8:445–467, 1998.

[402] J. Whitehead, Y. Zhou, J. Stevens, and G. Blakey. An evaluation of a Bayesian method of dose escalation based on bivariate binary responses. *J. Biopharm. Statist.*, 14:969–983, 2004.

[403] J. Whitehead, Y. Zhou, J. Stevens, G. Blakey, J. Price, and J. Leadbetter. Bayesian decision procedures for dose-escalation based on evidence of undesarable events and therapeutic benefit. *Statist. Med.*, 25:37–53, 2006.

[404] E.T. Whittaker and G. Robinson. *Calculus of Observations: A Treatise on Numerical Mathematics*. Dover, New York, 4th edition, 1967.

[405] P. Whittle. Some general points in the theory of optimal experimental design. *J. Roy. Statist. Soc. Ser. B*, 35:123–130, 1973.

[406] R.D. Wolfinger. Laplace's approximation for nonlinear mixed models. *Biometrika*, 80:791–795, 1993.

[407] H. Wolkowicz, R. Saigal, and L. Vandenberghe. *Handbook of Semidefinite Programming: Theory, Algorithms, and Applications.* Springer, New York, 2000.

[408] C.F. Wu. Some algorithmic aspects of the theory of optimal designs. *Ann. Statist.*, 6(6):1286–1301, 1978.

[409] C.F. Wu and Wynn H.P. The convergence of general step-length algorithms for regular optimum design criteria. *Ann. Statist.*, 6(6):1273–1283, 1978.

[410] C.F.J. Wu. Asymptotic theory of nonlinear least squares estimation. *Ann. Statist.*, 9(3):501–513, 1981.

[411] C.F.J. Wu. Asymptotic inference from sequential design in a nonlinear situation. *Biometrika*, 72(3):553–558, 1985.

[412] C.F.J. Wu. Efficient sequential designs with binary data. *J. Am. Statist. Assoc.*, 80:974–984, 1985.

[413] C.F.J. Wu. Optimal design for percentile estimation of a quantal-response curve. In Y. Dodge, V.V. Fedorov, and H.P. Wynn, editors, *Optimal Design and Analysis of Experiments*, pages 213–223. Elsevier, North Holland, 1988.

[414] C.F.J. Wu and M. Hamada. *Experiments: Planning, Analysis, and Parameter Design Optimization.* Wiley, New York, 2002.

[415] Y. Wu, V.V. Fedorov, and K.J. Propert. Optimal design for dose response using beta distributed responses. *J. Biopharm. Statist.*, 15(5):753–771, 2005.

[416] H.P. Wynn. The sequential generation of *D*-optimal experimental designs. *Ann. Math. Statist.*, 41:1655–1664, 1970.

[417] H.P. Wynn. Results in the theory and construction of *D*-optimum experimental designs. *J. Roy. Statist. Soc. B*, 34:133–147, 1972.

[418] H.P. Wynn. Jack Kiefer's contribution to experimental design. *Ann. Statist.*, 12:416–423, 1984.

[419] M. Yang. On the de la Garza phenomenon. *Ann. Statist.*, 38(4):2499–2524, 2010.

[420] K.C. Yeh and K.C. Kwan. A comparison of numerical integrating algorithms by trapezoidal, Lagrange, and spline approximation. *J. Pharmacokinet. Biopharm.*, 6(1):79–98, 1978.

[421] Z. Ying and C.F.J. Wu. An asymptotical theory of sequential designs based on maximum likelihood recursions. *Statistica Sinica*, 7:75–91, 1997.

[422] T.J. Ypma. Historical development of the Newton-Raphson method. *SIAM Review*, 37:531–551, 1995.

[423] Y. Yu. Monotonic convergence of a general algorithm for computing optimal designs. *Ann. Statist.*, 38(3):1593–1606, 2010.

[424] S. Zacks. Adaptive designs for parametric models. In S. Ghosh and C.R. Rao, editors, *Design and Analysis of Experiments. Handbook of Statistics*, volume 13, pages 151–180. Elsevier, Amsterdam, 1996.

[425] S. Zacks. *Stage-Wise Adaptive Designs*. Wiley, Hoboken, NJ, 2009.

[426] W. Zhu and W.K. Wong. Multiple-objective designs in a dose-response experiment. *J. Biopharm. Statist.*, 10(1):1–14, 2001.

Index

C_{max}, 199
E_{max} model, 158, 237, 254, 266, 270
T_{max}, 199
a priori distribution, 81, 148

adaptive design, 131, 132
adaptive Robbins-Monro procedure (ARM), 317, 319, 321, 322, 324
additivity of information matrix, 7, 9, 61
algorithm
    discrete design, 107
    exchange, 125
    first-order, 93, 101, 107, 108, 113, 115, 119, 125, 131, 133, 143, 152, 153, 188, 195, 203, 231, 302
    multiplicative, 108
    optimization, 17
approximate design, 63, 106
approximation
    first-order, 190, 194, 223, 231, 243
    second-order, 194, 211, 244
area under the curve (AUC), 189, 199
ARM, 317, 319, 321, 322, 324
atomized measure, 68, 94, 102
AUC, 199

basis function, 8, 121
battery reduction, 294, 300
Bayesian design, 59, 77, 81, 115, 129
best linear unbiased estimator (BLUE), 6, 8, 77, 78, 89
BI, 312, 314–316, 318, 322, 324, 325, 328

Carathéodory's Theorem, 64, 119
CIRLS, 30, 33, 39, 41, 48, 274
combined iteratively reweighted least squares (CIRLS), 30, 33, 39, 41, 48, 274
compartmental approach, 189, 199, 200
compartmental model, 189, 199, 202, 221, 231, 232
condition
    (Ψ, ω)-optimality, 123
    optimality, 65, 66, 82, 114, 118, 119, 121, 122, 146
confidence region, 6, 52, 53
constrained
    design measure, 122
constraints, 111, 117, 219
    cost, 111, 117, 219
continuous design, 62, 63, 106
convergence rate, 100
convex function, 61, 65, 66, 113, 148
cost function, 112, 133, 197, 198, 201, 226, 233, 249
coverage probability, 52, 53
Cramèr-Rao inequality, 21, 49
criterion
    A-, 54, 56, 58, 68, 80, 82, 90, 104, 105, 130, 132, 154
    D-, 53, 55, 56, 61, 68, 80, 84, 90, 94, 104–107, 113, 124, 133, 138, 154, 157, 253, 256, 302
    E-, 53, 55–57, 65
    I-, 58
    c-, 57, 156, 256
    convex, 61, 116
    homogeneous, 61, 106, 112
    linear, 54, 58, 65, 80, 90

minimax, 58, 81
monotonicity of, 61, 65, 106, 112

derivative
    directional, 65, 66, 68, 77, 79, 89,
        95, 113–115, 117, 130
    Gâteaux, 65, 68
design, 3
    A-optimal, 156
    D-optimal, 56, 70, 72, 74–76, 94,
        121, 148, 154, 158, 160, 174,
        192, 198, 203, 230, 231, 239,
        258, 262, 272, 275, 282, 302,
        312, 324
    T-optimal, 143, 145, 149
    c-optimal, 111, 156, 160, 258,
        272, 324
    adaptive, 129, 131, 132, 145, 155,
        252, 262, 268, 273, 289, 312
    atomized, 68, 117
    Bayesian, 59, 77, 81, 115, 129
    best intention (BI), 312, 314–316,
        318, 322, 324, 325, 328
    composite, 79, 115, 135, 262, 264,
        265, 268, 285, 287, 289
    continuous, 62, 63, 231, 295, 309
    cost-based, 111, 133, 191, 196,
        198, 203, 227, 233
    cost-normalized, 111, 114
    discrete, 62, 90, 106, 107, 303,
        309
    exact, 3, 21, 62, 106
    finite sample, 106
    locally optimal, 59, 128, 142, 152
    minimax, 81, 82, 129, 130, 302
    normalized, 62, 111, 301
    optimal, 50, 63
    optimal on average, 59, 81, 129
    penalized, 111, 113, 114, 165,
        168, 177, 183, 253, 275, 282,
        312, 315, 324
        adaptive D-optimal (PAD), 275,
        277, 279, 312, 315, 318, 319,
        328–330
    two-stage, 78, 79, 115, 116, 135

uniform, 74
weights, 51
design measure, 62
    constrained, 122
design region, 50, 94, 95, 152, 156,
        158, 192, 198, 231, 233, 237,
        257, 268, 287
    symmetrical, 52
directional derivative, 65, 66, 68, 77,
        79, 89, 95, 113–115, 117, 130
discrete design, 62, 106, 107
    algorithm, 107
discrete optimization, 62
dispersion matrix, 6, 294
distribution
    a priori, 81, 148
dose-escalation study, 256, 259, 262,
        314
drug combination, 180, 287

efficacy response, 161
eigenvalue
    maximal, 11, 55, 83
    minimal, 11, 55
elemental information matrix, 24–26,
        28, 136
ellipsoid of concentration, 6, 52, 55, 56
equivalence theorem, 70, 71, 91, 138,
        199, 234, 240, 258, 273, 303,
        307
    Kiefer-Wolfowitz, 70, 138
equivalent criteria, 148
estimator
    best linear unbiased, 6, 77, 78, 89
    iterated, 30, 34–36, 38, 48
    least squares (LSE), 4, 8, 20, 49,
        141, 142
    maximum likelihood (MLE), 20,
        31, 244
exact design, 21, 62, 106
exchange algorithm, 125

finite sample design, 106
first-order algorithm, 93, 101, 102,
        107, 108, 113, 115, 119, 125,

131, 143, 152, 153, 188, 195,
203, 231, 302
first-order approximation, 190, 194,
223, 231, 243
Fisher information matrix, 20, 136,
164, 190, 194, 231
forced sampling times, 197, 233, 237
function
basis, 8, 121
convex, 61, 65, 66, 113, 148
cost, 112, 133, 197, 198, 201, 226,
233, 249
homogeneous, 61, 106
quasiconvex, 113, 116
response, 17, 85, 141, 144
sensitivity, 69, 77, 79, 80, 94, 102,
117, 124, 130, 136, 137, 145,
153, 154, 157, 196, 199, 234,
240, 249, 258, 273, 275, 330
utility, 153, 312, 313, 316
weight, 13

Gâteaux derivative, 65, 68
Gauss-Markov Theorem, 6, 9
generalized inverse, 9, 79
generalized least squares estimator,
32
global (population) parameter, 38, 85

homogeneous function, 61

information
prior, 148
information matrix, 6, 10, 12, 19, 118,
156
additivity, 7, 9, 61
convexity, 64
elemental, 24–26, 28, 136
factorization, 95, 104
normalized, 61, 128, 131
set of, 63
singular, 8, 79
integration
Stieltjes-Lebesgue, 63
intrinsic variability, 222
IRLS, 13, 30, 33, 41, 244

iterative estimation, 14
iterative procedure, 119
backward, 100, 114, 136, 144,
153, 231, 249, 303
combined, 100
forward, 94, 100, 113, 131, 135,
144, 152, 153, 231, 234, 249,
303
merging, 101, 153, 182
iteratively reweighted least squares
(IRLS), 13, 30, 33, 41, 244

Kiefer-Wolfowitz equivalence theorem, 70, 138

Lagrangian, 147
theory, 119
least squares
combined iteratively reweighted,
30, 33, 39, 41, 48, 274
iteratively reweighted, 13, 30, 33,
41, 244
modified iteratively reweighted,
35, 36, 39, 41
least squares estimator, 4, 8, 20, 49,
141
Legendre polynomial, 73
Liapunov's theorem, 123
locally optimal design, 128, 142
Loewner ordering, 6, 61, 86, 92
log-likelihood function, 20, 31, 34,
137, 163
stationary points, 34
LSE, 4, 8, 20, 49

macroparameters, 233
matrix
g-inverse, 8
information, 6, 156
pseudo-inverse, 8
maximal concentration (C_{max}), 189,
199
maximin problem, 119
maximum likelihood estimator (MLE),
20, 31, 244

maximum tolerated dose (MTD), 161, 166, 312, 314

measure
  atomized, 68, 94, 102
  design, 62
  uniform, 74

MED, 166, 312, 314

merging procedure, 101, 153, 182

microparameters, 233

minimax
  criterion, 81
  design, 81, 82, 130

minimum effective dose (MED), 166, 312, 314

MIRLS, 35, 36, 39, 41

mixed effects, 85
  nonlinear, 188, 230

MLE, 20, 31

model
  E_{max}, 158, 237, 254, 266, 270
  binary, 139, 151, 154, 268
  bivariate binary, 140
  bivariate Cox, 151, 162, 164, 166, 275
  bivariate probit, 151, 162, 170, 282
  compartmental, 189, 199, 202, 221, 230–232
  Gumbel, 151, 162, 164
  logistic, 139, 151, 154, 158, 254, 266, 268, 270
  logit, 139, 155
  Michaelis-Menten, 232
  mixed effects, 85
  nonlinear mixed effects, 188, 230
  one-compartment, 202, 210, 222, 231, 232, 234, 235, 237, 241, 246
  partially nonlinear, 158
  probit, 155
  random effects, 85
  two-compartment, 191, 192, 232

model discrimination, 141

modified iteratively reweighted least squares (MIRLS), 35, 36, 39, 41

monotonicity, 61, 65

MTD, 161, 166, 312, 314

multiparameter logistic model, 158, 254, 266, 270

multiplicative algorithm, 108

multivariate response, 15

nested model, 144

noncentrality parameter, 142, 148

noncompartmental approach (non-parametric), 189, 199, 200

normal equations, 5

normalized design, 62

numerical integration, 207
  cubic splines, 209
  hybrid method, 209
  log-trapezoidal rule, 209, 213
  trapezoidal rule, 207

numerical procedure, 100, 105, 119, 125, 143

optimal design, 50, 63
  approximate, 106
  composite, 79
  continuous, 106
  convexity, 66
  on average, 81
  singular, 65, 69, 79, 105

optimal on average, 85

optimality condition, 65, 66, 82, 113, 114, 118, 119, 121–123, 146
  necessary, 106

optimality criterion, 51, 65
  convexity, 65
  monotonicity, 65

optimization
  discrete, 62

optimization algorithm, 17

PAD, 275, 277, 279

parameter
  global, 38, 85
  model, 189
  PK, 189, 199

population, 38, 85, 193
   space, 11
PD, 188
pharmacodynamic, 188
pharmacokinetic, 187
PK, 187
PK metric, 189, 199, 204, 211
   type I, 204, 206
   type II, 204, 206, 215, 218
   type III, 205
PK parameter, 189, 199
polynomial regression, 72, 106, 149
population model, 187
population parameter, 38, 85, 193
predicted response, 57
   variance, 57, 65, 70
principal components, 293, 294, 297, 304
principal variables, 294, 298, 305
prior information, 77, 148
probability measure, 62
pseudo-inverse matrix, 8

quasiconvex function, 113, 116

random effects, 85
random parameter, 85
regression
   polynomial, 106, 149
   random parameter, 85
   trigonometric, 74, 106
regularization, 8, 69, 79, 105, 144
relative deficiency, 176, 177, 183, 185, 264, 291
   penalized, 177, 186
relative efficiency, 56, 160, 169, 177, 195–197, 227, 236, 240, 264, 279
response function, 17, 85, 141, 144
rounding procedure, 105

sampling windows, 234, 237
second-order approximation, 127, 194, 211, 244
sensitivity function, 69, 77, 79, 80, 94, 102, 114, 115, 117, 124, 130, 136, 137, 145, 153, 154, 157, 196, 199, 234, 240, 249, 258, 273, 275, 330
Shannon information, 77
singular information matrix, 79
singular optimal design, 65, 69, 79, 105
sparse sampling, 204, 206, 218
spatial experiments, 122
stand-alone application, 230, 257, 268
steepest descent rule, 95–97, 102
step length, 95, 100, 102, 108, 303
Stieltjes-Lebesgue integration, 63
stopping rule, 101
support
   point, 9, 50, 51, 62, 63, 65, 66, 106, 107, 118, 121, 273, 284
   set, 62, 67, 114, 123, 149

Tchebysheff
   approximation, 148
theorem
   Carathéodory's, 64, 119
   equivalence, 70, 71, 91, 138, 199, 234, 240, 258, 273, 303, 307
   Gauss-Markov, 6, 9
   Liapunov, 123
time to maximal concentration (T_{max}), 189, 199
toxicity response, 161
trigonometric regression, 74, 106

uncontrolled variable, 84
uniform design, 74
univariate response, 15
utility function, 153, 312, 313, 316

variance-covariance matrix, 6, 9, 14, 17, 18, 148, 294

weight function, 13
weights, 51, 62
   optimal, 115